R E A D I N G S

NURSING TRENDS AND ISSUES

R E A D I N G S

NURSING TRENDS AND ISSUES

Carol A. Lindeman, RN, PhD, FAAN
Professor and Dean, School of Nursing
Oregon Health Sciences University
Portland, Oregon

Marylou McAthie, RN, EdD
Professor and Graduate Coordinator
Sonoma State University
Rohnert Park, California

Springhouse Corporation
Springhouse, Pennsylvania

Staff

Executive Director, Editorial
Stanley Loeb

Director of Trade and Textbooks
Minnie B. Rose, RN, BSN, MEd

Art Director
John Hubbard

Acquisitions
Margaret Belcher, RN, BSN; Elizabeth Steinmetz

Editors
David Moreau, Diana Potter, Nancy Priff

Copy Editor
Mary Hohenhaus Hardy

Designers
Stephanie Peters (associate art director), Matie A. Patterson, Lesley Weissman-Cook

Art Production
Robert Perry (manager), Heather Bernhardt, Anna Brindisi, Donald Knauss, Robert Wieder

Typography
David Kosten (manager), Diane Paluba (assistant manager), Liz Bergman, Joyce Rossi Biletz, Robin Rantz, Valerie Rosenberger

Manufacturing
Deborah Meiris (manager), T.A. Landis, Jennifer Suter

Production Coordination
Aline Miller (manager), Joy Dickenson

Editorial Assistants
Maree DeRosa, Elizabeth McBeath

Library of Congress Cataloging-in-Publication Data
Readings in nursing trends and issues/[compiled by]
   Carol A. Lindeman, Marylou McAthie.
     p. cm.
   Consists of reprints of articles from various sources.
   Includes bibliographical references.
   1. Nursing—Miscellanea.   I. Lindeman, Carol Ann.
   II. McAthie, Marylou.
   [DNLM: 1. Nursing—trends—collected works.   WY 16 R287]
RT63.R43 1990
362.1'73—dc20
DNLM/DLC   90-9407
ISBN 0-87434-232-5   CIP

Table of contents

Preface

Rapid and profound changes in the U.S. health care system have dramatically altered the nature and scope of nursing practice in the past decade. Rising health care costs, implementation of the prospective payment system, acute nursing shortages, a wider diversity of care settings and career opportunities, and technological advancements continue to influence the work that nurses perform—and thus the care their clients receive. Practicing nurses and nursing students alike must be well informed on these critical issues if they want to improve the status of their profession and enhance the quality of life for their clients.

Readings in Nursing Trends and Issues—a collection of timely articles written by prominent nurse practitioners and theoreticians—explores the major challenges and controversies facing the nursing profession. The authors address current issues not merely as problems to be solved but as opportunities through which nursing can increase its value to itself and to society.

In selecting the topics and articles for inclusion in this book, we conducted an extensive bibliographic search and literature review, considering not only the frequency with which a topic appeared in the literature but also the controversy surrounding the topic, its relevance to nursing practice, and the availability of quality articles published in the last few years. We purposefully chose to include material from a range of nursing journals and nonnursing sources.

Articles are grouped by themes within units. Each unit introduction establishes a historical context for the works it includes and explains the relationships among the articles. Chapter introductions explain each article's importance, relate it to other articles in the chapter, and, where appropriate, refer to ideas or themes in other chapters.

The five units in this book cover topics of vital interest to all nursing students and practicing nurses. Unit One, Nursing at the Crossroads: Learning from the Past, Growing Toward the Future, reviews the development of modern nursing and explores the nature and scope of nursing practice, educational preparation, and career development.

Unit Two, Discipline Issues: Nursing Research, Theory, and Practice, examines the nature of science, the relationship of theory and research to practice, and the role of the clinician in conducting and using research.

Unit Three, Health Care Delivery Issues, investigates four areas of particular interest to all nurses: health care financing, the nursing shortage, new career paths for nurses, and the role of technology in health care.

Unit Four, The Sociopolitical Environment and Nursing Practice, probes social and political forces currently affecting the profession, including access to health care by elderly and homeless persons, shifts in demographics, consumerism, and involvement of nurses in state and federal legislation.

Unit Five, Legal and Ethical Issues, examines an increasingly prevalent dilemma for nurses—the rationing of health care to poor or elderly clients—and addresses many other topics with legal and ethical implications, such as withholding treatment, questioning a physician's orders, and caring for terminally ill clients.

Readings in Nursing Trends and Issues includes practical aids that enhance the text's usefulness: introductions explain concepts, establish relationships, and provide historical contexts; study questions and additional assignments at the end of each unit promote content recall and encourage critical thinking. The questions can be used by the professional nurse as a self-test, by the student as a study guide, and by instructors as independent student assignments. Additionally, this well-rounded selection of current articles provides a starting point for further reading, the development of papers, and topics for research. (Selected references refer to hundreds of original articles, chapters, and books.) In short, this book is ideal for nursing students, practicing nurses, and nursing instructors and can be a valuable resource for administrators and researchers.

CAROL A. LINDEMAN
MARYLOU MCATHIE

Nursing at the crossroads: Learning from the past, growing toward the future

FOR MORE THAN A CENTURY now, nursing has been changing and growing — earning increased professional recognition and assuming ever-increasing clinical and administrative responsibility. But this change and growth have not been without a price. Change always generates some kind of resistance, and so it has been with nursing vis- à-vis the other health care professions.

As nurses carved out increasingly autonomous roles, developed and implemented baccalaureate and graduate degree programs, and structured a unique body of knowledge to make nursing a science as well as an art, their actions changed the traditional methods of health care delivery. Inevitably, other health care professionals (and even some nurses) resisted those changes, contributing to the critical issues of education and practice that confront nursing in its second century.

We view nursing's past and present with pride, but as the articles in Unit One remind us, we cannot fail to take the necessary steps to safeguard nursing's future. As long as issues of nursing's change and growth remain unresolved, nurses will continue to debate the actions needed to resolve them — and while we are debating, nonnurses will have the opportunity to dictate the direction nursing practice will take.

These are the key issues covered in Unit One:
• the continuing need for a definition of nursing
• the implications of the current changes in nurses' roles and in the practice and scope of nursing
• the development of criteria for entry into practice
• the drive to establish career advancement opportunities in support of nursing autonomy.

How these issues are decided today will permanently influence the future growth and direction of nursing. Where can nurses turn for counsel in making those all-important decisions? In part, of course, to the nursing leaders of today. But we must keep in mind that today's leaders are carrying forward the work of nurses of the past — nurses who courageously laid the foundation for today's complex structure of professional nursing. We should not go forward in deciding nursing's future without first recalling our early leaders' many contributions.

Nursing's three "founding elements"

According to Dock and Stewart, "We must know how our work of nursing arose...what lines it has followed, and under what direction it has developed best. Possessing this knowledge, each [nurse] may help to guide and influence its future in harmony with its historical mission."

Dock and Stewart also postulated that from its earliest roots in caring for others — mothering children and attending the sick, injured, elderly, and handicapped — nursing was founded on a strong desire to care for those in need. This humanitarian instinct is one of three elements Dock and Stewart cite to define nursing. The other two, products of recent times, are expertise attained through training and experience and knowledge based on science.

The beginnings of nursing

From prehistoric times, men and women sought to heal themselves and others through applications of plants and other substances believed to have healing powers. Through the ages, however, attending to the sick and injured evolved in two directions: caregiving and medicine-giving. Women tended to fulfill the caregiver role, while men tended the medicine-giver role. Along the way, men also assumed a monopoly on theoretical and scientific knowledge, as well as authority over their female caregiver assistants.

In the early Christian period (the third and fourth centuries), caring for the sick was considered an act of charity and a religious duty. (Nursing has always been influenced by religious beliefs and practices. Those who nursed tended to be either piously religious or remorseful and repentant, seeking to atone for their sins.) In Europe, religious orders provided nursing services and even founded the first hospitals.

By the end of the fifth century, medicine had developed into a science that incorporated the teachings of Hippocrates and was taught in European universities, which at that time were controlled largely by the Roman Catholic Church. For a while, medicine flourished in these centers of learning, but during the Middle Ages the Church's attitude toward medicine changed, and the practice of surgery was prohibited. Once again, the monasteries became the source of medical care.

Nursing's fortunes waxed and waned with those of medicine, but they were particularly affected by the Protestant Reformation in the 16th century. When religious and political upheavals forced the closing of Catholic churches, monasteries, and hospitals throughout Europe, nursing became more of a secular than a religious responsibility. As a result, what progress had been made toward creating a body of nursing knowledge fell by the wayside and, until well into the 19th century, nursing remained an ill-defined set of tasks that no one group was committed to perform.

In the early 19th century, most hospitals were overcrowded and unsanitary — places where the sick and injured were taken to die rather than to get better. This chaotic, unhealthy situation might have continued indefinitely but for the work of the woman universally acknowledged as the most influential force in the development of organized nursing: Florence Nightingale.

England: The legacy of Florence Nightingale

Born in 1820 to an English family of considerable wealth and high social standing, Florence Nightingale was educated, well traveled, and acquainted with most of the progressive thinkers of her day. While still a young woman, she became interested in becoming a nurse and concerned about England's lack of an educated and trained corps of nurses. Despite her family's opposition, in 1851 she attended a three-month nursing training program at the

Institution of Deaconesses at Kaiserwerth, Germany.

That was the beginning of Nightingale's lifelong devotion to nursing and nurses. In 1854, after a stint as superintendent of a London nursing home, she remedied the deplorable lack of nursing care and sanitation for the British Army during the Crimean War. By the war's end, her original group of 40 nurses had grown to 125 — and her prestige with the British government had grown accordingly. By 1860, using funds the government provided in her name for the education of nurses, Nightingale established the first nursing school in England. In the years that followed, many other nursing schools opened in England and elsewhere.

Nightingale's philosophy centered on the concept that competent and experienced nurses, not physicians or hospital directors, should educate, train, and discipline nursing students. Furthermore, she strongly believed that nursing's growth and the development of standards should be controlled through the schools rather than through government regulation. She also vehemently opposed the suggestion that nurses form a professional organization (although one was established in England during her lifetime).

Until her death in 1910, Florence Nightingale labored tirelessly to bring about improvements in hospital conditions, sanitation methods, and nursing standards in England and the British colonies. In doing so, she almost singlehandedly brought nursing into the modern era.

The United States: Nursing education after Nightingale

By 1873, graduates of Florence Nightingale's programs in England had made their way to the United States and were supervising the first hospital-affiliated nursing schools. This was a natural sequel to the burgeoning growth of U.S. hospitals and the many advances in medicine and sanitation that took place in late 19th century America.

What type of training did these early nursing students receive? On the whole, it was an on-the-job apprenticeship, with little or no classroom education. The students learned routine patient care — as it was practiced in the hospitals where they happened to train. There were as yet no state or national standards for nursing or for nursing education. After graduation, students tended to become private-duty nurses — and new cadres of students were recruited to fill their places in the hospitals.

But college- and university-based nursing programs were in the offing: The first collegiate school of nursing was established in 1909, the first baccalaureate programs in 1916. By the time associate-degree programs made their appearance in 1951, nursing school curricula had been standardized, post-BSN programs had become commonplace, and nursing specialization and administrative roles had begun to revolutionize health care delivery practices nationwide.

Portents of professionalism: The rise of nursing associations

The perceived need to prepare students not only to be nurses but to be teachers and leaders as well spurred nursing leaders of the late 19th century to organize nursing graduates into groups that met regularly to consider nursing issues. These meetings were held under the auspices of an organization formed in 1893 (with Isabel Hampton Robb as its first president) that in 1911 became the American Nurses' Association (ANA).

The ANA, the National League for Nursing (NLN), and other nursing associations formed in the first half of this century were instrumental in securing state licensing of nurses and standardization of nursing education programs. Just as important, they spearheaded the drive

Some landmark events in the growth and development of professional nursing

1909 University of Minnesota: establishment of first collegiate school of nursing

1911 American Nurses' Association (ANA) founded

1912 National Organization for Public Health Nursing (NOPHN) founded

1916 University of Cincinnati, Teachers College of Columbia University: inauguration of first baccalaureate nursing programs

1917 National League of Nursing Education (NLNE) report: "Standard Curriculum for Schools of Nursing"

1923 Committee for the Study of Nursing Education report: "Nursing and Nursing Education in the United States"

1926 ANA/NLNE/NOPHN committee formed to examine nursing school standards

1928-1935 ANA/NLNE/NOPHN committee reports: "Nurses, Patients, and Pocketbooks," "An Activity Analysis of Nursing," "Nursing Schools Today and Tomorrow"

1930 Third White House Conference: recommendation for advanced nursing training

1932 Committee on the Costs of Medical Care (independent group): recommendation for advanced nursing training and training of "nursing aides and attendants"

Association of Collegiate Schools of Nursing (ACSN) founded to develop and strengthen cooperation among nursing schools (first ACSN conference, 1933)

1934 Survey of public health nursing

1935 Federal Social Security Act: first government support of health care in United States

1937 NLNE report: "A Curriculum Guide for Schools of Nursing"

1941 National Association for Practical Nurse Education founded

1942 National Nursing Council for War Services (NNCWS) founded

1943 Federal Bolton Act: creation of U.S. Cadet Nurse Corps, scholarships for nursing education

1948 NNCWS-Brown Report: recommendations for further expansion of nurse's role into administrative and supervisory activities

Committees on Nursing Service Administration report

Committee on the Function of Nursing report: recommendation for extended nursing education focusing on professional issues and nursing research

1949 National Federation of Licensed Practical Nurses founded

National Committee for the Improvement of Nursing Service (formerly NNCWS) report: "Nursing Schools at the MidCentury"

1951 President's Commission Report: recommendations for establishment of more community colleges offering technical-level programs in nursing, dentistry, and medicine

Thesis, "The Education of Nursing Technicians" by Dr. Mildred Montag (Columbia University): introduction of concept of associate-degree nursing programs

Landmark events in nursing *continued*

1952 National League for Nursing (NLN) founded (combining NLNE, NOPHN, and National Accrediting Service)

NLN: establishment of a national testing service for accreditation of nursing schools

1952-1956 Eight community colleges implement associate degree nursing programs

1961-1964 Three-part monograph, "Newer Dimensions of Patient Care," by Esther Lucille Brown, proposes methods for individualizing patient care

1964 Federal Nurse Training Act: establishment of federally funded programs for nursing education and research, including graduate programs

1965 ANA recommendation of baccalaureate degree as minimum preparation for beginning professional nursing practice, associate degree for beginning technical nursing practice

Federal Medicare and Medicaid acts passed

1967 (final report, 1974) ANA/NLN (National Committee for the Study of Nursing and Nursing Education) report, "An Abstract for Action": recommendations for further nursing research, improved nursing education programs, clarification of nursing roles vs. other health care professionals, increased financial (particularly federal) support for nursing

1968 Renewal of Federal Nurse Training Act of 1964

1970 Surgeon General's report: "Toward Quality in Nursing"

NLN Committee on Nursing Perspectives: report on nurses' changing roles

1971 Renewal of Federal Nurse Training Act of 1964

Secretary's Committee to Study Extended Roles for Nurses (Department of Health, Education, and Welfare) report: recommendations for extending the scope of nursing practice

1979 Federal Nurse Training Act of 1979: mandate for Institute of Medicine (IOM) study on future federal support of nursing education, nursing practice issues

1980 National Commission on Nursing (Chairperson: Marjorie Beyers) begins study

ANA Congress of Nursing Practice report "Nursing: A Social Policy Statement": recommendations for nursing specialization

1981-1983 IOM study and report: many significant recommendations for changes in nursing practice and education

1982 ANA National Task Force on Nursing Practice established to promote implementation of BSN for minimum professional nurse preparation, ADN for minimum technical nurse preparation

1983 National Commission on Nursing report "National Commission on Nursing Summary Report and Recommendations": recommendations for innovations in nursing education, practice, and community relations; affirmation of ANA recommendations for minimum requirements for nurse preparation

Social Security Amendments: institution of the prospective payment system (PPS) for Medicare-reimbursed hospital costs

continued

Landmark events in nursing *continued*

1984 ANA/NLN/American Association of Colleges of Nursing/American Organization of Nursing Executives joint report, "National Commission on Nursing Implementation Project": recommendations for characteristics of future nursing education programs for two levels of nurses

1985 ANA House of Delegates: vote in support of title "registered nurse" for baccalaureate-prepared nurses, "associate nurse" for associate-degree-prepared nurses, with incorporation of practical nurses into "associate nurse" group

Western Council on Higher Education in Nursing report "The Preparation and Utilization of New Nursing Graduates": recommendations for defining competencies of two levels of nurses

1987 ANA Task Force on the Scope of Nursing Practice report "The Scope of Nursing Practice": definitions of two levels of nursing under one scope of practice, designed as guidelines for changing state nurse practice acts

1988 Secretary's Commission on Nursing (Department of Health and Human Services) report: recommendations for improvement in recruitment and retention of an adequate supply of RNs

Western Institute for Nursing report: recommendations for curriculum changes reflecting nurses' changing demographics and roles

---

toward nursing autonomy and professionalism by defining and broadening nursing roles, promoting nursing specialization and research, and widening nursing's scope of practice.

How should we define nursing?

After more than 100 years of nursing, the question remains to be answered: What is the definition of nursing? The ANA *Social Policy Statement* points to Nightingale's definition, that to nurse is to "have charge of the personal health of somebody....What nursing has to do...is to put the patient in the best condition for nature to act upon him."

About a century later, in 1969, Virginia Henderson defined nursing as "...those activities contributing to health or its recovery (or to a peaceful death) that [the individual] would perform unaided if he had the necessary strength, will, or knowledge...and to do this in such a way as to help him gain independence as rapidly as possible." The ANA definition

(1980) sums up today's direction in defining nursing: "Nursing is the diagnosis and treatment of human responses to actual or potential health problems."

Can the nursing profession expect to play a decisive role in defining the domain of nursing if it cannot yet define what nursing is? As the chapters in Unit One so dramatically demonstrate, little agreement exists among nursing leaders concerning a definition of nursing. With criteria for entry into practice still a subject of controversy, nursing's roles, functions — and particularly its professional status — will continue to be the subject of intensive debate throughout the health care delivery system.

The debate over nursing professionalism

Is nursing becoming a true profession? A number of nursing leaders have expressed their opinions. In general, most of them rate nursing high on social values, ethics, and motivation but low on community service, autonomy, educational commitment, and establishment of a unique knowledge base. Styles contends that to achieve professional status nursing must amass a unique body of knowledge, demonstrate a commitment to community service, establish a professional society, and achieve autonomy and self-regulation, presumably by adhering to a simple code of ethics.

Believing that nursing meets these criteria today, Styles considers nursing a true profession, despite the need for additional work in the areas of autonomy and establishment of a well-developed knowledge base. She cites in nursing's favor its concern for ethical issues and progress toward knowledge-base development.

In contrast to Styles's viewpoint, Etzioni and others feel that lack of autonomy and self-regulation places nursing at a subprofessional level. And so the debate continues.

Nurses' changing roles and scope of practice

As nurses assume more and more responsibility for patient care, this question increases in importance: What is the appropriate division of tasks between nurses and other health care professionals?

Parallel to major advances in medical care, major changes in delivery of health care services began taking place in the 1950s. With the advent of more and better treatments and sophisticated technology, more patients could be treated, and hospitals became increasingly complex workplaces for all health care personnel. In addition, nursing homes were growing in size and number, as were outpatient services and home care programs.

In this rapidly changing health care environment, however, nursing research did not keep pace with improvements in medical technology, especially in pharmaceuticals and electronic equipment. This was true even though the number of nursing schools of all

types continued to increase, and nursing leaders were expressing concern about the lack of progress in nursing research.

This situation began to change with passage and implementation of the Federal Nurse Training Act of 1964, which provided funds to ensure an adequate supply of nursing personnel through various routes, including nursing research and postgraduate education. This act, renewed in 1968 and 1971 (with an additional recommendation for funding to educate nurse practitioners), was followed by the Federal Nurse Training Act of 1979, with its mandate to the Institute of Medicine (IOM) for intensive study of the desirability of continued federal funding for nursing programs. Federal funding continues for nursing education.

The IOM's final report, published in 1983, made many recommendations for nursing education and practice. Overall, however, its effect was to remove nursing from the status of a national issue and nurses from consideration as national resources. The severe budget restrictions the report recommended appeared to signal an end to direct federal efforts to increase the supply of "generalist" nurses. Instead, the report recommended that the government provide the states with funding and technical assistance for "generalist" nurse education. (The IOM report did recommend federal funding for postgraduate nurse-specialist programs, however.)

Nursing's uniquely individual approach to patient care received national attention with the publication, between 1961 and 1964, of Dr. Esther Lucille Brown's three-part monograph, *Newer Dimensions of Patient Care*. In it, she analyzed the elements of planning for individualized patient care and assessed differing patient reactions to illness and to the experience of being hospitalized. Brown's influence on nursing practice was also felt in 1970, when she published her report — the result of discussions with the NLN-sponsored Committee on Nursing Perspectives — on the changes that the Medicare legislation of the 1960s was bringing to the practice of nursing.

At the crossroads: Criteria for entry into practice

Should a nurse be required to have a baccalaureate degree as the minimum requirement for professional status? A major issue today involves differentiating among the roles and functions of registered nurses who have graduated from the three types of nursing school programs: associate degree (two years of preparation), diploma (three years), and baccalaureate degree (four years). At issue, too, is what constitutes fair and adequate compensation for new graduates of the three programs. But the greatest controversy, of course, centers on the ANA's recommendation of a two-track educational system for nurses that will produce two nursing levels: professional nurses and technical nurses.

A pivotal year for nursing education and practice, 1965 saw passage of the Medicare and Medicaid acts and the promulgation of the ANA's landmark recommendations that (1) the BSN should be established as the minimum preparation for beginning professional nursing practice, with all professional nurses holding BSN degrees by 1985, and (2) the AD should be established as the minimum preparation for beginning technical nursing practice. (Under the ANA plan, practical nurses would become technical nurses, so only the two titles, "technical nurse" and "professional nurse," would exist.) Although these were only recommendations and had no immediate effect on nursing practice or on nursing licensure, their implications for the future of nursing set off a controversy that continues to this day.

In 1982, the ANA established the National Task Force on Nursing Practice to develop comprehensive recommendations for strategies to implement this program, which had also re-

ceived endorsement from the National Commission on Nursing. At this writing, some state nursing associations have started to implement the Task Force's recommendations by changing their licensing laws to encompass the two levels of nursing, professional and technical.

Nursing education programs are also affected. For example, in 1986 the North Dakota State Board of Nursing adopted administrative rules requiring that nursing education programs operating after January 1987 offer a curriculum leading to an associate degree for practical nurses and a baccalaureate degree for registered nurses. A number of commissions and committees have studied and are studying the ways the ANA plan would restructure nursing education.

Implementation of the ANA plan in the workplace is expected to continue slowly because work assignments traditionally have been made only on the basis of whether a nurse was an RN or LPN, not on level of education. In addition, deciding what competency levels are expected for each of the nursing levels is another important issue. In 1985, the Western Council on Higher Education in Nursing published definitions of the competencies expected from graduates of AD and BSN programs. Ultimately, the two groups will perform different tasks and receive different levels of compensation.

Impact of the prospective payment system

The Social Security Act Amendments of 1983 established what has become known as the prospective payment system (PPS) for reimbursing hospitals for patient care under Medicare. This system (discussed in detail in Unit Three), mandating a set price for hospital care of patients in specific diagnosis-related groups (DRGs), has revolutionized both hospital and home delivery of nursing services.

Nurses' workloads have increased under PPS within the hospital setting, according to Mitchell and Dibble, because the tendency is to admit patients only when they become acutely ill, then discharge them as early as possible in order to minimize the cost of their care. As a result, hospital nurses are caring for greater numbers of acutely ill patients, and home health nurses and nurses in long-term-care facilities are caring for sicker patients.

The PPS has also underscored the need for nurse-specialist education programs for hospital and home-care nurses. Kleffel reports that home health care agencies now have programs requiring specialty preparation in areas such as enterostomal therapy and respiratory therapy. Controlling the cost of patient care has led some hospitals to include specialized care as part of nursing functions in order to avoid the cost of maintaining, for example, separate respiratory therapy departments. Here again, the nurse's workload is increased.

Should the basic nursing curriculum be changed to prepare greater numbers of specialists? Should professional certification beyond the license to practice nursing be required to ensure a consistently high level of nursing care? The ANA thinks so and in 1980 outlined a certification process. Additionally, the ANA in *Nursing: A Social Policy Statement* (1980) and the Western Institute for Nursing in 1988 recommended revising nursing curricula to reflect the high level of competency required of today's nurses.

The clinical ladder concept

Our society's maintenance of an adequate supply of skilled nursing personnel will depend heavily on rewarding nurses for their excellence in clinical practice. One way to do this is through establishment of well-defined career advances — the "clinical ladder" concept. Although it is gaining favor slowly, this concept promises significant rewards for nurses who prefer patient care to administrative roles. Its

implementation will mean that nurses with higher levels of education can expect better pay for their clinical work, instead of having to be promoted into administrative positions to receive higher salaries.

The 1983 Institute of Medicine report supported the clinical ladder concept through its recommendation of standardized educational preparation for specific levels of nursing competency. Until this is accomplished, nursing job specifications, competency levels, and salaries will probably stay the same for all registered nurses.

Toward nursing in the 21st Century

In 1983, the independent National Commission on Nursing, chaired by Dr. Marjorie Beyers, fired an impressive salvo in the ongoing battle for recognition of nursing as both a profession and an indispensable part of modern health care. This commission, which included nurses from virtually every level and category of nursing, held a series of hearings throughout the country, beginning in 1980. The report of its findings, "National Commission on Nursing Summary Report and Recommendations," sets forth the major issues nursing will face as it heads into the 21st century:

• recognition of nurses' essential role in patient care
• recognition of nursing as a profession
• promotion of nurses' professional growth through provision of clinical and administrative career opportunities
• establishment of uniform qualifications to practice nursing
• involvement of nurses in policy development and decision making in health care agencies
• involvement of nurses in the management process
• compensation of nurses commensurate with their level of responsibility.

These and other major issues will occupy

the nursing profession for some time to come as it struggles to meld individual viewpoints and opinions into a collective voice. But regardless of where we as individuals stand in our opinions of today's professional problems and issues, we cannot do less than remain committed to developing our technical and intellectual skills and improving the quality of patient care. Nursing's professional evolution is in our hands; we are accountable to the nurses of tomorrow for the direction we give to nursing today.

CHAPTER ONE

Definitions of nursing

THE DIFFICULTIES IN defining nursing have existed since Florence Nightingale first described what she envisioned as the domain of nursing. The controversy has intensified since the publication of the American Nurses' Association's definition in 1980 in *Nursing: A Social Policy Statement:*

> Nursing is the diagnosis and treatment of human responses to actual and potential health problems.

The definition of nursing has shifted focus in the last decade. Although continuing to assist clients to attain and maintain health, nursing has increased its emphasis on health promotion and disease prevention. The nurse is no longer handmaiden to the physician; the nurse has the potential to become a scholar and an independent thinker capable of making critical decisions about client care.

An agreed-upon definition is necessary because of its guidance to the profession's practitioners. It provides necessary direction for professional education, for legal limits of practice, and for professional goals. Nursing also needs to reach agreement about the domain of nursing practice in order to develop further the knowledge base that is a key to its future.

A knowledge base specific to a field can build professional status. Nursing must support scholarly endeavors such as nursing research to ensure that knowledge development continues. Another determinant of professional status is control over practice.

Professional nursing organizations need to discuss and develop a definition of nursing that is acceptable to practicing nurses. The

ANA definition included in the *Social Policy Statement* is not acceptable to many nursing leaders and practicing nurses because of its narrow interpretation. The controversy continues to splinter nursing efforts, and it leaves nurses in dependent rather than independent roles.

All of the articles included in this chapter relate to the definition of nursing and to its mission and goals. Orlando, in "Nursing in the 21st Century: Alternate Paths," takes issue with the ANA definition, which she believes does not define the professional nurse's function or service objectives. This lack, she says, means the ANA definition does not distinguish between professional nurses and the lay public.

Schlotfeldt, in "Defining Nursing: A Historic Controversy," points out the congruence between Nightingale's definition of nursing and that of Henderson and contrasts this with what she sees as the ANA definition's ambiguity and lack of focus on health. After reviewing the development of conceptual models and frameworks by nursing theorists, Schlotfeldt discusses the perceived change in nursing's mission since the ANA's *Social Policy Statement* was approved. Finally, she suggests a new definition of nursing, one encompassing human beings' health status, health assets, and health potentials.

In "Nursing Comes of Age," Lynaugh and Fagin, writing from the perspective that our entire health care system has been built on the backs of nurses, focus on two major questions: (1) Is nursing a profession or simply a skilled occupation? (2) Should nursing continue to collaborate with medicine, or compete? This leads the authors to a discussion of five elements uniquely affecting the growth and development of nursing: mission, gender, women's issues, oppression, and preoccupation with professional status.

In "To Profess — To Be a Professional," Diers expresses the viewpoint that our task as nurses is not to defend our work but, instead, to recognize that the world has an outdated understanding of nursing and that we need to teach people what nursing is today. Defining nursing as "caring — primary, secondary, and tertiary," regardless of how those terms are defined, she goes on to describe her concept of what nursing is, what professionalism is, and why nursing is an important part of the health care system. The current situation is not a crisis in nursing, she says, but a revolution, with nursing's new professional responsibilities as the rallying point.

Nursing in the 21st century: Alternate paths

IDA ORLANDO, BS, MA

Introduction

OBVIOUSLY, I DO NOT have to be a Jules Verne or an H.G. Wells to consider alternate paths for nursing in the 21st century, because that is only 13 years away. On the other hand, I do have a crystal ball, and it has a rear view mirror in it. What I see is that there are only two paths. Neither path has changed, not for the 40 years I've been doing and watching nursing — its practice, teaching, supervision, research and the administration of nursing's service, educational and research programmes.

The two paths I see are marked with signs. One sign reads "dependent"; the other reads "independent." Both paths were possible in the past; both are possible now, but the independent path may not continue to be an alternate choice for our profession in the next century.

Nurses have walked both paths. The dependent path has been and continues to be paved by other professions and interests. The independent path can only be paved by our profession.

While nurses have walked both paths, the dependent path is growing ever wider. It has been so successful in fact that even those nurses who were on the independent path are increasingly switching over to a dependent one. I will first try to illustrate this point by sharing my vision of where we are in contrast to where we have been. I will then try to show the fundamental difference between these two paths and then discuss what our profession must do to get on, or get back on, and, in either case, stay on an independent path.

At a time called "then," hospital and university schools which trained professional nurses were all called schools of nursing.

Surely, this was a sign of perceived independence. Increasingly, over the last 25 years even the very best diploma programs have been closing down, and some university schools of nursing are being phased into schools with titles which do not include the word "nursing."

The nursing director of the hospital in which I trained was also the dean of our school of nursing. She was a registered professional nurse, yet, the very largest university school of nursing in New England, a little over 2 months ago, appointed an interim dean and this dean is not a nurse.

Roughly 16 years ago the Harvard Community Health Plan was founded. There were just a few members "then," but the director of nursing was organizationally equal to the medical director, and both were in a separate line relationship to the executive director of the plan. All nurses at the plan worked in a line relationship with the director of nursing. "Now" there are 200,000 members, and a nurse in a position called executive vice-president for nursing works in a line relationship with the medical director. There are no nurses in a line relationship with the executive vice-president for nursing. Nurses, instead, work under the direction and supervision of physicians in charge of the various services.

Nurses used to have their own agencies to provide care for individuals at home. All of them used to be called visiting nurse associations. "Now" they are increasingly being called health associations and the words "visiting nurse" deleted. I have a short story that goes with this switch.

As a youngster I always pointed with great pride to the Frontier Nursing Service in rural

Kentucky. It was founded, organized and controlled by professional nurses. In 1974 I heard the nursing director tell Barbara Walters, the then hostess of the TV *Today* show, on national television about her imminent retirement. Barbara Walters asked, 'What is the name of the nurse that will be taking your place?' I wept when the director replied it would not be a nurse; a physician would take her place instead. Nurses in the Frontier Nursing Service were not practicing medicine, at least not then. So why did they have to be directed by it? Surely, they were on an independent path and switched to a dependent one.

Nurses' work

Nurses used to say, "I will endeavour to assist the physician in his work." Now some nurses say, "I can do the physician's work, not only better but cheaper." Nurses used to say, "I can't give you aspirin; the doctor didn't order it." Now nurses and physician assistants can write and sign their own name to medicinal prescriptions, but of course under the overall supervision of a named physician. Paradoxically, in August 1985, the Massachusetts Supreme Judicial Court in the USA ruled that the "independent practice" of midwifery is legal by lay individuals but illegal by registered nurses. So nurses couldn't act like a physician "then" but can "now," and can't act as a lay person "now" but were able to "then."

"Then" nurses were prohibited from making a diagnosis. "Now" nursing diagnosticians are independently calling conditions like decubitus ulcers, "alteration in skin integrity"; cardiac insufficiency is "alteration in cardiac output"; varying degrees of paralysis are referred to as "impaired mobility," and the condition known as insomnia is called a "sleep disturbance."

"Then" it was against the law for a nurse to practice medicine. "Now," under Additional Acts Amendments in many states, some registered nurses are permitted to practice a little

bit of medicine but only with the permission of medical societies. Nurses who function in what is called the "expanded role" simply provide cost-effective assistance to the aims and goals of medicine. It is exceedingly worthwhile to be a physician's assistant; it just isn't nursing, and I'll try to show you why later. I fully acknowledge that some nurses in this role also do some excellent nursing, but only if they have the time.

I can remember when only the physician took a blood pressure reading. As the diagnostic need for ever more readings increased, nurses took them more and more. "Now" nurses and others not only take frequent readings, they do intravenous infusions, auscultation, resuscitation and just about anything else that only a physician used to do. These activities have increased exponentially, particularly since physicians started to pay attention to what social scientists were saying: "The physician is only concerned with the disease of the patient and has little or no concern for the patient who has the disease." Apparently, the social scientists just didn't know that professional nurses, in large numbers, provided patients with direct continuous care while the physician diagnosed and treated the patient's disease. Nor, did the social scientists know that nursing was and still is the only profession focused on the patient's need for care, and that nursing has been steadfast in responding as a collective whenever required 24 hours a day, 7 days a week or intermittently as required by a single professional nurse with the same full service.

Providers of care. It is nursing that provides care to individuals, in terms of the individual's experience, whether or not the individual has a diagnosed disease. I don't think anyone would question this statement. So, why has nursing continued to follow specialization defined by medicine? An individual is not a surgical, medical, obstetrical, neurological, oncological or psychiatric entity — diseases are! Individuals are infants, children, adolescents, young, old and very old adults. Individuals are mothers with and without partners, while pregnant or rearing children. Individuals can also be family members. Lastly any individual may or may not have a definable disease.

Why didn't nurses just continue to follow these individuals wherever they found them, whether in hospitals, clinics, homes, schools, workplaces or any other place service could be provided? Instead of following individuals needing care some nurses, as available assistants to the aims and goals of medicine, followed diseases and the prevention of them. That they have done so has increasingly freed physicians to follow the advice of the social scientists, and for several years I have heard this described as "holistic medicine."

So "now" we have some physicians doing marvelous nursing, and some nurses not only doing marvelous medicine but increasingly becoming certified to specialize in medical fields.

In spite of the marked variability, I have tried to illustrate where nursing was "then" and where nursing is "now." I insist that our "then" and "now" have maintained a single dependent path ever paved by others and non-nursing interests. This dependent path ignores the honorable independent past of our profession and may well by the 21st century succeed in extinguishing nursing as an independent profession.

Encounter between nurse and patient. I was thrilled in December 1984 to hear Dr. Lewis Thomas, president emeritus, Memorial Sloan-Kettering Center, New York, say at the dedication banquet for the Whitehead Institute in Cambridge, Massachusetts, the following, and I quote, "that for medicine, the disease is the main point of the encounter between the physician and the patient and the first task of the physician is to learn whether there is a disease,

then its nature and then what to do about it." More than anyone else, Dr. Thomas, however inadvertently on his part, validated for me that the main point of the encounter between the nurse and patient is to learn what care is required by the individual, with or without a diagnosed disease, then why the care is needed and then what to do about it. He further validated for me the necessity for nursing to take a radical independent path "then" and "now" and into the 21st century.

The question the nursing profession should ask is, why can't we get on or stay on an independent path? In order to answer the question, I would like to chart the path our profession has taken by employing a simple geometric principle. A single point can be used to represent where our profession is now. This single point is insufficient to chart a direction or path. An additional point is needed. The additional point represents where the profession has been. A line between these two points establishes the direction of the path the nursing profession has followed. The direction of this path may continue on into the indefinite future; it may stop, but the direction of this dependent path will never change.

The direction of the path cannot change unless a new point is charted, and this new point must represent a distinct function for professional nursing. The line between where we are and the point of our distinct professional function will firmly establish the independence of the path. This radical direction will guide us back to the fundamental nature of nursing, distinct from and independent of other professions. Thus, from here on anything which happens can be evaluated in terms of whether or not it causes practice to remain on the independent path.

The charting of a new point on the graph assumes that the distinct function of professional nursing has already been defined, and there are those who believe that the American Nurses' Association's Social Policy Statement of 1980 did just that. I don't and I would like to tell you why.

A definition of nursing. The definition being promulgated reads "nursing is the diagnosis and treatment of human responses to actual or potential health problems."

My first problem with this definition is that it does not permit a distinction between lay and professional nursing. An absence of distinction allows anyone to believe they are the same. A distinction must be made, and I can't make it unless you study with me a definition of what it means "to nurse." I learned about this transitive verb from my favorite dictionary (Funk and Wagnalls, 1935). "To nurse" means to encourage, to look after; to nourish, protect, and nurture; to give curative care to an ailment.

We all know that dictionaries over time conform to usage, but the transitive verb "to nurse" has remained stable. Definitions of the noun "nurse" have changed in two respects that I am aware of. Prior to 1954 Webster (1953) defined a nurse as "an assistant to physicians and surgeons." In 1963 I found Webster's emphasis change to "one who cares for the sick and infirm under the supervision of a physician" (Webster 1963). I used to blame Florence Nightingale for the usage Webster put in print because of one phrase in her pledge which reads, "I will endeavor to assist the physician in his work." I don't blame her anymore for the ever widening dependent path but wish her pledge had read instead, "I will endeavor to help the patient, even while a physician does his own work."

Lay nursing and professional nursing

Nightingale's pledge doesn't really matter. What matters is to differentiate a nurse and nursing from a professional nurse and professional nursing. Neither Webster (1953, 1963) nor Nightingale has done this, only our profession can.

Let us examine lay nursing first. All people

nurse themselves, or get nursed, or nurse others, a lot, if not most of their lives. All by themselves they give and find encouragement, nurturance, nourishment, protection and curative care with whatever personal, familial, social or public means are available. This is lay nursing and easy to do. Activities needed to accomplish the care are known and understood, and the self or another person is willing and able to perform the needed activity. In this context everybody is doing a lot of nursing and this is what heightens the importance of distinguishing lay from professional nursing.

While all this lay nursing is going on, individuals are forever reacting to immediate experiences. In ever so many of these experiences, the individual's ordinary and even extraordinary activity does not result in encouragement, nurturance, nourishment, protection and curative care. Instead, these individuals suffer distress because they are helpless. They do not know the "cause" of the inability "to nurse" themselves. In this circumstance, the lay individuals cannot ensure that the cause of the distress will be identified, nor can the lay individual ensure that the distress will be relieved. A nurse trained as a professional is needed for the following reasons.

1. The individual should but doesn't know why he or she is helpless. Stated another way, the individual doesn't know why he/she can't nurse the self.

2. The individual that doesn't know why he/she is unable to nurse the self is not able to communicate what the immediate need for help is.

3. The individuality of the distress cannot be observed directly even if the distress continues or escalates in intensity.

All that can be observed is what the individual says or what the individual's body does. Verbal forms of what individuals say can be grouped as complaints, requests, refusals, demands, questions and statements of any kind. Non-verbal forms include vocal sounds and the observable motor and physiological activity of the individual's body. Nothing else is known about the individual's experience at that moment in time, that is, not until the professional nurse's investigation is conducted. Thus, the nursing process must first find out the meaning to the individual of the behaviour the nurse observes. The meaning to the individual is available to the nurse because it is contained in what the individual already knows, that is, what he/she perceives, thinks and feels, says and does at any moment. As the investigation proceeds, the nurse finds out in sequential order whether or not the individual is distressed, and then why the individual is unable to nurse the self, which is what the distress is all about in the first place, As the cause and the individual need for help are identified, the professional nurse designs the activity to meet the need for help. This help relieves the distress and the individual's inability to care for the self is cured or ameliorated. Professional nursing does this; lay nursing does not, nor does lay nursing guarantee a result of curative care.

If we do not distinguish lay from professional nursing then we fail to recognize professional nurses who for as long as I can remember accomplished excellent results in restoring or improving the individual's ability to care for the self.

Function of nursing. A distinction between lay and professional nursing solves my first problem with the definition which reads, "nursing is the diagnosis and treatment of human responses to actual or potential health problems."

My next problem is that this definition does not attend to a distinct professional function, nor does it attend to the product our profession delivers to society. Before I continue I should

define the words "function" and "product."

By "function" I mean the noun. I do not mean the verb activity. The noun applied to nursing means: what is it that characterizes *every* activity of *every* nurse while practicing professional nursing? By product I mean: what is it that characterizes the outcome or result of professional nursing? I will discuss function first.

The definition being promulgated is too general for our or any other profession. It doesn't say anything to justify the existence of nursing as a distinct profession. Further, the amorphous generality does not permit understanding differences between nursing, other professions, and other people who also worry about "diagnosing and treating human responses to actual or potential health problems." Everyone is involved in this act! Further most people can be held liable if they do not attend to actual and potential health problems. Think for a moment of the essential, enormous contributions of sanitary engineers to the prevention of health problems, and the contributions of garbage collectors in terms of the frequency of service and the actual and potential response of most humans if the garbage is not collected.

Defining nursing as the "diagnosis and treatment of human responses to actual or potential health problems" cannot be the pivotal point, the central concern of our profession. It is too far removed from the inability of the individual "to nurse" the self. Distress resulting from this inability, its continuance or escalation in intensity, is what places distinct and critical importance on the work of our profession.

A definition of our distinct function should rather be related to what it is in fact: attending to individuals when in distress because they can't find their own encouragement; they can't look after themselves; they can't nourish, nurture or protect themselves; they can't give themselves curative care when they are ailing.

The definition being promulgated is therefore too general to give identity to our profession. It cannot therefore permit the plotting of a sharply defined point in order to create the radical direction of an independent path.

I might mention that in the September 1985 issue of *The American Nurse* I read that the American Nurses' Association's Board of Directors proposed adaption of four goals for our profession for the year 2000 (American Nurses' Association 1985). Defining a distinct independent function for professional nursing was not one of the goals.

My now 31-year-old rudimentary formulation of a distinct function for professional nursing reads "to find out and meet immediate need for help." I emphasize immediate need *for help*. While the need for help is highly individualistic and forever varied, it is distinctly different from human needs which we all share.

I don't much care what formulation of function is adopted by our profession, but I insist it must be distinct, to articulate and thereby justify having a distinct profession. A distinct formulation will provide the guiding statement not only for registered nurses to get on or stay on an independent path but will also guide consumers of professional nursing in selecting what service they require and wish to buy.

This ends my discussion of function. I will now discuss product.

Product of nursing. "The diagnosis and treatment of human responses to actual or potential health problems" says nothing about what professional nursing is supposed to accomplish as a product of service. You recall the product of service should answer the question: what characterizes the behavior of the person served after the professional function is carried out?

First, I'll dispense with my 31-year-old rudimentary formulation which reads "Improvement in the immediate verbal and non-verbal behavior when compared with the behavior of the individual before the immediate need for help was ascertained, and met." Before I continue I want to emphasize one aspect of the definition "to nurse," that is, "to give curative care to an ailment."

As a young nurse I thought that when I or the students I was teaching found immediate improvement in behaviors, some of these were medical and not nursing outcomes. I thought this because we were not working on signs and symptoms of disease, yet signs and symptoms of disease disappeared. Some of these included relief of pain, stabilization of blood pressure, reduction of fever, cessation of vomiting, swelling or distention, sudden progress in the healing of a wound or rash, etc. We were working on distress as experienced by the individual and finding out and meeting that individual's need for help in that situation. We were not working on signs and symptoms which disappeared.

Thus, cure of distress as experienced by the individual can take place. When it does the improvement is manifest in the verbal and non-verbal behavior after the immediate need for help is met. Behaviors which qualify as improved have been demonstrated in several publications (Orlando 1961, 1972; Gillis 1976). Of particular note are the published studies which emanated from the Yale University School of Nursing (Bochnak 1963, Bochnak *et al.* 1962, Tarasuk *et al.* 1965, Mertz 1963, Dumas 1963, Dumas & Leonard 1963, Dye 1963, Fischellis 1963, Rhymes 1964, Tyron & Leonard 1964).

My formulation of product could have been relevant to the definition being promulgated if a product had been stated. If the nurse "diagnoses and treats responses to health problems," is the product of the service "health"? I don't think so. Shouldn't the product be located in the response that the definition says nursing diagnoses and treats? I think it should be, but the promulgated definition doesn't say so.

What it does say is more like saying we are for motherhood and against sin.

I applaud what the nursing diagnosticians are trying to do because I think they are trying to classify nursing phenomena, but they are doing it in the dependent path. Moreover, the diagnoses developed thus far fall exceedingly short of fulfilling two meanings of the word "diagnosis." One meaning interweaves the word "diagnosis" with specific signs and symptoms, which allows labelling the signs and symptoms with a specific disease. The other meaning interweaves the word "diagnosis" with the investigation or analysis of cause. I emphasize analysis of *cause*. We know the nursing diagnosticians do not wish to copy medicine by labeling nursing phenomena with medicine's defined diseases, but the nursing diagnoses thus far do not attend to formulations of "cause." The formulations essentially ignore the question "why?." If someone has insomnia, it can also be called alteration in sleep, sleep disturbance, abnormal sleep, inability to sleep, disturbed sleep — it does not matter what you call it because none of these labels attends to cause and cannot therefore be called a diagnosis. If only the diagnosticians had started by collecting observable facts in nursing situations and then classifying these facts into categories such as (1) categories of observed verbal and non-verbal behavior which nurses respond to, (2) categories of distress resulting from the inability "to nurse" the self, (3) categories of causes of the inability "to nurse" the self, (4) categories of activity which meet needs for help and (5) categories of observed verbal and non-verbal behavior after the immediate need for help is met.

Conclusion

In this discussion I have tried to impress upon you the importance of articulating a product for our distinct professional function. It does not matter whether or not you subscribe to my formulations of function and product. Certainly your life will be easier if you don't. My formulations have not been popular or politically expedient. What matters is that a distinct formulation of function be articulated on a national scale and that it be stated in such a way that it makes reference to the phenomena of nursing's concern: distress caused by the inability to nurse the self, when the self alone cannot identify or get the needed help. The product of professional nursing should be formulated in terms of what professional nursing has and continues to accomplish, that is, the individual's restoration of or improvement in the capacity to care for the self.

A clear focus on a distinct function and a formulation of product will in turn provide the guidance for our research efforts. Our interventions in the phenomena of our distinct concern and the research data from them [are] all that can possibly create and maintain nursing on an independent path. Our interventions and the data from them will indeed show how individuals unable to nurse themselves alone, or with their own resources, whether or not they have a defined disease, affect their own or their family's sense of well-being. Our interventions will also show the progress of an individual's condition. Further, what we do in response to distress from helplessness will show an effect on the financial cost of individuals in continual distress and suffering. Lastly, our interventions will show an effect on the individual's willingness to comply or not comply with what is known as "doctor's orders."

I am compelled to digress and say a few words about who the doctor orders. We live after all in a free democratic society. Medical orders are for and directed at patients who are free to comply or not to comply. They may direct a physician's assistant but not a professional nurse. Our commitment is to the individual who may or may not require the nurse's care in response to the doctor's orders or in response to anything else. Helping the patient identify and meet immediate needs for help may result in the patient's more active participation by complying or not complying with the doctor's orders.

In connection with this, I ask that you study another transitive verb with me. That is, what it means "to doctor." I refer once more to my favorite dictionary (Funk & Wagnalls 1935). To doctor means: to treat medicinally, to repair, to alter with a view to deceive or adulterate.

I will not dwell on the wonderous benefits medicine continues to provide. I only wish to point out that "to doctor" does not mean "to nurse" nor does "to nurse" means just doing what a doctor orders or what a doctor does. To follow in the footsteps of the doctor or to function as the doctor's competitor maintains nursing in the dependent path. This [path] fails to provide guidance to struggling registered professional nurses in actively assuming independent authority to perform their independent function and behave autonomously in achieving the product of their service.

Authority to function as an independent professional is derived from the function of that profession. Laws already say we can function as registered professional nurses. The authority of physicians, institutions, agencies and health care policy has nothing to do with it, nor would anyone knowingly and publicly interfere with the whole purpose of providing professional nursing services in the first place. No chief executive officer, no physician, no official would publicly state "we don't care how much you suffer helplessness as long as we cure or prevent your disease." This is what our professional authority is all about. No one gives it to us; we assume legal authority to perform our function in order to produce our product.

I am not a prophet of doom when I say that in the absence of fully articulating our own functional authority, the medical authorities in hospitals and health maintenance organizations are moulding health care policy, legislation and nursing's educational programs. Ever new job descriptions are emerging which continue to push nursing into the dependent path while other jobs are being discontinued, which administered and ensured the continuity of the responsibility to provide and direct professional nursing services.

The choice. The choice is ours for the 21st century. We can choose the dependent path as assistants to physicians or as quasi practitioners of medicine, or we can chart the independent path. We did not "then," we have not "now," charted the critical point on the graph. Thus very few people really understand the functional importance of professional nursing. Others do not understand because we have not on a national scale articulated a distinct function and the product our profession in fact does deliver to society. We even keep the results of our excellent work a secret. Only collective clarity can give us the capacity to get on and stay on the independent path. This is the only path which will permit the independent organization and delivery of service anywhere it is needed, as well as the organization of educational and research programmes. Only this radical independent path in my view will cause health care policy makers to fully consider the importance of our professional services, whether anybody likes the image of the registered nurse or not.

If my crystal ball with the rear view mirror has any validity and the present dependent path continues, I defy Nightingale, nurses themselves and the heirs of Webster to give a clear definition to our profession now or in the next century. Charting the alternate path with a distinct function and product will protect consumers as well as the work and future of nursing as an independent profession.

REFERENCES

American Nurses' Association (1980) *Nursing: A Social Policy Statement*. American Nurses' Association, New York.

American Nurses' Association (1985) Goals for nursing, mission statement. *The American Nurse* 17(8), 14.

Bochnak M.A. (1963) The effect of an automatic and deliverative process of nursing activity on the relief of patients' pain: a clinical experiment. *Nursing Research* 12(3), 191-192.

Bochnak M.A., Rhymes J.P. & Leonard R.C.(1962) The comparison of two types of nursing activity on the relief of pain. In *Innovations in Nurse-Patient Relationships: Automatic or Reasoned Nurse Action*. American Nurses' Association, New York.

Dumas R.G. (1963) Psychological preparation for surgery. *The American Journal of Nursing* 63(8), 52-55.

Dumas R.G. & Leonard R.C. (1963) The effect of nursing on the incidence of post-operative vomiting. *Nursing Research* 12(1), 12-15.

Dye M.C. (1963) A descriptive study of conditions conducive to an effective process of nursing activity. *Nursing Research* 12(3), 194.

Fischelis M.C. (1963) An exploratory study of labels nurses attach to patient behaviour and their effect on nursing activities. *Nursing Research* 12(3), 195.

Funk & Wagnalls (1936) *Practical Standard Dictionary of the English Language*. Funk & Wagnalls, New York.

Gillis I. (1976) Sleeplessness: Can you help? *The Canadian Nurse* 72(7), 32-34.

Mertz H. (1963) A study of the process of the nurse's activity as it affects the blood pressure readings and pulse rate of patients admitted to the emergency room. *Nursing Research* 12(3), 197-198.

Orlando I.J. (1961) *The Dynamic Nurse-Patient Relationship: Function, Process and Principles*. G.P. Putnam, New York.

Orlando I.J. (1972) *The Discipline and Teaching of Nursing Process: An Evaluative Study*. G.P. Putnam, New York.

Rhymes J. (1964) A description of nurse-patient interaction in effective nursing activity. *Nursing Research* 13(4), 365.

Tarasuk M.B., Rhymes J. & Leonard R.C. (1965) An experimental test of the importance of communication skills for effective nursing. In *Social Interaction and Patient Care* (Skipper J.K. & Leonard R.C. eds). Lippincott, Philadelphia.

Tryon P.A. & Leonard R.C. (1964) The effect of patients' participation on the outcome of a nursing procedure. *Nursing Forum* 3(2), 79, 89.

Webster (1953) *Webster's New Collegiate Dictionary,* 2nd edn. G. & C. Merriam, Springfield, Massachusetts.

Webster (1963) *Webster's Seventh New Collegiate Dictionary*. G. & C. Merriam, Springfield, Massachusetts.

Defining nursing: A historic controversy

ROZELLA M. SCHLOTFELDT, PhD, FAAN

THE QUESTION ADDRESSED in this article is: To what extent are the definitions of nursing that are popular at particular times in history in harmony or in conflict with the profession's traditions and its generally sanctioned social mission? A further question is: will such definitions facilitate or impede progress in identifying phenomena that are of particular concern to nursing's practitioners and investigators, phenomena about which theories should be promulgated if nursing's body of knowledge is to be advanced?

Ideally, a definition of any field of professional endeavor gives guidance concerning the practice domain in that it identifies the goal and focus of practitioners' concerns and endeavors and the parameters of their work. It also gives direction to the educational preparation of professionals and identifies the phenomena about which professional knowledge should be continuously advanced. Definitions, thus, should be useful in stimulating theory generation for guiding research, the findings from which hold promise of improving practices. Unlike research in the basic disciplines, the link between knowledge discovery and its application in making practices ever more beneficially consequential is the imperative for clinical inquiry conducted by scholars in the service professions.

Definitions of nursing

Nightingale identified nursing's goal and practice domain by noting that nurses should use creatively that which she called "...the laws of health or of nursing, for they are in reality the same...."[1] She also anticipated nursing's scientific research agenda by observing that nature's laws of health were then largely unknown.

Henderson's definition of nursing evolved over time, as revealed by examination of early editions of a text she coauthored.[2] In 1960, members of the International Council of Nurses accepted the definition proposed by Henderson, thereby giving it positive, worldwide sanction. It is:

> The unique function of the nurse is to assist the individual, sick or well, in the performance of those activities contributing to health or its recovery (or to a peaceful death) that he would perform unaided if he had the necessary strength, will, or knowledge. And to do this in such a way as to help him gain independence as rapidly as possible.[3]

Nightingale's view and Henderson's definition of nursing surely are congruent. Both are based on the philosophic orientation that human beings inherently are magnificently endowed and goal directed. Both Nightingale and Henderson recognized the fact that, with rare exceptions, human beings have strengths, capabilities, and natural propensities to seek and to attain their goals, including health, and thus they are by nature health-seeking beings.

It is regrettable that Nightingale's observation that "nature's laws" governing human health, at the time largely unknown, did not result in the early development of nursing research designed to improve nursing practice. However, nursing's early leaders were preoccupied with the occupation's growth and with preparing sufficient numbers of practitioners to meet society's growing demands for their services. It is also regrettable that, as the occupation began to emerge as a profession, early investigators did not in large numbers pursue answers to research questions that could have been derived from Henderson's definition of nursing practice.

In a guest editorial celebrating the twenty-fifth anniversary of *Nursing Research,* Henderson observed that few nurses had engaged in research designed to improve nursing practice. She was cautiously optimistic about the seemingly developing trend toward investigators' involvement in research that holds promise of improving nursing practice.[4]

During the past three decades, nurses have demonstrated remarkably increased interest and involvement in scholarly endeavors that have derived from the profession's commitment to an enhanced research agenda and to identifying the components of the discipline underlying nursing practice. As Ellis noted, the question, "What is nursing research?," posed the more basic one, "What is nursing?"[5] In response to the latter question, some nursing scholars developed models, conceptualizations, and paradigms portraying nursing as a field of practice and systematic inquiry. Those frameworks have been proposed as perspectives within which to view nursing's world of work and of research that is designed to aid in advancing, verifying, clarifying, and organizing the body of knowledge, the discipline that underlies nursing practice.

Although there have been many calls for theory development, efforts of nursing's investigators to date have been devoted primarily to testing theories generated by scholars in the basic disciplines.[6] They have been less involved in theorizing about phenomena that are of particular concern to nurses and of which extant knowledge is minimal, contradictory, or lacking. It is, thus, particularly important that newly formulated definitions of nursing promote the identification of phenomena of which

more relevant, and verified knowledge is needed to make nursing practice ever more effective.

Nursing leaders following Nightingale and Henderson have agreed that nurses' central concern is to appraise and safeguard human beings' health and to promote their attainment of or restoration to optimal health states through the knowledgeable, humane, and ethical use of nursing strategies. There is widespread agreement that nurses serve those who are essentially well, but who need assistance in achieving additional knowledge, strength, and motivation to attain optimal states of health. There is also agreement that nurses care for persons who are ill, injured, impaired, and infirm and who are relatively or completely, temporarily or permanently, dependent on others, frequently nurses, to attain their health goals.

Generally, nurses accept the eudaimonistic interpretation of the meaning of health.[7] To them, health is a relative concept. Nursing's goal has traditionally been — and still is — to assist human beings attain, retain, or regain the highest possible levels of physical, physiological, social, and emotional function and comfort of which each is capable. In accomplishing this goal, nurses consider the current state of knowledge and do all possible to safeguard their patients' human dignity during their dependent states and at the time of their demise.

Whereas agreement persists among most nurses that the promotion of human health is their central concern,[8] evidence is mounting that the perspective of many nurses has changed. Nursing literature indicates that nurses' preoccupation with health problems, etiology, nursing diagnoses, and treatment has led to the belief that valid nursing science depends on a taxonomic classification of so-called nursing diagnoses, and theorizing about them. Diligent and persistent efforts have been made to develop approved lists of such diagnoses as a precursor to attainment of those goals.[9] These efforts reflect a remarkable shift in nurses' perspective of their mission, their world of work, and the phenomena about which theories are needed to guide research for the advancement of nursing science.

A change in perspective

Perhaps most influential in effecting a changed perspective of nursing's mission is the definition of nursing that was given official sanction by its inclusion in the American Nurses' Association's *Social Policy Statement:*

> Nursing is the diagnosis and treatment of human responses to actual and potential health problems.[10]

Is that definition in harmony with nursing's traditionally sanctioned mission? Is it likely to promote the identification and classification of natural phenomena about which nursing scholars should theorize?

The promotion of human health is not articulated as the goal of nursing care in the ANA's definition. Indeed, the term "health" appears only once, as an adjective that modifies the term "problem," thus conveying the message that the focus of nurses' concern is exclusively with persons who actually or potentially suffer from health problems. True, it focuses on human responses to health problems, but those responses are to be diagnosed and treated.

The commonly accepted definition of the term "diagnosis" is to identify the cause of that which is not normal, i.e., a pathologic state, especially when it is used in combination with the term "treatment."[11] The message conveyed is that human responses to health problems are not only to be diagnosed accurately but also to be treated, i.e., dealt with effectively to minimize, decrease, or eliminate their noxious or unfavorable nature and/or consequences. Logic, along with knowledge of the variety of responses that human beings

manifest when they experience health problems, lead one to question what nurses are to do when human responses are not troublesome, but are normal or beneficial. Consider, for example, temperature elevation, shivering, blanching and flushing of the skin, tensing of muscles over bone trauma and as a means to relieve pain, phagocytosis, vomiting, and self-protective, behavioral responses such as anxiety, withdrawal, and denial.

If responses are natural, normal manifestations of human beings' innate health-seeking mechanisms and behaviors, is treatment indicated? Moreover, is there agreement about treatments that should be instituted/recommended for human responses to health problems — all of them, all circumstances, and for all human beings, and thus considered to be good/usual nursing practice? Are there not multiple antecedents to persons' abilities to attain healthy states and to cope with and to overcome health problems? Should nurses not seek to assist individuals in maximizing their potentials in that regard?

Ambiguity and lack of clear logic also surround use of the phrase "...human responses to...potential health problems" in the ANA *Social Policy Statement*.[12] How do human beings respond to problems that are only potentially theirs and how do nurses determine which diagnostic and treatment modalities are relevant and appropriate?

If the appraisal and promotion of human health has traditionally been and still is the central concern and social mission of nurses, the ANA's definition is not only incomplete and in part illogical, but it is also in conflict with the long-standing conceptualization of the nature of nursing. The definition may delay or deter progress in theory development.

Advancement of science

Scientific theory development depends on identification of *natural* phenomena that are of particular concern to scholars in any discipline. For nursing scholars, those phenomena are human health-seeking assets — the mechanisms, propensities, behaviors, and powers with which they are naturally endowed and those they subsequently acquire, often with the assistance of knowledgeable, skillful, humane, and caring nurses. It is the responsiblity of nursing's scholars to advance, clarify, verify, and organize knowledge of those phenomena through promulgating and testing relevant and promising theoretical constructs. Nursing science will not be advanced by theorizing about "nursing diagnoses" for these reasons:

1. Nursing diagnoses are not natural phenomena. Valid science derives from testing and finding support for theories about natural phenomena.

2. The focus of nursing diagnoses is on *disability*, *dys*function, and human deficits. Theorizing about human deficiencies and disabilities denies the strengths, abilities, propensities, knowledge, and assets of the human spirit through which persons seek health.

3. Theorizing about labels attached only to human responses to health *problems* (nursing diagnoses) holds potential for precluding theory development and systematic inquiry that leads to knowledge of the gamut of health-seeking phenomena available to persons in all relative states of health, illness, and injury and the promulgation of theories concerning nursing strategies that are efficacious in assisting all human beings in various circumstances attain their health goals.

In contrast, nursing scholars should address pertinent questions that will guide observations and stimulate the generation of theoretical constructs about phenomena that are of particular or unique concern to nurses and worthy of testing. These questions are proposed:

1. What human phenomena, i.e., innate human health-seeking mechanisms and innate and learned health-seeking behaviors, are of particular concern to nurses?

2. How can those health-seeking mechanisms and behaviors best be named, classified, and characterized?

3. What universals govern/regulate those mechanisms and behaviors?

4. What factors promote and enhance and which ones disrupt and impede the regularity, function, and effectiveness of human health-seeking mechanisms and behaviors?

5. What nursing strategies are effective in preserving, protecting, regulating, and promoting the normal functioning and effectiveness of human health-seeking and behavioral mechanisms?

6. What nursing strategies are effective in bringing about constructive changes in the knowledge, beliefs, customs, commitments, motivations, and actions of human beings that lead them to avoid risks to their health status, assets, and potentials and to pursue life-styles and behaviors conducive to their attaining, retaining, and regaining optimal physical, physiological, social, and psychological function and comfort and the personal productivity, self-fulfillment, and dignity that are appropriate to their humanity?

Addressing those questions — along with thoughtful analyses of carefully and systematically recorded observations of human beings in laboratory and in clinical situations and the hard thinking and flashes of creative insights of scholarly nursing practitioners, scientists, and other scholars — will produce promising theoretical constructs. They will serve as guides to nursing investigations through which will come advancements in nursing's body of knowledge and improvements in nursing practice. A human health-seeking perspective is the appropriate focus of any definition of nursing.

Nursing can be accurately and succinctly defined to reflect its long-established social mission and goal, to guide the preparation of professionals, and to identify the phenomena about which theories are now and likely henceforth will be needed as:

Nursing is the appraisal and the enhancement of the health status, health assets, and health potentials of human beings.

NOTES

1. Florence Nightingale, *Notes on Nursing* (London: Harrison, 1860), p.6.

2. B. Harmer, and Virginia Henderson, *Textbook of the Principles and Practice of Nursing.* (New York: The Macmillan Company, 1939, 1955, editions 4-5).

3. Virginia Henderson, *Basic Principles of Nursing Care* (London: International Council of Nurses, 1960), p.3.

4. Virginia Henderson, "We've Come a Long Way, but What of the Direction?" (Guest Editorial), *Nursing Research,* 26 (May-June 1977):163-164.

5. Rosemary Ellis,"Theory Development in Nursing: The State of the Art," in *Nursing Theories: Sharing for Success,* Proceedings of a conference held at The Sir Mortimer B. Davis Jewish General Hospital, Montreal, Quebec, October 3, 1984, pp. 623.

6. Peggy Chinn, "From the Editor," *Advances in Nursing Science,* 6 (Summer 1984):ix.

7. J.A. Smith, "The Idea of Health: A Philosophic Inquiry," *Advances in Nursing Science,* 3 (April 1981):43-50.

8. Jacqueline Fawcett, "Hallmarks of Success in Nursing Theory Development," in *Advances in Nursing Theory Development,* ed. Peggy Chinn (Rockville, Md.: Aspen Systems Corp., 1983), pp. 3-17.

9. M. Kim, A. McFarland, and G. McLane, eds. *Classification of Nursing Diagnoses: Proceedings of the Fifth National Conference.* (St. Louis: C.V. Mosby Company, 1984).

10. American Nurses' Association. *Nursing: A Social Policy Statement* (Kansas City, Mo.: The American Nurses' Association, 1980), p. 9.

11. *Webster's New International Dictionary.* (Springfield, Mass.: G&C Merriam Company, 1966), p. 622.

12. American Nurses' Association, *op. cit.*

Nursing comes of age

JOAN E. LYNAUGH, RN, PhD; CLAIRE M. FAGIN, RN, PhD

WE WISH TO CELEBRATE a strange and paradoxical subculture in American society: a group whose conflicts internally and externally have been well recorded; a group that confronts barriers to advancement and even survival — barriers that stem from deep social, economic and professional ambivalences about its responsibilities and its privileges.

This essay is grounded in two historic realities: first, nursing is made up of individuals from heterogeneous class, ethnic and racial backgrounds; and second, the mission of nursing, giving care, is undervalued in our society. These two realities fuel contemporary debate and underlie the questions that we argue every day. Is nursing a profession or simply a skilled occupation? Does it matter? Should nursing continue to try to collaborate with medicine, or should we focus on competition? Can we succeed in attracting new nurses if we cling to our caregiving, altruistic mission? How does oppression of nurses as women fit into this story? Why is nursing reaffirmed as being crucial to society only in times of shortage and systematically devalued at all other times?

This confluence of paradoxes, problems and characteristics of nursing development and its current situation can be responded to in two ways. One is to bewail our failures and accept their inevitability in the face of an historically hostile environment. The other is to wonder at and celebrate the extraordinary accomplishments of nurses, mostly of the wrong sex and social class, who have the wrong history and education, who persist and achieve in spite of being held back by some of the most powerful forces in our society.

The perspective of celebration is vital. It would be supremely ironic if nursing and its public were to fail to recognize our victories. If we do not understand accurately where we are now, we will continue to fight the battles of yesterday and squander the resources that we need for addressing the problems of today and tomorrow. In this paper, we draw from the past and the present to propose a way of positioning nursing for the twenty-first century.

We identify some paradoxes of the nursing profession — enduring dilemmas — characteristics of our work that are, for nursing, both panacea and poison. We explore five fundamental and overarching descriptors and predictors of nursing's situation: nursing's mission — caregiving, nursing's fit with the economic system, gender — the women's issue, oppression, and our preoccupation with professional status.

A society that systematically undervalues care

The assumption in our culture is that nurses substitute for family members and servants. For 100 years, during those times when self-care and family care no longer suffice, we have experimented with ways to transfer the job of "caring for another" from the family to nursing. We cast our work in educational, assistive, empathetic, sustaining and managerial terms. We say that we "put the patient in the best condition for nature to act on him" (Nightingale 1860/1969) or that we "assist the individual...in...those activities...that he would perform unaided if he had the necessary strength, will or knowledge" (Henderson, 1966, p. 15). When nursing was invented (i.e., when women of the nineteenth century conceptualized how the substitutive function of nursing should be carried out), nursing was seen as assuring a safe environment, sharing moral and scientific knowledge and sustaining the whole person.

The idea that each specific disease should have a specific cure did not really take over until the end of the nineteenth century. Nursing, of course, was invented well before that — in the 1860s and 1870s. It was intended for American nursing to deal with the individual and collective problems created by dependence in the circumstance of illness. And, it is important to stress, the way nurses conceived of illness at the time was representative of the society at large; that is, although the sick hoped to be cured by medicine, they only hoped to be cured; they did not really expect it, the way we now expect a cure. Most individuals believed that health and illness depended on a balance between one's personal, inherited constitution and the surrounding environment. Nurses supported personal resistance to the ravages of disease and controlled the environment.

At first, most patients were persons who did not have family caregivers because they were poor and isolated through immigration or destruction of the family, or because they were a danger to their families as a result of contagion or insanity. By the end of the nineteenth century, however, more and more Americans were delegating their own care to nurses rather than to family members because they thought it was safer or more convenient and because they could afford it.

Just when the success of nursing as a substitute for family caregiving began to be realized, things began to change dramatically in health care. By the beginning of the twentieth century, an interventionist, specific disease model of medicine began to dominate. This model replaced older, more conservative, nineteenth

century "watchful waiting" approaches to sickness. With the success of the germ theory in explaining infectious illness, "disease" came to be the moral and logical organizing device for the payment for care. In the twentieth century encounters between health care providers and patients were justified by the existence of real or presumed disease (Rosenberg, 1987). As Rosenberg pointed out, "Specialization exemplified and exacerbated a more general tendency of medicine toward the reductionist and technological; its existence helped justify and act out the powerful image of the hospital as scientific institution" (pp. 174-175).

By 1900 the dilemma of how to constitute nursing's task of substitute caregiving in the face of these sweeping changes was confronted in hospitals most of all. In addition to the socially mandated task of substituting for the family, nurses were asked to assume the institutionally mandated task of substituting for the physician. The myriad tasks associated with diagnosis and therapy began to dominate the interior life of hospitals and the work day of nurses. Nurses, like other Americans, were captivated by the successes that disease-specific models of care seemed to achieve over the frightening toll caused by epidemic illness. For the first 60 or 70 years of the twentieth century, nursing essentially "tagged along" with this change in the way that health care was defined and delivered. Moreover, hospital nurses made possible many of the surgical and medical interventions that came to characterize care of the sick.

Now, as the twentieth century draws to a close, these acute care, interventionist models and disease-focused designs for payment for care seem to have become a problem. They fail to correspond in a functional way with our increasingly perceived need for providing care for children, the old, the chronically ill and the dying. There is heightening concern that these needs are in competition with each other for declining resources. We Americans believe that we have the best health care in the world, but we are unhappy and worried about the cost of the care as well as the number of people not receiving care, and we are uneasy about our individual prospects with respect to long-term and chronic care (Pokorny, 1988).

These concerns fit superbly with nursing's caregiving mission. Throughout its 80 years of collaboration with the acute care interventionist model, nursing has held on to its ideology of holism and family-based care. Let us celebrate what nurses have done to build that which is best about hospitals — caregiving, safety, competence and continuity where these ingredients are possible. Nursing continues to espouse the idea that illness affects persons and families, that care should be organized around individuals and families rather than diseases.

Person-based care has been practiced by nurses working in visiting nurse societies, in nursing homes and in private duty as well as in multiple other arenas of practice. Nursing has insisted on defining itself as the profession that assists ill persons without regard for their cure potential.

Recall that our discipline grew out of a public demand for knowledgeable caregivers. Nursing is a response to the insistence by modern society that dependent members not be abandoned to their fate and, beyond that, that the sick require informed and reliable care. We should celebrate the roles that nursing plays in ameliorating the harsher aspects of a highly individualistic, productivity-oriented society, the ideology of holism, adaptation favoring survival, reform rather than passive acceptance and altruism rather than the self-serving exploitation of others.

But we should also analyze critically our decisions about how those caregiving resources are used and to whose benefit they are applied. We need to be sure that nursing resources are applied first to the public good; vital nursing services should not be diverted to preserve institutions or support other professional groups.

Nursing and the economic system

Nursing has its origins in unpaid domestic work and powerful historic links with religiously inspired human services. Neither domestic service nor the religious sisterhoods are the route to individual financial success. Paradoxically, nursing also served as one of the most successful routes to respectable paid work for women. This is a complicated story; we will explore part of it.

Except for care of the insane and the infectious, the military and the very poor, there was minimal government involvement or investment in the care of the sick until after World War II. Nursing developed in the private sector, which, in the nineteenth century, attracted little public debate. What the private sector developed in the way of health care services was pretty much what the dominant middle class thought was important. Community leaders, businessmen and philanthropists wanted to buy, both for themselves and for those whom they thought worthy of their charity, those services that they thought counted for biological survival and freedom from pain or dysfunction.

It is important to remember that not much money circulated in the health care system before World War II. Neither hospitals nor physicians nor medical researchers, and certainly not nurses, resembled those of today, either in affluence or influence. For hospitals, a crucial crutch was the minimally paid pupil nurse. They subsidized American hospitals and made it possible for a labor-intensive business to survive and even grow in a cash-starved sector of the economy.

The pupil nurses were willing to trade their time, labor and sometimes their health for the title "graduate nurse" because nursing constituted paid work for women — and this was respected by society. The private duty practice that most of these graduate nurses entered offered an avenue of self-support, however unstable. By the 1920s there were nearly 2,000 traning schools churning out graduates into the private duty market. Most of these nurses worked in their patients' homes. Ironically, if the patients stayed home and paid the private duty nurse to care for them, they did not use the hospital. Thus the graduates of the hospital training school were in competition with their alma maters for paying patients (Reverby, 1983).

The patients were increasingly willing and able to pay for health care services. It is important not to lose sight of the attractiveness and significance to the American public of nursing care. Our predecessors had pride and confidence in their product. As individual practitioners, however, they experienced great difficulty in competing successfully with institutions. A second irony in this private duty-hospital competition is that the hospitals were led most often by other nurses. Christopher Parnell, the medical superintendent at University Hospital in Ann Arbor, explained in 1920 that hospital administration frequently attracted physicians who were "medical derelicts," whereas "the reason for the almost universal employment of trained nurses as hospital executives has been simply that a higher quality of intelligence could be purchased for the money than could be secured in the service of men in the positions" (Parnell, 1920).

A third element of this strange story is the unknown cost of nursing care. Except for private duty, nurses have been paid salaries by institutions that in turn sell their services either by renting beds by the day or selling nursing visits one at a time. Hospital-based nursing care was rarely singled out either as an expense or as a source of revenue. So, except for the earliest nurse-run hospitals, no one, including the nurse supervisor and the hospital administrator, kept track of the real cost of nurs-

ing, although it was the central service that the institution provided.

Perhaps because students were the laborers and because most hospitals were either benevolent institutions or tax supported, no "outsiders" demanded an accounting. Thus hospitals could and did operate under exceptionally simple and uninformative budgets. The outcome, however, was to hide the real costs of nursing care until the 1950s. Then, when student labor began to be withdrawn from the hospitals by the reformation or closing of diploma schools, pained outcries were heard. As long as retrospective reimbursement from insurers closed the gap, however, we still did not confront the real costs of nursing care. The distress over the cost of health care has made us begin to consider seriously accounting the actual cost and revenue of hospital nursing care; this belated concern was accelerated in 1983 by the prospective payment system.

During the 1950s, nurses also began to insist on improving their economic situation and turned to the tried and true methods of collective bargaining. Other workers in American society had organized much earlier, but for a long time nurses, isolated and altruistic, did not move. They tended to accept the economic facts of life as they were. Shirley Titus (1952), one of the founders of the movement to improve the economic plight of nurses, summed it up in 1952:

> As I have given thought to the situation, it has seemed to me that the nurse within the four walls of her job — and her job has practically constituted her whole waking life — has been like a sleeper who has slept serenely on while a great battle — a battle for human freedom and the rights of the common man — was being waged. But eventually the sleeper awakens (pp. 1109-1110).

The sleeper, 35 years later, is *almost* fully awake. We are learning to price our services in a way that is equitable both to the consumer and to the provider. We have learned that altruism and subsidization have too high a price; they devalue our work; they impair recruitment; and they burden unfairly a vital social service.

We have not touched directly on the impact of technology on the economic status of nursing. Nor have we brought public health and visiting nursing into the economic story. We will leave this question of economic fit by making only two points. First, nursing is a product that Americans have proved again and again that they want to buy. Second, Americans have no easy way of knowing what our services are worth or should cost. The reasons for this odd state of affairs rest in the hidden, intimate nature of nursing, in its altruistic and domestic origins and most of all in the great cultural reluctance to admit to the real costs of the nursing services we seem to want.

The creativity in hiding these costs is astonishing (Lynaugh, 1987). American ingenuity figured out how to use pupils instead of trained nurses to care for patients and created turnover (which we used to think was good) by refusing to employ married nurses. We kept salaries down by labeling women's wages "supplemental." We allowed hospitals to fix wages. We excluded nurses from direct insurance-based reimbursement. We argued that we could not afford to acknowledge the concept of comparable worth. (Feldberg, 1984).

Nursing has an essential product and our public is beginning to acknowledge this reality with economic rewards instead of kind testimonials. With help from consumers, we chip away at restrictions on third-party reimbursement. We are out from under the yoke of hospital domination of our educational system. Demand for our services drives entry-level salaries up even in these cost-conscious times, particularly when the spectre of shortage looms. Nurse-midwives, nurse practitioners,

psychiatric clinical specialists, nurse anesthetists, neonatal nurses and gerontology nurses prove their worth directly, and the purchasing public responds.

The American Nurses' Association (ANA) estimates that 20,000 American nurses have started independent business ventures, "and many more can be expected to embark on similar ventures in the future. Many nurses with capital for start-up costs have founded primary care clinics, birthing centers, or home health agencies" ("Perspectives," 1987, p. 3). Nurses are allowed in 25 states to bill private insurers directly for their services. The nursing lobby is pressuring federal lawmakers to remove Medicare restrictions that prohibit nurses from billing the government; nurse anesthetists and nurse-midwives are already there. Legislation introduced by Representative Richard Gephardt (D-MO) would allow nursing organizations to compete for Medicare risk contracts to provide certain Part B services to elderly beneficiaries. Senator Daniel Inouye (D-HI), a long-time champion of nursing, has offered multiple proposals for reimbursement of nurses and has protested when governmental health programs exclude proper utilization of clinical specialists. Many other members of Congress look favorably on a wide variety of proposals to expand the role and reimbursement possibilities for nurses.

All of these efforts are strengthened by the report of the Office of Technology Assessment (1986), which found that nurse practitioners were not being used to their fullest potential. The study concluded that, if their services were covered, access to care would be improved for underserved populations, and cost savings could be achieved. Currently, efforts are being made to find acceptable cost accounting systems for hospital nursing services, and several models have been developed and are being tested. We are documenting nursing interventions and costs so as to provide the data necessary for third-party reimbursement for nursing care in any setting (Fagin, 1986).

All of these economic accomplishments have been in the face of strong, organized opposition from the American Medical Association and, early on, from the insurance industry. Recently the insurance industry has changed its position, having recognized the possible cost savings of alternate health care providers, specifically nurses.

Gender — The women's issue

The history of nursing shows that women are dominated by the male values of American society and deterred from their goals by implicit and explicit acceptance of those values by the masses. Today 97 percent of Registered Nurses are women; while there have been, and continue to be, men in the profession who are major contributors, nursing's female image has deterred men from entering nursing in the numbers necessary to change its femaleness. How can nursing succeed unless we become a woman-valued work group? We have struggled with domination by male physicians, administrators and board members for almost all of our 100-year history. We have tried isolation, accommodation, isolation again, collaboration, demands for equality and negotiation. A woman's occupation with superb women leaders, yet dominated by men from other disciplines, is a paradox that is tied to the economic dilemma, but its complexity goes beyond economic equity.

Lavinia Dock lived and practiced across both centuries of our existence. She was an author, feminist and pacifist. Of all of the turn-of-the-century leaders, she probably understood best the American culture. She said it simply: "The status of nursing...depends on the status of women" (Dock & Stewart, 1920, p. 338). Nursing is a woman's profession because it is nursing.

There is another irony: Americans have an agenda of self-actualization and productivity. The vital role of nursing in relation to Ameri-

can social priorities has led to reluctance on the part of the public to come to grips with the worth of nursing, that is, to acknowledge how much it really costs to buy the freedom that nursing offers American families. As long as women were willing to subsidize the development of hospitals, high-technology care of the poor through their own low wages, America was free to expand these services at relatively low cost.

Nursing was born in the first women's movement in the midnineteenth century, bred in the second movement during the drive for the vote and will mature in the last years of the twentieth century. The renaissance of nurse-midwifery and the nurse practitioner movements can be seen as illustrations of nursing's sending out "pseudopods" of services desired by the public but left unattended through restrictions created by both medicine and nursing. These movements achieved the bringing together of nurses and consumers of nursing care. Nurse-midwives and nurse practitioners confronted the interdependence of medicine and nursing, which had been hidden by medical dominance. This was a painful and difficult process since it involved giving up the more comfortable strategy of isolation from medicine adopted by nursing in the 1950s and 1960s. In this new interdependence, the qualities that nurses value were allowed to influence overtly the interaction. Supportiveness, compassion, concern for others, concern for human relationships are qualities seen by some contemporary feminists as being essentially self-sacrificing (Blum, Homiak, Housman & Shaman, 1976). Nurses retained and continue to display these qualities despite value shifts that define "good" women's behaviors as those valued by men.

A critical mass of women leaders is found in all countries including those in the Third World — nurses working in practice and education as well as in associated health field roles in governments throughout the world. Reports at the quadrennial meeting of the International Council of Nurses in 1985 gave superb evidence of social reform and leadership in which all women could take pride and satisfaction. Hundreds of stories were told of nurses' taking leading roles in providing services to the unemployed, to people with AIDS and to other populations at risk. Nurses are at the front lines of care and the administration of health care in its vast variety of settings throughout the world. Many can now also be found in both the corporate world and law in positions that were anticipated by the "upward and onward" cliches in their high school year books.

The first case on comparable worth was brought by a group of nurses in Denver, Colorado, and one of the first suits brought by women faculty members seeking comparable salaries occurred at the University of Washington, stimulated by the faculty in the School of Nursing. The ANA served as amicus curiae in that case. More recently, in Illinois a case is being brought and a Pennsylvania suit was won (Holcomb, 1988). But, we still have trouble behaving like winners and we are some distance away from consensus on Melosh's (1982) call for a "generous and inclusive program [leading] toward expanded authority for all nurses" (p. 210).

Oppression

One explanation for fragmented group behavior may rest in the concept of oppression. Roberts (1983) argues that nursing can be considered an oppressed group because it has been controlled by forces outside itself that "had greater prestige, power, and status and that exploited the less powerful group" (pp. 21-22). Oppressed groups commonly feel self-hatred and low self-esteem.

Nurses are being targeted for a new public relations effort because it is apparent that we are caught up in self-flagellating and group-

flagellating behavior — the oppressors "blame the victim." Oppressed individuals are given to intragroup conflict, and this is often used by the oppressors to illustrate that the group cannot come together, cannot govern themselves, cannot organize. Examples of these two characteristics are found in the constant accusations that we are unable to speak with one voice. Our intragroup conflict is evident in any discussion about levels in nursing education; the current manifestation of this historic struggle is the 1987-1988 conflict between the ANA and several state nursing associations over who is entitled to membership in the profession's organization if professional nursing alters its credentialing requirements.

To remain oppressed, groups must be kept in their place. Only by behaviors that keep nurses "down" can the other players stay "up" (Myrdal, 1944). Nurses are ambivalent about protesting real or perceived threats and generally prefer accommodation. But nursing needs to examine the ends served by accommodation versus planning a coherent, strategic form of protest to conditions that, at the very least, threaten the performance of nursing. Individuals who protest may accomplish some important goals. One is to demonstrate that protest does not hurt and may even advance the protester. Group protest, of course, is much safer and certainly more potent, but so far it has been used insufficiently in nursing. Perhaps this is because, as Reverby (1987) suggests, "Occupational loyalty, the basic consciousness necessary to begin a professionalizing and standardizing effort, [is] difficult to elicit within nursing" (p. 122). Of the five discussed here, this dilemma is the most difficult to celebrate since the oppressed, though numerous, are far less representative than we would like of the group as a whole.

Profession versus occupation

All groups with special social functions (i.e., professions) are defined both by their social relevance and by their value orientations rather than by any empirical fact. Although the work of nursing continued to be important fundamentally, in the early part of the twentieth century something that presumably was better (i.e., cure and prevention of disease) was being offered. Our rhetoric remained unrelentingly holistic; it included the individual, the family and the environment and romanticized the view of the nurse as advocate for patients and their care during those times when the patients (clients) are unable to do those things for themselves. Retaining a holistic and romantic concept while seeking professional status through the university is yet another example of nursing's survival in a climate oppressive and antagonistic to both its basic essence and its belief system.

It seems strange that few among us are willing to relinquish the term "professional" from our identity — "strange" because it is irrational to consider that all registered nurses are professional no matter what their preparation. If we do, there does not seem to be much meaning to the term. If we could get the term "professional" out of our language, we might be better able to stratify and segment our group. Melosh (1982) believes that, "as a strategy for nursing, professionalization is doomed to fail; as an ideology, professionalism divides nurses and weds its proponents to limited and ultimately self-defeating values" (p. 16). In addition to the resistance to change created by moral and religious overtones and undertones, professionalization draws boundaries that may be resisted strongly by members of the group who are seen as outside those boundaries. When they are the clear majority, this opposition undercuts and often makes futile efforts to "upgrade," achieve power and achieve autonomy and other essentials of professionalization.

Early public health nurses came closer than any other nurses to claiming the privileges of professionals. Their work was relatively un-

confined; they were independent and they had an esprit de corps and a special identity. They did not make common cause with other nurses because they relished their own autonomy and their special relationship with philanthropic supporters (Buhler-Wilkerson, 1983). Later, when medicine challenged and succeeded in aborting this movement, their lack of common cause with the masses of nurses brought little support during the years of their demise. An interesting and contrasting case in point is the experience of nursing and nurse-midwifery. For decades the nurse-midwife group was shunned by nurses, and the feeling was mutual. For more than a decade now, this noxious and ultimately destructive situation has changed dramatically. Nurse-midwives are very much a part of nursing and its leadership and support and are supported by other nurses in their quest for independence, autonomy, power and access to the reimbursement stream. Yet nurse-midwives are facing new pressures both within and outside of their group as their own fragile professionalism is just being achieved. Their problems mirror the larger questions of power, control, occupational loyalty and group cohesion.

Achieving professionalism for a caring discipline with a holistic philosophy, predominantly female and oppressed, with limited access to the funding stream may be a laughable objective. But celebrate what we have accomplished.

Most national nursing organizations have endorsed the baccalaureate degree as the minimum entry-level credential for professional nursing. The W.K. Kellogg Foundation-supported National Commission on Nursing Implementation Project (NCNIP), composed of a broad spectrum of nurses and other educators and health professionals, recommends differentiated practice with clear delineation of professional and associated nurse roles. The most recent survey of the American Hospital Association (AHA) (1988) shows that almost 60 percent of hospitals in this country prefer to employ the baccalaureate graduate in entry-level staff positions. This survey also indicates a 25 percent vacancy rate for master's-prepared clinical specialists. That such findings would occur from an AHA study of hospitals rather than from a guild of nursing educators may amaze some audiences, but it seems to be a clear indication that the marketplace would advance nursing's goals of professional preparation.

The acceptance and desirability of the clinical specialist in all modalities of treatment and care are extraordinary indicators of achievement of professional status. Nurses appear to be the providers of choice in case manager roles. The data show that nursing affects patient outcomes and contributes to the goals of a competitive health care system (OTA, 1986). Convincing evidence for hospitals' and physicians' support of professional status are such studies as the one completed at George Washington University, which compared the outcome (mortality) of 5,020 patients in intensive care at 13 hospitals. In intensive care units that had the lowest mortality, nurses operated with a high degree of autonomy, were the best educated and had independent responsibilities (Knaus, Draper, Wagner & Zimmerman, 1986).

Several foundations have been instrumental in enhancing the professionalism of nursing. A major initiative was the Robert Wood Johnson Foundation Teaching Nursing Home Project. This program proposed to improve the quality of care provided in nursing homes through linkage of selected nursing homes to university schools of nursing. It was also intended that nursing students might be attracted to long-term care as an attractive career opportunity because of the role modeling of expert clinicians. Now completed, the project is being evaluated and by all accounts appears to have been successful in improving the quality of

care in the nursing homes involved and increasing the professional status of the carers (Aiken, Mezey, Lynaugh, & Buck, 1985; Joel, 1986; Mezey, Lynaugh, & Cartier, 1988).

The most important reason to celebrate achievements in nurse professionalism are the extraordinary accomplishments of nurse researchers in conducting research that focuses on patient care and systems improvement. The frequently cited study of Brooten (1986) is a case in point. Brooten et al. studied the effects of early discharge of low birth-weight infants when the family was supported by a perinatal nurse clinician according to a specific regimen. The results were positive for the families, and the cost benefits were significant. Publication in the *New England Journal of Medicine* brought a great deal of attention to the team and to the nursing profession, and, like the study on intensive care cited above, provided additional credibility for the effectiveness of the credentialed nurse specialist.

As nursing comes of age, no achievement seems as paradoxical as the establishment of the National Center of Nursing Research, which recognizes and supports the professional status of nursing at the uppermost level, while the occupational membership refuses to come to terms with preparation for such status at the entry level.

Moving to coming of age

Biologist and philosopher Rene Dubos made clear that biological success in all its manifestations is fundamentally a measure of fitness (and he meant fitness to survive); fitness requires never-ending efforts of adaptation to the environment, which is ever changing (Dubos, 1959). So, we will try to develop a picture of the environment and the fitness of nursing now and in the coming decades — an epidemiologic picture.

According to Olshansky and Ault (1986), epidemiologic scholars outline a four-state historical sequence of events, beginning with the age of pestilence and famine, when infectious diseases such as infant diarrhea, tuberculosis, and small pox killed children and young adults frequently and at young ages. This was followed by the age of receding pandemic — an era of falling death rates from infectious illnesses, probably resulting from rapid improvement in sanitation and nutrition in the nineteenth century and creating a redistribution of death from the young to the old. Midway into the twentieth century, we reached a plateau — the age of degenerative and man-made diseases, when the major causes of death were heart disease, cancer and stroke; life expectancy reached into the seventies. Now, in the waning years of the twentieth century, a rapid decline in mortality signals a new era — the age of "delayed degenerative diseases." Nursing's current and future priorities must reflect this epidemiologic reality.

Although it is important that we continue our concern about the care, treatment and prevention of acute illness, our experience teaches us that acute infectious illnesses do not very often kill our children. Lack of prenatal care and violence do. Our parents no longer succumb early to acute pneumonia, the "old man's friends," but recover to face an uncertain future and need help with everyday living. A nation that places all of its resources in cure-oriented diagnosis and treatment of disease shortchanges the growing part of the population who require care and support. All health care providers must explore and adapt their educational and service structures to meet the needs of the current era. Nursing, the most adaptable of all the providers, conceives its future and chooses among socially and ethically sound alternatives to accommodate to this "age of delayed degenerative diseases."

Conclusions

We have explored five enduring dilemmas or paradoxes affecting nursing since its origin in

this country. In each instance we illustrated, if not pure "panacea," at least extraordinary accomplishments yielding more than enough reason to celebrate where we are in 1988 and giving us confidence to plan for the future.

The entire health care system has been built on the backs of nurses — first on the training-apprentice model of free service, then on the poorly paid masses of service-oriented, educated, but mainly female workers. We can celebrate thousands of nurses and leaders at multiple levels. There are hundreds of experiments in innovative models of nursing practice, which address the structural problems that diminish the participation and effectiveness of nursing; these are new examples of managed care and differentiated practice and creatively responsive services for the elderly in nursing homes and in the community. Nurse entrepreneurs are at the leading edge of market developments in health care. Nurse researchers are exploring issues ranging across the entire spectrum of patient care as well as the social and biological sciences. In many cases this research has significant cost implications. Nurses are in distinguished, elected and appointed positions nationally and regionally, and nurse lobbyists are considered to be among the most effective in Washington.

Many nurses are "at the table" of decision making at local and national levels in governmental and private groups that customarily are closed to women. We believe that this shows that nurses have much greater access to power than we recognize. The concern that many men express about possible conspiratorial behavior when women collect is an indicator of the potential power of women and nurses to foster change. Clearly it is one reason for the continued opposition of the AMA and the AHA to upgrading nursing education for the masses. After all, with more education, we might have even more articulate movers and shakers and be even more dangerous to the status quo.

Coming of age requires that we look beyond the splendid minority in our group and recognize that within our unrecognized and invisible majority are many extraordinary contributors to the lives of individuals who must be brought into visibility within the profession and to the public. The accomplishments of our leaders have meaning only when they support, sustain, make sense of and forward the work of those for whom the leaders speak and act.

In clarifying the persistent and pervasive paradoxes of the profession, we must ask how we have accomplished so much in the century of our existence. We believe that is the common link to caring that brings nurses together. It is the link that brought us all to this great field of oppression and opportunity; it is this which keeps us persisting despite the seduction of less problematic fields or work.

It doesn't take a horticulturist to know that a beautiful tree has a very limited life span when the roots are unattended. It is crucial to include all nurses in our pursuit of autonomy, authority and development. Our leading thinkers must collaborate in solving the problems of the two thirds of nurses who work in hospitals. We need new organizations of work to enhance the position of all nurses and patients in the special modern institutions created for care of one group through reliance on the other. Together we can ensure that there is enfranchisement and expanded authority for all nurses while we struggle to agree to a different and more unified future. We can learn from each other, build our broad base for action through mutual respect, recognize and cherish our diversity and come of age as a profession by using to its fullest our unusual combination of caring, ambition, initiative, smarts and true grit.

REFERENCES

Aiken, L., Mezey, M., Lynaugh, J., & Buck, C. (1985). Teaching nursing homes. **American Geriatrics Society** 33, 196-201.

American Hospital Association (1988 in press). **Survey of hospitals.** Chicago: AHA.

Blum, L., Homiak, M., Housman, J., & Shaman, N. (1976). Altruism and women's oppression. In C. Gould & M. Wartofsky (Eds.), **Women and philosophy.** New York: Putnam.

Brooten, D., Kumar, S., Brown, L., Butts, P., Finkler, S., Bakewell-Sachs, Gibbons, A., & Delivoria-Papadoponlus, M. (1986). A Randomized Clinical Trial of Early Hospital Discharge and Home Follow-Up of Very-Low Birth-Weight Infants. **New England Journal of Medicine,** 315, 934-939.

Buhler-Wilkerson, K. (1983). False dawn: The rise and decline of public health nursing in America, 1900-1930. In E.C. Lagemann (Ed.), **Nursing history, new perspectives, new possibilities** (pp. 89-106). New York: Teachers College Press.

Dock, L. & Stewart, I. (1920). **A short history of nursing.** New York: Putnam.

Dubos, R. (1959). **Mirage of Health.** New York: Harper and Row.

Fagin, C. (1986). Opening the door on nursing's cost advantage. **Nursing and Health Care,** 7, 356-358.

Feldberg, R. (1984). Comparable worth: Toward theory and practice in the United States. **Signs: Journal of Women, Culture and Society,** 10, 311-328.

Henderson, V. (1966). **The nature of nursing: A definition and its implications for practice, research and education.** New York: Macmillan.

Holcombe, B. (1988, June). **Ms. Magazine,** 78.

Joel, L., (1986, November 14). **Comparison of clinical outcomes.** Paper presented to the conference, Teaching Nursing Home Program: a Perspective on Education/Service Collaboration, Rutgers College of Nursing. Newark, NJ.

Knaus, W. A., Draper, E., Wagner, D., & Zimmerman, J. (1986). An evaluation of outcome from intensive care in major medical centers. **Annals of Internal Medicine,** 104, 410-418.

Lynaugh, J. (1987, June 9). **Riding the yo-yo: The Work and Worth of Nursing in the 20th Century.** Paper presented to the conference, Nurses for the Future, Philadelphia, PA.

Melosh, B. (1982). **The physicians hand: Work, culture and conflict in American nursing.** Philadelphia: Temple University Press.

Mezey, M., Lynaugh, J., & Cartier, M. (Eds.) (1989). **Nursing homes and nursing care: Lessons from the teaching nursing home.** New York: Springer.

Myrdal, G. (1944). **An American dilemma.** New York: Harper and Row.

"News" (1985, September, October) **International Nursing Review.** 32, 131-137.

Nightingale, F. (1860/1969). **Notes on nursing: What it is and what it is not.** New York: Dover Publications.

Office of Technology Assessment (1986). **Nurse practitioners,**

physicians assistants and certified nurse-midwives: A policy analysis. Washington, DC: U.S. Government Printing Office.

Olshansky, S.J., & Ault, A.B. (1986). The fourth stage to the epidemiologic transition: The age of delayed degenerative diseases. **The Milbank Quarterly,** 64, 355-391.

Parnell, C. (1920). The selection and organization of hospital personnel. **Transactions of the American Hospital Association,** 1920. Chicago: AHA.

"Perspectives" (1987, May 11). **Medicine and Health,** 3.

Pokorny, G. (1988). Report card on health care. **HMO First Quarter,** 3-10.

Reverby, S. (1983). Something besides waiting: The politics of private duty nursing reform in the depression. In E.C. Lagemann (Ed.), **Nursing history, new perspectives, new possibilities** (pp. 133-156). New York: Teachers College Press.

Reverby, S. (1987). **Ordered to care: The dilemma of American nursing,** 1850-1945. Cambridge, London and New York: Cambridge University Press.

Roberts, S.J. (1983, July). Oppressed group behavior: Implications for nursing. **Advances in Nursing Science,** 5, 21-22.

Rosenberg, C. (1987). **Care of strangers: The rise of America's hospital system.** New York: Basic Books.

Titus. S.C. (1952). Economic facts of life for nurses. **American Journal of Nursing,** 52, 1109-1110.

To profess — To be a professional

DONNA DIERS, RN, MSN, FAAN

IT IS A GREAT PLEASURE to talk about professionalism and about nursing as a profession. I will take the posture that we are no longer searching for our profession; we already have it.

I begin this paper by turning to the dictionary, for much as I think I know what the words "profess" and "professional" mean, it is always good to be grounded by Webster. Among the meanings of the infinitive "to profess" is "to lay claim to some belief insincerely." That may be what we are accused of doing in nursing — simply claiming we are a profession when others may think not. We may feel forced to be ambivalent about nursing, about being a nurse, and we may feel defensive in explaining nursing to others, or embattled as others attack. We have been thought to be mere pretenders to professionhood.

I would propose that the problem with nursing in today's world is really quite simple, and like everything else in nursing, quite complicated. The bottom line is this: the problems with nursing, as we hear them, are *not nursing's problems*. That is, there is nothing seriously wrong with nurses or nursing. What is seriously wrong is that we — nurses and nursing — have changed a lot over the years and the world has yet to catch up with us.

Thus the trouble nursing seems to be in, or that nurses feel so badly about, is good trouble and is not our problem. The world simply has an outdated view of nursing, and our task is not so much to defend our thoughts or our work but simply to yawn and patiently teach people what nursing is today. Seeing the task that way makes it a whole lot easier, for the pressure is then not on nurses to interpret so that others can understand us and our issues; it is on others to understand for they are so pitifully unknowing.

All of us get dumb questions from time to time. We are asked, for example, what is the difference between medicine and nursing. Sometimes that throws us into a fit because it is so hard to define for the unknowing what nursing is. But if one simply considers that question dumb, or at least uninformed, then it can have a snappy answer: doctors are authorized by the states to practice medicine, which is to diagnose, treat, prescribe and operate — on disease, not people. Everything else is nursing.

A colleague of ours, a distinguished nurse dean, was recently put on the spot at an interdisciplinary national meeting by the dumb question, "Is there really a body of knowledge universally accepted as nursing? What is nursing research anyhow?" She replied, correctly I believe, that she found the question insulting. Had the questioner read any of the nursing literature? Of course not. Well, had he read any physics lately, or economics, or cell biology? There is hardly universal agreement in those fields either, so why should he expect a higher standard for nursing?

A male student in my school was asked by friends, when he announced his intention to go to nursing school, "Why do you want to be a male nurse?" His reply, which I cherish, was, "I already know how to be a man. What I want to be is a nurse."

A colleague and I have collected the responses one gets when one is introduced as a nurse at a social gathering, or when one introduces oneself as a nurse to the stranger in the next airplane seat. The responses fall into four categories: (1) "Oh, really, how nice. Excuse me, I need another drink"; (2) a rambling story about the other person's experience with hospitals, surgery, birthing or an aged parent; (3) a random pass, as if one were automatically an available, experienced sexual partner; (4) "Oh, I could never do that, all those bedpans and blood and all."

These kinds of visceral responses make the nurse feel strange, to stand there in one's best basic black and try to make polite chatter. Indeed, it can make one feel as if one doesn't belong in this social situation, as if one has egg on one's blouse, a tattooed Nightingale lamp on one's forehead, or a red "RN" on one's chest. It takes a while to realize that the reactions one gets in polite social conversation are not the problem of laymen who simply do not know how to deal with nurses outside the institutional setting, where we can be set apart by uniform or role or function.

Nursing as metaphor

Nursing is metaphor, meaning that the nurse is not real, in these kinds of social settings. The nurse is merely symbolic and reacted to as a symbol.

Nursing is metaphor for the class struggle, for example, and in more recent times, for the struggle of women for equality. True or not, nurses are thought to be maids or domestics. While domestic service is a perfectly honorable way to earn a living, one does not ordinarily run into servants as guests at cocktail parties.

Nursing is also metaphor for motherhood. Nurses are the archetypical mothers, and it makes some people nervous to have awakened in a social scene the regressive feelings of being a child.

Nursing is also metaphor for the kind of power the Amazons used, or Lysistrata. Thus nurses evoke in others an atavistic fear of

women, based on the remembered or fantasied experience of lying in bed with a woman in white towering over us, helping to do the kinds of intimate and personal things that, if we were well, would be done in the privacy of our house behind a closed door.

Nurses are thought, and quite correctly, to know the kinds of secrets that scare the layman. Nurses have confronted death; have heard the late night secrets; have been present at birth; and have seen mutilation, pain, terror, agony and hope. Those who have seen such things are untouchable, for their knowledge is frightening and makes others feel weak, timid, or naive.

But at the same time, nurses are thought to be mindless, even in the choice of profession. Bright nurses are thought to have simply "settled" for being a nurse, either out of lack of ambition to be a physician or lack of money for the training. It is rarely thought that nurses might *choose* nursing over the mystical opportunity to be a doctor, a lawyer, or whatever the other upscale choices are.

The cocktail party is a stereotype of the social setting in which nurses encounter the middle-class lay public. We are there pinned by conflicting images, all of which we are supposed to embody. We are simultaneously weak, strong, motherly, castrating, dumb, smart, powerful, warm, cold and any other contrasts you wish to add. And when we feel legitimately confused with this kind of feedback, we tend to think it is our fault, that there is something inherent either in our profession or in our inarticulateness that does us in. But it is impossible to be quick, graceful, smooth and clever when the metaphors about nursing contradict each other and do not match the reality.

So that we do not profess insincerely, we need to be reminded every now and then what nursing is and does and where it is going.

There is no point to nursing unless it is to serve. Indeed, there is no point to nursing education unless it prepares for service and no point to nursing research unless it guides, documents, reinforces and informs practice.

It is of interest to me that within the past two years, several university-based professions have realized what nursing long ago discovered: that practice professions are not like the humanities and the liberal arts in which knowledge is sought for its own sake. An engineer who knows the theories of stress and mass will build bridges that fall unless his knowledge is built also in the vicissitudes of practice, where winds do not always behave and human error is an eternal possibility, and shortcuts make a joke of architectural drawings or job specifications. A lawyer who learns the practice of law only through a cram course before taking the bar examination may be a legal scholar but is unlikely to be helpful to a client with a mundane but personally crucial problem. A minister who knows the history and theories of sacred theology will not inspire a congregation to higher moral or ethical behavior unless he is also trained in applied psychology and human behavior, for the ministry, too, is a practice profession. And knowing — having the knowledge — to practice is a very complicated thing, more so in nursing than in any other profession because the sheer scope of our social mandate is so huge.

Caring

Nursing is primary care, secondary care and tertiary care, no matter how those are defined. Nursing is health care and sickness care, prevention, health promotion and rehabilitation. Nursing is community care, home care, institutional care, mental health care, and increasingly, self-care. Nursing is there at the beginning of life and the end. Nursing treats individuals, families, groups, communities, and where it is practiced as administration, institutions. Nurses observe, listen, test, assess, diagnose, monitor, manage, treat and cure. But above all, nursing is caring.

As a profession, we have any number of divisions among us, divisions of training, gender, education, philosophy, state, organization, setting and regulation. But the one thing upon which nurses agree is that the essence of the practice, and thus the knowing, is caring.

In the first place, it is not easy to care for people — any people — any time, anywhere. It is especially difficult when there are no ties of blood or common interest that bind the nurse and the patient. In nursing, caring requires authentic altruism that must be titrated precisely so as not to overwhelm on the one hand, nor be lost on the other. Caring takes enormous energy, even when genuine liking is present, for it is impossible to care equally for or about everyone. Yet that is precisely nursing's assignment.

Caring cannot be forced. It may be built through the luck of a happy childhood; fostered through friends, family, teachers; nurtured by direct learning; and crafted, finally, through application. One's quantum of caring is diluted and then replenished but must always be there. The nurse must find it in herself if it has drained away in the pressures of an unrewarding position, in a corrupting institution, in a bleak and confusing world. When the spark of caring is gone, the nurse is truly burned out.

Nursing done right is physically, emotionally, and intellectually fulfilling. Many people think nursing is simple — just take nice people and turn them loose. But to be caring, to deliver tender loving care, is exquisitely difficult. If being tender and loving were merely inborn characteristics, there would be no need for psychology, sociology, or the humanities. Sensitivity trainers, psychiatrists and social workers (to say nothing of police) would be out of a job. Nursing, practically alone among the human service professions, deliberately tries to train its young in empathy, sensitivity and compassion. Nursing goes far beyond that because those attributes alone aren't enough either.

Nursing provides its students with ways to tool, hone, sharpen, deepen, and direct the tenderness and love with which most people are equipped. Indeed, nursing realizes that care which is simply technical or merely procedural and not tender and loving is not quality care. Similarly, care which is simply tender and loving but not thoughtful and planned is not good care.

Caring for and about people cannot be dismissed as merely intuitive. But intuition has been defined as "unconscious intelligence." Nursing is not just comfort, care, coordination, collaboration, or just applied psychology, physiology, sociology, anthropology or diluted medical science. Nursing is all of these things and more. It requires an effort of considerable intellectual acuity — which looks to an outsider like intuition — to thread one's way through all the knowledge, technique and tenderness one has and to come out with the right action to serve the patient's particular need.

Caring is not restricted to the situation in which one nurse is alone in a room with one patient. It is also an exercise of caring to manipulate a budget so as to provide enough staff to handle the patient load. It is the application of the concern for caring that makes a curriculum change to include more carefully analyzed clinical work, buttressed by selected readings, self-study and validation by examination. It is caring to help a community organize to mount an immunization program, or provide school lunches, or construct a rape crisis center, or promote an alcohol counseling program. And it is caring that fires nursing up to change legislation to make needed resources available not only to the people but to nurses themselves.

Grace DeSantis, a sociologist at DePaul University, has made a significant contribution to our understanding of professionalization in nursing. Her major point is that nursing has

chosen to try to professionalize the field through higher and higher education, as if requiring doctoral preparation would make the field more professional. She argues that professionalization will come only when *practice* is professional, improved over what it is today by intelligent caring, not through simply credentialing individuals. She cites Friedson to the effect that having one's occupational claims of expertise acknowledged is the first step in the pursuit of professionalism. She says that the significant flaw in the decision to raise educational standards lies not in advanced education per se but in the absence of a monopoly over the work that will be performed once the training and education are completed.

Three kinds of knowing

I suggest there are two ways in which the professionalization of nursing will happen, following DeSantis' notions. The first is determining what kinds of knowledge will best serve the development of a monopoly over the work. The second is realizing that the long-desired monopoly is just about to fall into our hands and we should be ready for it.

There might be three kinds of knowing to be prescribed for nursing as a profession of practitioners. First, there is the kind of knowing that prepares one for civilized life — the content and experience that allow one to participate in the life of one's times, with an appreciation for history, ideas, the studies and sciences, the explorations and the frontiers of thinking. Because nursing's social mandate is so large and the need for nursing's contribution to the reform of health service delivery so apparent, an argument can be made that this kind of knowing is basic.

Yet, this kind of knowing may also suggest that the students be more experienced in life than nursing's new students generally are. This kind of knowing has been called the liberal arts, but liberal education has become so pre-professionalized that it is not the civilizing influence it once was. Perhaps this kind of knowing is something that should come later in one's nursing education rather than earlier, for I doubt that late teenagers just coming out of their own personal developmental crises are able to truly appreciate the great ideas, the philosophies, the grand schemes of the past or future. Perhaps such material is useful after, rather than before, one has learned and experienced the world of work — when one feels more of a need to be able to place professional identity and gifts in a larger framework of society; when one knows enough to be able to find a place in political science, economics, sociology; and when one has seen enough human behavior under stress to want to know history, psychology or group process.

Also, the notion that liberal education is confined to the undergraduate years or the first 2 years of a BSN program does not give enough credit to the liberalizing effect of graduate education. We might think of how to make more of that point.

The second kind of knowing is most conveniently labeled science. There is a growing realization that nursing education, in its efforts to carve off a piece of turf and call it exclusively nursing, may have gone too far and neglects to provide students with knowledge of the human body and how it works.

The advances in human science over the past quarter century suggest that now it may be easier, rather than harder, to teach all of the science students need. We know so many more of the principles of physiology, cell biology, or biochemistry that it is no longer necessary to force students to learn by rote and memorize things that now have conceptual explanations. The sciences of human behavior have developed to the point at which it is no longer even interesting to seat nursing students in a survey course on psychology, when social psychology has whole bodies of knowledge directly pertinent to the phenomena of nursing.

Psychiatry has moved from the analytic to the biologic, and a psychiatric nurse who does not have a grasp of the dopamine theory or who does not understand the relationship between the limbic system and behavior is simply not prepared for practice. A pediatric nurse who is not fully grounded in clinical child development will be unable to practice to the potential limits of patient or parent need. A nurse in a cancer setting will be unprepared if she does not have enough of a grip on cell biology to interpret particular chemotherapeutic regimens when the patient asks.

The content of science, however, is now too huge to be encompassed by any single human mind. What now needs to be learned and known are the processes of human body and mind, so that new content discoveries can be linked to past learning.

We are still conceptually young in nursing. Where nursing education has not been closely tied to practice, some intellectual excesses have produced education which fits people for no kind of practice at all. Opal Hipps has argued magnificently and amusingly that some so-called integrated curricula do not well prepare a student to deal with patients who are not integrated. I would argue also that some attempts at nursing theory, when they come out of the armchair rather than the practice field, do not help us advance. Self-care theory, for example, useful as it may be in some situations, does not seem to work when the patient is the high-risk newborn, the comatose individual, or, perhaps, the floridly psychotic. And when we use an intellectual process — taxonomy — as if it were a political process, and believe if we can just find new names for nursing phenomena we will have a profession and be recognized, we are dreaming. There seems to me to be no particular advantage to calling "pain" alteration in comfort, potential or actual, if we do it just to prove we are not doing medicine or using medicine's words.

There is, then, a third kind of knowledge or knowing, and it is called nursing. I mean the process of patient care, the diagnostic process, the application of all kinds of knowledge to the immediate situation, the discovery and assessment of patient condition and the uses of information for decision making. I also mean the kinds of knowing we used to call nursing process, the therapeutic use of the self, the nurse-patient relationship. I also mean the techniques and talents of physical care which, along with many other things, have washed out of some nursing curricula. The kind of knowing called nursing is learned in its exercise, though it may be planned and analyzed in the conference, tutorial or classroom.

The three kinds of knowing will be basic to the future practice of nursing in ways that have not been required of nurses in the past. It will be essential that nurses know the methods and processes of scientific explanation of the human body. It is necessary now, in some situations, such as intensive care. In trauma centers, once the patient has been treated for the fractures and shock, he is transferred to the hands of the primary nurse. She adds or subtracts oxygen as she repeats blood gas levels; she adds or deletes intravenous medications; she preserves skin integrity and prevents infection, which in these compromised patients would be fatal. The nurse in this situation must know a great deal about cells and fluid balance and electrolytes and pressures of blood and spinal fluid, about neurons and permeable membranes and synapses and the neurophysiology of consciousness. The technology of monitoring the body is already with us, and the possibility of preventing complications in any patient with impaired physiological processes is already here.

The job of nursing now and increasingly in the future will be to know the range of ways in which the human body and its workings can be controlled by machinery and medication. Even now, nursing is in the position of making decisions about when and how to use the results of technology and chemistry. We are especially in the position of limiting the use of devices, capsules, pills and machines when their use is questionable or when the patient has been subject to so many specialists' orders and prescriptions that the care becomes uncoordinated because no one is in charge. Nurses of the future will be.

Nursing's authority

Things are about to change for us, not so much in the work itself, but in the visibility and authority of it. Without even asking, the health care system is being forced to confront nursing as central, powerful, and reimbursable. There already have been changes in institutional reimbursement under Medicare. Hospitals will now be paid for their services under a prospective, rather than retrospective, reimbursement system.

When health economists or public policyniks discuss these phenomena, as Paul Starr has done in his book *The Social Transformation of American Medicine,* and in a conference I attended recently, it is amazing how little account is taken of nursing. Starr and others simply assume that nursing will fall into line with the decisions being made by others. While he was at some pains to point out some of the consequences of new reimbursement patterns on nursing, such as cutting hospital nursing staffs, he has not grasped the point.

The point is that the new system of hospital reimbursement transfers the power of decision making — economic decision making — into the hands of nursing. The only reason for the existence of the modern hospital is to provide nursing care. That is why hospitals were created and why they are the social institutions they are today. Thus, the service provided by hospitals, and billed to Medicare or other third parties, is essentially nursing service. Now, the Health Care Financing Administration has said that hospitals are costing too much, and so they have proposed to fix it through a system of charges with nationally referenced standards.

The Diagnostic Related Group formulas (DRGs) for pricing hospital costs was invented to control the behavior of institutions and physicians, not nurses. Yet, we already hear that nursing will have to suffer; staff will be cut; and we should realize what this issue is.

For way too long, nursing has been buried in the hospital bill along with brooms, breakfast and building mortgage. It has not been in the interest of institutions to treat nursing as a revenue center, and so nursing has been economically invisible. Under the new system of reimbursement, that will stop. That may well be painful for nursing, but we will have little choice. Since hospitals were designed to deliver nursing service, it will be in their interests to figure out just what that service is and how much it costs. DRGs in their present form are used to pay hospitals on the basis of case-mix by diagnosis. Yet nurses have long known that it is not the diagnosis alone that determines what kind of nursing service is needed; that is especially not true in cancer nursing. Therefore, it will become an institutional interest to have nursing define the care given and thus why it costs whatever it does.

In an economic climate in which institutions will be forced to justify expenses and in institutions in which a large chunk of the expenses are called nursing, we will finally be brought out from under the bushel to say what we do and spend our time on. And that will force us, usefully I think, to make our care more directed and precise, while not eliminating the social conversation and easy dialogue that makes patients feel cared for and secure that somebody knows what they are doing.

There is an inexorable chain of logic here. If institutions will be pressed, as they already are, to justify their costs, and the largest chunk of the noncapital costs in hospitals is nursing, then the eyes will be upon us.

At first, the eyes will turn to us because it is inconvenient or uncomfortable or politically unwise to look elsewhere — at ancillary services, or other contributions to the bill. But eventually, if not immediately, it will become clear to hospital economists and financial managers that they will need to depend on nursing to help the institution survive economically.

If we are clever about it, we will be standing there poised to be helpful. Already, we know how important nursing has become to decisions about hospital discharge. Since length of stay is the unit of analysis on which prospective rates are set, we are in the policy mainstream right now. Nobody but nursing has the data that will be desperately needed for institutions to plan their prices and reflect not only minimal care but *quality* of care.

The next step in the logic, at least as we might shape it, will be to separate nursing costs from other direct and indirect costs. The instant that happens, nursing will suddenly be in a position of authority we have longed for. If we are going to be responsible for the costs of care, we must also have the authority to determine how these costs will be defined, controlled, monitored, and accounted.

The reimbursement tinkering to date has concentrated on what had to happen first — a way to define quantity of care as a factor in hospital costs. Whether DRG system survives or some other comes in is not very relevant; something like it will be with us for a long time simply because it makes so much sense. The greater the quantity of care given (so long as it is appropriate), the more it costs, and thus, the higher the price to the third party insurers.

The next step will be, however, to add to the measures of quantity some measures of quality. For it is simply logical that if care is better, it ought to be priced higher. That's the American capitalist way and there is no reason to think the health care industry will work any differently from any other.

No one but nursing can define and decide upon measures of quality of institutional health care, for nobody else is there all the time.

What we are in, then, is not a health care crisis but a revolution, and one of the things it is already accomplishing, whether we like it or not, is returning nursing to the central role it had in the old days. In this revolutionized health care system, nurses will not only be seen as essential and central but will have to be rewarded for that centrality as well, whether the rewards come through money or through increased ability to participate in public policy.

With these new kinds of professional responsibilities, nursing will have the authority we have been saying for years that we wanted. We will also have a visibility that we have never had before and that in itself will get us over the hump to being considered one of the "learned professions." The future is already with us and we cannot hold it back.

As a new high holy days prayerbook, put together a couple of years ago by the Reform branch of Judaism, says:

> There was that law of life, so cruel and so just, which demanded that one must grow or else pay more for remaining the same.

C H A P T E R   T W O

Changing roles and the scope and practice of nursing

DEVELOPMENTS IN TECHNOLOGY and in methods of reimbursement for health care services have changed nursing's roles. Consequently, nurses have had to acquire new knowledge and skills to assume new functions and responsibilities. The profession, which must ensure that individual nurses are adequately prepared and competent to care for those entrusted to them, uses RN licensure and self-regulation to fulfill its responsibilities.

In 1985, the House of Delegates of the American Nurses' Association (ANA) directed the ANA's Cabinets on Nursing Education, Practice, and Services to develop a joint statement delineating the scope of practice for nursing. The resulting report, approved by the ANA in 1987, describes a single scope of clinical nursing practice based on the core of nursing practice, also described.

Within this single scope of nursing practice — which includes a legal definition of nursing — the report defines the knowledge bases for professional and technical nurses and relates their different roles specifically to their different levels of educational preparation. For example, the report states that the depth and breadth of the professional nurse's practice are not limited by the type of client population or practice environment, whereas the technical nurse's practice is limited to defined patient populations.

Unfortunately, the ANA's scope-of-practice concept has apparently had little impact on clinical nursing practice: To date, very few institutions have differentiated the roles of baccalaureate-prepared nurses from associate degree nurses, even though the drastically changed roles and functions of nurses in general would seem to support this differentiation.

"Nurses Fight Back," by Holcomb, vividly underscores the lack of control many nurses have over their practice. The author cites the way nurses are floated from unit to unit regardless of whether they are prepared for the tasks they face, and she points to the use of temporary staff as a source of problems in providing quality patient care. She also discusses how issues such as these have led to nurses' strikes in some parts of the country.

According to del Bueno, in "The Promise and the Reality of Certification," the drive toward requiring advanced education plus certification for nurses working in specialty areas is gaining momentum. However, in her opinion, little or no evidence exists to support the belief that certified nurses give better care or service or have better patient-care outcomes than noncertified nurses.

In "The Nursing Scene: A Need for Specialists," Grimaldi highlights the many options open to nurses and asserts that there is a growing need for more nurse specialists. From traditional registered-nurse preparation to master's degree programs, she lists the educational requirements for the various clinical specialties; reviewing them, the reader is given insight into the problem of implementing the ANA position on specialization.

Peplau, in "American Nurses Association's Social Policy Statement: Part 1," explains her position in relation to specialization: She supports the need for nurses prepared at the master's and doctoral levels to fill specialty roles as well as the need for certification through professional nurse-specialist organizations. Peplau also indicates her support for the

ANA's definition of nursing as set forth in the *Social Policy Statement*.

Spitzer and Davivier discuss the changes anticipated for the future of nursing in "Nursing in the 1990s: Expanding Opportunities." Citing the growing need for nurse managers and the increasing involvement of nurses in policymaking and in managing nursing practice, they urge nurses to exercise courageous leadership and make positive changes in the delivery of health care. Although these authors do endorse nursing specialization and see an increasing need for nurse-specialists, they question the need for "two-tiered" (professional and technical) licensure.

Nurses fight back

BETTY HOLCOMB

HEART ATTACK VICTIMS are no longer guaranteed a bed at the University of Mississippi Medical Center in Jackson, Mississippi. People severely injured in car accidents and stroke victims may also be turned away. The problem is not that the hospital is full: only about half the beds on its intensive care units are being used. But the hospital has been short as many as 100 nurses — almost one third of the nursing staff it needs if it is to run at full capacity.

"There are more and more days when we just don't have enough nurses to care for any more patients," says David Bussone, hospital director at the medical center. "It's no longer uncommon for us to divert ambulances to other hospitals."

So far, Bussone believes, no one has died for lack of space in his hospital. One of the other four hospitals in Jackson has accepted the emergency patients he had to turn away. "What I'm afraid of is the day when all the hospitals in town go on ambulance diversion. Then what's going to happen?" Bussone asks.

Bussone is not the only one asking that question. A growing shortage of registered nurses across the country is creating serious questions about patient care.

Nurses who remain on duty face nearly impossible demands, both physically and emotionally. Some nurses are working as many as three double shifts a week. Translated, that means working 16 hours a day, sometimes three days in a row, often in emergency rooms or on floors that are overflowing with patients.

"I could see things were going to explode on me if we didn't do something," says Jamie Miller, head nurse on the neonatal intensive care unit at Bussone's hospital. On some days last fall, nurses there were caring for six or seven very sick babies at a time, triple the normal caseload. By Miller's calculations, each baby was getting only four to six hours of nursing a day when they needed 17 to 24 hours of care.

Bussone agreed to close nearly half of the 55 neonatal beds and began a high-profile campaign to recruit and retain nurses. More often, though, nurses say their concerns are ignored. "Many hospitals are placing nurses in impossible situations," says Anne Schott, director of communications for the New York State Nurses Association.

"A nurse can come on duty at night and be told she'll have to be the only nurse caring for 20 or 30 very sick patients. Those patients may be on respirators, may be incontinent, may not be able to walk by themselves. If she's lucky, no more than one patient will need her at one time." Otherwise, she will have to choose between them.

The New York association now encourages nurses to file official reports saying they are working under protest, whenever they are required to work a shift so short of nurses that they believe it threatens patient care. The association has received scores of such forms, from nurses all around the state.

"The fate of nurses and patients is inextricably intertwined," says Mary Foley, R.N., chair of the Cabinet on Economic and General Welfare of the American Nurses' Association (ANA). "I'm not sure if the public quite understands that yet."

A national crisis

Today, nearly 80 percent of the nation's hospitals report an acute shortage of registered nurses in the most sensitive areas of care — in the intensive care units, in emergency rooms, and in operating rooms. It is a shortage affecting major medical centers and tiny rural ones, and it takes its toll on nurses, patients, and their families.

The nation has weathered chronic nursing shortages in the past, but this one is decidedly different: the demand for the most highly trained, highly educated registered nurses is exploding, while the number of people choosing the profession is steadily declining. If nurses' concerns are not addressed, hospitals could face a permanent, crippling shortage of skilled nurses.

Revolutionary changes in medicine have created the nearly insatiable demand for registered nurses. They are the most highly trained of all nurses, with at least two years of postsecondary education from a college, hospital-sponsored nursing school, or community college. An increasing number of them — about one third — have bachelor's degrees from a university. By contrast, a licensed practical nurse or nurse's aide may have only a high school diploma or a few quarters of schooling after high school.

Hospitals today need nurses who are knowledgeable about medications, their side effects and interactions, nurses who can operate heart monitors and interpret their results, nurses who understand dialysis and the complications of kidney failure. Already, the number of R.N.s in hospitals has jumped from 33 percent of nursing personnel in 1968 to 58 percent in 1986.

Radical changes in the Medicare payment system are also resulting in increased work for nurses. Starting in 1983, the federal government capped payments for Medicare patients and established a flat fee that creates an incentive for hospitals to discharge patients as quickly as possible. The idea is to save billions of dollars as hospitals care only for the most severe phases of illness and let patients recuperate at home. "Hospitals today are like one big intensive care unit," says Helen Feigenbaum, assistant clinical director of medical nursing at Yale–New Haven Hospital in New Haven, Connecticut.

These trends have accelerated the demand for nurses. In 1975, the average hospital used 50 nurses for every 100 patients, compared to 91 nurses for every 100 patients used today.

The demand for nurses outside the hospital is also exploding. An ever-increasing number of elderly people with chronic diseases need skilled care at home and in nursing homes. Patients discharged earlier from hospitals need nursing supervision at home. A booming home health care industry now competes actively with hospitals for a limited pool of registered nurses. Corporate health programs, insurance companies, and freestanding medical clinics are also aggressively recruiting nurses. And a new breed of R.N.s is also creating new options for themselves in independent practice. Yet even as the need for nurses grows, fewer women than ever are interested in the career.

The number of people applying to nursing schools has been dropping for the last five years. In 1986, for the first time ever, the number of college women who wanted to be doctors outstripped the number of women wanting to be nurses. That same year, a survey by the University of California showed that five times as many first-year college women planned to enter business as planned toenter nursing. "Talented, bright people go into law, business, or computers." says Donna Richardson, lobbyist for the American Nurses' Association. "They can make a lot more money, have more status and more autonomy." Today, the average SAT scores for high school students most interested in nursing are "well below average" for college-bound students, according to a recent article in the *New*

England Journal of Medicine. By contrast, in the 1950s, the brightest women were attracted to nursing, because it was one of the only options available.

The long-range solutions to the nursing crisis are no mystery. In the last decade, nursing leaders and blue-ribbon commissions of health care experts have warned that the nursing profession must be overhauled. Salaries need to be upgraded, especially for nurses with experience. Nurses need more autonomy over their work and opportunity to use their skills and expertise. More money needs to be channeled into nursing education.

Nurses themselves are fighting hard for change, waging impressive and creative battles on many fronts. Some are engaged in political action; others are walking picket lines. Some have joined lawsuits to challenge the historical pattern of sex discrimination in pay.

The nurses' struggle is one with implications for all women, for it is a struggle for the recognition of the value of women's work and a struggle against sex discrimination. "To my mind, nursing is a logical standard-bearer for all women," says Margretta Styles, president of the ANA. "Nursing is 97 percent female, and the problems we face are typical of those faced in women's professions, especially low pay and low status."

Indeed, nurses can be seen as the leading edge of a new wave of feminism, one with the potential to give women's work the pay and status it deserves. Many of them hope the current shortage will provide the leverage they need to secure lasting change in their profession. But profound obstacles still remain: a reluctant medical establishment; entrenched economic interests of hospitals, doctors, and other health professionals; and powerful sexual politics. "This is definitely a boy-girl issue," asserts Pamela Maraldo, executive director of the National League for Nursing. "Make no mistake about that."

"Disposable-nurse syndrome"

A key obstacle to attracting bright, young people to the nursing profession is pay and lack of any obvious career path. A staff nurse fresh out of school, with as little as two years' education from a community college, can start at a good salary — somewhere around $21,000, and sometimes even more in major cities. But within five to seven years, she reaches her maximum earning power — which is often only a few thousand dollars more than where she started. Even world-famous facilities such as New York University Medical Center in New York City, which boasts of a "career ladder" for nurses, pays a staff nurse with seven years' experience only about $6,000 more than a nurse with no experience at all.

"I call it the disposable-nurse syndrome," says Claire Fagin, dean of the school of nursing at the University of Pennsylvania. "They bring you in for a couple of years, wear you out, and throw you away." Fagin warns that entry-level replacements will get harder and harder to find.

Unlike most industries, hospitals also fail to compensate nurses adequately for overtime, night, or weekend work. It is simply an expected part of the job.

Many nurses working on critical care units today have at least a bachelor's degree, and sometimes even a master's degree in their specialty. By the time she arrives at a patient's bedside, an R.N. is likely to have studied basic sciences, psychology, sociology, and even communications. Her goal is to speed recovery, prevent relapse, and teach a patient to care for herself. She learns how to use and run the high-tech machinery in today's hospitals — in many cases, she is the one who orders it. She consults with the family, when needed, and draws up a plan for care once the patient is discharged. She often teaches interns and residents the business. "A lot of physicians come out of training overwhelmed by the responsibilities of caring for patients," says Mary Lewis Sheehan, an R.N. with advanced training in mental health, who now works in private psychiatric practice. "They want you as the nurse, the person who's been there all the time, to make it easier. Nurses would correct their orders and clean up the emotional mess they'd leave hanging with the family." Yet nurses earn less than most men in unskilled labor. Several years back, nurses in Denver were outraged to learn the city paid them less than the average tree-trimmer. The *Washington Post* reported last summer that staff nurses in Washington, D.C., earn about $23,753, which is less than the average hospital maintenance worker. A 1983 study commissioned by the Illinois Commission on the Status of Women looked at historic patterns of wage discrimination against women in female-dominated professions. The study revealed that electricians — whose duties include fixing refrigerators and air conditioners — earned $8,600 more than registered nurses — who must make life-and-death decisions about critically ill patients. "You have a minute, maybe two to react when you see a patient is not getting enough oxygen," says Irene Downs, head nurse in the recovery room at New York University Medical Center. "Otherwise, there can be brain damage."

"Our society places a lower value on nurturing and caring roles, which are very integral to the work of nurses," says Joyce Clifford, nurse-in-chief at Beth Israel Hospital in Boston. "It's seen as women's work, and it's undervalued, just as the care of children and the elderly is undervalued."

Yet it is not just the pay. Nurses also say that a lack of control over their practice often drives them out of a hospital. Pediatric specialist nurse Jamie Miller from Mississippi, for example, left her previous job after she was rotated into an adult intensive care unit. She

was supposed to assist two other R.N.s who knew the unit well, but neither had showed up for duty. Miller, fresh out of school, was suddenly the most senior person on the unit.

"I was the only R.N. with 18 patients," she recalls. "I had never even laid eyes on some of the equipment on the floor, and I was supposed to supervise four or five licensed practical nurses and technicians. It was scary." She had been warned in the past that she could be fired for refusing an assignment. But she still balked. "I called nursing administration and said, 'You have 15 minutes to get me an experienced nurse or I am walking out the door.' The hospital sent another R.N. to the floor."

But Miller's experience is far from unique. The practice of "floating" nurses from unit to unit is quite common in most hospitals, especially during the current shortage. The practice is one of the reasons why 3,000 nurses employed by the county of Los Angeles went on strike in late January for the first time ever in that county. "Many of our nurses are concerned about indiscriminate assignments," says Sandra Delahoussave, a supervisory nurse in the hospital and spokeswoman for the local unit of the Service Employees International Union, which represents the nurses. "They feel they are being treated as robots."

Systematic surveys of the way hospitals use nurses bear out nurses' own impressions that they are moved about like cogs in a wheel. In a recent study in the *New England Journal of Medicine*, Linda Aiken, professor of nursing and sociology at the University of Pennsylvania, revealed that in a move to cut costs, hospitals have generally reduced their hiring of licensed practical nurses, nurse's aides, and other support personnel, apparently expecting registered nurses to pick up the slack.

"Hospitals are willing to use them as all-purpose employees who can stand in for anyone — a secretary, a nurse's aide, or a hospital manager after hours," says Aiken, who believes such practices have both exacerbated the nursing shortage and added to nurses' workloads.

Ann Van Slyck, a Phoenix, Arizona, nursing administrative consultant who visits scores of hospitals a year, reports that it's not unusual to discover that registered nurses spend 50 percent or less of their time in direct patient care. "When I start asking questions, I find out that they're running to the lab, or running to the pharmacy, because someone forgot to get the medications up to the floors." She says: "If you take 1,000 nurses and figure that they spend 35 percent of their time on less-skilled labor, that's a waste of a big pot of money." The current nursing shortage has only made nurses' workload more difficult. Many hospitals routinely ask nurses to care for more patients per shift. "We try to maintain a ratio of one nurse for every four to five patients on our medical surgical floors, but now we're having to extend that to one nurse for every six or even seven patients at times,"says Susan Bode, senior vice president at St. Luke's Medical Center in Milwaukee.

Many hospitals are using temporary staff — usually nurses from private agencies — to fill the gap. But that often creates as many problems as it solves. "I had nurses coming on duty who didn't know anything about the emergency room — not even where the syringes were. I was trying to supervise them and deal with emergency asthma patients who couldn't breathe, patients in cardiac arrest, and AIDS patients in great suffering," says a head nurse in a busy New York City hospital, who asked that her name not be used. She also had to supervise young interns and residents with little familiarity with the emergency room who rotated into her area every few months.

"I used to love my job. We were a team, and it was exciting every day. My adrenalin was pumping," she recalls. But as other nurses burned out and quit, and the load fell increasingly on her shoulders, "it got to be too much responsibility. I came home every day ex-

hausted and angry." Last November, she switched to the hospital's visiting nurse service. She took a slight cut in pay, but she can now keep regular hours, as she cares for patients recuperating at home. "I don't think I could ever be happy working in a hospital again," she says. "The thought of a hospital makes me shake."

Still, while hospital administrators can be responsive to nurses' key concerns, Van Slyck rubs up against some resistance. "I met with a hospital administrator a few months ago, and he started off by telling me that retention of nurses is a serious issue, and he wanted to do something to reduce turnover," she recalls. "I was excited, so I asked him what he thought we should do to start. 'Paint the nurses' lounge pink,' he said." Van Slyck almost laughed, until she saw he was dead serious.

"A damn good nurse"
Nurses find it is hard to get taken seriously outside the hospital as well. Indeed, the poor image of nurses has been frequently cited by nurses and health care experts as yet another cause for the current nursing shortage. In the era when careers on Wall Street have been romanticized and women are urged to compete in such professions as law and medicine, its been tough for nursing to recruit. "Face it, who wants to go into a profession that's seen as powerless?" asks Maraldo from the National League for Nursing. And even though the Women's Movement has fought for comparable worth and for better recognition of the value of women's work, many nurses resent the message that grew out of the 1960s feminist movement: Be a doctor, not a nurse. How many times have you heard that and never stopped to think how it denigrates nursing?" asks Maraldo.

"I go to a party and say I'm a nurse and people either walk away or say, 'Why do you want to empty bedpans and clean up vomit?'

They rarely bother to find out what I really do," says Linda Rahn, head nurse of coronary and medical intensive care at New York University Hospital.

"I've been advised to tell people I'm an educator, not a nurse," says Betty Jackson, assistant director of nursing research at Montefiore Medical Center in New York City, who has landed several grants to do research into nursing practice. "It makes me angry when people say that. Don't they know that when you're in a hospital what you need is a damn good nurse?"

If nurses were in charge

Still, many nurses are more hopeful than ever about the future of their profession. Not only are they in demand, but their services offer a cure for what ails the American medical system: steadily increasing costs, and inappropriate care. Nurses, even if decently paid, provide relatively inexpensive care for the chronic incurablediseases of aging, from arthritis to heart disease. With the number of people in America over the age of 85 growing at six times the rate of the general population, and the Baby Boom headed toward middle age, care by nurses is an increasingly attractive alternative to doctors.

Hospital spending has tilted toward high-tech, highly interventionist treatments since the mid-1950s. In some cases, such as neonatal intensive care units, the payoff has been enormous. "The babies we take care of would not have survived 20 years ago," says nurse Miller in Mississippi.

But the technology can also lead to treatment that is ineffective and at the same time painful and invasive. "Right now, we operate on a medical model that tries to cure people of diseases that are incurable," says Vivien Deback, R.N., director of the National Commission on Nursing Implementation Project. "We are shunting people through hospitals acting as

if we have a cure, when we have none. Why not spend our money on caring for them, teaching them to care for themselves?"

That question has been asked with increasing urgency by legislators eager to trim health care costs, at both the state and national level. Between 1962 and 1980, for example, as the proportion of the average hospital budget dedicated to staff dropped from 66 percent to 50 percent, spending for new medical technology swelled. Each piece of technology generated new costs: blood analyzing equipment generated the use of more blood tests. Brain scanning equipment generated orders for routine brain scans. By 1986, medical costs were outstripping inflation by more than six to one, and everyone was looking for relief — for more appropriate, less costly care.

Increasingly, nurses are seen as one important and viable alternative. The new Medicare payment system was created just to get patients out of the expensive, high-tech hospital environment and into the home, where there could be cared for by nurses. A recent study from the University of Pennsylvania shows such a strategy is right on target when skilled nurses are available. The hospital discharged babies from its neonatal intensive care unit an average of 11 days sooner than usual to be cared for at home under the supervision of nurses. Their care cost about $18,000 less, and they recovered just as well as babies who had been kept in the hospital longer.

A landmark study from Congress' Office of Technology Assessment in 1986 concluded that nurse practitioners — registered nurses with advanced training in primary care — were often as good, and sometimes even better, than physicians.

Twenty-five states now recognize nurses as independent health practitioners, who can practice on their own, and bill insurance companies directly. "Not every nurse wants to rush out, hang up a shingle, and go into private practice, but it does open up another career path for nurses, one that gives them autonomy and satisfaction they might not find in a hospital or might want after they've worked in a hospital," says Patricia Ford-Roegner, R.N., political director for the American Nurses' Association.

Nurses fight back

Nurses are working hard to take advantage of their newly recognized value to the nation's health care system, and use the ever-growing shortage of hospital nurses as leverage to secure long-term change in their profession. From inside the hospital and inside the political system, they are fighting for autonomy, better pay, and an improved image.

Perhaps the most significant fight is one to gain an equal footing with physicians, to be paid just as physicians are, directly by insurers. In most cases today, a nurse cannot be paid — nor can her hospital, nursing home, or clinic be paid — unless the services of a nurse have been ordered by a physician.

In December, nurses won a key victory in this area. Congress passed legislation championed by then-Presidential hopeful Richard Gephardt, which will establish the first health centers to be run by nurses directly reimbursed by Medicare. "It means physicians will no longer be gatekeepers to every health service," says Rich Miller, lobbyist for the ANA. So far only four demonstration centers have been funded, but it is still an important symbolic victory. The centers will provide a broad range of services, such as preventive care, nursing for chronic diseases, and helping patients recuperate.

Congress also voted to establish a Center for Nursing Research with the prestigious National Institutes of Health and authorized $19 million to get it up and running, despite opposition from the American Medical Association and a veto from President Reagan. It is a measure of nurses' growing political clout.

"When I first came to Washington a decade ago, we only had three people on staff and all we did was react to things," says Pat Ford-Roegner. The ANA's political action fund has grown from $30,000 in contributions to political campaigns to $350,000 in 1986. Not a huge war chest by Washington standards. The American Medical Association, for example, spends more than $2 million a year. But the PAC represents nurses' growing sense of power, with 25,000 donors. Ford-Roegner claims that 10,000 nurses also worked in Congressional campaigns in the last election. "Now we can initiate action, and we are seen increasingly as a force to be reckoned with. We are consulted and called on to help write language for legislation."

The ANA, as a founding member of the National Committee on Pay Equity, has led the way in the battle to pay women and men equally for work of comparable value. The Illinois Nurses Association is currently suing the state of Illinois in the second-largest pay equity suit ever. Last year, Pennsylvania nurses won a $16 million settlement for some 3,000 nurses, based on the principle of comparable worth.

Many nurses are also rising to positions of authority within hospitals, and using those positions as a springboard for change. Annette McBeth, director of nursing at Lake Region Hospital in Fergus Falls, Minnesota, for example, has started billing patients and insurers directly for nurses' services. It sounds like a small thing, but it is revolutionary in the hospital business. "Nearly all hospitals include nursing services under 'room and board,' which means that no one puts much value on nursing care," says McBeth. Yet by her calculations, nurses generate 50 to 60 percent of the hospital's revenues. "Up until now, nurses were always seen as a cost, not as a profit center," she says, "Just recognizing them on the bill made a huge difference in how nurses are valued by the organization."

The practice, now in place in about 100 of the nation's 5,728 hospitals, "also makes it easier to go into budget negotiations and force everyone to recognize the true value of nursing services," says consultant Van Slyck. "Face it, there wouldn't be hospitals without nurses. Most patients are put in the hospital for nursing care. But no one ever stopped to really look at what nurses do, and calculate what it was worth."

Many nursing administrators are also striving to establish more autonomy for nurses. At Beth Israel Hospital in Boston, nurses practice what is known as "primary nursing," that is, they are responsible for 24-hour planning for a patient, just as physicians are, and they follow those patients from admission to discharge, in collaboration with the physicians. Beth Israel also pays nurses well — a staff nurse can earn as much as $51,000 — and gives the nursing function unusual recognition within the hospital. Joyce Clifford, a vice president for nursing and nurse-in-chief, is given equal rank with the hospital's chief of medicine. Beth Israel has more applicants than it needs. "We draw on the same pool as everyone else, but because of what we offer nurses in their practice," says Clifford, "we get them more easily and they stay with us."

Nurses at the New England Medical Center hospitals, also in Boston, are taking autonomy one step further. They began a "case management" system of nursing three years ago. "We are reorganizing the whole hospital around patient-centered teams, which will be coordinated by nurses," says Karen Zander, director of consultation services at the Center for Nursing Care Management in the medical center. A patient is admitted to an attending physician and nursing group. Eventually, the teams will work like a group practice, referring patients to each other, and to other health facilities in the city.

"Politically, this puts nurses on a new foot-ing within the health care system. They are in charge of allocating health resources, of managing the care. Nurses have always done this, of course, but not up front. Now we're claiming what is ours," says Zander.

But there is still formidable resistance to nurses' goals, especially from organized medicine. The American Medical Association, for example, adamantly opposes legislation that would allow nurses to be reimbursed directly, without a doctor's explicit order. "If nurses want to be doctors, they should go to medical school and get a license," asserts James Sammons, the AMA's executive vice president. At least part of doctors' resistance to increasing roles for nurses stems from basic economic interests. The health care environment is increasingly competitive, with doctors, nurses, and other specialists all vying for patients and the dollars they bring in.

Most nurses say, however, that they are not out to compete with physicians, but to work collaboratively with them and be recognized as an equal part of the team. "Nursing focuses on the process of prevention, healing, and recovery, not on the medical process," says nurse researcher Jackson. Some nurses joke that sometimes doctors "practice nursing without a license," too.

Most hospitals offer only shortsighted solutions to the nursing crisis: some are boosting starting salaries, paying a one-time bonus to recruit new nurses, or offering free tuition, a benefit generally used by nurses in the early stages of their career. But few are giving any attention to establishing career ladders or giving nurses more control over their practices.

Many hospitals are simply hiring temporary help from private nursing agencies. Use of these agencies grew by about 31 percent last year, according to the American Hospital Association, despite the fact that such nurses cost more than a staff nurse, and many people believe the practice only makes the nursing shortage worse.

In the worst cases, hospitals are turning their backs on American nurses altogether and spending money to recruit abroad. Ten percent of all hospitals in the U.S. are recruiting nurses from foreign countries, according to Connie Curran, executive director of the American Organization of Nurse Executives. "American nurses fear that hospitals are saying, 'Hey, if you won't put up with this, we'll just find someone more desperate or docile enough who will,'" Curran says.

The failure to address the concerns of nurses can only continue at a terrible cost not just to nurses, but to all Americans. There is the waste of money. Turnover, for example, eats up health dollars that might be spent to improve and expand health services. It costs $20,000 to recruit and train a new nurse. Last year, hospitals spent more than $3 billion on this rotating door, according to Curran.

At the very least, hospitals could hire more aides, clerks, and licensed practical nurses to lighten the load for registered nurses. Sharon Ness, staff nurse in the critical care units at St. Joseph's in Tacoma, Washington, quit after 16 years because the hospital failed to respond to her requests for more staffing. "If I had felt that what I was doing was respected, if I had felt that when I needed more staff I'd get it, I'd probably still be at St. Joseph's Hospital," says Ness.

The promise and the reality of certification

DOROTHY DEL BUENO, RN, EdD

EVERY YEAR ANOTHER vocational, professional or specialty group initiates certification for its members. Dietary managers, medical stenographers, insurance underwriters, association executives and even those who make their living giving speeches have already developed a certification process. Others such as trainers and educators are still considering it. Each of these groups including nursing specialties claims that its primary motivation is protection of the public from fraudulent, unsafe or unprofessional practices. For licensed individuals such as nurses and physicians, certification is an additional means to acquire formal recognition or distinction in their own and the public's view. Certification is not only an "in" process but is gaining momentum as a mechanism for credentialing that has both worth and value. This article reviews the important issues, benefits and costs related to what has been promised and what has thus far been achieved.

Trend or fad?

Fads receive a great deal of publicity, are highly visible in the literature, media or lecture circuit and rapidly become hot. They are novel, capture people's attention and appeal to the imagination. Conversely, trends evolve much more slowly, gathering support from both the avant-garde and traditionalists. Often modified in response to individual or group needs, trends become an enduring part of belief and practice systems (del Bueno, 1985).

Certification has been addressed extensively in a variety of publications including newsletters, professional journals and the lay literature and has recently received a great deal of publicity even though physicians have been board certified for more than 70 years. The American Association of Nurse Anesthetists is the nursing group with the longest history of certification, having initiated the mechanism in 1946. It is only in the past five years that a plethora of other groups have developed and implemented certification for their members.

The inauguration in 1975 of the National Commission for Health Certifying Agencies (NCHCA) (1985), a voluntary agency whose goal is to promulgate standards for certification, reflects an increased interest in this process. By 1987, 29 organizations had joined NCHCA. At least 23 nursing organizations, some of them members of NCHCA, offer certification. Fickeissen (1985) estimated that more than 85,000 nurses have already been certified. This number appears impressive until we remember that there are almost 2 million registered nurses.

A recent telephone survey of 20 of the several hundred health-related organizations listed in the *American Hospital Association's Guide to the Health Care Field* (1985) revealed that 13 (65%) of the selected sample have had a certification process in place for a range of time from 2 to 20 years. The remaining 7 (35%) did not have and were not contemplating a certification process. If publicity and proliferation were the only criteria used to judge the status of an innovation, certification would certainly qualify as a trend. However, a more important criterion may be practical utility. Many exciting, popular, conceptually sound or logical ideas and innovations do not prove to be economical, useful or cost effective — variables associated with practical utility. Those ideas and innovations that do meet this definition of practical utility will survive and be adopted or adapted — characteristics of a trend.

To determine whether or not certification has practical utility, several other questions must be considered.

Who benefits?

A common definition of certification is that it is a process by which a nongovernmental organization grants recognition of individual competence based on achievement of specific predetermined criteria (Lee, 1986). Certification has also been described as a process that publicly attests to the achievement of specific qualitative or quantitative attributes or characteristics. Implicit and/or explicit in most descriptions of certification is the belief that it will, like spinach, be good for the consumers or clients served by the certified individual. Although such claims are a standard "party line," some groups have been more candid about their vested self-interests and how these are served by certification, for example, the Association of Management Companies (1986):

> The biggest benefit [of certification] is that it segregates the best by proving their expertise. It also has a psychological effect on people, making them more professional. This in Turn benefits the profession. (p.44)
>
> And in an article in *Convention World* we believe that a new professionalism will evolve from the Certified Meeting Professional Program that will set every CPM at a level above those who are not yet certified...the certified individual will go on to be the director of meetings in a corporation or the director of a meetings department in an association. ("Bright Future," 1986, p. 1)

The American Nurses' Association initially proposed certification as a vehicle for recognizing and encouraging personal achievement and superior performance in nursing (Fickeissen, 1985). Some hospitals pay certified professional nurses a differential that is added to the base salary; others offer the certified nurse a one-time bonus; still others reimburse the nurse for both the time and expenses incurred in becoming certified.

At the present time certification as a credentialing process appears to have great practical utility for the certifying agency and perhaps for the individual who has been certified. However, in spite of the rhetoric, there is little or no evidence to support the notion that certified individuals provide better care, give better service or achieve more desirable or higher quality outcomes than do noncertified individuals (Warren, 1987). Opportunities abound for evaluation and research studies to test or validate such assumptions and claims made or implied by certifying groups. Certification may indeed be in the public's best interest, but it behooves those who espouse, implement and promote it to demonstrate for whom it has practical utility and whose best interests are really being served — yours, mine, ours or theirs.

Logistical issues

Many of the issues related to certification center on questions such as, what criteria should be evaluated and how often? What methods of evaluation should be used? What constitutes success or failure on the selected criteria? Who should control the certification process? Haladyna (1987) outlines 19 important recommendations for organizations presently considering certification. Several of these recommendations address the logistical questions identified. First, what should the certification process measure? The process, or examination, should sample the domains of knowledges and skills that are desired by the certifying group and are typical or representative of competent performance. By using a job analysis or role delineation it is possible to identify the knowledge and skills needed to be competent. It is also possible to refine the job analyses by selecting the frequent and critical skills and knowledge required to achieve subsequent or ultimately desirable outcomes and responses. Multiple problems occur, however, in attempting to resolve the measurement question: What methods can or should be used to evaluate performance? Measurement of knowledge, facts, concepts and principles is relatively easy. Although there may be problems such as ambiguity of phrasing, length of items, relevance and cognitive level associated with developing test items, it is possible to select and train content experts in the science of writing reliable and valid knowledge questions. Performance skills, however, can be reliably measured only by direct observation, a process that is both difficult and expensive. Thus most certifying processes use knowledge testing exclusively. A few agencies use other methods such as a review of the candidates' work experience and education complete with transcripts, statements of qualification from employers and instructors and personal references. The American Society of Civil Engineers also interviews candidates for certification in their offices, and the American College of Nurse Midwives uses a written three-part case study essay in addition to the multiple-choice examination.

These examples, however, are the exception rather than the rule. The cost and logistical difficulties inherent in testing actual or simulated performance are considered prohibitive by most certifying agencies. Therefore the agencies that use written tests make an assumption that if individuals select the correct answer, they not only are knowledgeable but probably also possess the ability to perform. Although this assumption may be true, it represents an inferential leap, based thus far on

faith alone. As previously suggested, comparison of hypothetical test performance to actual performance in a simulated or clinical setting, albeit highly desirable, has yet to be done by most certifying agencies.

Claims about the content validity of written certification exams can in most cases be supported, but predictive validity, a highly desirable criterion that reflects the test taker's subsequent performance on the job or in the profession, cannot be claimed. Neither on-the-job performance of unsuccessful test takers nor the test-taking ability of persons evaluated as being incompetent has been measured. Thus competent practitioners could either pass or fail the certification examination, and successful test-takers could be either incompetent or competent on the job.

Another thorny logistical question is, how often should an individual be recertified? The certification examination may measure possession of desired knowledge at the time of testing, but it does not guarantee retention of the knowledge for any length of time. Some certifying organizations stipulate an arbitrary period of time before certified individuals must either be retested or submit evidence of continuing education and knowledge update. Thus it is possible that the individual would continue to be recertified even though they could no longer pass the original test. Recertification requirements, therefore, should ideally be based on studies that identify actual retention rates, a costly and time-consuming process.

Another logical question is, how often should the test be revised? Advances in technology, knowledge obsolescence and knowledge expansion give cause to wonder at the ability of any written test to reflect changes in the knowledge base needed to maintain competent performance. Employers and consumers may be lulled into a false sense of security thinking that an individual certified three, five or even one year ago still has current knowledge relevant to the vocation or profession.

For instance, in 1984 the National Commission on Certification of Physician Assistants (NCCPA) required recertification of their members. Individuals who did not meet the standards required by the second examination received a two-year rather than a six-year renewal of their certification status. (One wonders why they were recertified at all.) The NCCPA examination results revealed that first-time physician assistants did better than recertificants. The NCCPA (1985) therefore concluded, based on three years of retesting experience, that the examination did not address the crucial issue of valid examination of the experienced practitioner's competence.

Another difficult question is, what constitutes examination success or failure? There has been severe criticism of the practice of setting passing or cut-off scores based only on the subjectivity of an identified point on a numerical scale. This arbitrary number theoretically separates the "competent" from the "incompetent." If the test truly represents the important knowledge that competent individuals should possess, it seems more logical that the examinee be required to answer correctly all items. If some test items are redundant or repetitive, the cut-off score should be based on answering correctly the important items. "The paradoxical situation often arises that a person scoring exactly at the passing score is judged competent, whereas a person scoring one point lower is judged incompetent" (Haladyna, 1987). This decision is based on the assumption that all items have both the same ability to discriminate between competent and incompetent performers, an assumption possible to test but, like actual performance or predictive testing, it is both time consuming and costly.

Control of the certifying process carries both implementation and legal implications. The implementation implications of control are related to the selection of expert consultants and staff to initiate and maintain the ex-amination process, to develop policies and procedures for fees and to determine testing site locations and frequency of test offerings. Legal implications of the control question are related to decisions about eligibility, retesting and opportunity to appeal. For example, some certification programs include specific educational and/or experience requirements to qualify for testing. These requirements could eliminate or exclude competent and knowledgeable individuals or groups who are unable to acquire the credential simply because of their ineligibility. Locus of the responsibility for making these decisions could result, purposefully or inadvertently, in legal liability for the certifying agency.

Legal liability

Potential or actual legal liability involved in the certification process relates to conflict-of-interest, restraint of trade and discrimination:

> Because failure to pass a credentialing examination is the most disputed and tangible basis for denying a credential, such examinations have come increasingly into public awareness and criticism. Recent legal challenges have raised questions about job relatedness and fairness of such examinations, especially when they are primarily in the written and multiple choice mode. The validity of credentialing must be viewed in terms of the extent to which these examinations simulate job-related performance and permit appropriate judments of competence. (D'Costa, 1986, p. 138)

The major decisions made by courts in cases involving certification have evolved from antitrust law and constitutional issues of discrimination and restraint of trade, or the inability to pursue one's profession. It is clear that courts want assurance that any examination does in fact measure the knowledge, skills and abilities required to perform the job competently and that the exam differentiates between those who are and are not competent (O'Brien, 1986).

Although most definitions of certification include explicitly or implicitly the concept of voluntarism, incorporation of certification requirements and procedures into licensing or legal credentialing is not uncommon (Geolot, 1986). Certification requirements can affect nurses who wish to be acknowledged officially as nurse practitioners and may therefore promote or hinder nurses' ability to obtain a specific position. In Pennsylvania, for example, a nurse wishing to be recognized as a certified nurse practitioner must have attended a program approved by the State Board of Nursing. Thus nurses already certified by the American Nurses' Association can be denied the right to call themselves certified nurse practitioners if they did not attend an approved program. These nurses deemed "competent" through certification by one agency may be ineligible for a job that requires certification based on another agency's criteria.

Many state courts have held that, when a voluntary professional association makes determinations about a member's ability to practice the profession, the association must observe principles of fundamental fairness. The basic requirements related to fundamental fairness are: (a) private bodies cannot restrict membership rights and privileges on an arbitrary or discriminatory basis, and (b) members must be afforded proper notice and opportunity to be heard (Massaro, 1986). Voluntary self-regulatory bodies including certification agencies therefore need guidance as to what due process and other safeguards they can institute to insulate themselves effectively from antitrust liability (Peplau, 1987).

Another potential legal problem is related to truth in testing. This concept requires that the examinees have access to test questions, answers, forms, rules and policies. Proponents of truth-in-testing legislation have been trying to include licensing and certification examinations in such disclosure law:

> Members of the licensing and certification community cannot afford to be sanguine about this issue. If the legislation passes, it will have profound effects on those involved in developing, administering, and using the results of licensing and certification tests (Shimberg, 1987, p. 1).

All of these legal and logistical questions may be indicative of a much broader issue: public distrust of testing in general. People are becoming increasingly aware of the important role that tests play in their lives and often feel powerless when it comes to the critical decisions made about their lives based on test results. Test takers also often have misgivings about the accuracy of the scoring and question whether or not the keyed answer is the correct answer (Shimberg, 1987).

Even if they were correct, however, would the questions be relevant to actual practice? A paradox in psychometrics is the inverse relationship between objectivity and relevance. A truly objective test is context free; life is not. The conditions and circumstances in which individuals perform their vocations and professions affect and influence the acts themselves. Objective tests can determine what individuals know, but they cannot reflect the guided intuitions, holistic sensitivity or richness of experience that proficient and expert practitioners use in managing patients and clients. Most examinations trivialize competent and expert performance to a structured, formalized set of facts, rules, principles and theories. Possession of these is not undesirable or unnecessary to practice — it is just not the complete story.

Conclusions
Those who develop, promote and implement certification programs have desirable and rele-

vant intentions and goals. The reality thus far, however, does not seem to match that which has been promised or is anticipated.

> Some hospitals responding to the unfortunate fact that certification and licensure have not addressed hospitals' need for specific and continuing competence have instituted their own skill validation and employee credentialing. (Bradley, 1985, p. 2)

Employers, practitioners or consumers may feel as negative about certification and its benefits; however, there is a paucity of either subjective or objective data to demonstrate specific client or patient benefits from certification. There are also considerable costs both in real dollars and lost opportunities associated with the certification process. When done rigorously and correctly, installation, implementation and maintenance of certification programs are costly. Fees paid by the examinee or the employer may not cover the actual costs of the certification process; thus the costs will have to be passed on to patients, clients or organization members. Dollars may have to be diverted from other income sources or costs subsidized by profits from other activities. Salary increases or bonuses given to certified individuals may be passed on to patients or clients.

The time, money, energy and effort spent on certification activities may indeed be worthwhile and justifiable, in spite of the lack of evidence demonstrating real benefit to customers, if those within the professions and vocations value both the credential and the process necessary to acquire it. Those who value it,

then, should bear the burden of costs. Conversely, certification may be a passing fad that will be replaced by another process, credential or expectation that has both promise and practical utility for patients and clients.

REFERENCES

American Hospital Association (1985). **Guide to the health care field.** Chicago, IL.

Association of Management Companies, Inc. (1986). Certification is a national pastime. **Elected Leader**, 5(3), 39-44.

Bradley, D.K. (1985). Employee credentialing at some hospitals fills a gap. **NCHCA Newsletter**, 6(1-2), 9.

Bright future ahead for CMP program (1986). **Convention World**, (5), 1.

D'Costa. A.G. (1986). The validity of credentialing examinations. **Evaluation and the Health Professions**, 9, 137-169.

del Bueno, D.J. (1985). Bandwagons, parades and panaceas. **Nursing Outlook**, 33, 136-138.

Fickeissen, J.L. (1985). Getting certified. **American Journal of Nursing**, 85, 265-269.

Geolot, P.H. (1986). The relationship between certification and practice. **Nurse Practitioner**, 11(3), 55-58.

Haladyna, T.M. (1987). Three components in the establishment of a certification testing program. **Evaluation and the Health Professions**, 10, 139-172.

Lee, C.(1986). Certification of trainers. **Training**, 10(11), 56-64.

Massaro, T.M. (1986). Continuing competency-regulatory alternatives. **Issues**, 7(4), 8-10.

National Commission for Health Certifying Agencies (1985). Mandatory recertification in the P.A. profession. **Newsletter**, 6(1-2), 7-8.

O'Brien, T.L. (1986). Legal trends affecting the validity of credentialing examinations. **Evaluation and the Health Professions**, 9(2), 171-185.

Peplau, H. (1987). Is nursing's self-regulatory power being eroded? **Journal of the New York State Nurses' Association**, 18(3), 13-17.

Shimberg, B. (1987). Truth in testing for the professions. **Issues**, 8(4), 1-6.

Warren, L. (1987). NSNCO meeting report. **American Association of Diabetes Educators News**, 13(2), p. 1.

The nursing scene: A need for specialists

CAROL A. GRIMALDI

A BABY BOY born prematurely battled silently for life inside an incubator in the neonatal intensive care unit of a large hospital. His lungs were so undeveloped that he needed extra oxygen in the air he breathed. The machine provided the necessary concentration of oxygen and, by means of wires attached to tiny sensors on the baby's body, monitored his breathing and heartbeat. A registered nurse (RN) with special training in critical care read the incubator's gauges carefully, and checked the wires and sensors.

Two floors below, attendants wheeled a middle-aged woman — the victim of a traffic accident — into the emergency room. The patient was unconscious. A team of physicians and nurses went into action immediately. A certified registered nurse anesthetist (CRNA) carefully inserted a breathing tube in the patient's airway, then gently pushed a needle connected to an intravenous (IV) line into a vein. One of the physicians quickly determined that the woman had a concussion and instructed the CRNA to give medications through the IV to reduce the swelling of the patient's brain.

In a small town miles away, a registered nurse welcomed a young woman into the RN's office. The nurse performed a routine physical examination on the patient and then counseled her on the importance of breast self-examination. The RN was a nurse practitioner in private practice.

Greater specialization

The critical care nurse, the CRNA, and the nurse practitioner represent a major trend in the rapidly changing profession of nursing — specialization in the work of registered nurses. RN's make up just one of two large groups of people licensed to practice nursing. The other consists of Licensed Practical Nurses (LPN's) and Licensed Vocational Nurses (LVN's), individuals who practice under the supervision of RN's. This article discusses career opportunities for registered nurses.

The most numerous group of RN's are hospital personnel who have a wide variety of job specialties, but whose job title — staff nurse — does not reflect their specialization. According to a November 1984 survey conducted by the U.S. Department of Health and Human Services (HHS), there are 1½ million RN's employed in nursing in the United States, and about 1 million of them work in hospitals. About 73 per cent of the hospital RN's are staff nurses.

Many hospital staff nurses specialize in the care of patients who have certain types of illnesses or special needs. Oncology nurses, for example, work with cancer patients. Other staff nurses work in special locations such as emergency rooms, operating rooms, obstetrical units, critical care units, and hospital outpatient clinics.

Registered nurses who acquire additional education or training may hold other job titles and credentials. In hospitals, the most numerous of these highly trained nurses — about 16 per cent of all hospital RN's — are supervisors, head nurses, and administrators, and their assistants. The remaining 11 per cent of hospital RN's include instructors, clinical nurse specialists, CRNA's, nurse clinicians, nurse practitioners, nurse-midwives, and researchers.

Clinical nurse specialists are RN's who have a master's or doctoral degree with specialization in such areas as medical-surgical nursing, maternal and child nursing, or psychiatric-mental health nursing. The title *nurse clinician* was commonly used in hospitals in the 1970's for RN's who performed special functions, regardless of the extent of their education. The present trend is for special titles to reflect defined levels of education or experience.

Growing demand — and growing supply

RN's with all levels of education and experience in all areas of specialization are in great demand. According to the HHS, there were 1.9 million RN's in the United States in 1984. The 1.5 million employed in nursing represented 79 per cent of the total, a high participation rate.

Furthermore, the unemployment rate for RN's is astonishingly low. The Bureau of Labor Statistics of the U.S. Department of Labor reported in June 1987 that the average unemployment rate for RN's in 1986 was only 1.6 per cent, compared with 7 per cent for the civilian labor force as a whole. In December 1986, hospitals throughout the United States reported that 13.6 per cent of their positions for RN's were vacant — twice the vacancy percentage reported a year earlier. The demand for RN's is expected to outpace the supply into the next century.

The salaries of RN's also are increasing. In 1976, the average annual starting salary for a hospital staff nurse was $10,440. This grew to $16,116 in 1981 and to $20,340 in 1986. The average maximum pay for experienced hospital staff nurses rose from $13,200 in 1976 to $21,408 in 1981 and to $27,774 in 1986. Registered nurses in certain specialties can earn much more — over $40,000 for CRNA's and about $45,000 for top administrators.

Job openings and average salaries have in-creased despite the fact that the number of RN's has been growing steadily. The total increased by 35 per cent from 1977 to 1984, according to the HHS study.

Effects of new cost-consciousness

Changes in health-care financing have altered the employment patterns of RN's in the 1980's. In 1982, the federal government changed the reimbursement policy for the Medicare health-care program for the elderly. The government stopped reimbursing hospitals on the basis of the cost of treating patients and established payment levels for various categories of illness called *diagnosis-related groups* (DRGs). Hospitals received only a certain amount to treat patients with a specific illness, regardless of how much the treatment cost the hospital. Thus hospitals would lose money on patients who cost more to treat than the amount set by the DRG. On the other hand, hospitals could make a profit on patients whose care cost less than the fixed rate of reimbursement for a particular ailment.

Cost-conscious hospitals began laying off staff, including RN's. The American Hospital Association (AHA) reported that U.S. hospitals reduced their staffs by about 70,000 employees nationwide in 1984 and again in 1985, though about 10,000 jobs were restored in 1986.

Hospitals also reacted to the cost pressure by limiting the amount of hospitalization patients receive. Patients were sicker when they were admitted to hospitals, and they faced shorter stays. The average length of stay declined steadily from 1981 to 1985 before inching upward 0.7 per cent in 1986, according to the AHA. This "sicker and quicker" policy meant that hospital patients needed more care, leading to greater demand for RN's, particularly in specialty areas such as critical care, operating room nursing, and discharge planning.

The policy also increased the typical RN's

workload substantially, but nurses received no increase in pay or benefits for the additional responsibility, according to the American Nurses' Association (ANA), the national professional organization for RN's, based in Kansas City, Mo. As a result, many nurses left hospitals to work for other types of institutions, including health maintenance organizations, home health agencies, and hospices. Some nurses established their own practice.

Fewer women, more men in nursing

The shortage of nurses in hospitals is aggravated by the fact that fewer women are choosing nursing as a career. Until about the mid-1970's, high school guidance counselors often directed career-minded women into traditionally female-dominated professions, primarily nursing, teaching, and secretarial work. Since that time, however, increasing numbers of women have pursued male-dominated professions, becoming business executives, lawyers, and physicians.

An ongoing, nationwide study begun in 1966 by the University of California at Los Angeles (UCLA) and the American Council on Education documented the shift away from nursing. Each year, UCLA's Higher Education Research Institute polls 300,000 full-time freshmen at two- and four-year colleges. In 1974, 10.4 per cent of the women polled said that nursing was their career choice, the highest percentage ever recorded in the study. By 1986, the figure had plunged to a record low of 5.1 per cent.

As women are moving away from nursing, increasing numbers of men are entering the profession, according to the National League for Nursing (NLN), an organization that accredits nursing education programs. At present, 3 per cent of the RN's in the United States are men. During the 1985-1986 school year, 5.2 per cent of the nursing education students were men.

Education and licensing

Currently, three kinds of education programs qualify individuals to take state examinations for RN licenses — community college or vocational school programs leading to an associate degree, college and university programs leading to a bachelor's degree with a major in nursing, and hospital-based programs leading to a nursing diploma. All three types of programs require a high school diploma or its equivalent for admission.

An associate degree program takes two school years to complete. The curriculum is divided between nursing courses and classes in the sciences and liberal arts. In the 1985-1986 school year, full-time nursing students enrolled in two-year programs at public schools paid an average of $781 in tuition and fees. Students in private schools paid an average of $4,025. Almost 97,000 students enrolled in associate degree programs in 1985, a 7.8 per cent decline from 1984.

Bachelor's degree programs in nursing take at least four school years to complete. The curriculum includes a minimum of 64 credit hours in nursing and 68 hours in science and liberal arts. The average annual cost of tuition for full-time students in four-year programs in the 1985-1986 school year was $1,330 for public universities and $5,257 for private colleges. Just over 91,000 students were enrolled in such programs in 1985, down 4.2 per cent from the previous year. In addition, 43,000 individuals who had already received RN licenses were studying for bachelor's degrees.

Diploma schools of nursing require three calendar years of study. Two-thirds of the course work consists of nursing studies, and the remainder covers the sciences and liberal arts. The average annual tuition in 1985 was $1,773 at public hospitals and $2,552 at private hospitals. Slightly more than 30,000 students were enrolled in diploma schools of nursing in 1985, down 19 per cent from 1984. This decline reflects a 20-year trend among hospitals to cut costs by closing their schools.

After completing an approved course of study in nursing, a prospective RN must pass a licensure examination conducted by a state board of nursing. Since 1982, all 50 states have used the same test, the National Council Licensure Examination.

To meet the demand for larger numbers of RN's who are prepared to meet the complex and rapidly changing health-care needs of the nation, the ANA recommends new professional standards. The ANA has urged the states to establish two levels of clinical-practice nursing personnel — a technical level requiring an associate degree and a professional level requiring a bachelor's degree. In January 1986, North Dakota became the first state to revise licensing requirements in this way. Other states are pursuing changes in educational requirements and licensure.

Some nursing specialty fields

Specialist RN's find special joy — and special frustrations — in their jobs.

Nurse anesthetists. Terry Piere, a CRNA at Truman Medical Center in Kansas City, Mo., enjoys the independence and variety his job provides. He receives his surgical schedule the day before the operations take place. This gives him time to interview each patient so he can detect problems that might occur during surgery. Of particular concern are the presence of allergies and the abuse of drugs, including alcohol, that might interfere with the action of the anesthetics or otherwise cause complications during surgery.

After the patient is brought to the operating room, Piere inserts an IV line through which a nutritive liquid will flow. He then administers the anesthetic by means of a mask or by injection. Sometimes, he gives the patient a muscle relaxer to prevent muscle spasms and ensure that the surgeon will have good access to the site of the operation. He also may administer antibiotics to prevent infection. Throughout surgery, he monitors the patients's vital signs, including pulse and breathing rate, and informs the surgeon of significant changes. After the operation, Piere checks the patient for nausea, pain, and other responses to the anesthetics and the surgical procedure.

According to Piere, studying to become a CRNA was demanding and time-consuming. After earning a bachelor's degree, he completed a two-year program leading to a master's degree in nursing. On the job, the demands have continued. "You must be on call, usually staying in house (in the hospital) during a long shift, to respond to emergencies," he says.

Operating room nurses. These nurses, also called OR or perioperative nurses, are part of the surgical team. Many OR nurses find their work rewarding because their efforts are highly visible and important to the effectiveness of the team. They also have the opportunity to take part in advanced procedures, such as organ transplants and surgical techniques involving lasers.

Rebecca M. Patton, an OR nurse at University Hospitals of Cleveland, rotates between serving as a scrub nurse and a circulating nurse. The scrub nurse works with the operating surgeon inside an area called the *sterile field*, which surrounds the operating table. All personnel within the field must be scrubbed, gowned, and wearing sterile gloves, and all equipment must be sterilized. The circulating nurse who manages the OR, moves about outside the sterile field, handling responsibilities requiring more mobility.

"You see wonderful things in this job, and you see horrible things," says Patton. "You may work on a case in which a 1-year-old child has tumors, but because of early diagnosis and surgery, that baby has a chance of growing up and living a normal life. As a nurse, you feel you're partially responsible for that."

As a scrub nurse, Patton derives particular satisfaction from cases in which she and the surgeons do not need to speak during an operation. "It's as much experience as it is my ability to anticipate their needs," she says.

Patton is excited about research that nurses can do in the OR. She and her colleagues, for example, have been collecting data indicating that mastectomy patients who undergo laser surgery experience a better recovery than do patients whose tissue is cut with scalpels.

Public health or community nurses. These nurses provide care for a wide variety of patients in schools, community health and social agencies, visiting nurses' associations, home health agencies, shelters, day-care programs, discharge-planning units, and outpatient facilities. Public health nurses enjoy the independence of their practice and the wide variety of services they can provide in caring for families and other groups. Some are frustrated, however, by low salaries that are common in many public-service jobs.

Barbara A. Blakeney, a public health nurse at the Long Island Shelter, a facility operated by Boston's Department of Health and Hospitals, works mostly with homeless and elderly people. Blakeney says, "Being poor is very hard, and many of these people have physical and psychological problems. They often crumble emotionally and physically from poverty."

Blakeney's colleagues include nurse practitioners, psychiatric clinical nurse specialists, and specialists in drug and alcohol abuse as well as other public health nurses. "We essentially run a nursing clinic and provide care on-site," she says. "This shelter alone may have as many as 1,200 visits a month, and we attempt to take care of most ongoing health problems of the homeless. You and I would be able to go home and rest in bed after we were hospitalized. The homeless can't do that."

"The nice thing about public health nursing is that you can do something like this," Blakeney adds. "There is relative independence. The people we see need nursing care. We are their link to the health-care system, the case manager. We are pivotal in meeting these health-care needs. That is an excellent role for nurses."

Nurse practitioners and clinical nurse specialists. These nurses provide a full range of health-care services, including health assessment, health maintenance, patient treatment, patient and family education and counseling, medication management and review, and referral to other health-care professionals. They work in the fields of family health, maternal and child health, adult health, gerontological health, school nursing, community health, and women's health. As many as 20,000 nurse practitioners and clinical nurse specialists practice independently.

Nurse practitioner programs were developed 20 years ago to provide care in rural and inner city areas where physicians were in short supply. Duvall, Wash., is such a place. This town of about 1,000 people is located about 18 miles (29 kilometers) northeast of Seattle and has no physician.

Since 1982, nurse practitioner Ted Ritter has operated the Duvall Family Health Clinic. He sees an average of 14 patients per day. He has a general family practice, treating patients with upper respiratory and urinary tract infections, monitoring individuals who have chronic disorders such as diabetes and high blood pressure, and providing well-baby checkups, immunizations, and school physicals.

Ritter frequently refers patients to medical specialists such as allergists, urologists, cardiologists, and orthopedists. "I enjoy a good relationship with physicians and other health-care providers in the area," Ritter comments. In fact, he has been granted hospital privileges at one institution.

Why does Ritter work so hard in a place

whose economy is not strong enough to attract a physician? "Nurses who practice in underserved areas don't do it for the money," he says. "My compensation is at a couple of levels. Monetarily, I get by, but being my own boss and being an important part of the community are great rewards."

Nurse consultants. These nurses provide an expert opinion about problems pertaining to nursing. These specialists work with hospitals, home care agencies, schools of nursing, and manufacturers of pharmaceutical and health-care products. Some operate their own businesses, conducting education programs, providing formal reviews of health-care services, acting as recruiters of nurses, and even supplying entire nursing staffs for various organizations.

Lieutenant Colonel Barbara Jo McGrath is the nurse consultant to the commanding general of Hanscom Air Force Base in Massachusetts. She keeps the general informed about how well the base's nursing staff meets Air Force requirements, identifies problems experienced by the staff, and suggests solutions for the problems.

McGrath also has worked as a civilian nurse consultant. She says that consultants follow the same process, whether they work with a military or a civilian organization, and whether they are employed by that organization or by an outside firm. The consultant first identifies problems, then analyzes the functions of individuals who work in the problem areas. He or she then recommends solutions, helps carry out the recommended changes, and evaluates the effectiveness of the measures. "As a consultant, you might recommend changes in the organizational structure, or in the functions or duties of units and personnel," says McGrath.

Nurse consultants will have plenty to do through the 1990's just to keep their employers and clients abreast of changes in the nursing profession. Nurses will become better educated, with larger numbers of them earning advanced credentials. As health care progresses technologically, new skills will be required, and the nursing profession will provide them. And the services of RN's will continue to be in great demand, assuring young men and women who enter the profession of steady employment and plenty of opportunity for advancement. To experienced observers, the outlook for careers in nursing has never seemed brighter.

American Nurses' Association's social policy statement: Part 1

HILDEGARD E. PEPLAU

In 1980, the American Nurses' Association (ANA) published Nursing: A Social Policy Statement *(SPS), a pamphlet with far-reaching implications for the advancement of the nursing profession. Peplau discusses major points of the SPS in the following excerpt.*

IN 1971, THE New York State Nurses' Association put forth a radically new definition of nursing, which became part of the Nursing Practice Act of New York State in 1972. Nursing was defined as "the diagnosis and treatment of human responses to actual and potential health problems. "This definition provided the keystone — the missing piece — that was essential for the full professionalization of nursing. For the first time in nursing's history, a phenomenological focus for nursing practice was specified. It is this definition of nursing that is contained in the SPS. The task force believed that there was a growing consensus, within nursing and among the public, that this definition best expressed the essence of nursing. This consensus was seen as inherent in the fact that about one third of the states had, by 1980, adopted identical or very similar definitions in their nursing practice acts. These states obviously had a substantial number of nurses and legislators — representatives of the people — who were in agreement that the delegated social responsibility of nurses, in health care, should be focused on "human responses to...." For the SPS to suggest some other definition would most likely be viewed — and rightly so — as denial of this obviously mounting consensus.

The SPS presents the view that society owns the professions, that there is a social contract between society and a profession. That contract implies a defined, socially delegated responsibility, one that is mutually beneficial and is in the public interest and that entails a reciprocal responsibility and obligation on the part of nurses and society. The social responsibility delegated to nurses, in nurse practice acts, carries with it the authority with regard to the defined domain. There are also expectations. Society expects nurses — indeed all professions — to provide essential services; to research, generate, and refine knowledge related to the profession's domain; to teach the public what the profession knows will maintain the health of citizens; and to regulate its members in the public interest.

In return for meeting these expectations, society takes on the obligation to provide the resources essential for the profession to execute its responsibilities. This obligation, however, is not fulfilled automatically but rather requires the professions to press their claims to society's resources through the political process.

The central feature in the social contract between nursing and society is the phenomenological focus for the profession's work. All professions have a phenomenological focus or core — it is the only unique feature because knowledge, technology, client data, activities, and so forth are often shared among professions. The phenomena of concern to a profession, specified in its definition, constitute what needs particular explanatory theories and where practices should be directed to produce beneficial effects for the client. These phenomena, for example, are central to other professions: for medicine, disease and injury; for law, injustice and grievance; for theology, soul, spirit, and a person's relation to God; for architecture, the function and form of buildings; for economics, resource distribution; and for nursing, human responses to actual and potential health problems.

The definition of nursing in SPS constitutes a major paradigm shift — a new way of looking at nursing (e.g., paradigm: the world is flat vs. the world is round). This shift is inherent in reformulation of the question from "What do nurses do?" to "What do nurses fix, correct, seek to change, relieve, or ameliorate?" in the direction of health and healthy living for persons. It is the answer to this latter question, "human responses to...." that pinpoints the core, focus, essence, and target for nursing practice, nursing research, and the content of nursing education and health teaching for patients and the public.

Human responses are behaviors, clusters or sets (patterns) of such behaviors that a nurse observes, or obtains from the subjective reports of a client. Such responses can be physiological, psychological, sociological, and so forth. They can be intrapersonal, interpersonal, or systems responses.

This domain of "human responses to..." is a very broad net. It is sharpened and partially delimited by two qualifiers: "actual and potential health problems." It is being further refined by the developing classification of nursing diagnosis. Nursing diagnosis has thus far had only 14 years of development; other professions have been identifying, refining, and revising phenomena contained in their classification systems for hundreds of years. So, nursing has a very long way to go in classifying the contents of its turf, in determining the theoretical explanations for each phenomenon, and in identifying and testing phenomena in relation to specific practices in nursing. Diag-

nosis, of course, is mere naming of a phenomenon; professionals are expected to exercise ability to go beyond the surface (the name) and to grasp theoretically the basic working of a phenomenon. Complex processes have an order, a regularity that can be made known, particularly through research. [Currently], much more is known about physiological bodily processes than about behavioral and environmental system processes. Nurses are beginning to think diagnostically, and nurse researchers are beginning to lay out theories of behavioral and systems processes.

ANA's SPS lays out a structural model — a paradigm for practice (ANA, 1980, pp. 14-15). It combines the nursing definition, nursing process, and nursing standards. There are advantages to a structural as opposed to a content model for practice. A structural model shows the components of nursing practice to be taken into account in providing services to clients (ANA, 1980, pp. 14-15). It suggests relations among those components. It is a general (holistic) model. Presently, various theoretical models are being proposed. In contrast to a structural model, theoretical ones have disadvantages. Those that are global, intended as models for all of nursing, give no direction for direct practice to particular clients. They often are used as ideologies rather than as explanations. Theories also follow fashions and become outmoded if not disproved. Theoretical models tend to impose theory upon phenomena, point to vague rather than specific phenomena, or limit their applicability. They suggest that theory rather than phenomena is the starting point for practice.

The ANA model conveys the idea that the starting point for practice is the identification of those phenomena to be fixed, corrected, changed, relieved, ameliorated, and at the very least brought into the client's awareness. Historically, nurses have been taught to think in terms of medical phenomena — disease, defect, or injury. In staking and defending a claim to a domain of nursing phenomena, a shift in thinking is required of nurses. Nursing actions related to medical phenomena are prescribed by physicians. Nursing actions in relation to nursing phenomena require, as a first step, identifying, that is, diagnosing, those concerns of clients. This cognitive effort includes diagnoses and is followed by the nurse's intellectual effort to recall or otherwise obtain a theoretical understanding of the problem. This is theory application — a nurse performance that goes beyond mere naming (diagnosing) and becomes the basis for determining the required corrective nursing actions. Theory application at the practice level consists primarily of the use of concepts and processes defined so as to interpret data about the client's problem and used to provide an explanation or understanding of that problem. Interference is used when diagnoses or theories are unavailable and in effect are hypotheses — in the sense of "this problem may be...."

In other words, thinking theoretically — when the ANA model is used — becomes a major dimension in nursing practice and takes precedence over an activity orientation. What nurses do will be derived from what nurses know in relation to diagnosed nursing phenomena.

There is a great deal of work to be done in clarifying theories useful in nursing practice. A diagnosis of a nursing phenomenon merely describes, enunciates, or names the problem. The most useful theories applied to explain, interpret, or understand the nature of that problem would include, in each defined concept or process, what the origins and functions of the phenomenon are, how it works, and how it may be corrected as suggested by the theory. Such theoretical information can be drawn from any basic or applied science or generated through nursing research.

The other three papers in this series are each addressed to theory about a clinical phenomenon seen in nursing practice. Phenomena and theory are interrelated. Theory — in the form of concepts and processes in the head of the nurse and available for recall — is used during observation and data collection and in diagnosing in the sense of hypotheses. Is it anxiety; is it shame; is it envy? The indicators of diagnostic concepts are theoretically based, but these are merely cues to identify a diagnostic category rather than to explain and to understand it. Professional practice requires going beyond naming a problem, which means having a theoretical understanding of its natural history — of the regularities and steps in the evolution of that problem as seen in most people. Theory, then, serves the nurse as a map for reviewing the particulars of a problem in the individual case.

Theory also serves as a framework for the nurse to decide nursing actions. Many nurses think of intervention as doing something, but in the case of behavioral change — an elusive, difficult goal — the nursing action is most often asking a question. Those human responses having to do with behavioral change more often than not are best served when the nurse's aim is to assist patients to notice and to become aware of problematic behavior. Being aware of behavior patterns and their variations is the only viable basis a person can have for self-change.

In the ANA structural model for nursing practice there are four defining characteristics. So far, phenomena, theory application, and nursing action have been discussed briefly. The fourth characteristic, *effects*, refers to the short or long-term outcomes resulting from nursing actions taken in relation to particular diagnosed phenomena. Evaluation — outcome studies — are expected of professionals. Professional services are supposed to have beneficial, that is, remedial, effects. Whether such results occur can be made known by testimonials, periodic evaluations, and by research studies, which obviously provide the soundest basis for evaluation of effects of nursing actions on diagnosed conditions.

The ANA SPS also addressed the matter of scope of practice. Efforts to do so had been underway for 2 decades. The task force saw the scope question in terms of core, dimensions, intersections, and boundary. The *core* of nursing is its phenomenological domain — its area of socially delegated responsibility as stated in the definition of nursing in the nursing practice act in a given state. Nursing has legal authority to practice, teach, and research the contents of its domain — its phenomenological focus. Knowledge derived from scientific sources or nursing research gives further nursing authority.

The *dimensions* of nursing include philosophy and ethics, functions, roles, skills, and technology, in fact everything that impinges or is relevant to core, that is, domain.

Intersections characterize the areas in which nursing is adjacent to or overlaps the work of other health professionals. The task force conceptualized health care as a large pie having wedges representative of all of the health professions. This concept of health care as more than medical care is a recent one, no more than 2 decades old. It is possibly an example of a current shift away from hierarchical systems of all kinds and toward recognition of interdependent, collaborative systems. Health care is rapidly coming to be viewed as being comprised of many segments, with each autonomous professional segment having its own definite characteristics and independent functions.

This concept of health care is likely to give rise to interprofessional disputes, particularly between medicine and nursing but with other professions also. Medicine's domain is well established; nursing is only at the beginning of identifying and defining its phenomena. Moreover, all professions have access to and in their work may use any published theoretical knowledge or apply any publicly available technology; in these areas of shared expertise there tends to be and probably in the future will be more areas of overlapping function. Except for highly esoteric knowledge and know-how — cardiac surgery, for example — only the phenomenological domain identifies the unique turf of a profession, that turf being contained in the profession's diagnostic classification system. The domains of medicine and nursing, although separate, are complementary, that is, when both physicians and nurses diagnose and treat their separate phenomena and interrelate their work, a higher quality of care will be provided to sick patients. Yet, it is at this intersection of the two domains that the use of commonly shared knowledge or technology is often disputed or challenged. Moreover, at the intersection of nursing and medicine, there also is overlapping function. Historically, physicians taught nurses about diseases — their symptoms, course, prognosis, and treatment. Physicians also passed on to nurses those procedures — taking temperature, pulse, respiration, blood pressure and giving injections — that were formerly medical procedures. Nurse practitioners, in particular, have extended their practices still further into medicine. Consequently, there is, and no doubt will continue to be, a gray area where overlapping occurs in all aspects of care.

The fourth aspect of scope of practice has to do with boundary. The task force viewed boundary as an outer perimeter that is fluid and amenable to *expansion*. Such expansion occurs as a profession responds to new social needs, as these arise, and by claiming new phenomena arising from changing and emerging social needs. All professions expand this way: (a) A new social concern is noticed; (b) the problem is claimed, that is, named, diagnosed, and included into the profession's diagnostic classification system; (c) theoretical explanations are worked out; (d) theory-derived treatments are tested; (e) services are offered; and (f) the public is advised of the new development. Similarly, any new theoretical knowledge generated in nursing research or in any scientific field can lead to new developments that expand a profession's boundary. Thus, the task force distinguished between *intersections,* borders between professions, and *extensions* into these health care professions — medicine, dentistry, social work, and so forth. Nursing is the largest slice of the health care pie. As pointed out earlier, the unique feature of a profession is its phenomenological focus — all else, scientific knowledge, technology, philosophy, goals, ethics, is shared although they may be stated or applied in somewhat different ways. In the case of nursing and medicine, there is a large gray area of overlap. It is at this interprofessional intersection that most lawsuits occur, but as a judge in Missouri ruled, that thin boundary line cannot be identified.

The scope of nursing also has to do with its outer boundary. Many nurses had hoped that this boundary could be a hard and secure one. The task force saw it as flexible, ever expanding outward as nursing responds to changing social needs. Thus, nursing expands its autonomous service outward and also extends into the medical field.

The SPS also addressed the matter of specialization in nursing. The present picture of specialization virtually confirms the validity of the concept of keeping the outer boundary of nursing fluid. A review of the NLN brochure, which describes specialty programs in some 100 graduate programs, shows a very wide spread of interests in specialization in nursing. The SPS does not address what areas of specialization in nursing there should be. Specialization at the graduate level is less than a half century old. The idea, however, has been around since the turn of the century. Between 1900 and the 1940s the term was used for pri-

vate duty nurses, "specialing patients," and for advanced basic hospital-based programs in mid-wifery, operating room nursing, communicable diseases, and psychiatric and tuberculosis nursing. When university-based programs started in 1943, they tended to continue the use of these medical disease categories for program titles. Now there is a movement in nursing away from the medical model toward a nursing model. The SPS points out that a nursing model will lead to nursing specialty categories drawn from clusters of phenomena within nursing's domain. In other words, the classification of nursing diagnosis needs more time — several decades at least — to develop to a point where groupings of phenomena become clearer than now.

The SPS did define specialization (ANA, 1980, pp. 23-25), along the following lines: (a) It is a narrowed focus on a part of the whole phenomenological core of nursing. (b) The educational preparation occurs in a university at the graduate level — master's and doctoral. (c) It includes theory pertaining to that of the field-indepth knowledge. (d) Faculty in the program hold graduate degrees, preferably higher than that for which the program prepares. (e) Upon graduation, the graduate should be eligible for certification in that specialty.

The SPS suggested that specialty programs should be research oriented and include theory testing, that is, does a particular theory explain phenomena to which it pertains and guide practice, and such programs should include empirical research, that is, theory generation.

The SPS advocated that the role of clinical specialists should not be standardized into job descriptions with regard to institutional employment. Instead, all specialists before employment should negotiate their work role so as to make full use of their particular competencies and interests. Specialists should be of the growing edge of the profession and therefore should conduct a systematic study of particular phenomena and then write and publish their findings. This is their contribution to the advancement of clinical nursing.

The SPS briefly addressed some important reasons for certification as a form of self-regulation within the profession and as the profession's way of assuring the public that a nurse's claim of being a specialist is true.

The SPS identified two criteria for specialists — completion of graduate education in the specialty area and eligibility for certification. In reviewing trends, the task force (TF) believed there were three categories of nurses: generalists, mostly in small hospitals and rural areas; generalists practicing in specialized areas; and specialists.

The complexity of health care today is such that most generalist nurses, on the basis of experience and due to interest and job availability, become generalists in specialized areas. They are, however, not ipso facto specialists.

The TF did not pursue the ramifications of this development.

The SPS is an answer to the question "What is nursing?" It is an answer for now, for this time, not for all time. The report was written by a committee that met five times, so the time limitation is reflected as a content limitation. There was only one forum — 2 hours — for open discussion of a draft of the report. Regional forums would have been desirable, but ANA membership dues income did not support such forums. The report has had only limited published critique, which is regrettable. There are several universities using SPS as a basis for curriculum. All departments of ANA, with the exception of the academy, have discussed implementation of SPS. The SPS will probably be revised, I hope, in the next century and not before.

REFERENCE

American Nurses' Association. (1980). *Nursing: A social policy statement*. Kansas City, MO (pamphlet).

Nursing in the 1990s: Expanding opportunities

ROXANE B. SPITZER, RN, MA; MARYANN DAVIVIER, PhD

AT OUR RECENT strategic planning session, held every year off campus for our top nursing executives, we discussed some of the current trends in the health care industry and in the nursing profession specifically.

Basic trends

Prognosticators abound in the literature of today with many and varied views of nursing's future, some positive, some perhaps not so positive. It seems, however, that there is some general agreement among them such that, barring a major economic disaster in the next few years, some basic trends emerge on which planning can be based.

Economic stresses. Cost containment is and will continue to be the most widely used buzzword in the industry. Cost containment is here to stay. It is an enduring fact of life that nursing must assume as a given basic to all decisions, plans, professional career objectives, and educational programs. To ignore this feature of today's economic climate would be fatal.

All payers today are trying to control costs and are instituting measures to reduce patients' use of services. These conditions will not change in the 1990s or even beyond. *Hospitals* predicted that employers and third party payers will collaborate to control costs by substantially increasing the employee-paid portion of health care coverage by the year 1990.[1] This translates to reduced use of facilities and shorter lengths of stay as well as increased deductibles for employees.

Medicare and Medicaid are also striving for reduced utilization and shorter lengths of stay, with the result that many poor and elderly pa-

tients are going home "sicker and quicker" or are waiting longer before seeking aid. Medicare patient-days dropped 6.1% and 7.96% in the first two quarters of 1985 while outpatient visits increased 15.21% and 12.69%.[2]

Proposed government budget cuts together with the potential effects of the Gramm-Rudman-Hollings Act and the Consolidated Omnibus Reconciliation Act of 1985 will result in more out-of-pocket payment by Medicare patients as well as higher monthly premium rates. This is creating a strong trend toward increased use of home care services and outpatient facilities, not to mention increased acuity of inpatient care, a trend from which nursing can most expeditiously prove the worth of costing nursing services and have an impact on net revenue.

Reducing the length of hospital stays may be desirable but is placing greater stress on nursing home and home health care services, which are not being adequately funded and currently cost Medicare recipients five dollars a visit. In fact, a recent study in Washington state indicates that health care visits have increased as much as 45.7% in urban areas and 12% in rural areas, while professional in-home nursing visits have increased 37.1% in urban areas and 17.8% in rural areas.[3] This report also stated that home health agencies are being pressed to their limits to meet these demands. This, of course, has encouraged 75.5% of the hospitals across the country to expand their home health services.[4]

A survey of chief executive officers (CEOs) by Kurt Salmon Associates, Inc., in 1985 found that 85% felt that a drop of up to 20%

from 1984-level inpatient days could be expected during the next few years. This expectation of shrinkage in inpatient days has provided considerable incentive for hospitals to expand services in several areas, in addition to increasing home-health services. It was reported that 75.1% are planning to expand outpatient surgery (in-house), while 61.4% are increasing or adding wellness and health promotion programs and outpatient diagnosis centers (in-house). Cardiac rehabilitation units are being increased by 44%, oncology services by 41.4%, industrial medicine services by 40.8%, and women's medical services and programs by 40.2%.

These data give nurses clear evidence that there are new worlds to conquer, new horizons to approach, and new, exciting roles to assume as the health care industry moves through its current transition into a new age of redefined health care services and new modes of patient care delivery.

Demographic trends: Population shifts.
Hand-in-hand with these economic stresses, the U.S. population is experiencing some rather dramatic alterations. For one, the increase in life expectancy together with the aging of the baby-boomers is resulting in a "senior-boom" of major proportions. By the year 2000, 50% of all health care expenses will be related to the care and treatment of people aged 65 or older. Those over age 75, who now constitute 38% of the senior population, will account for 45% while those over 85 will constitute 12%, hitting a peak of 4 million by the end of the century.[5]

Ken Dychtwald, psychologist and gerontologist, asserts that "we are presently witnessing the birth of a powerful 'gerontocracy'; larger, healthier, better educated, more politically savvy, and more economically secure than any previous generation of elders anywhere."[6] As a consequence, signs of changes are evident throughout the culture, including, for example:

• shifts of health care focus from childhood diseases to age-related diseases, with emphasis on prevention and life extension;
• growing concern for Medicare and Social Security;
• increased awareness of mid-life crises;
• emergence of older media stars and public heroes;
• increased emphasis on leisure and recreation for the mature consumer.

These areas give nurses exceptional opportunities for expanding their roles, their contributions, and entrepreneurial expertise if they are so inclined. In 1980 the over-55 households accounted for more than 80% of all savings in the country and spent 30% of all discretionary money — nearly that of the under-34 crowd,[7] making it quite clear that a sizable market is available to be tapped.

In conjunction with this trend, a recent report on life care centers describes explosive growth that will continue over the next few years at least.[8] Data from a study conducted by Laventhol & Horwath indicate a need for more than 2,000 new life care facilities, each with a self- contained nursing facility providing nursing care at a prescribed package rate for apartment dwellers when they need it.[9]

Shifts in trends. Another interesting aspect of shifting trends can be seen in the increased numbers of women in the job market, the proportion of families headed by women, the expansion of career options for women, and an even more extraordinary change — the increased number of women medical students. This phenomenon will have a major impact on the health care industry in the next two decades.

Because women as guardians of their families' health tend to make major decisions about health care, women's medicine is now seen as an important new field, a field to which nurses are clearly the heirs apparent. Many hospitals, particularly those in the 200-

to 400-bed category, are instituting programs developed, marketed, and managed by enterprising nurses. Approximately 40.2% of all hospitals are planning to expand soon into women's medicine.[10]

Coincident with this change is the dramatic increase in enrollment of females in medical school, a phenomenon being branded the feminization of health care. This promises to alter the work environment for nurses and may result in a qualitative shift in the relationship between doctors and nurses. It may well be that our dream of a collaborative partnership between the two professionals will result from this extension in women's career options.

Health care marketers are eyeing a growing trend toward fitness and health promotion as a source of revenue. Wellness programs are springing up all over the country, especially in the Midwest; 34% of midwestern hospitals, 32% of northwestern hospitals, and 24% of those in the West report wellness programs.[11] Many more (21% overall) are planning them, suggesting still another opportunity for nursing entrepreneurship.

Concurrent with this trend in health care marketing is a focus on occupational health programs, now offered by 31% of U.S. hospitals. Presumably employers are finding a favorable trade-off between the cost of these programs and savings achieved through fewer absences due to illness, fewer job-related accidents, lower insurance premiums, and increased productivity. A twelve-month projection indicated a 21% increase in these programs overall and an increase of as much as 32% in the smaller (100-199 bed) hospitals.[12]

Alternate care. Any number of competitive alternatives to hospitals are springing up, including surgicenters, urgent care centers, HMOs, outpatient rehabilitation centers, skilled nursing facilities, hospices, and outpatient dialysis centers. Sleep disorder, eating disorder, pain control, and birthing centers top the list of new

and promising opportunities for nurses, nurse practitioners, nurse entrepreneurs, and health care educators to ply their trade, not to mention the unlimited opportunities for nurse managers and executives who would like to branch out in new directions. In fact, one of the exciting aspects of today's changing health care climate is the wide variety of managerial opportunities to be developing during the nineties. As Leah Curtin declares, "Many of the (new) roles haven't been invented yet. We, you and I, will have the opportunity to invent them. What an *interesting* time to be a nurse — and what a *fantastic* time to be a nurse in a leadership position."[13]

Changing roles. An interesting study recently performed by Wett Associates, Oakbrook, Illinois, disclosed that nurses are quite happy in the executive role. It indicated that "nurses are being allowed to manage; they believe they are making a difference to the well-being of patients, staff, and their institutions and that their jobs offer variety."[14]

In line with recommendations by the 1983 National Commission on Nursing (NCN) that hospitals give nurses greater roles in policy making, managing nursing practice, and setting quality standards, Connie Curran, vicepresident for nursing, American Hospital Association (AHA), points out that nurse executives are no longer considered just department managers but are among the top hospital executives. In fact her own newly created position is highly indicative of the changing role of the nurse executive in hospital policy making.

Actually it comes as no surprise that nurses do well as executives and seem so satisfied in their work. Considering the primary responsibilities that nurses have shouldered for so long, what do nurses do better than solve problems and manage people?

Changing roles means changing issues. The hottest issues ahead of us in the coming decade will be the two-tiered nursing system and peer review. These derived, of course, primarily from alternative-site care, emphasized by prognosticators as important to nursing's future, such as home health care and occupational health care. Certainly peer review is essential to maintain the quality of care we have come to expect. The desirability of two-tiered licensure may be questionable, although with today's technological advances and the greater independence and responsibility inherent in the changing health care climate, two-tiered licensure seems inevitable. Moreover, it may be necessary to include graduate requirements for some clinical applications. The role of nurses is no longer simplistic, and as it becomes increasingly complex so will requirements and procedures for licensure.

In fact, AHA's cabinet on nursing research recently stated that graduate education will be essential to prepare specialized practitioners for technologically complex care of the critically ill. At the same time, they stated that nursing will continue to experience an accelerated rate of change in clinical therapeutics and that nurses will need specialized knowledge to care for the critically ill, acutely ill, and chronically ill in technologically sophisticated treatment centers.

Still another set of issues coming to the fore in the next decade will be the role of nurses as patient advocates and the participation of nurses on ethics committees concerned with the patient's right to die, the question of a "duty-to-die," euthanasia, bioengineering, and robotics. It has been suggested that nurses will fill the gap between technology and the consumer and that robots will take over technical tasks. In fact there are currently available for home care robots that understand speech, can take and deliver messages, dial a number, and sense body heat; soon robots will be able to perform other monitoring tasks such as reading heartbeats and determining skin tone.[15]

Nursing's role. Now as never before in the history of our profession, nurses have virtual carte blanche to develop new roles and define their own future. Nurses can either sit back passively and become victims of technology and economics or can be active in seizing opportunities to design the future according to particular values, concerns, and interests.

What are the obstacles to this utopian dream? Can nurses control the forces that seem to be relentlessly reshaping our world? In which direction should nurses exert their influence? These and other such questions will be examined repeatedly during the coming decade. Some will answer themselves; some will cause uncertainty for a time; some will test nurses' mettle and push them to the limits of their creativity and ingenuity. One thing is certain, nurses will grow stronger and wiser from it all and will become the inspired leaders of tomorrow. Furthermore, nurses have an obligation to do so. Leadership today is floundering, unable to determine the proper course to follow or control the forces influencing that course. Health care is in danger of falling prey to the Madison Avenue approach, which may or may not create the world we desire. Its track record in other industries has not been that good.

Overcoming obstacles. One obstacle nurses have to overcome, if courage and leadership are to emerge, is a history of submissiveness and deference to authority figures, especially those that are male. We must learn "to reach for and obtain power, authority, and control over (our) own destiny."[16] Another obstacle was pointed out so clearly in a recent article in *Nursing Outlook* that states: "Nurses must change society's sexist perceptions of Nursing. Seeking a change will require nurses to alter *their own perception* that it is immoral to care for oneself or to further one's own interests."[17] Also, the stereotype of the "intellectual (male) physician and the nurturing (non-intellectual) nurse (female) persists"[18] and must be eradicated. The stereotype of nurses as doing "women's work" or as domestic "housekeepers for the sick" must be superseded by the new model of clinical expert, knowledge-based professional practitioner, and aggressive business manager, if nurses are to fulfill their potential. Only then can nurses be at the forefront, the veritable cutting edge of change, within the framework of a modernized, 21st century health care system.

Effecting change. Nurses can effect positive change in the delivery of health care in a number of ways:

• Nurses can conduct research to determine consumer needs and design services to meet those needs.

• Nurses must play a major role in developing programs, coordinating interdisciplinary efforts to provide services. They must be instrumental in making these effective.

• Nurses must gain the authority and flexibility to maximize use of resources, efficiency, and cost containment.

• Nurses must realize and fully capitalize on their position as public relations representatives for their institutions.

• Nurse managers must become marketing directors, both inside and outside their institutions.

• Nurses can use community education programs and home care services to market nursing services.

• Nurses must add business knowledge to their clinical skills.

• Nurses should remember at all times that high quality care gives a competitive edge.[19]

Future-speak

At a recent seminar in Los Angeles entitled "Nursing 2020," various futuristic scenarios were discussed. They were nicknamed (1) "Earth to Nurse," high-tech health in space, (2) "SuperNurse," competition and conglomerate, (3) "Boss Nurse," the disciplined

society and reregulation, and (4) "Barefoot Nurse," the wellness surge. These are fun to speculate about but are probably far too limited in scope. Present trends indicate that health care and specifically nursing in the 21st century will be far more highly differentiated than even this. Nursing will be "high-tech" in acute care facilities, surgicenters, home health care, and other areas not dreamed of yet. The major trend will be toward greater independence in practice, greater authority and control, more public/community contact, and increased specialization. Many new titles or license designations may develop in keeping with these specialties. The geriatric nurse may be the most prevalent and widely needed resource for available health care services. If that is the case, appropriate educational support must be planned now before the crisis hits. Certainly the occupational health practitioner and wellness eduator are here to stay and will play an increasingly important role in tomorrow's society.

Some of the trends identified during the seminar included:

• Reduction of size and function of the hospital, which would serve basically as an ICU for inpatient services;

• More family responsibility in caring for their sick and especially for the elderly;

• A strong need for nurses to train patients in self-care and caregiving;

• Deinstitutionalization and more home care, especially among the elderly;

• Acceptance and legalization of euthanasia.

These are challenging times, times that try souls but in which nurses will thrive. Nurses who do not seize opportunities as they develop have no one but themselves to blame. As Nancy Higgerson, president of the Association of Nurse Executives stated, "Although nurses now are under a phenomenal amount of stress, it is also a time of tremendous opportunity. There has never been a more exciting time for nursing practice."[20] Stress is often the prelude to major strides forward in any endeavor. Nurses working together can ensure that adversity will again serve that noble purpose.

REFERENCES

1. "Many CEOs Say U.S. Faces Health Care Crisis: Survey." *Hospitals* 59 (November 1, 1985): 36-37.

2. *CHA Insights* 9 (1986).

3. *Hospitals* 59 (June 16, 1985): 70.

4. *Hospitals* 59 (December 16, 1985).

5. *Health: United States*. 1978, Washington, D.C.: U.S. Department of Health and Human Services, 1978, p. 148.

6. Dychtwald, K. "The Senior Boom." *Hospital Forum* 28 (May-June, 1985): 64.

7. Ibid.

8. "Life Care Industry Grows Despite Costs." (December 1, 1985): 95.

9. Ibid.

10. Moore, W.B. "CEO's Plan Resource Shift for 1986." *Hospital* 59 (December 16, 1985): 69.

11. "Occupational Health, Wellness Plans Grow." *Modern Health Care* 15 (December 20, 1985): 50.

12. Ibid.

13. Curtin, L. "Nursing in the Year 2000." *Nursing Management* 17, no. 6 (1986):8.

14. Gallivan, M. "Nurse Executives Surprisingly Happy in their New Roles." *Hospitals* 60 (April 5, 1986):92.

15. *Outbreak* (January-February 1986): 8.

16. Chaska, N.L. *The Nursing Profession: Views through the Mist.* New York: McGraw-Hill, 1977, p. 368.

17. Vance, C., et al. "An Uneasy Alliance: Nursing and the Women's Movement." *Nursing Outlook* 33 (November-December 1985): 282.

18. Ibid., 283.

19. Spitzer, R. "The Nurse as Product-line Manager." American Hospital Association Seminar, Boston, May 19-20, 1986.

20. Gallivan, M. "Nurse Burnout: A Cooling Issue." *Hospitals* 60 (March 5, 1986): 95.

CHAPTER THREE

Entry into practice

MEMBERS OF THE nursing community have long been trying to agree on the educational requirements for a professional nurse. Florence Nightingale initiated nursing training in schools associated with but not controlled by hospitals. The Nightingale model served for the first schools of nursing in the United States. Unfortunately, the standards of educational practice in the English programs were not maintained as nursing schools proliferated in large and small hospitals across America. Nonetheless, the hospital-based diploma program for nurses became the norm. Not until the 1940s did baccalaureate programs expand, and not until the 1950s were associate degree courses developed in community colleges.

The three levels of entry into nursing have created confusion among the members of the profession and in the agencies where nurses practice and are employed. This confusion led to the ANA's decree in 1965 that the entry level into professional nursing should be the bachelor's degree. The 1965 policy statement had little effect; therefore, the ANA reaffirmed the position in 1985. Major nursing organizations supported the ANA, and in 1987 the ANA further defined professional and technical nursing practice in *The Scope of Nursing Practice*.

One problem with the 1965 ANA position was that its policy was embraced before a plan of implementation had been devised. One of the major controversial issues currently being debated is which level of nursing will continue to use the title "Registered Nurse" and its initials (RN). Another issue is whether one li-

censing examination can be used for bachelor's, associate, and diploma graduates or whether two are needed — one for bachelor's graduates and another for associate degree and diploma graduates. Complicating the issue is that licensure changes will have to be initiated in each state and territory. One state, North Dakota, has instituted such action.

Schlotfeldt, in "Resolution of Issues: An Imperative for Creating Nursing's Future," takes the stance that the current registration procedure for nurses should be left unchanged. She suggests initiating new nurse practice acts to license professional nurses. Schlotfeldt also expresses her concern that political control of nursing has thwarted and defeated efforts to establish the nursing baccalaureate degree as the minimum credential for entry into registered nurse practice.

If no nurse would agree to teach at less than the baccalaureate level, says Christman in "A View to the Future," the nursing profession could have entry at the baccalaureate level immediately. Furthermore, he states, to function effectively in the future, all nurses will need to have clinical doctorate degrees — by age 26! — in order to begin their practice at the same age as other doctorate-degreed professionals.

"An Analysis of Entry Into Practice Arguments," by Warner, et al., is the report of a study analyzing the North Dakota experience in standardizing requirements for two levels of entry into nursing practice. Acknowledging the dilemma that arises when two opposing points of view are both supported by valid arguments, these authors conclude that nursing education and nursing licensure are separate issues and should be dealt with separately.

The suggestion by Roberts that nurses should qualify for a series of licenses, similar to the way airline pilots are qualified, is a feature of "Nurses for the Future: The Yo-Yo Ride," which discusses a number of issues and gives support to preparation of nurse specialists at the baccalaureate level. Also in this article, Lynaugh points out that whenever entry into practice issues are discussed, cost seems to be the main consideration rather than the pursuit of solutions to the problems.

Resolution of issues: An imperative for creating nursing's future

ROZELLA M. SCHLOTFELDT, PhD, FAAN

Issues in nursing education and its control

PROGRAMS OF TECHNICAL education are, by definition and in concept, different from programs of professional education. They differ in qualifications required of applicants to programs of study, in the subject matter of curriculums and their organization, and in the rigor, difficulty, and length of time consumed by preservice, basic preparation. They further differ in the socialization processes through which graduates are prepared for remarkably different types of work and responsibilities, and in the qualifications of faculty members who socialize the trainees.

Technicians are required to partake of minimal general education, and their technical preparation is task oriented, requiring mastery of scientific knowledge sufficient to rationalize the tasks that graduates are prepared to execute, upon assignment by and with surveillance of professionals in their respective occupational fields. Technicians are not independent, autonomous practitioners.

Applicants to professional schools are typically broadly educated through college level, liberalizing education in the several fields of human knowledge prior to their seeking professional preparation. They are mature learners, judged to be capable of mastery of vast amounts of professional knowledge and capable of developing attitudes and interests required of those who devote their lives to service, continuous learning, and professional careers. They are expected to become competent, self-confident practitioners and to use their professional knowledge and skills selectively, creatively, wisely, ethically, and humanely and with the exercise of exquisite judgment. They are fully accountable, not only for their own practices but also for all practices accomplished by those assisting personnel to whom they delegate the performance of technical tasks.

Unfortunately for nursing, and for those served by nurses, unresolved issues (some largely political) have prevented nursing from clearly differentiating its professionals from their technical assistants, the preservice programs that prepare those kinds of practitioners, and the credentialing systems that grant them the privilege to practice.

Similar to other human service endeavors, nursing emerged to professional status as a consequence of two factors: 1) society's recognition of the essential, consequential nature of professional nursing services provided for all members of society at particular times in their lives; and 2) nursing leaders' recognition of the need for professionals to have preservice preparation that qualifies them as independently accountable practitioners who have mastered a distinctive body of professional knowledge, skills, and values. Despite the facts, nursing remains essentially an other-directed and controlled occupation, rather than a self-directed profession. The direction and control of basic nursing education come primarily from political, not professional sources.

Nursing leaders' efforts to upgrade the nature and quality of preservice education for practitioners and to insure reasonable comparability in the preparation of nurses began in the late 1800s and early 1900s.[1] That was a time when nursing was a relatively new occupation and when the number of schools was growing at a phenomenal pace. Control of nursing education by an appropriate society of qualified professionals was then either not an option or deemed to be impossible by early leaders in the field. The compromise they adopted was likely seen as the only effective control available; they opted to place control of all of nursing, including nursing education, within the state regulatory boards, beginning in 1903.[2] It has remained in the political arena, subject to the vagaries of politics internal and external to nursing ever since. The issue is: Will nursing leaders active in the period just prior to the beginning of the 21st century continue to relegate control of basic education of professionals to governmental appointees who are subject to political pressures, or will nursing leaders act to insure that basic nursing education will be guided and controlled by qualified professionals within the field of nursing?

There can be no question that a crucial ingredient for preparing professionals is identification of a body of knowledge that is fundamental to professional practice and about which there is agreement by a cadre of qualified professionals. However, as yet there is no consensus among qualified professionals in nursing concerning the *subject matter* that should represent the intellectual armamentarium of professionals called nurses, although the recently published final report of a study to establish essentials of education of professionals in the field is a monumental step in that direction.[3]

Because the work of professionals is consequential, it is also expected to be beneficial. Because it also holds potential for being harmful, if attempted by ill-prepared, incompetent, or impaired practitioners, the privilege of professional practice is typically restricted to those who hold valid, current licenses and is denied to all others. Licenses are granted by agents of state government, namely state regulatory boards whose members typically ad-

minister the license procedure and monitor and control the practices of licensed professionals. The license examinations are typically prescribed by representatives of designated professional societies, based on the assumption that only qualified professionals have the necessary expertise to determine the subject matter that must be mastered by those who seek to enter professional practice. The official credentialing procedure for registered nurses differs remarkably from the norm.

Nurses are currently registered, not licensed, and the examination (when passed) permits candidates to enter undifferentiated registered nursing practice. The registration examination used by the several state regulatory boards has been judged to be a valid test of current nursing practice.[4] A relatively high percentage of that practice is accomplished by registered nurses graduated from preservice programs that require a minimum of two years of post-secondary school study, that generally considered to be technical training. The issue is: Will corporate nursing continue to settle for undifferentiated, registration of nursing personnel, or will professionals act to establish a license procedure for its clearly identified professionals?

Nursing, with few exceptions, has appropriately placed the preparation of its specialists within the nation's system of graduate education. Although some recent legislation has broadened political control over nursing (to include "advanced" nursing in a few states), those changes are generally considered to be ill-advised. There is currently agreement that control of specialty preparation and certification of specialists are responsibilities of the profession.[5] There is, however, little agreement concerning what nursing's specialties are, the preparation that is appropriate for each specialty, and the knowledge and skills that particular kinds of specialists should demonstrate.[6]

In summary, major issues in nursing education relate to the proper identification, preparation, credentialing, and control of professionals, as contrasted with professionals' assisting personnel and the role of the profession in identifying and keeping current the body of knowledge that is fundamental to generalized practice of professional nursing and that which is fundamental to each of nursing's recognized specialties. Resolution of those issues and others previously identified is an imperative for those nursing leaders who seek to create a nursing future appropriate for the 21st century.

Creating the future

...The mission of professionals in nursing is to appraise and to optimize the health status, health assets, and health potential of human beings and to safeguard human dignity during their dependent states and at the time of death. That statement is succinct, properly focused, and establishes nursing's enduring, stable goal. It anticipates changes in means to attain that goal that logically derive from advances in knowledge, the development of new technologies, and the design of new nursing strategies. Such a mission statement would provide an appropriate definition of nursing to propose for new nursing practice acts in states that develop a license procedure (in contrast to registration) for qualified professionals in the field.

Recent efforts to change existing nurse practice acts in order to establish the baccalaureate in nursing as the minimal credential for entry into registered nursing practice have often been thwarted and sometimes defeated in the political arena. It is proposed here that consideration be given to a different approach.

The current registration procedure for nurses should be left unchanged. New nursing practice acts that would license professionals should be established. Such a change would require that (a) designated society(ies) of qualified professionals would need to take responsibility for identification and structure of the subject matter that comprises the professional knowledge that is fundamental to generalized professional nursing practice. A licensing examination valid for testing professionals could then be made available to state boards for testing candidates graduated from schools of professional nursing and holding the minimal academic credential acceptable to the profession (currently, the BSN). The profession would need to decide whether currently registered nurses who hold baccalaureate and higher degrees in nursing would be eligible to take the licensing examination, or to be "grandfathered" as licensed professional nurses.

The proposed change holds promise of removing professional nursing education from the vagaries of political control. It poses no threat to the status of currently registered nurses nor to those who henceforth would earn credentials that now qualify them to become registered nurses. It eliminates the threat of "grandfathering" unqualified practitioners as professionals and thus fulfills the primary mandate of credentialling, namely that of protecting the public. State regulatory boards would obviously continue to hold responsibility for administering the license and registration examinations and for monitoring and controlling nursing practice. A crucial ingredient for implementing the proposal is identification of a professional agency or society comprised of qualified generalist and specialist practitioners, educators, administrators, investigators, theorists, and testing experts who, in the aggregate, have the necessary talent, knowledge, and skills to develop and keep current forms of tests that are valid for professionals in nursing. Identification, structure, and agreement about the body of knowledge that is fundamental to generalized nursing practice is a prior agenda item.

Resolution of issues concerning nursing's specialities could be a simple matter once agreement is reached concerning the professional's body of basic knowledge. Based upon the assumption that newly developed specialities are legitimate when specialists must have command of knowledge and skills that surpass those had by generalists, two criteria are proposed: 1) each specialty must be demonstrated to require mastery of knowledge that is more extensive and more narrowly focused than is general nursing knowledge and require skills that are more complex; and 2) each specialty must be demonstrated to require mastery of knowledge and skills that are different from those required for all other nursing specialties.

Investigators of the future will continue to be prepared through programs of doctoral and post-doctoral study, primarily in nursing, but also in relevant disciplines. Nursing will always have need for well-prepared basic and clinical scientists, philosophers, historiographers, educators, and administrators. Upon them will fall responsibility for continuing to advance knowledge relevant to improving all practices in the field.

It is impossible to make precise estimates of what the future holds. Leaders in nursing have experienced a long and difficult struggle to fulfill generally accepted criteria for the profession many nurses have long claimed nursing to be. There is likely now a critical mass of able, well-educated, dedicated, and determined leaders who have the capacity to envision the future that nursing can have, along with strategies necessary for its creation. Surely the resolution of long-standing issues will permit the creation of a brilliant nursing future that is essential to the well-being of all human beings.

REFERENCES

1. Nutting MA: The preliminary education of nurses. Am J Nurs 1:416-424, 1900

2. Proceedings of the Sixth Annual Convention 1903. Am J Nurs 3:871-873, 1902-1903

3. American Association of Colleges of Nursing: Essentials of College and University Education for Professional Nursing. Washington, D.C., AACN, 1986

4. Dvorak E, Kane M, Laskevich L, et al: The National Council Licensure Examination for Registered Nurses. Chicago, Chicago Review Press, 1985

5. Liaison forum seeks ways to promote action. The American Nurse Jan 1987, p 8

6. Williamson J: Masters education: a need for nomenclature. Image: The Journal of Nursing Scholarship 16:99-101,1983

A view to the future

LUTHER P. CHRISTMAN, RN, PhD, FAAN

DESCRIBING THE FUTURE in a time of intense, widespread and massive change is as difficult as grasping a handful of fog. Further, it is likely that the predictions of changes and developments will be understated to a considerable degree. It is, nonetheless, the province of both the sage and the fool, and only time distinguishes one from the other.

Each profession and discipline has followed an historical behavior pattern in its responses to change in the external and internal environments. The stronger professions have had more proactive styles in making efforts to shape change. The weaker follow accommodation patterns that are more reactive and less imaginative.

Much has been written about change. From generalists such as Toffler and Naisbitt to more specific foreseers of the future, such as Lesse, each in his own way stirs the imagination, creates a state of intellectual excitement and almost forces each reader to do a self-inventory of personal abilities to cope with highly unpredictable and uncontrollable changes.[1-3]

It is futile to dwell on the missed opportunities that nurses spurned when each of the several insightful studies was conducted on the profession.[4-8] Inactive and passive resistance to the alerting signals for accommodation to general professional norms indigenous to American society at the time of each study was a cue to how strongly nurses resist proactive change. Contrast this to the way the leaders in the medical profession responded to the Flexner report and how effectively they steered a proactive course.[9] A similar comment can be made about the teaching profession. At a time when university-educated teachers were in a minority, their leaders directed what was, at that time, a dramatic change: a baccalaureate degree as the entry level for a qualified teacher. Their opposition included school teachers who were normal school graduates, administrators and faculties of normal schools, many school board members and school superintendents who believed they would be unable to staff the schools, and many taxpayers who believed teachers' salaries would become unaffordable. Despite opposition of this magnitude, the change was made. In both instances, society benefited by the change. Also, both groups increased their social stature.

To resist changes that ultimately benefit society may border on the unethical. The rapid expansion of science makes it possible for all the clinical professions to provide sophisticated care with more certainty. However, this means that each group must consistently upgrade the basic education of its respective constituency. This rationale leads to the conclusion that teaching in a program that is below the university level borders on unethical practice. No one can use knowledge he or she does not have. Nursing education programs that prepare students at less than the university level are depriving patients of the full benefit of science. This appears to be a deliberate action. It raises ethical questions. If this premise is substantive and true, it is unethical to recruit students into programs of less strength than those of other clinical professions. The nursing profession could have entry at the baccalaureate level immediately if no nurse would teach at less than that level.

Professional responsibility requires that one put the welfare of the group above oneself. How can nurses keep pace with other care providers unencumbered by this artificially created barrier? Science and technology will not wait for us to use them. Nonusers will be bypassed. The ability of nurses to serve patients is diluted by the ratio of the less well prepared to the more fully prepared. The ethics of preserving an obsolete system will one day be questioned; who will accept responsibility?

Although no one has fully analyzed the history of the profession, it may show that the faculty of each specific era have been the critical deterrent to change. Those in schools targeted for closing may have had more interest in keeping their faculty roles than in seeing patients better served. When a graduate degree becomes the mandated entry level, one can predict rear-guard skirmishing by those who are unqualified.

A professional stance is highly dependent on the cohesion of its members. Taking advantage of opportunity requires solidarity of purpose. A startling example of inability to rally around an opportunity is evident in the aborted attempt to provide a center for nurses in Indianapolis. The combined efforts of a private foundation, the Indianapolis Chamber of Commerce, and the city government to construct a center that would house all the nursing organizations in the country at no cost to nurses went awry because of the lack of commonality of purpose among nurses. An unwillingness to set aside individual and petty self-interests for the good of the profession was clearly evident. The public goodwill and social benefit of such a center may have been lost forever. Furthermore, the potential catalytic effect of such a center for speeding the development of the profession was negated.

What can nurses expect of the future? Science and technology will drive the world of work. In all likelihood, more changes in clinical practice will occur in the next two decades than in all of previous history. The clinical model of applied science as the central motif will be the driving force to achieve competence in practice. The various conceptual models of nursing practice will undergo the same erosion as the Freudian model. The utility of applied science cannot be denied. Superficial constraints cannot be imposed for very long; imagination cannot be constrained. The rigorous use of the methods of science will dominate and prevail. Thinking and behaving in this fashion will become fully intertwined. The harnessing of artificial intelligence through computer-assisted care and other technology will accelerate. Thus, the exploration and insightful use of the basic sciences will be the keystone of all scholarly enterprise. Patient care programs not only will be planned with exquisite precision but also will be enhanced by the ability of every clinician to search rapidly through the whole network of care protocols in the country (or the world) for the newest techniques in the clinical management of patients with any particular diagnosis.

To function effectively in this milieu, a clinical doctorate will be the required minimal level for all practitioners. Nurses will learn that rich clinical preparation is the one means of professional survival. They will emulate the other powerful professions by obtaining professional rather than academic doctorates. The chief way of using sophisticated artificial intelligence will be asking the right questions. The clinical doctorate has the most potential to provide the scientific underpinnings needed to function in this fashion.

Many nurses will find it useful to obtain, in addition to the clinical doctorate, a doctorate in a field of basic science closely tied to specialty practice. Both the DNSc-PhD and the MD-PhD training will be commonplace. It will be one way of staving off obsolescence. This strong preparation will raise the management of patient care to previously unachieved heights. The use of this dyad as the keystone for care and clinical research will enable both nurses and physicians to stay on the cutting edge of the new and innovative.

Imagination precedes doing. Those who think big do big things and those who think in a constrained way do small things. All the clinical professions will integrate the subrole functions of care, education, and research into one holistic professional role. This development will help reduce the divisiveness in nursing. Cost-effectiveness also will emerge as a byproduct of competence. Thus, it can be predicted that all nursing education will occur in universities. The number of nursing schools will be reduced drastically and probably will be limited to those in sophisticated, vertically integrated medical centers. These settings will become centers of excellence in nursing.

The introduction of computer-assisted patient care, robots, telecommunications and other technology will reduce the demand for health care professionals of all types. Competition for career opportunities will be keen. Only outstanding clinicians will be secure. The technology used to care for patients will be programmed to screen and evaluate the competence of providers. Each person's clinical ability will be on record and, hence, easily evaluated. Those who cannot outlast this form of scrutiny may not survive. The elimination of the retirement age in combination with much better health maintenance will substantially prolong the work life of each person. The need for replacements will be reduced.

Every prognosticator envisions many fewer hospital beds. Much patient care will be outside the hospital. The various competitive forms of out-of-hospital care will require considerable competence on the part of all the staff for these designs of care to stay viable. Most of the clinical effort will be focused on illness prevention and health maintenance. Health maintenance concepts will be incorpo-

rated in curricula from kindergarten through college. Many will use their personal computers to identify the latest in scientific knowledge. Thus, everyone will be able to collaborate intelligently with clinicians. Illness will evidence itself primarily as a byproduct of genetic loading, accident or personal neglect. Research investigators will find solutions for everything from schizophrenia to coryza.

Self-governance of a high order will embrace responsibility and accountability for all scientific, clinical, ethical and humanistic events. Separate medical and nursing staff self-governing organizations will be merged into one self-governing professional staff. If any semblance of the present professional ratio persists into the future, nurses will be the most numerous members of the staff. This provides an interesting but awesome responsibility as a chief component of assuring the quality of care. The full and useful exploitation of the clinical model — not the medical or nursing models — will be in place. Close collaboration rather than territoriality will be the operating design.

The profession will become fully democratized in its composition. Instead of remaining 90 percent white female, nurses will emulate the other major professions in vigorously recruiting the best talent. No one sector of society holds monopolies on intelligence, imagination or sensitivity. Men and nonwhite women will have to be recruited constantly to ensure that the nursing profession obtains its fair share of desirable candidates. A more democratic constituency that reflects the composition of society will provide easier articulation, both with patients and with the other professions.

Now is not the time for posturing, haranguing, stereotyping or blaming others. The issue is clear cut. Do nurses want mediocrity or a place on the influence scale similar to the powerful professions? Many changes in attitude and structure are necessary if nurses aspire to the latter. Knowledge is a free marketplace available to all who can pay the price in time and money. Everyone can partake of the storehouse to the degree each desires and can afford. Perhaps there would be more unity among nurses if they all had earned doctorates. No one is preventing nurses from reaching this stage of development except themselves.

The future is with the young. They have the potential for achieving the ultimate if they are strongly encouraged to have their clinical doctorate by about age 26. Thus, they will be starting as peers with those obtaining professional doctorates in other fields. Their socialization into the profession will be dramatically different. When a large number attain this level of competence at an early age, the very ethos of the profession will change. The previous unachievable will become possible. Nurses will contribute in more visible and fruitful ways to breakthroughs in health care. Who knows, some may even become Nobel laureates.

REFERENCES

1. Toffler, A. *Future Shock.* New York, Random House, 1970.

2. Naisbitt, J. *Megatrends: Ten New Directions Transforming Our Lives.* 6th ed. New York, Warner Books, 1983.

3. Lesse, S. *The Future of the Health Sciences: Anticipating Tomorrow.* New York, Irvington Publishers, 1981.

4. Committee for the Study of Nursing Education, Josephine Goldmark, secretary. *Nursing and Nursing Education in the United States.* New York, The Macmillan Co., 1923.

5. Brown, E.L. *Nursing for the Future: A Report Prepared for the National Nursing Council.* New York, Russell Sage Foundation, 1948.

6. Committee on the Function of Nursing. *A Program for the Nursing Profession.* New York, The Macmillian Co., 1949.

7. Bridgman, M. *Collegiate Education for Nursing.* New York, Russell Sage Foundation, 1953.

8. National Commission for the Study of Nursing and Nursing Education, J.P. Lysaught, director. *An Abstract for Action.* New York, McGraw-Hill Book Co., 1970.

9. Flexner, A. *Medical Education in the United States and Canada: A Report to the Carnegie Foundation for the Advancement of Teaching.* New York, The Foundation, 1910.

An analysis of entry into practice arguments

SANDRA L. WARNER, RN, PhD, CS; M. CANDICE ROSS, RN, PhD; LORI CLARK, RN, BSN

A DILEMMA EXISTS when opposing views about an issue are both supported by valid arguments. Entry into nursing practice qualifies as a dilemma because it is an emotionally charged issue with political, social, economic and professional ramifications (Glick, 1985; Maraldo & Solomon, 1987; Stevens, 1985; Waters, 1986). Some leaders feel that education and licensing will be the most critical issues in nursing over the next few years (Mallison, 1984), while others, according to Maraldo & Solomon, feel that it is unwise to focus on a single issue to the exclusion of current marketplace opportunities or the nursing shortage. Whichever, the entry issue is too important to ignore; survival of nursing depends on the quality of its practice, which in turn depends on the quality of its educational underpinnings.

History and significance

Confusion about titles and nursing education abounds. Traditionally, graduates from a community college with a two-year Associate Degree program, from a hospital with a three-year diploma program, and from a university with a four-year baccalaureate degree program may obtain by successful examination the title, "Registered Nurse" (R.N.).

Nontraditional ways to attain the title of R.N. are relatively recent innovations in nursing education. The New York Regents External Degree Program (REDP), established in 1972, was expanded in 1976 to include baccalaureate as well as associate degree candidates. Upon successful completion of specific college-level tests and performance examinations, graduates sit for the R.N. licensing examina-

tion (Grippando, 1986). The doctor of nursing (N.D.) degree, similar to the doctor of medicine (M.D.) was established in 1979 at Case Western. The Research College of Nursing in Kansas City, Missouri, established the first hospital-based baccalaureate program in 1980. Nursing programs designed for college graduates exist at Yale, Pace, the University of Tennessee at Knoxville and Massachusetts General Hospital Institute of the Health Professions. Each program requires a college degree for admission; education occurs at the master's level, and graduates are able to sit for State Board Examinations although at different stages in the educational process (Ellis & Hartley, 1988; Wright, 1988).

In 1964 the American Nurses' Association (ANA) specified that baccalaureate education be required for entry into professional practice by 1985. In 1984, a more realistic time frame was adopted: 5 percent of the states by 1986, 15 percent by 1988, 50 percent by 1992 and 100 percent by 1995 (Hood, 1985). In 1985, the ANA urged the State Associations to establish (a) a baccalaureate in nursing as the minimum educational requirement for licensure to practice professional nursing and retain the title of R.N., and (b) an associate degree in nursing as the educational requirement for licensure to practice technical nursing (Lewis, 1985).

After weathering battles in the executive, legislative and judicial arenas, North Dakota became the first state to standardize educational requirements for two entry levels of practice. The process used to effect this change is chronicled by Wakefield-Fisher, Wright and Kraft (1986). Part of that process included open hearings where testimony related to the proposed changes in the Rules and Regulations was presented to the North Dakota Board of Nursing. An analysis of that testimony can provide useful information related to the entry issue.

The study
The purpose of this study was to analyze the North Dakota testimony and identify, define, categorize and tabulate the arguments by prevalence, direction and selected demographics. Answers to the following questions were sought: What kind of arguments inherent in the entry issue were presented to the North Dakota Board of Nursing to oppose or support the proposed changes in the Rules and Regulations? Who testified or wrote letters? Which arguments were favored by nurses representing different educational backgrounds, by those who lived out of state and by those living where specific nursing programs were located?

Findings
There were 479 persons from North Dakota and 107 persons from out of state who expressed their views on the entry issue. More than 80 percent of the sample were nurses, followed by clinical administrators, some of whom were nurses (7%), consumers (5%), college administrators (3%), and others (3%). The others included lawyers, schoolteachers, dieticians and social workers. The inherent threat within the proposed changes to the continuance of diploma programs and state reciprocity probably explains the fact that approximately 40 percent of the testimony came from cities where diploma schools were located and 20 percent came from out of state.

There were 6,346 arguments within the 586 coded testimonies used to influence the Board's decision. The nonissue category was dropped from the original taxonomy and further analysis because it was used only 35 times. Of the remaining 6,309 arguments,

2,427 (38.5%) favored the status quo and 3,882 (61.5%) favored change. After hearing the testimony, the North Dakota Board of Nursing voted to accept the proposed changes in the Rules and Regulations and thus effected new educational requirements for entry into nursing practice.

Lewin's (1951) theory would predict change if driving forces were stronger than were restraining forces. Assuming that the frequency of an argument were to equal its valence, then specific categories of arguments had stronger valences for driving forces (Societal/Professional Expectations; Dated and Time-related Evidence; Curricular Concerns and Marketability); while arguments from the Resources, Legal Processes and Evaluative Responses had stronger valence for restraining forces....

Out-of-state concerns. Out-of-state testimony favored restraining arguments in all categories except Curricular Concerns. Letters and Western Union Mailgrams, often with multiple signatures, represented the 107 testimonies. Representative restraining arguments from the Societal/Professional Expectations, Resources, and Dated and Time-related Evidence categories might be written as follows: The current licensure system ensures the safe practice of all nurses, including A.D. and diploma nurses. These graduates have proven to be effective care givers and have scored higher than have B.S. graduates on the NCLEX, a test of minimal standards. There is no evidence to prove the professional superiority of graduates from any program and no existing research to support the proposed change. This change would limit mobility of nurses, increase nursing shortages, close nursing schools and cause nurses to leave the profession. There will be great discertainty among states in terms of trade restrictions, reciprocity and supply limitations.

Arguments by educational preparation. Students, graduates or faculty members from a particular type of program were coded as A.D., B.S. or diploma. Nurses who did not identify their educational background were classified as R.N.s. Driving outnumbered restraining arguments in all categories for B.S. nurses, while A.D. and diploma nurses favored restraining arguments in the Resources and Legal Processes categories.

B.S. nurses. B.S. nurses supported the change and argued that standardized education housed in institutions of higher learning would benefit patients, the health care system, nursing students, nurses and the profession. They believe that this change is necessary because of the need for complex, independent clinical judgments associated with advanced technology, older and sicker patients, innovative practice settings, expanded roles and evolving practice autonomy. Typical arguments included:

1. Decreasing confusion among patients, physicians, other nurses and clinical administrators about titles and practice competencies, which in turn protects everyone including nurses from unsafe practice and potential liability.

2. Protecting future nursing students from the high cost of diploma education at the outset, which, if upgraded, would be compounded by the financial, emotional and time cost of repeating nontransferable credits.

3. Protecting future students from being less competitive and marketable (ads read "B.S. only") for the armed services, public and community health positions and read "B.S. preferred" for many other jobs).

4. Offering a curriculum with the depth and breadth to provide the knowledge and foster the skills (critical thinking, decision making and leadership ability) associated with practice concerns such as management, ethics, research, theory, advocacy and politics.

5. Promoting the professional status of nursing by upgrading to the minimal credential required by evry other health care profes-

sional, thereby giving the interdisciplinary recognition required for successful patient advocacy.

6. Decreasing the professional fragmentation and disunity caused when individual nurses put personal and specialized organizational concerns before professional concerns.

Diploma Nurses. Recurrent themes included:

1. Validation of worth as evidenced in their success on Licensing Examination, their clinical competencies and their presence at the bedside, so critical to the staffing of hospitals.

2. The lack of evidence to support the change or negate their professionalism.

3. The students' need for choice in educational pathways in lieu of individual constraints related to finances, time, family and geographical accessibility.

4. The closing of diploma schools in terms of potential community impact (financial, political and social).

5. The decreased supply of nurses in terms of graduates and reciprocal agreements between states.

6. The emotionalism and negative feelings (anger, fear, frustration) linked to displeasure with the hearings and mistrust in grandfathering.

7. The cost of educational upgrading in terms of time, money and stress.

Some diploma nurses/students and their parents felt angry, cheated and betrayed by these added costs and supported the change to protect parents and future students from similar experiences.

In spite of the legal protection of title and license for A.D. and diploma nurses (grandfathering), many nurses felt threatened because they perceived their professional status devalued and their educational preparation negated. It was difficult to admit that educational credentials often take precedence over title in the marketplace. There is no tangible target for the anger and frustration they feel when penalized today for valid decisions made yesterday. One nurse likened her diploma program to a dinosaur — the biggest and the best in its day but becoming extinct because it won't adapt to the needs of the student consumer, the marketplace and an ever-changing health care system. This analogy is supported by 1985 statistics reflecting the closure trend (13 states and 1 territory had no diploma schools; 5 states had 1 remaining diploma school; and 9 states had 2 left). It is the hospitals who chose to close these schools because of declining enrollments and increased maintenance costs.

A.D. Nurses. The A.D. arguments, which focused on titling concerns, were similar to those of diploma nurses. Both A.D. and diploma nurses objected to the technical rather than the professional label. Some did not wish the two-year graduate to be known as a licensed practical nurse and opposed North Dakota's choice to link the L.P.N. to the two-year associate degree, contrary to national trends. Some suggested that the nurse with an A.D. degree remain the professional nurse and let the four-year graduate invent some new title or require the master's degree as the professional entry degree. Recurrent themes in the A.D. arguments included:

1. The merits of college-based A.D. programs over hospital based diploma programs such as an emphasis on education rather than on service and the relative ease in upgrading credentials by transferable credits.

2. The merits of an A.D. education in light of the current trend in hospital hiring practices (i.e., replacing L.P.N.'s with an all-R.N. staff).

3. The need to explicate competencies to ensure proper utilization of A.D. graduates since titles are identical but educational preparation is not.

4. Emotional reactions (anger, fear, disgust) to threats or changes in marketability, career expectations, liability and professional or legal status.

5. The fact that many hospitals and service settings offer the A.D. nurse, who has invested less money and time in education by half, the same salary as the B.S. nurse.

Arguments by location of specific nursing programs. Again, the predominant driving arguments across all sites were from the Curricular Concerns, Societal/Professional Expectations and Marketability categories, while the predominant restraining arguments were from the Resources and Legal Processes categories. Site 2, cities with both B.S. and diploma programs, may best illustrate a statistical reflection of the issue. The ratio of driving over restraining arguments was approximately 3:1 (244/76) for Societal/Professional Expectations and 8:1 (82/10) for Marketability, and the ratio of restraining over driving arguments was approximately 9:1 for both Resources (192/83) and Legal Processes (222/26). These ratios reflect the proportionate valence for arguments on each side of the issue. Manpower needs, titling, grandfathering, dissatisfaction with the process of the hearings and reciprocity are very strong restraining forces, while the need to upgrade professional standards and educational requirements to better serve society (consumers, students, patients, hospitals, marketplace demands and the profession) and better meet the increased intellectual, technical and judgmental demands required by the expanded roles inherent in current nursing practice are strong driving forces.

Discussion

Documenting trends and/or changes in an issue will be facilitated if a consistent system of classification is used over time. For example, the nursing shortage was just emerging at the time of the hearings. The juxtapositioning between the current nursing shortage and the initial success of North Dakota in standardizing educational requirements for professional practice is fortunate for those wishing to maintain the status quo and unfortunate for proponents of change. This study provided a classification system and descriptive data related to the concerns inherent in the entry issue in the Fall of 1985.

Resolution of the entry issue will evolve through iterative interactions between the states, nursing organizations, societal needs and marketplace demands. It is obvious from the North Dakota testimony that certain components of the entry issue need to be resolved by the players on the force fields of individual states, and nationally acceptable parameters will evolve and become operative over time. For example, a nurse who passed the Ohio State Boards with a score of only 350 in 1962 could not practice in Michigan, a state with higher standards. It took a while for all states to standardize the passing score on state boards.

It is obvious from a national perspective that the largest group of practicing nurses comes from the A.D. pool. Questions such as how to license and title nurses who are educated at the technical and professional level, how to explicate the expected competencies of a technical and professional nurse, how to increase the upward educational mobility and how to maintain interstate reciprocity for nurses licensed and titled under present systems will be answered over time by the process just described. Answers will often be partial but will contribute to the final resolution.

The education of nurses and licensure of nurses are two separate issues. A commitment from the National Council of State Boards to test the unique content offered in the B.S. curriculum would provide a first step in documenting educational differences and expected competencies. The data from the present study suggest that Educational Accessibility, a component of Curricular Concerns, had a strong valence for both driving and restraining forces; hence discussions focusing on mutual needs and shared concerns in this area may have the potential for resolution of the issue. Finally, the willingness of national and state nursing organizations to compromise and put societal concerns before self-serving organizational and individual concerns will hasten the discovery of solutions, answers and consensus within and among the states. It would be ironic if the current cohesiveness of national nursing organizations prompted by the Registered Care Technologist proposal were to effect a beginning resolution of the entry issue.

REFERENCES

deRivera, J. (1976). **Field theory as human-science.** New York: Bardner Press, Inc.

Ellis, J. & Hartley, C. (1988). **Nursing in today's world: Challenges, issues and trends.** Philadelphia: J.B. Lippincott Company.

Glick, M. (1985). Educational entry level into nursing. **The Journal of Continuing Education in Nursing**, 16(6), 185-188.

Grippando, G. (1986). **Nursing perspectives & issues.** Albany, N.Y.: Delmar Publisher, Inc.

Hood, G. (1985). At issue: Titling and licensure. **American Journal of Nursing**, 85(5), 592,594.

Lewin, K. (1951). **Field theory in social science.** Westport, CT: Greenwood Press.

Lewis, E. (1985). Taking care of business: The ANA house of delegates, 1985. **Nursing Outlook,** 33(5), 239-243.

Mallison, M. (1984). Time to talk about licensure [editorial]. **American Journal of Nursing**, 11, 1353.

Maraldo, P. & Solomon, S. (1987). Nursing's window of opportunity. **Image: Journal of Nursing Scholarship**, 19(2), 83-85.

Rasch, R. (1987). The nature of taxonomy. **Image: Journal of Nursing Scholarship**, 19(3), 147-149.

Stevens, B. (1985). Does the 1985 nursing education proposal make economic sense? **Nursing Outlook,** 33(3), 124-127.

Wakefield-Fisher, M., Wright, M., & Kraft, L. (1986). A first for the nation: North Dakota and entry into nursing practice. **Nursing & Health Care,** 7(3), 134-141.

Waltz, C., Strickland, O., & Lenz, E. (1984). **Measurement in nursing research.** Philadelphia: F.A. Davis Company.

Waters, V. (1986). Restricting the RN license to BSN graduates could cloud nursing's future. **Nursing & Health Care,** 7(3), 143-146.

Wright, M. (1988). **Field analysis of nursing education models designed for college graduates.** Unpublished Dissertation. University of Texas at Austin.

Nurses for the future: The yo-yo ride

Joan Lynaugh: A yo-yo is an appropriate symbol for the history of nursing. As you know, yo-yos are powered by strings that make them rise and fall. Yo-yos also spin a lot if you don't know how to control them.

One face of the symbolic yo-yo is our American social priorities over the last century — to transfer the care of the sick from the home and family into an institution and to responsible professionals; to use biomedical interventions to ease the burden of morbidity and mortality; and to sustain the image of our so-called "healthy society" through public health.

The second face of the yo-yo concerns society's feeling that health care should be low cost, and so should education for caregivers. In America, we first relied on the free labor pool of women who went into hospital schools of nursing. They were paid minimally during their two, and later three, years of training. Afterwards, they were not paid at all in hospitals; they graduated and went into private duty.

Another assumption has been that there should be an abundant supply of what we might call "the disposable nurse."

The idea of a disposable nurse starts with the satisfactory arrangement that made pupils in the hospital schools caregivers who would pass through the system and leave. Then we found it satisfactory to have women enter nursing training, practice for short careers, and leave when they married.

The string that powers this nursing yo-yo — this oscillating relationship of nursing with society — is much more complicated and not very visible. One way to characterize the string that powers nursing is society's image of nursing as concerned with reform and usefulness.

Another powerful factor is the nurses' views of themselves, complicated by this business of upward mobility that we equate with higher education.

Another characteristic of this "string" — the oscillating relationship — is the American preference for a quick technological fix. Americans are impatient people who don't like to think about mortality and are, therefore, interested in getting things fixed — an interest in which nursing, too, has been absorbed.

There is no doubt that the work of nursing is extremely vital, so vital that we must be much more assertive in stressing the value of our profession than we have been in the past. We must make it absolutely clear that nursing is about humane care, about being humane to one another; that nursing is about care that is available and about care that is oriented toward the people receiving it.

We need to find effective and economical nursing systems to deliver that humane care. We need a consensus on what professional practice should be, and we need nursing education that will meet those standards.

And finally, I want to say something about this best and brightest tag we are using in this conference. We need to decide the best and the brightest of what. We Americans are fascinated by royalty and celebrities; at the same time, we are very, very touchy about elitism and deny class differences when we can. I want to remind you that our nursing ancestors expressly eschewed Florence Nightingale's insistence on a class orientation for nurses.

American nursing has always operated on the pretense of a classless nursing collective. The question really is one of nursing's getting really good people to do good work.

Discussion and comment

Rosemary Stevens: I decided I should talk about power and romance. And I am serious. I would like to start by jumping us back 75 years because by jumping us back, I want to pick up some of these points and bring us forward again.

From our 1980s vantage point, nursing in the early days was a profession with grim working conditions. Hospitals were overcrowded; nursing residences were unsanitary and uncomfortable. Overworked nurses suffered from chronic fatigue, poor food, and often were in poor health. Many worked a 10-hour day, and then had to study on their own time. Nurses also worked a 50-week year; they had to make up sick time on an hour-by-hour basis.

My purpose in reviewing this history is to ask why were conditions in nursing so appalling?

Joanne Ashley has written a study that views the history of nursing from the perspective of hospital exploitation. Another hypothesis has to do with sexism — the relationship between physicians and nurses. Clearly, the health care system has discriminated against nurses as women.

But beyond these two hypotheses, I return to the questions of power and romance and suggest yet another hypothesis for the conditions that persist in nursing: duplicity within the nursing profession itself.

It puzzles me why a profession that accounts for the largest percentage of workers in the health care field, and that, therefore, is theoretically the most powerful, has not exerted its power. For most of this century, hospitals have been primarily nursing and surgical institutions.

At the beginning of this century, nurses were powerful figures. Nurses, not physicians, were responsible for taking pulse rates and temperatures, measuring blood pressures, preparing dressings, even serving as anesthetists.

My question is, why did these women go along with this sense of deference, this sense of powerlessness, that has distinguished the history of nursing until recently? Nutting, for example, in 1912 quotes a nursing school superintendent who says, "12 hours a day is not too many hours if there is plenty of good, nourishing food."

My point is that nursing's own past has much to do with the assumptions and stereotypes that may be inhibiting nursing roles and nursing leadership today. These assumptions and stereotypes are powering the string of the nursing yo-yo. It is the weight of domesticity, the burden of deference, and the image of nurse as a generalist that distinguish the profession's history.

Consideration of nursing's many contemporary roles leads me to the conclusion that nursing must be articulated in different ways today. The first step is to move away from the idea of generalism that has infused nursing all along. Why not educate nurses in terms of distinct and separate professional roles?

Different educational tracks do exist, but why not sell nursing in terms of those different educational programs? Why not build nursing's image on specialties within nursing schools? Professional differentiation in nursing has already been suggested.

I am also concerned that efforts to jettison stereotypes regarding the social worth of nursing may produce another stereotype: the nurse as entrepreneur. I am uncertain whether moving from an image of nurse as a generalist to that of a money-making entrepreneur is necessarily what nursing really wants to do.

My final point about power is that nurses are potentially extremely powerful, and much of this power is concentrated in the hospital setting. If nurses remove themselves from hospitals and into some other type of organization, they may be setting the stage for the same kind of confrontation that has dogged the medical profession and hospitals for so long. Before nursing jettisons the image of romance for the image of money, I hope there will be careful consideration of just what the implications might be.

Joan Lynaugh: A recurrent issue in our discussions about nursing is our "invisibility," or the fact that people don't know what nursing is and what nurses do. Then, if we skip immediately to organizational systems and entrepreneurship without first defining what nursing is and what nurses do, we are accused of abandoning our mission. That's another current issue.

Vivian DeBack: The problems arise when we confuse *what* nurses do for clients and *where* they do it. The point is nurses provide services for the ill and the well in a number of different settings — from hospitals to nursing homes, HMOs, factories, and schools.

One reason that nursing has had neither power nor sex appeal is because we have not defined the business of the role as separate from the business of the place. Our failure to distinguish between the two makes it appear that we don't like certain roles in nursing. But talk of entrepreneurial activities does not mean that nursing plans to abandon its roles in hospitals, nursing homes, and so on.

Thelma Schorr: I want to follow up on what Vivian DeBack said. I think we are confusing the distinction between the generalist and the entrepreneur.

What hospital nurses are saying is that they want more control over their own practice. To get that control, many of them are becoming entrepreneurs and that has nothing to do with being a generalist or a specialist. It has everything to do with nurses who are educated for the profession, know what they are doing, but

who have little autonomy in their practice.

Leonard Laster: Statistics indicate that some time in the next 30 years, I am probably going to be sick. I may go to an intensive care unit, after that to some intermediate unit, and then home. Now, I am going to spend 10 percent of that time with my physicians. But the other 90 percent of the time I am going to spend with nurses.

I don't know what the best and the brightest means. I just want them to be damn good. When I'm sick, I don't want, as a friend of mine had, a nurse sitting at the bedside, talking about how much she hated nursing and wished she had gone for her MBA.

Eli Ginzberg told us society hasn't solved any of its big problems. We are not going to solve this nursing issue today, for no economists or people-power experts, or government leaders have ever solved the yo-yo phenomenon.

I think nursing is going through one of those cycles common to service professions in that today's young people are finding other career choices more attractive — and it has everything to do with today's value system.

Now, some might think me a relic, but I think we are due for a change. Just as the tragedy of AIDS is making us rethink the sexual revolution, the "yuppification" of our society is going to make us rethink our revolution in values.

I'm old-fashioned and romantic enough to believe that we are going to start putting value on giving to each other again. In the meantime, I want to be sure there's a nursing profession these young people can come back to. It bothers me when we talk about the medical industry, the nursing industry, the health care industry. I didn't bust my gut to become a physician so that I could go into an industry. And when I'm sick, I don't want to be a client. I don't want to be taken care of by entrepreneurs who are worried about market patterns and PR.

For crying out loud, nursing is something really wonderful. Whatever strategies you come up with, keep that in mind so you don't lose it.

Claire Fagin: I want to second what Len Laster has said about the meaning of the best and the brightest. It means that we recognize that nursing requires brains, self-esteem, self-respect, self-knowledge, and respect from society for what nurses do.

Unless we have a system that supports and enhances the self-respect of nurses, we are not going to be able to attract people to this profession.

When we talk with 16-year-old high-school juniors, they tell us they have already heard from nurses in the field all the reasons why they shouldn't be nurses. The system must change; it must become more possible for nurses to practice; then nursing schools will be able to attract nurses.

Mitchell Rabkin: In the old days, when nurses worked 10 hours a day and some had to cook and clean as well, there was no statement about burnout. Nurses indeed were burned out, but it wasn't articulated.

Today, at least, the question is one of capacity to avoid burnout, which is due not only to hard work but, as Thelma Schorr pointed out, the capacity to exercise some control over the environment.

Myrna Warnick: I read the yo-yo paper with a great deal of interest for it pinpointed many current problems in nursing. For instance, patients have certain expectations of us as nurses: they want us to care for them and to care about them, their families, their visitors, their dog, whatever. Patients also do not want to leave any environment in worse condition than when they came. So it is up to us to prevent problems and infections.

We are also advocates, acting on the patient's behalf so that what needs to be done gets done and vice versa. We are competent in using sophisticated technology in intensive care and when the physicians finish their procedures, we are the ones who clean up.

On top of all that, the hospital expects us to do what we do and not lose them money in the process.

Now it takes time to prepare a person to perform so many roles and perform them well. Last week, I attended a shortage task force meeting in California. They showed a videotape of a nurse who was burned out in three years. Why? Because there are unrealistic expectations regarding all the roles a nurse plays, given the short time for preparation.

So what we are seeing is, number one, the two-year programs claim to be 72 credit hours, but they are really 100 to 110 hours. Number two, once their graduates are faced with the obligations of the hospital setting, they simply can't perform. In six months, they are trying to take charge of an intensive care unit, and in three years we lose them and we say, "That's the breaks; let's increase again."

Nursing education needs more than the quickest, cheapest way. The clinical practice discipline requires more money than chemistry courses at the university setting. I think there has to be a major restructuring.

Marc Roberts: As an outside observer, I find it baffling that very different educational tracks lead to the same professional qualifications. In any other profession, different tracks would lead to different qualifications and, consequently, to more stratification and specialization.

I would like to suggest, as a provocative example, airline pilots. Pilot licensing is the opposite of nursing licensing. You get a whole series of different licenses that allow you to fly different aircraft under different circumstances, perform different procedures. There is also continual recertification; use it or lose it.

Joan Lynaugh: We have evolved in our system of nursing certification a specialized certification that parallels the evolution of specialization in the other health professions. Beginning in the mid-fifties, nursing developed a certification mechanism that excludes people from certain specialty practices but, hopefully, assures the public that they can have confidence in nurse midwives, nurse anesthetists, and all of the other nurse practitioners.

I would argue that economics is the reason for so many entry points into nursing. Whenever society begins to think about regulating entry to nursing practice, we count the cost and back away each and every time. This has been going on since 1912. The expense of standardizing nursing is a difficult issue to confront. For example, it took from 1890 to 1925 to standardize medicine.

CHAPTER FOUR

Nursing practice: Autonomy, compensation, and advancement

THE RAPID EXPANSION of technology in medical care and the advent of diagnosis-related groups (DRGs) have profoundly affected nurses and their roles and functions. As indicated earlier, nurses need to be involved in decision making and in control of their practice domain to ensure high quality, skilled patient care. Correspondingly, nurses need compensation that is commensurate with their job assignment, education, and clinical competence.

Many hospital pay salaries based upon advancement in the clinical setting. Predetermined criteria define each rung on the clinical ladder so that practicing nurses can document those accomplishments that make them eligible to move to higher levels of functioning, autonomy, and salary. This approach to salary setting contrasts with that of the union concept of collective bargaining. There, contracts for pay and benefits are negotiated for the individual through a union shop. Persons with similar job titles usually receive similar compensation.

Where salaries and advancement are linked to predetermined educational and performance criteria, the institution must be open and decentralized. (The average health care agency is highly bureaucratic, with centralized decision making.) The concept of shared governance embraces the participation of nurses at every level of decision making in the organization. Accountability, control of practice, and authority are apportioned. Decisions involving such procedures as staffing, assignments, and scheduling are made by staff nurse councils or committees. This concept requires professional and personal commitment and accountability by every staff member.

Job satisfaction and the opportunity for professional advancement are important personal ingredients for anyone committed to nursing. In return, the nurse has a responsibility to be academically prepared and a competent practitioner. The profession also has a responsibility to provide support and opportunities for career mobility. Health care institutions also have responsibilities to provide nurses with career advancement programs and to aid nurses who wish to pursue advanced education programs.

Some of the authors in this chapter agree with one another, others disagree, but all reflect current thinking. Tribulski, in "How You Can Use That Federal Report on Nursing," highlights four of the sixteen recommendations of the report by the Commission on Nursing. (The Commission had solicited comments from nurses and nursing groups in hearings held throughout the United States.) The significant recommendations endorse preserving the nurse's time for direct patient care by providing adequate staffing levels in clinical and non-clinical nursing services; increasing compensation and improving nursing career orientation; supporting the nurse's participation in governance, administration, and management in health-care organizations; recognizing the decision-making authority of nurses in relation to other health-care professionals. The report is responsive to the positions taken by authors in this chapter and in Chapter Two (see Spitzer and Davivier).

An approach to establishing shared governance is described in "Moving to Shared Governance" by Ortiz, et al. These authors provide an overview of the methods used at the University of Rochester Medical Center, Strong

Memorial Hospital, Rochester, N.Y., where the philosophy of nursing managers is to encourage self-actualization of each staff member. Allen, et al., in "Making Shared Governance Work: A Conceptual Model," support autonomy and responsibility as central goals in attaining professionalism in nursing. They propose a conceptual model of shared governance and assert a relationship between its use and job satisfaction, performance, and the reward system (pay, recognition, and promotion).

O'Grady, in "Shared Governance: Reality or Sham?" also supports the idea of "ownership" and shared governance in an organization, arguing the importance of commitment by all staff members. He indicates that traditional collective bargaining as practiced in unionized organizations "falls away" as nurses move to decision making and shared governance.

In a speech presented to the Wisconsin Nurse's Association, Miller, an industrial relations professor, provides a view of shared governance and collective bargaining that differs. He takes issue with O'Grady and others, arguing that they discuss power — power to control, to decide, and to administer — whereas the old forms of power are no longer effective and may be counterproductive.

McNerney, a professor in management and the former president of the Blue Cross and Blue Shield Association, provides still another perspective on nurses' involvement in management and medical staff affairs in "Nursing's Vision in a Competitive Environment." He supports recognizing nurses for service and leadership through career advancement programs, but he notes that in many instances such programs do not exist. Yet autonomy of practice can be maintained within institutional

and professional guidelines. He further states that the envisioned roles of nurses as providers of service, knowledge developers, executives, diagnosticians, and professional intervenors will have to be earned and not proclaimed. He doubts that the vision of nurses as more autonomous, more independent, and mastering a wider scope of functions is feasible in today's competitive world. He predicts that the nursing profession must develop structure for and skill in decision making to survive in a competitive market place.

Hougaard, in "Clinical Ladder Program Builds Self-esteem," describes how the clinical ladder has benefitted the nurse, patient, and hospital and has enhanced nurses' self-esteem. Hartley and Cunningham, in "Staff Nurses Rate Clinical Ladder Program," report on the program at St. Mark's Hospital in Salt Lake City, Utah, where the evaluation revises and strengthens the clinical ladder options.

Wintz, in "Career Paths of Nurses: When Is a Nurse No Longer a Nurse?" claims that the future of nursing rests with pioneers who create new career paths. Since the health care system is in flux, new positions and competencies will be required. Wintz identifies specialized roles that are emerging and urges nurse students to plan their careers while in school. Nurse executives should give career guidance to young nurses and build career advancement programs in health care agencies.

Nursing leaders support programs that increase the scope of nursing practice, participation in decision making and shared governance, and career opportunities. Individuals outside nursing but involved in health care warn that the profession is not distinguishing clearly between nursing roles and management practices.

How you can use that federal report on nursing

JEAN A. TRIBULSKI, RN, PhD, CNA

THE FEDERAL COMMISSION on Nursing clearly paid attention when nurses across the country spoke before it last year. The 16 recommendations in the panel's final report are right in line with what nurses have been saying for years and what coalitions of national, state, and specialty organizations have been pounding home in recent months.

If the report holds no surprises, why then is it important? For one thing, it helped focus national attention on the nursing shortage, proclaiming with the voice of authority that it's real; it's dangerous; and it could become a lot worse. "More intense efforts on the part of nurses have so far staved off major negative effects of the shortage," acknowledged Carolyne K. Davis, RN, PhD, who headed the commission.

With increasing attention from the media, the public has become more aware of the seriousness of the situation. This, in turn, creates a climate in which change becomes possible.

Change won't come about, however, unless nurses mount convincing arguments for it within their own institutions. The commission report can help in two ways: First, it puts the weight of the federal government firmly behind nursing efforts. Second, it provides a focus for those efforts.

You can obtain a complete copy of the commission report by writing to Office of Public Affairs, U.S. Department of Health and Human Services, 200 Independence Avenue SW, Washington, D.C. 20201. Here are the four recommendations most crucial to advancing nursing's goals.

Health care delivery organizations should preserve the nurse's time for the direct care of patients and families by providing adequate staffing levels for clinical and non-clinical support services. Recommendation No. 1

The commission members quickly got down to specifics. They want administrators to "provide non-clinical support services on a 24-hour, seven-day per week basis," and they want those services to cover a broad range: "telephone, paperwork, other clerical support; maintenance of and ready access to supplies; maintenance of a hygienic environment; transport of patients, specimens, equipment and documents; and the processing of admissions, transfers and discharges."

They also want other clinical services — respiratory and physical therapy, pharmacy, radiology, laboratory — staffed during off-hours. The report notes that the practice of having nurses fill in for personnel on these services has increased the overall demand for nurses, exacerbated the shortage, and contributed to high stress, high turnover, and poor job satisfaction.

What strategies can the staff nurse use in response? You can start by translating the report's general statement into the specifics of your own institution. Keep track of services you're performing that could be provided more appropriately by other workers or departments. Document the time you spend carrying specimens to the lab, ordering meds, moving patients back and forth to X-ray, tracking down lab reports. Look for the document patterns in the shifts and days of the week when your non-nursing load peaks.

Yes, this means extra paperwork now, but consider it as an investment in potential power. When you and your colleagues have amassed some hard data, you can take it up your chain of command, citing the commission report for support.

At the same time, some of us must consider whether the real pressure to perform many of these extra functions comes from within ourselves. Does the need to be needed sometimes skew priorities? It is exemplary to want to give the best care to patients, but is it essential to jump in and perform these other functions? Weigh the value of these tasks against time lost for teaching, providing emotional support, and exercising the full range of nursing knowledge. Which will make the bigger difference in our patients' healing?

Health care delivery organizations should increase RN compensation and improve RN long-term career orientation by providing a one-time adjustment to increase RN relative wages targeted to geographic, institutional and career differences. Additionally, they should pursue the development and implementation of innovative compensation options for nurses and expand pay ranges based on experience, education, performance, and demonstrated leadership. Recommendation No. 5

Here, the commission focuses on resolving the wage compression issue. That means expanding the pay range between entry level and the maximum to move it into line with other professions. The report also recommends a one-time salary increase to establish equity among hospital, nursing home, and home care nurses.

Bringing this recommendation to reality demands collective action through state, specialty, and other nursing associations. Many of these groups have already gathered the financial data necessary to make salary comparisons with other professions. They also have es-

tablished ties with legislators, state and federal commissions, and other organizations whose power can be tapped to help convince administrators to boost salaries.

When faced with pay-hike petitions, however, hospitals are likely to cry that they have no extra money to give nurses. Even an insider can counter that argument: Connie Curran, RN, EdD, FAAN, who was a vice president of the American Hospital Association and represented the group before the commission, suggested in her testimony that hospitals take a closer look at how they use their money: One source of funds for a pay raise might be the nearly $20,000 it costs to replace a nurse who leaves for greener pastures.

In a parallel recommendation, No. 6, the commission itself suggests a way to fund pay hikes for nurses: federal legislation providing for a one-time increase in Medicare hospital rates specifically ear-marked for nursing salaries. The commission, furthermore, recommends that states and private payors keep Medicaid rates and reimbursement schedules at levels high enough to permit health-care facilities to recruit and retain nurses.

Salary is not the only compensation issue the report addresses. It calls for hospitals to offer more and more flexible benefits as well, particularly child and elder care.

Individual nurses can push for such changes by becoming active on the human resource or recruitment and retention committees at their institutions. Again, use the federal report to add weight to arguments for innovations like cafeteria-style benefit programs that allow employees to spend a set amount of benefit dollars on the programs they need most.

Employers of nurses should ensure active participation in governance, administration, and management of their organizations. Recommendation No. 8

The report makes a strong case for involving nurses at all levels of decision-making: They are the largest group of health-care givers, provide a substantial proportion of patient care services, have a unique knowledge of the patients, and interact extensively with all departments in the hospital. The commission's idea of involvement is active participation and full voting rights on committees.

Hospitals — and the doctors who traditionally run them — are unlikely to voluntarily give away such power, so individual nurses will have to seek out membership on committees. They'll also have to be ready to spend their time attending meetings and following through on committee assignments.

Nurses who want to expand their knowledge in business principles, quality assurance, labor relations, and similar management areas before assuming committee responsibilities can take CE courses or enroll in classes at local colleges. Tuition reimbursement may not be available, but the expense is an investment building on the momentum of the commission's report.

> Employers of nurses, as well as the medical profession, should recognize the appropriate decision-making authority of nurses in relationship to other health care professionals, foster communication and collaboration among the health care team, and ensure that the appropriate provider delivers the necessary care. Close cooperation and mutual respect between nursing and medicine is essential. Recommendation No. 9

Autonomy is a key issue, according to the commission, and a few specific questions will show whether your own hospital is serious about giving nurses appropriate decision-making power. Is there a joint practice committee, for instance, and does it function on an institution-wide or at a unit or speciality level? How do staff nurses become involved in the committee? What kinds of decisions does it make? Who's responsible for implementing those decisions?

Do nurses write nursing orders and make decisions about basic activities of daily living for their patients? Must they have a doctor's order to give a patient a shampoo or let him take a shower? Can a med/surg nurse assess for bowel sounds and advance a postop patient's diet as a nursing order?

The answers to these and similar questions will help you outline the changes needed at your hospital to meet goals set by the commission.

Translating autonomy into financial terms was one issue where the commission faltered, however. The specific question involved direct reimbursement for nurses who certify and recertify Medicare and Medicaid patients for long-term care.

When doctors certify patients, Medicaid or Medicare pays them directly for the job. In 1987 Congress authorized nurse practitioners and clinical nurse specialists to do this work, as long as they were not employed by the facility providing the care. After extensive lobbying by organized medicine against the concept, though, Congress did not authorize direct payment to nurses. In other words, physicians will be paid to certify the need for care, whether they do the exam or not.

The commission report fails to address this inequity, even though a number of private health insurers have already decided that it makes sense to pay nurses directly. The commission does recommend, however, that nurses other than NPs and clinical specialists be allowed to certify and recertify.

Four other commission recommendations are important to the staff nurse, although they offer no immediate help for solving the shortage. Recommendation No. 2 notes the need for innovative staffing patterns that appropriately utilize the different levels of education, competence and experience of nurses. Though not specifically mentioned in the report, this certainly would discourage the notion that "a nurse is a nurse is a nurse" who can be floated to any unit.

Recommendation No. 3 speaks to the need for automated information systems and other labor-saving technologies. The commission cited testimony from its hearings to support the need for computers: Hospitals allot only some 2% of their annual operating budgets for information technology, while other service industries spend as much as 11%. Nurses spend 30% of their time handling information, and computerization could reduce that by 70%. The time saved could total as much as an hour and a half per RN per shift.

Recommendation No. 10 calls for financial assistance to both undergraduate and graduate students. The commission suggested service payback loans. These can be forgiven by working in practice settings or clinical specialties — hospitals in low income areas and gerontological nursing, for example — where the nursing shortage is most acute.

Recommendation No. 13 charges the nursing profession to take responsibility for promoting a positive accurate image of its members. The report outlines strategies for national organizations, employers of nurses, and the business community, but individual nurses can take part in this work also. One simple way: Write letters objecting to any negative or inaccurate depiction of nurses and nursing. Additionally, most hospital public relations offices will think it very much in their own interest to help nurses find forums for spotlighting positive aspects of the profession.

The remaining recommendations dealt with costing and budgeting methods that track nursing resources, government reimbursement, putting nurse members on accreditation bodies, improvements needed in nursing school curricula, recruiting nursing students from non-traditional segments of society, and maintaining nursing resources through research, an advisory commission, and a data bank.

The Commission on Nursing has outlined an exciting agenda. But will its report become a dust collector, another collection of good ideas going nowhere? That depends on nurses, individually and collectively. Nothing will happen if all they see is an other stack of papers. Anything can happen if they seize a new tool for advancing the profession.

Moving to shared governance

MARLAINE E. ORTIZ, RN, MS; PHYLLIS GEHRING, RN, BSN; MARGARET D. SOVIE, RN, PhD, FAAN

DESPITE OUR STRIDES toward greater professional status and recognition, the full spectrum of power that some other professions exercise still eludes many nurses. Nurses frequently complain that as employees within a hospital organization, they do not influence decisions about their practice.

Traditionally, nurses have worked in bureaucratic agencies. Nurse administrators have held the major responsibility for developing practice standards and making decisions —frequently without soliciting staff nurses' input and participation. In fact, nurses often have had to struggle for professional autonomy.[1]

At the University of Rochester Medical Center, Strong Memorial Hospital, we have established a professional nursing organization so that practicing nurses can participate in the business of nursing and health care delivery. Our 1,500 nurses have integrated practice, education, and research according to a unification model established in 1972 [2]. Licensed practical nurses, aides, and technicians make up 6.5 percent of the nursing staff of our 741-bed hospital.

We have five inpatient services (medicine, surgery, pediatric, psychiatry, and Ob-Gyn) and a cancer center, each administered by a clinical nursing chief. The clinical chief reports both to the associate director for nursing and to the director of nursing. The associate director and director also hold the university positions of associate dean and dean for nursing practice.

Building from our base

Our philosophy of nursing management is that *each* staff member should be encouraged to-ward full self-actualization. We recognize each staff member's right to express his/her own view, to participate in decision making, to be provided with information about fiscal management of patient care, to practice in an environment conducive to learning and open to an exchange of ideas and peer support, and to engage in collegial and collaborative relationships with nurses and others.[3]

We have practiced participative management since 1977. With participative management, decision making involves staff nurses as well as administrators. Staff nurse advisory boards (SNABs) and the staff nurse executive committee (SNEC) are key components of participative management. The SNAB for each service — established in 1981 — promotes and supports staff involvement. Elected staff nurse representatives from each patient care unit serve one-year terms on the SNAB. (An alternate is elected in case the representative is unable to attend scheduled meetings.)

SNABs address practice issues and concerns or problems specific to the service, such as new patient care programs, standards of practice, and quality assurance reports. The SNABs meet twice a month with the clinical nursing chiefs. These meetings are open to all nurses within the service.

The staff nurse executive committee (SNEC) is composed of the chairpersons of each SNAB and meets monthly with the associate dean for nursing practice. The SNEC addresses issues that concern all practice areas and establishes the agenda for the nursing update forums held every other month for the entire nursing staff. The SNABs and the SNEC have introduced:

- a clinical advancement program,
- a longevity benefits program,
- nursing forums held every other month,
- strategic planning,
- a day-care program,
- outstanding nurse awards.

The most ambitious project — the development of the professional nursing organization model — resulted from staff nurses' responses to a questionnaire that asked: Where do *you* want nursing to be in the year 1990?

Themes emerged from the responses: image; staffing, recruitment, and retention; politics; computers and technology; inservice education, continuing education, and formal degree programs; research; budget and reimbursement; relationships with administration; RN/MD relationships; practice; support services; and benefits. A major theme was shared governance with professional recognition and autonomy.

Working with the associate dean for nursing practice, a task force set out to develop bylaws creating a professional nursing organization as part of a shared governance model. Incorporating recommendations from nursing staff, legal counsel, university personnel officers, and hospital administrators, the bylaws were approved by the hospital's executive committee and the university's board of trustees in June 1984. They describe the professional nursing organization as a guide to the continuing development of nursing practice at our hospital. Its purpose is to:
- provide an integrating structure for professional nursing affairs,
- participate in the development of nursing practice standards,
- promote quality nursing care,
- influence, contribute to, and support the professional education of students and staff,
- encourage and support scientific inquiry for the continual improvement of nursing practice and health care,

- promote the continuing development of professional nursing,
- address the practice needs of all members of the nursing staff.[4]

Once approved, the bylaws were distributed to all staff. A staff development instructor became responsible for educating the nursing staff about the new organization and shared governance. She also helped conduct the election of the organization's first executive committee.

The bylaws task force designed the educational processes and provided advice on the election process. Sessions with each group included discussions about the concept of participative management and shared governance functions, composition of the professional nursing organization and its standing committees, and executive committee functions.

Starting the professional organization

The executive committee is a 43-member governing body. The director of nursing, the associate director, and the immediate past chairperson sit on this committee with 40 elected members. The number of representatives from each area is based on the number of full-time–equivalent positions. Eight members are faculty; 22 are staff nurses; and 10 are nurse administrators.

The chairperson of the professional nursing organization is also a voting member of the hospital's executive committee, as is the chairperson of the medical staff organization.

The executive committee of the professional nursing organization meets monthly. The committee's agenda includes reports on nursing acuity and census, on the standing committees, on the hospital's executive committee, and on other nursing and patient care issues. Executive committee minutes are posted on each unit throughout the hospital.

Like the executive committee, nine standing committee memberships include staff, faculty, and administrators. Thus, in keeping with our unification model, each committee has input from each nursing constituency. The standing committee chairpersons are members of the executive committee. The standing committees meet monthly or every other month, depending on their objectives.

We have learned that change takes time. So far, the *research committee* has designed a resource book that lists current and completed research projects, resources, and tips on planning clinical research projects. The committee plans to offer in-service programs on research.

The *career advancement/development committee* assessed staff continuing education needs. Based on those findings, we offered a physical assessment series and a stress management program. Monthly programs have also been planned. This committee has also explored ways to provide certified nurses with the continuing education units that they need for recertification.

The *public and institutional relations committee* has developed programs to promote professional nursing. One such program was a unit-based open house for each service to provide an overview of the specialized work of each service and also to support matrix staffing (floating). This committee also works with the SNEC to design and organize National Nurses' Week activities.

The first general membership meeting was held in March 1986. General membership meetings, held quarterly, provide open discussion among staff. What makes nurses want to attend? An agenda that they perceive as important and related to their concerns:

• updates on new clinical programs, such as the birthing center or bone marrow transplantation,

• nursing budget changes,

• JCAH and state inspection reports,

• committee reports.

Although the professional nursing organization is just two years old, we predict it will become a major driving force in nursing practice — a dynamic, integrating mechanism for all nurses at Strong Memorial Hospital. From concept to reality, shared governance is a giant step forward.

REFERENCES

1. Bixler, G.K., and Bixler, R.W. The professional status of nursing. *Am. J. Nurs.* 59:1142-1147, Aug. 1959.

2. Sovie, M.D. Unifying education and practice: one medical center's design. Part 1. *J. Nurs. Adm.* 11:41-49, Jan. 1981.

3. School of Nursing and Hospital. Nursing Practice. *Philosophy of Nursing Practice Management*: 1977 (Revised 1982).

4. University of Rochester Professional Nursing Organization. *Bylaws* 1983.

BIBLIOGRAPHY

Bopp, W.J., and Rosenthal, W.P. Participatory management. *Am. J. Nurs.* 79:670-672, Apr. 1979.

Carson, F.E., and Ames, A. Nursing staff bylaws. *Am. J. Nurs.* 80:1130-1134, June 1980.

Christman, L. The autonomous nursing staff in the hospital. *Nurs. Adm. Q.* 1:37-44, Fall 1976.

Cleland, V.S. Shared governance in a professional model of collective bargaining. *J. Nurs. Adm.* 8:39-43, May 1978.

Kimbro, C.D., and Gifford, A.J. The nursing staff organization: a needed development. *Nurs. Outlook* 28:610-616, Oct. 1980.

Lebreton, P.P. A council of staff nurses: a proposal. *Nurs. Health Care* 2:261-266, 285.

Sovie, M.D. The economics of magnetism...a composite representation of a magnet hospital. *Nurs. Econ.* 2:85-92, Mar.-Apr. 1984.

Making shared governance work: A conceptual model

DAVID ALLEN, RN, PhD; JOY CALKIN, RN, PhD; MARLYS PETERSON, RN, MSN

INCREASED AUTONOMY AND responsibility are central goals driving nursing's quest for professionalism.[1] Many publications address the actual and potential conflict between these goals and the organizational settings in which nursing is practiced. In recent years, nursing literature has increasingly advocated decentralization, participation in decision making, and shared governance or similar strategies as means for making organizational structure and professional practice more complimentary.[2-10] In general, however, participation remains an ideal, and there are few research-based guidelines for how to accomplish productive participation.[11-16] One reason for this gap between reality and participatory ideals is that nurses at all levels of the organization are not clear about the mechanisms or pathways by which participation achieves its highly touted effects.

Clearly there is no single system of implementing participation in decision making (PDM) that will fit every situation. Change agents (be they staff or administration) will be more likely to achieve their goals if they have a solid understanding of what PDM is, the effects it has had on organizational members, and the processes which mediate those effects. This article synthesizes a broad range of empirical research on PDM into a model which may help nurses decide how to design a participatory intervention which will accomplish their goals.

Research on participation ranges over a plethora of alternative models and the boundaries shift from study to study. The level at which participation occurs moves from individual jobs (enrichment) through small groups up to the company level (codetermination) and input into national policies. Similarly, the subject matter of participative decisions includes wages and economic issues, employment conditions, productivity, cost reduction, and strategic decisions. Participation also varies in degree, from joint consultation where management makes the final decision, through the consensus of joint decision-making to worker control. It occurs in settings where capital and labor come from separate sources and in worker-owned enterprises (like producer cooperatives).[9-19]

Figure 1 represents our conceptual model. The discussion which follows will explicate the model and suggest some implications for nursing. The model was synthesized from a review of more than 100 research reports on PDM in a variety of organizations — some were health care organizations, many were not.

The direct arrow from PDM to satisfaction represents an almost universal relationship: in virtually every setting and for all levels of employees, increased PDM led to increased satisfaction.[20-24] Insofar as satisfaction is an end in itself, PDM is an effective intervention. The relationships among satisfaction and other desirable goals (e.g., performance, turnover) is very complex and is influenced by a variety of intra- and extra-organizational factors (such as whether the employee perceives other viable and attractive alternatives).[25-27]

Though PDM increases satisfaction, some people involved in PDM are more satisfied than others. The bulk of our model is designed to explain these variable effects: what makes some people respond more positively than others to participation?

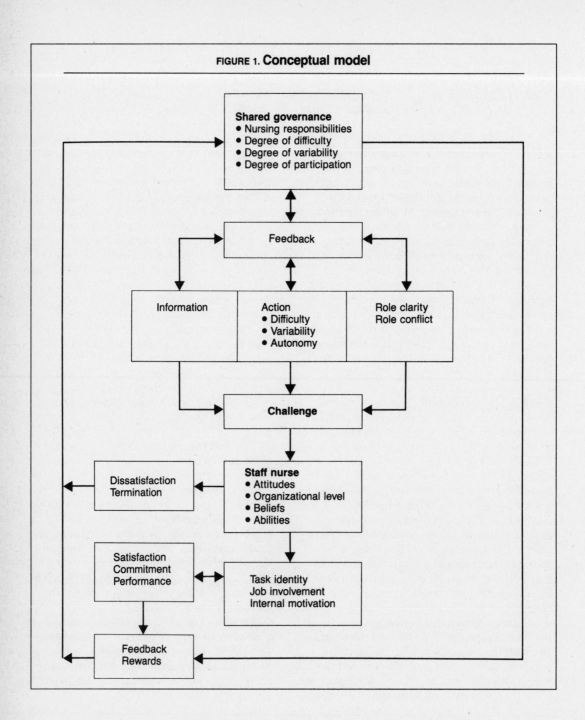

FIGURE 1. **Conceptual model**

First, of course, there are just differences among people (indicated on our model as staff nurse values, attitudes, and abilities). One such grouping of individual characteristics which appears related to PDM is called Growth Need Strengths (GNS).[20-31]

The GNS is an index of the kinds of challenges people prefer from their work. Those who desire a lot of autonomy and responsibility respond more favorably to PDM than those who do not place as high a priority on those qualities. It is important to note that virtually all previous studies have been cross-sectional, that is, the organization has been studied at only one moment in time rather than over a period of months or a year. We expect that people exposed to PDM over time will come to value growth more highly. A more specific measure is simply how much employees desire participation.[32-37]

Those who want and have a lot of PDM or desire little and have little will be more satisfied than will be employees for whom there is a large gap between the desired state and the current situation. This relationship may even hold for specific decisions: that is, someone may want a lot of participation in decisions regarding scheduling but not want to be involved in decisions about patient assignments.

These and other individual differences have an impact on the relationship between PDM and satisfaction. To offer just one example from our model, the presence of role conflict (having incompatible expectations from different parts of one's job — such as trying to please administrators and physicians when they disagree over what you should be doing) leads to tension, and tension is negatively related to satisfaction. But for individuals who enjoy or can ignore conflict — in other words, experience it as a challenge — there may be minimal negative impact on satisfaction.

Apart from these individual differences, what factors mediate the relationship between PDM and satisfaction? Our model identifies two basic pathways: an information component and an action component. Though there is some interaction between the two components, separating them makes analysis easier.

The information pathway is concerned with the quantity and type of information one has about one's work. Various sources of information are usually present: policies and procedures about how to do one's job, supervisors, co-workers, and the work itself.

This information is increased through increased participation — PDM gives one more access to work-related information. One can use this information to reduce two troublesome role characteristics: role conflict and role ambiguity (or at least reduce their negative consequences). Role conflict, as we noted above, occurs when two expectations that are part of one's work role are incompatible.[38,39]

Experientially few nurses need much explanation of role conflict: they often answer to two bosses, administrators and physicians. Administrators may expect nurses to hold down costs by questioning physician's orders for excessive laboratory studies whereas physicians expect unquestioning obeisance. A number of studies of nurses have found both causal and correlational relationships between role conflict and satisfaction. By having an active voice on decisions about one's job, one can gain information to help make those conflicting expectations more apparent and negotiate a situation where the demands are reconciled or eliminated. The same holds for role ambiguity (positively stated as "role clarity" in our model).[40-42]

When one is unsure what one is expected to do or how one fits into the organization as a whole, one is experiencing role ambiguity (again, nurses are no stranger to this phenomenon or to its negative impact on satisfaction). PDM provides opportunities to clarify ambiguous dimensions of one's role. But even in cases where conflict or ambiguity cannot be eliminated or reduced, having gained more knowledge through PDM makes people less uncomfortable or dissatisfied with the residual conflict or ambiguity. For example, when employees know which dimensions of their roles are conflictual or ambiguous, PDM apparently gives them more control over how much energy is directed toward ambiguous functions or the ability to redirect rewards to be based on performance of nonconflicting expectations.

Another crucial area on the information pathway is the relationship between performance and reward.[43-45] If one believes there is fairly little linkage between how well that person performs and the organizational rewards she/he receives, then PDM will not have as great an influence on satisfaction. In other words, if a nurse believes that the hospital will not alter his/her rewards (pay, recognition, promotion) regardless of how well or how poorly he/she delivers nursing care, then for that nurse, the opportunity to participate will influence his/her satisfaction less than for a nurse who does believe rewards correspond to performance quality. Alternatively, increased PDM can help employees clarify or create a link between performance and reward, thus heightening their satisfaction. A nurse who participates more may discover that the organization does reward quality performance.

Notice on the model that one arrow leads from challenge to a cluster of three concepts: job involvement, task identity, and internal motivation. These concepts refer to attitudes toward one's work and together and separately they account for part of the relationship between PDM and satisfaction.

Task identity is the perceived importance of one's role in the delivery of the service or creation of the product by the organization.[46,47] When the hospital takes in a patient with angina, chronic fatigue, and potential or actual myocardial infarction and discharges someone with improved coronary perfusion well on the way to rehabilitation, can each nurse see the contribution he or she has made to that process? Increased participation facilitates awareness of that contribution, leading to increased satisfaction.

Job involvement includes three dimensions: (1) how important the job is to the employee; (2) the ambition and energy associated with the job; and (3) the willingness to work apart from extrinsic rewards.[48-52] PDM leads to increased job involvement (and to organizational involvement). More involved employees are more satisfied. PDM contributes to this process by tapping more of the employee's abilities (as we will see when we discuss the action pathway), by engaging him or her on more levels.

Internal motivation is a function of how one's feelings of competence, growth and self-esteem are affected by one's performance.[53-55] Internal motivation is strengthened by PDM in part because the information pathway permits more feedback and facilitates the employee's awareness of the importance of his/her contribution.

The feedback (from supervisors, co-workers, and observing the work process itself) makes it easier to attempt and evaluate changes and performance, and the latter's connection to rewards.

All three of these variables are even more strongly influenced by the action pathway to which we will now turn our attention.

As we have seen, what one knows about one's job affects how satisfied one is with that job. PDM increases the amount of information one has about one's work. But the nature of the work a person does often has an impact on how positively one responds to participation (and, conversely, participation itself changes the quality of one's work).

The two action or task characteristics that have been most researched relative to participation are task difficulty and variability.[56-58] Closely tied to these two is the notion of autonomy or discretion (i.e., how much freedom a nurse has to determine what nursing procedures or methods he/she will use). Task difficulty is usually regarded as a function of the *analyzability* and *predictability* of one's work. When it is fairly easy to know both the nature and sequence of actions to be performed in accomplishing one's goal, the job scores high on analyzability. Doing good skin care on a well-hydrated, conscious, 50-year-old woman hospitalized for an appendectomy is more analyzable than skin care on a confused, cachexic, 90-year-old man with painful bony metastases. Predictability is the degree to which one can anticipate the outcome of a specific series of tasks. Raising the head of the bed, hyperventilating, and administering an osmotic diuretic will usually lower a patient's intracranial pressure. It is not as predictable that information about tomorrow's surgery will lower a patient's anxiety: sometimes it will, sometimes it won't.

Variability reflects the number of exceptions encountered in one's work or how many different tasks one must perform in an average day's work. If each of the surgeons who admit abdominal surgery patients to a unit has a different set of orders regarding dressing changes, then the nurses' work is more variable that if the surgeons agree on a certain protocol.

Autonomy or discretion is a measure of the freedom an employee has to define his or her own tasks or projects, the methods or procedures used to accomplish those tasks, how problems or exceptions will be handled, and what criteria will be used to evaluate performance. This is an important dimension of "professionalism." Depending on the type of shared governance or PDM system being implemented, an individual nurse may gain more discretion (perhaps through a primary nursing system), or a unit may be able to develop its own policies and procedures that reflect the skills and interests of the staff and the nature

of the patient population more accurately than hospital-wide policies.

Together, these three characteristics (difficulty, variety, autonomy) and the role dimensions of conflict and clarity constitute a dimension of "challenge." In other words, when an organizational change leads to nurses' work becoming more difficult, having more variety, and permitting them more autonomy or discretion, their work will be seen as "challenging." When these qualities are present in a mixture that "fits" the individual's abilities and desires (e.g., GNS), the challenge is viewed as a positive dimension.

The arrow from role clarity to challenge reflects the fact that if a role is sufficiently ambiguous, the work can be more frustrating than challenging. In other words, when nurses are unable to gain a clear understanding of their role, they are not likely to see their work as challenging — regardless of the presence of difficulty, variability, and autonomy.

Task identity is a term that, while derived from assembly line type work, still has important implications for nurses. It refers to the ability of someone to see the positive impact of his/her work on the final product. When a patient leaves a unit in better health than he/she entered it, task identity is present for a nurse if he/she can see how nursing care contributed to the patient's improvement.

Task identity seems to be a summary of the individual's evaluation of and reaction to the meaningfulness and importance of the job. As such it is causally dependent upon the degree to which the job provides autonomy and stimulates and involves the occupant in the process of enhancing and acquiring skills and abilities.[59]

Jobs enriched by PDM provide these qualities and also lead to increased internal motivation.

Even setting aside the individual differences discussed earlier, the effects of PDM are different at different organizational levels.[60] Any particular shared governance system is experienced differently by staff nurses, head nurses, and supervisors.

The conclusions about how PDM affects different organizational levels remain unclear. This is largely because participation itself varies by organizational level. For example, if one institutes a model of shared governance that involves a decentralization of decision making to the unit level and measures the impact on, say, staff nurses and head nurses, the two groups may have different reactions. While staff nurses have *more* voice in determining unit policies, the head nurse may find she/he is suddenly only one vote among many rather than being the final arbiter. Middle and upper level managers who feel they are already involved in making many decisions may be either relieved or threatened by the prospect of turning some of these decisions over to others. Top level administrators may have the predictability of their work increased as the impact of actual or potential decisions becomes more apparent through discussions by employees.

In summary, a significant increase in decisional participation can be expected to produce a number of positive outcomes for the employees and the overall organization. When employees are participating in decision making, their satisfaction increases. They can be expected to become more involved in their jobs; their work will become more important to them; they will be more internally motivated and more committed to the organization.[61] These relationships will be stronger for those with strong desires for achievement, responsibility, and autonomy, for those who perceive themselves as decisionally deprived, and for those whose work is more difficult and variable. Over time a reinforcing process can be anticipated: people may come to value autonomy and responsibility more highly and to find their jobs more challenging.

An important caveat, however, is the notion of *significant* participation. The research provides a number of indicators about which work-related variables need to be impacted if a program aimed at achieving PDM is to be effective.

The information pathway reinforces the necessity of the free flow of information *in all directions*. For this to be achieved, members of the organization must have trust that communications with peers, supervisors, and subordinates will be handled in an open, constructive fashion. It must be possible, for example, to air perceived conflicting expectations without fear of defensive or retaliatory responses.[62] People must perceive that their participation has an impact. Most importantly, role conflict and ambiguity should not be resolved through increased routinization — an all too common tendency in our opinion. Routinizing work leads to decreased variety, difficulty, and autonomy, ultimately defeating the central purposes of increased participation. The connection of information with performance cannot be overemphasized: the employee must understand the relationships between performance and reward, how their role contributes to the organization and its services. A participative program cannot expect positive results.

The action pathway emphasizes the importance of challenge. A participative program can increase challenge if it impacts on employees' autonomy (their control over determining methods, tasks, goals). If the intervention promotes variety, taps more of the nurses' abilities, helps them develop new skills, it can also make their work more challenging and hence more satisfying. It is likely, however, that these dimensions must be seen as integral to their work and not just as an overload unrelated to performance and reward. This implies, among other things, that it is essential that staff participate in those decisions which they perceive as being most important to them.

There is little question that given the tremendous differences among health care institutions and the broad range of individuals who work in them, a plethora of creative strategies can be implemented to increase PDM. The research we have summarized here suggests there are a number of exciting gains from implementing PDM programs. Staff nurses and administration can use PDM to create a true "win-win" situation while enhancing professional practice. Though our model of Shared Governance emphasizes both structural and procedural revisions and, we believe, is applicable to a broad range of institutions, *any* intervention directed at promoting participation will more likely produce positive outcomes if it impacts on the organization factors identified in our model.

REFERENCES

1. Allen D. Professionalism, job segregation by gender, and the control of nursing. Women and Politics 1987; 6(3):1-24.

2. Can A. Staff participation in management decision making. Nurse Focus March 1981;2(7):217.

3. Vickenson M. Employee participation in decision making in a hospital organization. Lamp November 1976; 33(11):27-33.

4. Floyd G., Smith B. Job enrichment. Nurs Mgr May 1983; 14(5):22-25.

5. Hatfield B. Participative management. Hospital Topics Jul/Aug 1982; 60(4):6,32,42.

6. Porter-O'Grady T. Creative nursing administration. Rockville, MD: Aspen, 1986.

7. Porter-O'Grady T., Finnigan S. Shared governance for nursing. Rockville, MD: Aspen, 1984.

8. Stevens B. The nurse as executive. 3rd ed., Rockville, MD: Aspen, 1985.

9. Cherniss C., Egnatios E. Participation in decision making by staff in community mental health programs. Am J Community Psychol 1978;6(2):171-190.

10. Althaus JN, Hardyck NM, Pierce PB, Rogers MS. Nursing decentralization: The El Camino experience. Wakefield, MA: Nursing Resources, 1981.

11. Peterson M, Allen D. Shared governance: strategy for transforming organizations (2 parts). J Nurs Adm 1986; 16(1):9-12 (part 1); 1986; 16(2):11-16 (part 2).

12. Cleland V. Shared governance in a professional model of collective bargaining. J Nurs Adm May 1978; 8(5):39-43.

13. Kelley CA. Quality circles in the hospital setting: Their current status and potential for the future. Health Care Mgt Rev 1987; 12(1):55-59.

14. Wellington M. Decentralization: How it affects nurses. Nurs Outlook 1986;34(1):36-39.

15. Aumiller L., Rudloff G. Decentralization reduces absenteeism. J Nurs Adm 1986;16(1):23-27.

16. Fanning JA, Lovett RB. Decentralization reduces nursing administration budget. J Nurs Adm 1985;15(5):19-24.

17. Strauss G. Worker's participation: A symposium. Industrial Relations 1979;18:247-261.

18. Loveridge R. What is participation: A review of the literature and some methodological problems. Br J of Industrial Relations 1980; 18(3)297-317.

19. Gardell B. Worker participation and autonomy: A multilevel approach to democracy at the workplace. Int J Health Services 1982; 12(4):527-558.

20. Alutto J, Acito E. Decisional participation and sources of job satisfaction. Academy of Management Journal 1974; 17:160-167.

21. Cooper M, Wood M. Effects of member participation and commitment in group decision making on influence, satisfaction and decision riskiness. J Appl Psychol 1974; 59:127-134.

22. Dewar R., Werbel J. Universalistic and contingency predictions of employee satisfaction and conflict. Administrative Science Quarterly 1979; 24:426-448.

23. Meadows I. Organic structure, satisfaction, and personality. Human Relations 1980; 33:383-392.

24. Wood R. Participation, influence, and satisfaction in group decision making. J Vocational Behavior, 1972; 2:389-399.

25. Calkin J. Effect of task and structure on nurses' performance and satisfaction. (Doctoral dissertation) University of Wisconsin-Madison, 1980.

26. Lawler E. Job attitudes and employee motivation: Theory, research and practice. Personnel Psychology 1970; 23:223-237.

27. Price J, Mueller C. Professional turnover: The case of nurses. New York: Spectrum, 1981.

28. Abdel-Halim A. Employee affective responses to organizational stress: Moderating effects of job characteristics. Personnel Psychology 1978; 31:561-579.

29. Hackman JR, Oldham G. Development of the job diagnostic survey. J Appl Psychol April 1975; 60(2):159-170.

30. Oldham G, Hackman JR, Pearce J. Conditions under which employees respond positively to enriched work. J Appl Psychol 1976; 61:395-403.

31. Pierce J, Dunham R, Blackburn R. Social systems structure, job design, and growth need strength: A test of a congruency model. Academy of Management Journal 1979; 22:223-240.

32. Bartol K. Individual versus organizational predictors of job satisfaction and turnover among professionals. J Vocational Behavior 1979; 15:55-67.

33. Bartol K. Professionalism as a predictor of organizational commitment, role stress, and turnover. Academy of Management Journal 1979; 22:815-821.

34. Ivancevich J. High and low task stimulating jobs: A causal analysis of performance/satisfaction relationships. Academy of

Management Journal 1979; 22:253-269.

35. Alutto J, Belasco J. A typology for participation in organizational decision-making. Administrative Science Quarterly, 1972; 17:117-125.

36. Alutto J, Vredenburgh D. Characteristics of decisional participation by nurses. Academy of Management Journal 1977; 20:341-347.

37. Cherrington D, England J. The desire for an enriched job as moderator of the enrichment-satisfaction relationship. Organizational Behavior and Human Performance 1980; 25:139-159.

38. Rizzo I, House R, Lirtzman S. Role conflict and ambiguity in compelx organizations. Administrative Science Quarterly 1970; 15:150-163.

39. Schuler R. Role perceptions, satisfaction, and performance moderated by organizational level and participation in decision making. Academy of Management Journal 1977; 20:159-165.

40. Beehr T. Perceived situational moderators of the relationship between subjective role ambiguity and role strain. J Appl Psychol 1976; 61:35-40.

41. Kahn R, Wolfe D, Quinn R, Snoeck J, Rosenthal R. Organizational stress: Studies in role conflict and ambiguity. New York: John Wiley & Sons, 1964.

42. Lyons T. Role clarity, need for clarity, satisfaction, tension, and withdrawal. Organizational Behavior and Human Performance 1971; 6:99-110.

43. Dunham R. Reactions to job characteristics: Moderating effects of the organization. Academy of Management Journal 1977; 20:42-65.

44. Podsakoff P, Tudor W, Skov R. Effects of leader contingent reward and punishment behaviors on subordinate performance and satisfaction. Academy of Management Journal 1982; 25(4):810-821.

45. Schuler R. A role and expectancy model of participation in decision making. Academy of Management Journal 1980; 23:331-340.

46. Sims H, Szilagyi A. Job characteristics: Individual and situational moderators. Organizational Behavior and Human Performance 1976; 17:211-230.

47. Moch M. Job involvement, internal motivation, and employee integration into networks of work relationships. Organizational Be-

havior and Human Performance 1980; 25:15-31.

48. Lawler E, Hall D. Relationships of job characteristics to job involvement, satisfaction, and intrinsic motivation. J of Appl Psycho 1970; 54:305-312.

49. Lodahl R, Kejner M. The definition and measurement of job involvement. J Appl Psychol 1965; 49:24-33.

50. Patchen M. Participation, achievement, and involvement on the job, Englewood Cliffs, NJ: Prentice-Hall, 1970.

51. Ruh R, White K, Wood R. Job involvement, values, personal background participation in decision making, and job attitudes. Academy of Management Journal 1975; 18:300-312.

52. Siegel A, Ruh R. Job involvement, participation in decision making, personal background, and job behavior. Organizational Behavior and Human Performance 1973; 16:318-327.

53. Hackman R, Lawler E. Employee reactions to job characteristics. J Appl Psychol 1971; 55:259-286.

54. Hackman J, Pearce J, Wolfe J. Effects of changes in job characteristics on work attitudes. Organizational Behavior and Human Performance 1972; 15:467-505.

55. Mitchell T. Motivation and participation: An integration. Academy of Management Journal 1973; 16:670-679.

56. March J, Simons H. Organizations. New York: John Wiley & Sons, 1958.

57. Perrow C. A framework for the comparative analysis of organizations. American Sociological Review April 1967; 32:194-208.

58. Van de Ven A, Ferry D. Measuring and assessing organizations. New York: John Wiley & Sons, 1980.

59. Walsh J, Taber T, Beehr T. An integrated model of perceived job characteristics. Organizational Behavior and Human Performance 1980; 25:252-267.

60. Szilagyi A. An empirical test of causal inference between role perceptions, satisfaction with work, performance, and organizational level. Personnel Psychology 1977; 30:375-388.

61. Hrebiniak L, Alutto J. Personal and role related factors in the development of organizational commitment. Administrative Science Quarterly 1972; 17:555-573.

62. Driscoll J. Trust and participation in organizational decision making as predictors of satisfaction. Academy of Management Journal 1978; 21:44-56.

Shared governance: Reality or sham?

TIM PORTER O'GRADY, RN, EdD, CNAA

THE CURRENT SHORTAGE is sprouting a new crop of short-term, but often short-sighted, solutions. While they do sometimes attract nurses who are looking for work, short-term "Band-Aids" do nothing substantive for nurses who are toughing it out long term in one place. Further, these solutions have nothing to do with preparing nurses for the expanded roles they're sure to assume in future professional practice.

Enter shared governance for nursing — the model that offers nurses not just participation but *ownership* in the organization. Nurses at every level play a role in the decisions that affect nursing activity throughout the system. Authority and accountability are shared in a systematic format among all members of the nursing department.

The structure of a shared governance system varies with the institution and with the model it chooses to develop. Usually, councils, congresses, cabinets, or executive groups are created, filled, and chaired by both leadership and nonleadership nursing staff. Through these key groups, clinical staff define, delineate, create, approve, and evaluate all nursing-practice activities and assume full responsibility and accountability for such activities. (For a detailed example of how nurses developed one system, see "Moving to Shared Governance," *AJN,* July 1987, pages 923-926.)

Successful shared governance demands the commitment of every nurse in the organization. Nurses belong to key decision-making groups that deal with issues of practice, quality of care, personnel issues (such as salary and quality of work), staffing, scheduling, recruit-ment, education, and evaluation. They do not need to present their ideas to management; they themselves have the power to implement their decisions in the clinical arena.

Nurse managers move out of their traditional industrial-model roles into a systems model, becoming moderators of the service process as well as facilitators of the nursing process. The staff builds the system for nursing practice, but the manager assures that the system is working.

Usually a structure of rules or bylaws helps to define the system. After the nursing staff passes the rules, the hospital's board of trustees typically approves them, and they become the operating rules of the nursing organization. In some more integrated governance systems, the chief nurse officer of the system's highest congress may also be a member of the board of trustees. A shared governance system also includes management decision-making forums for issues that support practice, such as finances, use of resources, interdepartmental conflicts, and problems with delivery of care.

Shared governance builds on trust — trust in the commitment to high-quality nursing care, trust in the belief that all nurses in the organization constantly seek the very best for their patients and for the profession, and trust in the managers' commitment to keeping the resources, tools, and supports essential for good nursing care in place. Management and clinical teams work closely together to find mutual solutions to care-delivery problems.

Reliance on traditional collective bargaining strategies and on "us versus them" behaviors falls away as all nurses move into the de-

How can you tell the real from the imposter?

REAL GOVERNANCE	THE IMPOSTER
Staff controls practice.	Management defines practice.
Staff are elected by peers to leadership roles.	Management appoints or approves staff leadership.
Staff roles are based on accountability.	Management encourages staff to participate in what managers control or influence.
The nurse executive shares in decision making; does not have or use veto.	The nurse executive has final authority for all decisions in the department.
Staff has a formal organizational structure of control and authority.	Managers chair all formal bodies affecting the nursing department's work.
The nursing organization has a conceptual model (theory base) that clarifies nursing values.	The nursing organization's belief system is undefined; few in the organization value such a process.
The organization is guided by operating bylaws that have been developed by staff and are staff-controlled. They have also been approved by the hospital's board of trustees.	Staff can develop bylaws but they are not both staff- and board-approved and are thus subject to arbitrary change or deletion.
Potential exists for a nursing staff member to represent nursing interests by serving on the board of trustees.	The nurse executive remains the sole representative to the formal leadership, including to the board of trustees.
Staff plays a role in, or has direct input into, issues of wages, budgeting, staffing, and quality of work life.	Salary, staffing, and working conditions remain the exclusive prerogative of management.
Staff has the authority to change its areas of accountability and to enforce its decisions.	Staff advises managers, who may take staff recommendations into consideration. The managers make the decisions or approve the staff recommendations.

cisional mainstream of shared governance. As has been true in the business sector, financial compensation for these nurses will eventually be based less on static wage programs and more on the value of actual service delivered and on productivity.

Ultimately, shared governance structures will enable nurses to shed dependent, voca- tional roles. Instead, nurses will operate and manage their practice as do other front-line professionals. As nurses take strong control of their individual practices, they can approach the policy table with well-defined and well-structured roles and expectations, ready to help write the script for excellent health care delivery in the twenty-first century.

Staff nurse councils, shared governance, and collective bargaining

RICHARD U. MILLER, PhD

Introductions

THE FIRST POINT I want to make this morning is that I am not Barbara Nichols as some of you perhaps expected as the speaker. Barbara has gone off to Geneva for a meeting of the International Council of Nursing, and I agreed to pinch hit. Since my background as an Industrial Relations professor equips me more to deal with collective bargaining issues than Nurse Councils and Shared Governance, I found myself scrambling this week to learn about these subjects.

Among others, I discovered some interesting facts.

For example, it seems almost impossible to find a nursing journal, magazine, or book which doesn't make some reference, in one fashion or another, to shared governance. It is a hot topic to say the least. What's more it also seems to be a panacea for what ails the nursing profession. You want to beat the nursing shortage? Shared governance will do it. It is an antidote for nurses' sense of powerlessness. It is miraculous. It is a dream.

If you forced me to take a position on this, I would probably agree with the dreamers.

What is shared governance?

I found also that as people talk about shared governance there is a babel of tongues — a confusion of terms. Few writers bother to attempt a precise meaning of the term and whether the meaning is expressed or implied, they are often at odds with each other in its coverage or application.

For example, Tim Porter-O'Grady, writing in a book titled "Shared Governance for Nursing" argues that, in the context of professional practice control, shared governance is accountability with control, authority, and autonomy over factors related to the professional's work. In an effort to "smash the organizational pyramid," Porter-O'Grady conceives of a series of functionally based nurses' councils covering such activities as education, practice, quality assurance, and management. The councils establish an organizational base for accountability and control.

What is the role of nursing administration under shared governance as defined by Porter-O'Grady? It becomes "centralized and directed specifically to assure appropriate support for the nursing staff." That is, to provide the resources and assistance required by the staff; to carry out the mandates of the clinical councils; and to incorporate their decisions into operational activities.

Others such as Jeffrey Hill *(Georgia Nursing,* Sept.-Oct. 1986) contend that shared governance is:

> based on a decentralized organizational structure which concentrates increased emphasis on principles of participatory management and the accountability of each individual nursing practitioner in those areas related to both the governance and practice of nursing.

By the way, Porter-O'Grady would dispute the notion that participatory management is consistent with shared governance. He specifically excludes participation in management from his concept of shared governance.

Still others talk in terms of participative decision-making systems which relinquish control and develop adult to adult interactions

(M.E. Peterson, *Nursing Administration Quarterly,* Winter 1983).

And there are still others who see shared governance as self management, self governance, or democracy on the job.

A review of the difference definitions and organizational schemes thus reveals a great variation in concepts, forms, and motivations. Lawrence McLachlan, Labor Counsel for ANA, views nearly all of these approaches with some skepticism, concluding, "There is little clarity, consistency, or uniformity in either the definition or the intended purposes of the melange of concepts collectively identified as 'shared governance.'" Variations in the application range from utopian to a forthright admission (that the primary purpose is) preventing employees from exercising statutory rights of collective bargaining" (*SNA Legal Developments,* Special Report, May 20, 1988).

McLachlan goes on to say, "If the essence of government is the ability to govern rather than to suggest, then, with one exception, shared-governance shows itself to be neither governing nor shared."

Shared governance and power
Whether you accept McLachlan's evaluation or not, it is clear that what we are talking about here is power: power to control; power to decide; power to administer.

Shared governance in all its permutations, and, depending on your point of view, is a system to transfer power from the governors to the governed; from nursing management to staff nurses — or conversely to block that transference of power. Whichever way you are going the name of the game is power.

Collective bargaining and power
We have not mentioned collective bargaining up to this point — but clearly it too is a power game. That is, to transfer power to the union or at least share it under some set of specified circumstances. The primary, if not single, objective for the union in exercising power has been job control. This is such as basic and consistent trait that some observers of American unions have labeled this behavior as business unionism or pure and simple unionism.

Collective bargaining is different from the systems of shared governance briefly mentioned above. While those approaches often obscure or sugarcoat power, in collective bargaining power is made manifest. In nearly every bargaining situation, the forms of power are evident in one manifestation or another: strikes, lockouts, picketing, boycotts, demonstrations, etc.

Traditionally in the U.S., collective bargaining has epitomized adversarial relationships. The old maxim of Management manages and unions grieve sums it up well.

Collective bargaining also has possessed a narrower perspective in the sense that generally the subjects for shared power have been limited to those matters derived from the employment relationship. That is, and this by law, to wages, hours, and other terms and conditions of employment. Shared governance schemes would clearly go far beyond this narrow vision.

For these and similar reasons, collective bargaining and trade unionism have been viewed at best ambivalently by nurses. For example, it is a common belief that collective bargaining is incompatible with professionalism. Some years ago a writer in the *American Journal of Nursing* argued that unionizing nurses made as much sense as unionizing mothers.

Recent changes in labor management relations
Present day collective bargaining is changing however. Unions must now confront tough employers, a world economy in which the hallmark is competition and a labor force by

age, gender, education, and occupation which bears little resemblance to the workers' unions traditionally organized.

One change, however, parallels the movement for shared power in nursing. That is, the recognition that the old forms of power are often ineffective or counterproductive. This realization has led to new attitudes and a search for new forms. As adversarialism and job control unionism have given ground, we now find a proliferation of experiments going on under such names as Quality Circles, Quality of Work Life programs, not to mention a variety of employee involvement and participatory management schemes that are resulting in a radical restructuring of such companies as General Motors, Ford, and Xerox among others.

For example, at the main Pontiac plant of General Motors, work teams have replaced traditional assembly line operations; supervisors have now become team facilitators; and the top level plant administration is a shared responsibility of the union and the former plant manager. For its new Saturn Corporation, under construction in Spring Hill, Tennessee, the United Auto Workers were invited by GM management to jointly design a new system of employee relations. Least we forget, these are the same union and corporation who previously were virtually at war with one another for nearly 50 years.

In Wisconsin, the Harley-Davidson Company is a major local success story of employee involvement as a strategy for survival.

And speaking of Wisconsin, labor management cooperation is now being actively supported by Governor Thompson. In part through his efforts and support, regional labor-management councils are now operating in various parts of the state including one each in Green Bay and Fox River Valley.

Not all organizations, however, have accepted power sharing in any of its guises as witness to the recently settled strike at the International Paper plants, the Cudahy strike, the long bitter strike at Stoughton Trailers, among others. The policy of these companies is union avoidance, and, I have no doubt, the avoidance of power sharing by any name.

The prospects of shared governance in health care

The lessons to be learned from the private sector are clear.

1. In most cases power sharing must be forced over the objections of a reluctant management.

2. Where management has voluntarily and sincerely agreed to power sharing, it has been a deathbed conversion. The very survival of the organization was at stake.

3. The systems have worked only in conjunction with strong and stable unions. In that respect, power sharing beyond job control unionism requires new union attitudes and new management structures that accept and integrate the union into the management structure.

How does this translate into shared governance for nursing?

1. Hospital administration attitudes have frequently and rightfully been characterized as a plantation mentality — overseers dealing with aborigines. Perhaps because of its origins in the old diploma nursing programs together with the high proportion of young, female employees management systems have tended to be paternalistic, authority oriented, and extremely status conscious. The "Docs," of course, strongly reinforce these attitudes. In view of this latter point, I found it curious that, in the various articles I read, little was said about how to get the doctors to agree to giving up their rights and privileges — that is to say, to share power or, as Porter O'Grady would have them do, capitulate completely to a series of nurses' councils.

2. In a similar fashion the typical hospital organizational structure does not seem to lend

itself to nurses' self-management. Power, authority, and control are divided between the medical staff, the administrative group and the trustees. Where does a nurses' council fit into this structure? Which, if any of these other units in the organization, will willingly share, or cede, its power to the nurses?

3. Next, one must consider the emergence of the multiunit, "for-profit" hospital corporations in any evaluation of power sharing or transference. Corporations like HCA, Humana, and the like, are themselves mass, centralized concentrations of power in which return on earnings and the price of stock is, indeed, the bottom line. What of the dream of nurses' self-governance under these circumstances?

4. Finally, there are the HMOs, PPOs, and related prepaid medical organizations where cost control and efficiency are the watchwords and where power may be wielded by an administrative clerk. One quickly gets a lesson in HMO power politics from a brief conversation to the Doc who has been reprimanded for ordering too many tests or prescribing too much medicine not subject to the HMO's approval. The weight of bureaucratic rules, standards, and controls is the source of power in these health care organizations. As such, by what process or structure will this power to govern be shared with others, particularly when they may not even possess full employee status?

Is there hope for shared governance?
Despite the efforts to hold the line in the cost of health care through the HMOs, PPOs, the system of DRGs and the like, the price of treatment and caring continues to climb at a rate far surpassing that of other goods and services. It was recently announced in Wisconsin, for example, that health insurance premiums would go up more than 40 percent for standard plans and 25/30 percent for many Health Maintenance policies. Moreover, the circumstances of many Americans with no health insurance grows worse.

Health care providers thus stand on the brink of economic and regulatory disaster no less severe than that experienced by counterpart organizations in such industries as electronics, automotive manufacturing, etc. This situation offers to nurses both a challenge even to the existing distribution of power as well as an opportunity to achieve a basis for a more equitable sharing.

On the one hand, the opposition of many health care managers to whatever form power sharing might take, unionized or otherwise, will harden. Healthcare is already an industry which, particularly through management consultants, has bitterly fought the ANA, other Nurse organizations and traditional unions from acquiring representation rights among its workforce. The managers will see the current economic and regulatory climate as one which will necessitate complete unilateral control of nursing practice, staffing, compensation, and education matters. Change will come only through force that few health care employee associations or unions can now muster.

On the other hand, opportunities for change will also present themselves. As experience in the private sector reveals, this will probably occur in conjunction with strong nursing organizations whose leaders, and those of management, are ready to discard combative attitudes.

It is unlikely, however, that what results will bear much resemblance to councilar systems of nurses' self management as advocated by Porter-O'Grady. First of all, I do not think these models are feasible for reasons already pointed out. Secondly, even if they were, they would be counterproductive in the long run. It is an irony that the councils represent a form of job control which few unions, even in their heyday, were able to achieve. The councils embody job control that is now being rapidly abandoned elsewhere in the face of the need for workforce flexibility and efficiency.

More probable than the councils will be a series of more modest steps embodying such employee involvement devices as the Quality Circle jointly created by the SEIU and administrators at Booth Memorial Hospital in Flushing, New York. In many cases also participatory and shared governance systems will grow from existing patient care committees, staffing pattern committees, professional practice committees, and the like.

While these steps lack the glamour of their more radical power sharing models, they also are more likely to succeed in the long run. Particularly when these steps are institutionalized and protected within a collective bargaining environment, they provide a means by which adversarial attitudes can change; decision making skills can be learned; and both staff nurse and manager integrate their efforts for the betterment of all concerned.

Nursing's vision in a competitive environment

WALTER J. MCNERNEY

GREAT STRIDES HAVE BEEN made in patient care in the past 10 years, and nursing clearly has played a prominent role in these advances. Nursing serves an essential function equal to that of the best of the professions. The role of the nurse has grown in importance with the advent of new technology and new delivery sites (home care, extended care, etc.). This role requires more sophisticated and better-educated practitioners.

In many institutions morale among nurses is not what it should be, and there are fewer applications to schools of nursing. Although many causes can be cited for this situation, I believe it can be attributed in many cases to poor governance and management. Too often, communication links are weak among the Board of Trustees, hospital administration, medical staff and nursing. Administrators, who often are preoccupied with costs, downsizing, restructuring, mergers, diversification, and so on, have lost sight of the basics, including the pervasive importance of a sound nursing program.

Nurses should become involved strategically in board, executive management and medical staff affairs. Not only should nurses be on the cutting edge of quality assessment, risk management and other new programs, but also they should be given the responsibility for managing key resources required to provide high-quality patient care. In addition, nurses should be recognized for service and leadership through career advancement programs. In too many cases, these conditions do not exist.

Professions can prosper in an institutional environment. Management structures and professions are compatible, given the right amount of discipline and leadership, and in fact, a well-managed institution can unleash more energy through synergism than individual or small group efforts, even though at times this does not seem to be the case.

Comments on visions of nursing's future

Some nurse leaders assert that nurses operate with autonomy of practice (*not* as MD assistants or administrative agents). This assertion is appropriate if the autonomy is maintained within institutional and professional guidelines. All of us are autonomous in this sense, but it does not follow that nurses are *per se* autonomous.

I doubt seriously that institutional arrangements will evolve to a few dozen national or international companies. Health is and will remain, essentially, a local and regional "business." The shift to for-profit companies will not be pervasive, but both for-profit and not-for-profit institutions will be brought under closer surveillance as will the entire subject of MD conflict of interest. We will have not only stronger buyer voices, but also better-informed voices. The projected role for the nurse as a provider of services, developer of new knowledge, care manager and executive, and diagnostician and professional intervener is aggressive and bold; however, perhaps it should be made clearer that whatever evolves with have to be earned, not proclaimed, in the pragmatic world of what works and what does not.

There has been reference to nursing's "exclusive knowledge base." I am uncertain what is meant by that, but I am sure that the public is increasingly wary of territorial aspirations by professionals or others. Although professionals must be prepared in self-governance, as opposed to self-management, I have reservations if this is interpreted as becoming autonomous, instead of self-reliant. Some nurses believe that reimbursement systems should pay directly for nursing services through contracts and that such payments will validate the nurse's "worth." I am not certain what this assertion means. Many professionals are paid salaries; in fact, the number is increasing, but certainly, professionalism does not equate to direct payment.

A preferred vision of the future that suggests that the nurse should be more professional, more autonomous, and more independent and should perform a wider scope of sophisticated functions, acting as the primary pathway for patient interaction, is problematic. I question the feasibility of a profession asserting itself this grandly in today's competitive world.

Projections for economic, social, and political change

In the early '80s, the health care field began in earnest the transition from a cottage industry to a more dynamic, competitive one. Frustrated by major cost increases, public and private institutions paying for health care services became more cost conscious. The President effectively dismantled planning programs, favoring deregulation to open market entry, and encouraged competition. As the territory became more precious, competition increased, and more sophisticated buyers were able to choose among a growing number of options. Segmentation and some market shake-outs started to occur.

In search of economy of scale, access to capital and better control, providers integrated vertically and linked horizontally, generating new enthusiasm for managed care and often linking delivery and financing of care. Multihospital systems grew in number, spanned by holding companies. Inevitably, price sensitivity increased and, in conjunction, use of the most expensive facilities and services (inpatient care) dropped. Armed with a better data base, the buyer assumed control, looking upon providers more as vendors subject to a new variety of buyer specifications than as public functionaries.

There are few signs on the horizon to indicate that this trend will abate significantly. No major legislative reforms are in sight, and public and private buyers of care feel that there is still water in the system; further, providers have been "demythed." The mood of the country, which shifted away from the great society programs in the '70s, still supports market as well as selected regulatory forces.

Competitive forces are driving the field in three directions: vertically integrated and horizontally linked health systems at the local and regional levels; niching institutions seeking special market advantages, e.g., birthing centers, reference labs or home nursing corporations; and modifications of traditional configurations. Behind each strategy there is an impelling force. To cite one example, hospitals that are vertically integrating are seeking income to compensate for losses of inpatient revenue. They are reaching out to solidify old territory or acquire new, such as through strategically positioned primary care centers or physicians' offices.

Further, they are hedging against market shifts (and thus, becoming more attractive to bond markets) and are paving the way for HMO or PPO development. The shifts we have seen and some of those that lie ahead have basic market roots. They are not a fad. They have upset old pathways and created higher risks for all players. Consequently, they have produced considerable anxiety among the professions.

The implications for health institutions are increasingly clear. Governance and management must boldly pursue their initiatives, based on aggressive strategic planning, human resource planning, marketing, quality assurance programs, management information systems, productivity efforts and other initiatives. Loose, collegial links tying physicians to hospitals must be strengthened through physician representation on boards, more full-time and part-time positions and joint ventures. Collegiality has palpable limits in a competitive world. Under cost reimbursement and UCR (usual, customary and reasonable) payments, in which the inefficient and efficient were rewarded equally, it was a different matter. Increasingly, physicians with multiple appointments will be required to choose sides as the plans of individual institutions on systems become more proprietary and privileged.

While the odds favor strong market forces in the years ahead, there are unresolved issues that could signal a return to more regulations and less competition. It is a matter of balance. We are making poor progress against the large numbers of underserved. Medicare pays only a portion of the bill for the aged, and Medicaid covers less than 40 percent of those whose income falls below the poverty line. The number of uninsured individuals is increasing, and few retirement health benefit plans are funded. Long-term care for the elderly is poorly financed and often poorly administered, and concerns about quality of care are growing. Tort liability has affected doctor/patient relations. Also, difficult ethical questions have arisen out of our increased ability to preserve life. Because there is some ambivalence about whether to treat health care as an economic good or as a social good, escalation of any one of the above issues could affect the current balance between competition and regulation.

In any event, the less demanding days of the '60s and '70s are over. Under any reasonable scenario, health care institutions will have to be governed and managed more rigorously.

Professionals will have to become more sophisticated about survival and growth under new ground rules.

Implications for nursing

There are many lessons inherent in what is happening in the health field today. A few of these particularly deserve note in the context of the vision of a preferred nursing future.

First, it is essential for all professionals to make the transition emotionally from a cost-reimbursement environment, an era of being all things to all people and of wish lists, to a competitive, price-sensitive world. The differences between a world dominated by the provider and the profession and one dominated by the buyer are critically important. We must keep in mind that markets are much crueler task-masters than professions are.

Not all leaders are meeting the challenge. The turnover rate among hospital administrators, deans, nurse directors and leaders, and physician leaders is high. Many simply can't cope with the risks and uncertainties of the new market. In the '60s and '70s, many became used to defining their own future. Often money was of little importance. There was room to expand all disciplines, including nursing.

In this vein, we must all learn to accept that it is critically important to understand that the doctor and nurse are no longer on a pedestal; the power has swung toward emerging health systems. Health care is becoming more institutionalized and, to a certain extent, commercialized and privatized. Pathways to the patient are being challenged from several directions, and no profession can take its territory for granted. Competitive markets are more open to new entries, particularly where economies can be affected. Professionalism is respected but results count more; if the elite nurse or physician or others fail, they will be replaced by new skills or technologies with fewer barnacles attached.

Increasingly sophisticated buyers are shopping for value; however, they will not abuse quality in the process. In fact, it is highly likely that quality of care will improve as cost increases decelerate. The buyer will be considerably aided by new data bases that will probe not only institutional costs of medical procedures but also variations in a variety of use or cost patterns. Arguments over whether all-RN staffs are more efficient will be testable, and some balloons will be punctured in the process.

Still in this vein, we must understand that *all* professions within the health field are being bruised as competition increases. Furthermore, injury is not confined to the health field. College presidents competing for students have had to become concerned with merchandizing. In recent years, businessmen have had to struggle to meet sharp domestic and foreign competition.

In turn, many businessmen blamed government or trade barriers for their problems and only now are they facing the fact that better management and higher productivity are the only sure ways to gain their way back into the market. Like business, the health field is on the edge of blaming others, both within and outside of the field. It is important that we get through this zone of paranoia as quickly as possible, or bad decisions will result.

Second, we must accept the fact that in a competitive environment, it is essential that the mission be rooted in an environmental analysis of buyer needs, competition analysis and legislative analysis, rather than in individually projected needs. And, process must be paid as much attention as direction. It is essential to set a course, plan strategically, manage aggressively, be bold about new initiatives, and take some risks. The focus must be on effectiveness, not on status. The buyer wants to save money, but more than that, he wants to transfer risk through incentive payment, including capitation. This will, per

force, drive a greater provider interest in productivity as well as quality, which is turn will require *management*.

Currently, nursing is excessively tied up with form rather than substance. An increasing number (some 40 or more) of national associations reflect different prejudices and opinions on education, credentialing, standards of practice and defining the profession. Much creative energy is being grounded debating these differences, as if each point were immutable or precise solutions existed. In institutions that finance and/or deliver care, short-term solutions will increasingly be found in the light of everyday patient or buyer needs or coping with competitors.

Third, a word of caution about moving to a more strategic orientation: The changes called for require considerable skill and courage to implement. Often such changes are blocked actively or passively by the fearful and inefficient who offer various excuses about red tape and the rights of professions or simply refuse to respond. The shift from collegiality to a more businesslike format is viewed like a surgical intervention.

After the transition to a strategic orientation is made, many people tend to treat missions and goals as unchangeable when, in fact, they should change as conditions change, because they are rooted in demand and consumer needs. Strategic planning should be a dynamic management process, not one bogged down in bureaucracy.

Fourth, as implied above, it is important to stop looking for answers mainly from national perches. Hospitals and health systems vary considerably by locality and region, as do the markets they serve. Thus, there are varying configurations of structure, management, vertical and horizontal integration, HMOs, PPOs, and entrepreneurial niche players. Varying emphasis is placed on health promotion, acute care, extended care, dying care and maintenance care, and these programs are linked in different configurations. Furthermore, various forms are evolving constantly in response to changing market demands.

Such an environment of change calls for good grounding in the basics and flexibility. It underscores the need for a liberal education and an overlay of nursing practice education which links such disciplines as organizational behavior, management and health policy. Experimentation with different educational models and evaluation is needed to assure maximal adjustment of new graduates to the job.

Intercourse between various disciplines such as what has been done with combined MBA/MD and MPH/MBA programs is necessary. Master's degrees and doctorates should be sought in other departments as well as in nursing per se, or in new degrees that create bridges between nursing and others. Clearly, continuing education to keep nurses up-to-date assumes new importance.

Various patterns of nursing practice and administration should be tried out and evaluated. Neither in education nor in practice will orthodoxy be beneficial. The demand for sophistication and flexibility will increase.

None of my comments above is intended to imply that a floor isn't needed under the professional nurse. Nurses will be needed to manage patients, units and programs, to make patient evaluations and to prescribe courses of action. Such nurses will clearly require baccalaureate preparation, given the demands of management, the pace of technology, and the sophistication required for independent judgments. Added training in specialized areas will be needed.

Nurses with less education can continue to provide support and make technical contributions. However, to view both levels as the same is to ignore the fact that professional nursing must compete for the hearts and souls of young persons against medicine, law, engineering and business. A higher floor is needed

for the professional nurse both because the job demands it and because such a level is necessary to attract the talent capable of doing the job. At the same time, strategies for more challenging career paths and appropriate pay scales must be implemented; the professional nurse will have to become a more integral part of management, governance, and medical staff affairs. The signals are unmistakable. Talented women are not applying to nursing degree programs in large numbers, and it is increasingly clear that high-morale hospitals involve the nurse liberally at all levels.

The variable pattern locally will provide room for the entrepreneurial nurse who, individually or collectively, sells his or her services to, for example, hospitals or home care institutions. Other skills will find similar niches, for example, within ambulatory surgical units owned by physicians.

Fifth, tomorrow's environment will call for more teamwork (use autonomy) at every level. Physicians have started the institutionalization process. Approximately one-half are on salary full- or part-time. Solo practice is phasing out and physician groups are moving in. Many are joining hospitals in marketing health services. A growing number of HMOs are demanding predictable, organized care. As incentive payment grows, the need to link institutions, doctor and nurse productivity will increase. For reasons of efficiency, quality assurance, liability, and access, the tight-rope nurses walk between physicians and management will become easier to handle. Nurses who want to leave management and become practitioners should do so, but it is increasingly clear that the majority will be institutionally employed. Focus should center on how to make that employment productive.

In a broader context, nursing won't solve its problems by debating about what 2010 will bring precisely or what impact technology will have. No one is able to gauge the future with certainty. Rather, it will be necessary to make long-range assumptions and to examine them periodically.

To cope with change, nursing will have to learn better how to manage change at both the institutional and association levels and to re-gear the profession accordingly. Just as the AMA and AHA are rethinking their structure and roles, so should nursing. Currently, some factions in nursing are debating role apart from first-class strategic planning, keyed off those who will be served (or who pay). This approach is self-serving and fails to meet mar-ket demands and needs where the rewards lie.

Young women and men will not be at-tracted to a fortressed profession. More than ever before, young people are seeking oppor-tunity and creative outlets per se, not opportu-nities for self-denial and orthodoxy. They place more faith in professionals and institu-tions that can manage change than in those that react against it.

The hurdles ahead are not insurmountable. Although an increasing supply of doctors and other skilled professionals will result in more territorial concerns, nurse practitioners and midwives and others are slowly gaining a foot-hold state by state. Buyers are demanding requisite skills, at minimum costs; many doc-tors are overtrained and too expensive for what they do. Insurance companies are opening up to new professions and are lessening hurdles such as physician management and/or supervi-sion. In effect, they are more inclined to allow market forces and consumer satisfaction deter-mine courses of action. Progress is being made, but achieving a more professional status will take time.

An increasing number of female physicians and more full-time, security-minded medical practitioners will blunt the male/female factor and blur the distinctions between doctors, nurses and others. Patients will be open to more objective appraisal of service and cost. Although the nursing shortage may give the nurse some leverage, in no way will it over-come the need for productivity and response to market demands. The need for the specialized skills of nursing will increase, with greater emphasis on care of patients with diseases of middle and advanced age and dealing with ex-panding technology.

Nursing is clearly achieving success, as can be seen in the recent establishment of the Cen-ter for Nursing Research. Nursing expertise is being sought in identifying ways to improve the quality of home care (IOM study), and sev-eral nurses are being appointed to key posi-tions. But, much work remains to be done.

Conclusion

Let me underscore the fact that none of my remarks, which heavily emphasize manage-ment of change, is meant, in any way, to drain nursing of its ideals or its service orientation. A good nurse or a good physician must be compassionate and empathetic. However, we must understand also that the best of our ef-forts in a competitive market will require a structure for and skill at decision making. Without these tools, any professional group will become increasingly vulnerable. It may not be too brash to assert that without structure and discipline, the best of intentions and most compassionate claims can become ineffective if not unrealistic.

Clinical ladder program builds self-esteem

JUDY HOUGAARD, RN, MS

IMPLEMENTATION OF THE clinical ladder completed the list of goals I set for the Department of Nursing at St. Mark's Hospital, Salt Lake City, when I accepted the position of assistant administrator nine years ago.

This goal has been achieved, the culmination of efforts of many people. For the most part, I have been pleased with the results and believe our objectives have been met. Since we are in the evaluative phase of our program, these remarks will explain how I think the clinical ladder has benefited the nurse, the patient and the hospital.

Benefits for the nurse

One of the most positive outcomes of the program is the pride nurses feel when they advance to a higher level. The portfolios the nurses have prepared about their work have been excellent, much more detailed and complete than we had expected. By documenting their practice in portfolios, the nurses have been forced to recognize their accomplishments, a process enhancing the self-esteem of nurses who have chosen to "ladder."

Another benefit is the change I see in the perspective of the nurse. As nurses choose to move up the ladder, their perspective becomes much broader. This reminds me of the change in myself between the time I gained the B.S. in nursing — and thought I was as smart and capable as a master's-prepared nurse — and the time I entered graduate school. In the master's program, I did not necessarily gain a much larger body of knowledge, but I gained a broader perspective on nursing, and that broadened my scope of resources. Nurses moving up the clinical ladder are also achieving a new perspective.

The third important benefit I call professional behavior. Nurses who have "laddered" have a much higher level of professionalism than before. As many of us know, the negative attitude of just one nurse can disrupt an entire unit. A nurse seeking advancement must demonstrate and encourage cooperation with peers, management and interdepartmental units, a criterion that leads nurses to create a supportive, positive attitude.

It would be wonderful to say I have been pleased with every aspect of the program, but I must express my disappointment that nurses generally do not support each other. When a nurse tells me she does not want "Clinical Nurse II" on her name badge because her peers ridicule her or tell her to take all the hard patients because "you're making more money and you're a Clinical Nurse II," it is disheartening.

Benefits for the patient

The clinical ladder program provides nurses an incentive to perform at a higher level in delivery of care, a major benefit to the patient. A review board studies the portfolio of each nurse wanting to move up the clinical ladder. Sitting in on a meeting of a review board, I was amazed at the portfolio of an operating room nurse who completed a beautiful patient teaching plan based on adult learning principles. Often, many of us look at operating room nurses as very task-oriented, but this nurse went well beyond what was expected, with a successful patient outcome.

The clinical ladder program also clearly defines the expectations of nurses by providing distinct, measurable criteria. Nurses know exactly what is expected and have a detailed guide for carrying out the nursing process. This must result in more effective care.

Benefits for the hospital

The major benefit for the hospital derives from the way nurses in the clinical ladder program are reimbursed. Financial rewards for the nurse are based on performance and productivity, as well as the nurse's contributions to the organization by serving on committees, completing projects and/or representing the hospital in community service. Traditionally, rewards have been based on tenure rather than performance and productivity.

The hospital also benefits from the public relations mileage that comes from having a successful program. I receive calls almost daily about some aspect of the program.

In this time of nursing shortage, the hospital benefits because the clinical ladder program focuses on key elements in job satisfaction — payment and recognition — thus promoting retention of nurses. The program also helps the hospital keep skilled clinical nurses at the bedside by rewarding those nurses who choose to remain in clinical nursing rather than rewarding them only if they move on to management or some other form of nursing. The nurse has an incentive to advance in clinical nursing as a professional career option.

With the implementation of the clinical ladder program, all my original objectives were met, but the importance of evaluation cannot be overstated. Once implementation has begun, evaluation must begin. Our success will continue only as we evaluate and refine our program to meet the needs of nurses in the changing hospital environment.

Staff nurses rate clinical ladder program

PATRICIA S. HARTLEY, RN, MS; DIANE CUNNINGHAM, RN, MS

THE CLINICAL LADDER has been in place at St. Mark's Hospital, Salt Lake City, for about a year. As explained in the July-August 1988 issue of *The American Nurse,* the clinical ladder has four levels of practice, with Level 1 encompassing the entry level staff nurse and those who meet minimum practice requirements. Progress to further levels is voluntary. In this article, the term "leveled" applies to nurses who have advanced beyond Level 1; they are actively using the clinical ladder.

As part of the evaluation process, integral to the program, staff nurses were asked how the clinical ladder was working to meet their needs. Personal interviews were conducted with staff nurses who had leveled and those who had not yet advanced beyond Level 1. A representative sample was chosen from each group for the interview process.

Staff nurses who have advanced on the clinical ladder were eager to talk about their experience, offering insight into problems they had faced with the review process. In general, they supported the program and readily discussed its strengths. This group included some staff nurses who were on the review board determining whether nurses could advance on the ladder. The board members were the program's most enthusiastic supporters.

Non-leveled staff, those not using the ladder, gave mixed reactions to being interviewed. One refused to be interviewed because she had negative feelings about the clinical ladder. Since they were not advancing in the program, some wondered why they were being interviewed, but most agreed to the interview once its purpose was clear. In general, the non-leveled staff were not well informed about the program. On some units, no one has leveled; however, some are now in the process of leveling.

The accompanying chart shows the interview questions and summarized responses. The answers from both nurses using the ladder and those not using it have given us an excellent foundation to work from in the process of evaluation. We plan to revise and strengthen the program in the following ways:

• Extend the interviews to all nursing staff through formal questionnaires.

• Revise generic and unit-specific criteria to reduce redundancy and clarify expectations.

• Plan in-service sessions and handouts to help direct staff who want to advance on the clinical ladder.

• Streamline the evaluations required by peer reviewers.

• Encourage the development of unit-based support groups.

We are encouraged that staff have gained so much from this program and that the results have been consistent with our original program goals. The interviews have given us feedback and direction for the future. Our focus on staff involvement has proven essential to the continued success of our program.

Staff nurses' assessment of the clinical ladder

	NURSES USING THE CLINICAL LADDER	NURSES NOT USING THE CLINICAL LADDER
How is the clinical ladder beneficial to you as a staff nurse?	• Improves my ability to communicate with patients, explain what I do as a nurse and why. • Stimulates me to be more professionally involved, more aware of and active in the work of the nursing department. • Makes nursing more professional. • Helps me gain more clinical expertise. • Gives me an opportunity to advance my career and stay at the bedside. • Improves my charting and better reflects what I do for patients. • Provides recognition, acknowledges going "above and beyond" having a job, more like having a career.	• Increases the salary potential. • Increases professionalism. • Provides a mechanism to update my nursing practice. • Symbolizes status. • Improves my patient teaching skills. • Not worth the time and effort.
How does the clinical ladder benefit the patient?	• Increases awareness by nurses of avenues to help patients get the care they need and want. • Encourages nurses to extend themselves to meet patient needs (individualized care). • Provides more knowledgeable nurses who administer care with greater expertise. • Gives patients more awareness of services being provided and the expertise involved in the nursing profession.	• Provides more knowledgeable caregiver. • Stimulates better patient care. • Encourages more patient teaching. • Makes no difference because there are good nurses who haven't "laddered" yet.
How does the clinical ladder benefit the hospital?	• Increases satisfaction with care, which reflects well on the hospital. • Stimulates nurses to become more familiar with policies and procedures. • Attracts to the hospital nurses who want a career at the bedside. • Promotes loyalty to the institution through recognition activities and financial rewards.	• Increases the professionalism of nurses. • Creates a more dynamic learning atmosphere. • Serves as a good recruitment and retention tool. • Shows that the hospital is progressive. • Provides more opportunities for nurses.

continued

Staff nurses' assessment of the clinical ladder *continued*

	NURSES USING THE CLINICAL LADDER	NURSES NOT USING THE CLINICAL LADDER
What are your plans concerning the clinical ladder?	• Nurses who have moved up the ladder plan to stay involved in the program. Some plan continued advancement; others are happy with their current level. Some plan to advance in six months.	• My timing problems have been addressed and I plan to "ladder" the next time. • I have been at the hospital a long time and was making a good salary, so the program didn't seem worth it to me. However, the salary range has been increased and that is appealing to me. • I am not going to "level" unless I top out at my level. The money isn't a motivating factor to me. If I am going to advance, I'll do it for my professional growth, not the money. • It's not worth the time and effort. It doesn't measure whether I'm a good nurse or not. • I am embarrassed to ask my peers to review me.
What are the clinical ladder program's strengths?	• Promotes integrity of the review process, fair to all. • Provides the opportunity for nurses to have career advancement and stay at the bedside. • Encourages competence and gaining more knowledge. • Encourages professional involvement. • Makes us nurses more informed about expectations and the nursing profession. • Provides a good advancement tool.	• Focuses on the things you need to do to keep current and be a better nurse. • Provides leveling opportunities twice a year. • Demonstrates a good peer review process. • Provides a wide salary range. • Encourages nurses to participate in patient teaching. • Allows nurses to advance in nursing without leaving the bedside. • I can't think of any strengths. • It doesn't force nurses to "level"; it is a professional issue.
What are the clinical ladder program's weaknesses?	• The required evaluation forms ask redundant questions (the most consistent criticism). • Puts peer reviewers in a tough spot—they don't want to be responsible if someone is not promoted. • Involves too much paperwork for promotion. • Requires refining to reflect all that we do. • I can't think of any.	• I resent having to prove to someone else that I am a good nurse. • Too much paperwork. • Some people aren't honest in the peer review process because they are afraid of repercussions. • Timing process for salary adjustments. • Doesn't accurately measure the quality of patient care.

Staff nurses' assessment of the clinical ladder *continued*

	NURSES USING THE CLINICAL LADDER	NURSES NOT USING THE CLINICAL LADDER
How would you change the clinical ladder program?	• Promote it to other staff through mechanisms to help them with the process. • No change needed. The program was thorough.	• More efficient documentation. • Anonymous peer review process. • Only coordinators should pick the peer reviewers. • Change the amount of work peer reviewers have to do. • Streamline the paperwork in general. • Have some kind of test we can take.
Would the clinical ladder be a factor in seeking a position at another hospital?	• I would ask if another hospital had a clinical ladder, but don't know how much a factor it would be in my decision to work there. • Most hospitals have clinical ladders now.	• Not unless I had topped out in my salary range.

Career paths of nurses:
When is a nurse no longer a nurse?

LEIGH WINTZ, RN, BSN

WHEN DOES A NURSE cease to be a nurse and become something else? Is Sheila Burke, Senator Dole's Chief of Staff, an "ex-nurse" as a recent *Washington Post* headline[1] would have us believe? Has her career path carried her beyond the boundaries of her role as a nurse? From another perspective, is the Vice President for Nursing Services still a nurse or is she an administrator of nurses? If the Vice President for Nursing becomes Chief Executive Officer of the hospital is he/she still a nurse? Is it appropriate for nurses to aspire to this position as a nursing career goal?

What are the boundaries of nursing?

The literature reveals our uncertainty about the boundaries of nursing. Robinson-Smith[2] states that one of the advantages of a nursing career is the wealth of options for work, including the following alternative or nontraditional careers in nursing: private practice, home care agency nurses, nurse editors, nurse recruiters, advertising/sales representatives, and continuing education nurses. Today's health care system also provides nurses with careers in quality assurance, utilization review, risk management, materials management, and HMO administration. Powell[3] proposes that nurses are in an excellent position to identify, develop, and market services or products to meet consumer needs in a "high touch-high tech" environment. These opportunities will combine skills in nursing, administration, marketing, and entrepreneurship. Scott[4] claims that the time is right for nurses to move into senior management.

The future of nursing rests with pioneers who forge new career paths by extending their responsibilities beyond the traditional limits of nursing administration, education, research, and clinical practice. Will these nurses still have careers in nursing?

Several authors[5-8] discuss career planning, but only Morrison and Zebelman[9] attempt to define a nursing career. They arrived at their definition by combining definitions of career with an unspecified philosophy of nursing. Nursing career was defined as "a life-long professional commitment to excellence in practice in which the individual nurse can be flexible in meeting the needs of work, self, and family as these needs vary throughout adult life." The authors present a framework for examining the stages of the career process. Their view of nursing, however, seems narrow, and their framework is applied only to providers of direct patient care.

How far can nurses roam from the bedside and still be considered to have a career in nursing? Nursing theorists such as Johnson, King, Orem, Roy, Rogers, Travelbee, and Paterson and Zderad[10] describe nursing as interacting with individuals or groups concerning their health state. Their definitions do not allow nurses to pursue a career path that strays very far from direct interaction with the patient, client, or consumer. Would these theorists include the nurse who designs computer software packages for nursing care plans or patient classification systems? How about nurses who are hired as lobbyists, health care policy analysts, or employees of Nursing Associations? Would the authors of community health texts that state nurses work to improve the health of target populations include or exclude these roles from nursing practice?

With health care delivery systems in a state of flux, nurses need to shape new positions and develop competencies in fields that will be in high demand. Without thought to the profession, nurses attempting to forge new careers in this turbulent environment run the risk of confusing peers and consumers even further about the role of nursing. Nursing will be an integral part of the new health care delivery system, but as Coleman, et al. ask, "Will nurses be caught in giant corporate webs or become principals in spinning them?"[11] Nurses following nontraditional career paths could benefit from knowledge that their profession considers them to be contributing, active members, not lost sheep who have strayed from the fold.

Developing nursing career paths

Smith[12] supports the belief that career development in nursing is a professional as well as an individual responsibility if we are to fulfill nursing's role in the planning and delivery of health care services. Unfortunately, little has been written about nursing career paths, so one must look to sources outside the profession for guidance.

Dalton et al.,[13] in their study of professionally trained employees (scientists, engineers, accountants and professors), identified four distinct career stages that seem to apply equally to men and women in a variety of professional fields.

Stage I involves mastering basic tasks and learning both formal and informal channels of communication. In this stage, the employees' primary relationship is that of being a subordinate. Employees most successful at this stage adopt a mentor that becomes a role model and learn to deal with the fact that there is much boring, routine work in any job, even for a professional. Nursing has formalized this mentor role in many institutions with preceptor programs.

Stage II finds the professional making the transition to independence. Peer relationships assume greater importance. It is during this stage that the decision to specialize may be made. Technical competence is the most important task to be mastered, and the professional's reputation established at this stage affects any future advancement. Kramer, in her book on reality shock,[14] describes this stage as "social integration." Some people never move beyond this stage of technical competence. Their orientation to work becomes that of a job rather than a career over time. Many nurse administrators are all too familiar with staff members who fit this description. We have even nicknamed them "appliance nurses" because they are only working to purchase a new appliance, make home improvements, or send a child to college. They show little interest in clinical ladders or in-service programs that expand their professional horizons.

In Stage III, the employee becomes a mentor for others and finds his interests and capabilities broadening. At this level, the employee deals with people outside the organization for the benefit of those within the organization. Stage III people often find themselves being pulled away from technical work, sometimes with real ambivalence. How far from technical work should one move? What further preparation is needed if they assume new nontechnical roles? Most of us probably know several nurse managers who demonstrate this ambivalence by continuing to work an occasional shift at the bedside, "just to keep their hand in."

Stage IV people are influential, key people throughout the organization. These professional people were found by Dalton et al. to play at least one of three key roles: manager, internal entrepreneur, or idea innovator. The work these people do and the decisions they make shape the organization, or at least a key part of it. They develop future influentials, and they are heavily involved in strategic external relationships that benefit the organization. Successful transition to this stage is dependent on relinquishing close control of day to day operations and being comfortable with using power to shape the future (a task often difficult for women). Most nurse executives will find themselves at Stage IV, but they need to be alert to identify and use other influential professionals to expand nursing's domain within health care organizations.

The entry level for any nurse's career path is the basic, general body of knowledge gained in the nursing program. The next step, choosing a career path and acquiring that combination of education and experience necessary to successfully travel this path, is less clear for nurses today than in years past. The traditional path was staff nurse, charge nurse, head nurse, associate director, and director. Now there are a multiplicity of specialized roles and what steps one is to follow on a given career path are less clear. For instance, how can an aspiring nurse plan a career in quality assurance? Even for the novice aspiring to the current equivalent of the traditional Director of Nurses, the Vice President for Nursing Services, the steps are unclear. Previously, the career path in nursing management required longevity, loyalty, and expert clinical skills. Now, many hospitals are requiring master's degree preparation, business skills, and experience in other institutions for promotion to any managerial position. Job descriptions and requirements are changing rapidly, making career planning problematic.

Career planning should begin while still in school. Educators are beginning to address the idea of career planning for nurses. Once baccalaureate education is firmly established as the entry level for professional nurses, perhaps we can once again consider the idea of creating specialty tracks within baccalaureate generic preparation. Not a new thought for nurs-

ing, this model is used by other professions. Engineering students are taught the same basic body of knowledge during their first one-two years of education and then choose a specialty area (e.g., chemical, electrical, civil engineering) that directs their remaining baccalaureate entry-level preparation. Law pursues a similar approach for its entry-level practitioners. Nurses in their senior year could choose to specialize in an area of clinical expertise, preparing them for entry level within a broad clinical area such as maternal/child health. After practicing and achieving Stage I and II in career development as described by Dalton et al., nurses would return to graduate school to prepare for positions described in Stage III.

Many of the nurses who have pursued successful nontraditional nursing careers in the past have opted for advanced educational degrees outside of nursing. Many nurses saw them as turning their backs on the profession. Another perspective is that traditional educational programs were unable to provide a means for that nurse to continue her career development. Today's challenge is for graduate nursing education programs to adapt and offer preparation for nurses to shape new roles in today's rapidly changing world.

A program in nursing administration that offers management and business courses outside of nursing and relevant nursing electives such as quality assurance, ethics, and law allows a nontraditional nurse to pursue a meaningful curriculum and network with other career-oriented nurses who are planning both traditional and nontraditional career paths. Hospital nurse executives have felt pressured to pursue degrees in business or law because their nursing graduate degree did not adequately prepare them for their role or because nursing administration degrees were unavailable. Nurses who already feel estranged from the profession because of a chosen career may perceive that earning a degree outside the discipline is the definitive step outside the boundaries of nursing. If education is one way to define who is a nurse, we may be losing some of our best to other fields.

Implications for nurse executives

The nurse executive in the traditional setting needs to be aware that many of her entry level practitioners look at their work as a career but are unclear about how to plan a career path that maximizes use of their talents within the organization. Guidance on career development, an important management function at all levels, can be built into inservice education. Programs such as clinical ladders that increase technical skills as well as help staff plan and set career goals are valuable to both employee and employer.

Nurse executives in nontraditional settings need to be especially aware of their presence at the cutting edge of the profession. They need to analyze health care issues, share their experience with others, and advise nurse educators on curricular modifications necessary to help students to assume these nontraditional roles.

Nurse executives in both settings need to proactively assist novice nurses in their career planning. In an editorial on nursing career development, Keough stated, "It seems reasonable to assume that nursing as a profession will gain strength from practitioners who view their careers as desirable and worthwhile."[15] If this is so, nurse executives must foster attitudes that are sensitive to individual goals as they pertain to career paths.

In their book, *Creating Excellence,* Hickman and Silva[16] stress the importance of sensitivity in promoting a corporate culture that allows employees to meet individual needs. Nurse executives desiring to assist their employees with career planning will need to master this sensitivity if they are to help the novice nurse articulate her career goals. Ground-

ing in a nurturing, caring profession such as nursing should make this task easier for the nurse executive than the average corporate executive for whom Hickman and Silva wrote. These attitudes may help to halt rapid staff turnover. A study conducted by the National Association of Nurse Recruiters in 1980 showed that among the factors contributing to the nursing shortage were a lack of career mobility for nurses, a low professional image, and lack of professional recognition.[17] The same factors are probably applicable today.

Will the nurse executive in a traditional setting want to assist the novice nurse in career planning if the career path leads outside the setting? We must recognize that nurses pursuing nontraditional career paths may spend a year or two in the hospital just to acquire clinical background. Sensitive nurse executives, concerned with the profession, will accept this trend and help these nurses design meaningful career paths as well.

Another way to assist others in career development is for the nurse executive to recall her own steps in career development. What moves along your career path were the most valuable? What experience and/or education did you have that allowed you to progress in your career development? What roles did mentors or peers play in your career? Being able to articulate the essential steps of your career path will help you guide aspiring nurses appropriately.

Nurse executives need to examine performance evaluations and promotion policies that may hinder aspiring employees by being too rigid or by requiring that particular milestones be met within that institution before advancement can occur. Policies should support employees who pursue formal or continuing education or seek relevant experiences outside the work place. Recognition of the value of community service experience, even if it may not be directly applicable to their current situation, is important. Managing a budget, writing a plan, or supervising people remains a valuable experience whether performed in a hospital, a Senator's office, or as a volunteer in a community setting.

Very little is known of nurses' careers beyond adjustment to reality shock and factors associated with burnout. Nurse executives need to know what the career expectations are of today's beginning practitioner. What career paths did nurses in nontraditional roles follow? Having planned to become nurses, what were the factors that turned their feet from the traditional path? Answers to these questions will enable nurse executives to support and encourage nurses who desire to pursue meaningful careers in today's health care environment.

Summary

When is a nurse no longer a nurse? Lillian Wald established the first settlement house. Elizabeth Kinney founded the discipline of physical medicine. These nurses saw a need and used their nursing knowledge and experience to fill that need. Did these innovations make them ex-nurses? Florence Nightingale did not stop considering herself a nurse when she began the discipline of biostatistics. Modern nurse pioneers will not only define but expand the boundaries of nursing. You can take the nurse out of the profession, but it seems unlikely that you can take the profession out of the nurse.

REFERENCES

1. Spencer Rich. Ex-nurse tackles new challenge as senate leader's chief of staff. Washington Post, Feb. 18, 1986, p. A-17.

2. Robinson-Smith G. Alternative careers in nursing. Imprint 1984; 30(5):23-24.

3. Powell DJ. Nurses: "high touch" entrepreneurs. Nurs Econ 1984; 2(1):33-36.

4. Scott PP. Executive career planning. Nurs Econ 1984; 2(1):58-63.

5. Dunkelberger JE, Aadland SC. Expectation and attainment of nursing careers. Nurs Res 1984; 33(4):235-240.

6. McBride AB. Orchestrating a career. Nurs Outlook 1984; 33(5):244-247.

7. Miller MM, Shortridge LA, Woodside DJ, et al. Career planning and professional development: a unique course for nursing students. Nurs Educator 1984; 9(3):40-42.

8. Lenz ER, Waltz CF. Patterns of job search and mobility among nurse educators. J Nurs Ed 1983; 22(7):267-273.

9. Morrison RS, Zebelman E. The career concept in nursing. Nurs Adm Q 1982; 7(1):60-68.

10. Walsh YB, Yura H. The nursing process: assessing, planning, implementing, evaluating. Norwalk, CT: Appleton-Century-Crofts, 1983; 56-60.

11. Coleman JR, Dayari EC, Simms E. Nursing careers in the emerging systems. Nurs Mgmt 1984; 15(1):19-27.

12. Smith MM. Career development in nursing: an individual and professional responsibility. Nurs Outlook 1982; 30(2):128-131.

13. Dalton GW, Thompson PH, Price RL. The four stages of professional careers: a new look at performance by professionals. In: Morgan MA, ed. Managing career development. New York: D Van Nostrand Co., 1980.

14. Kramer M. Reality shock. St. Louis: CV Mosby, 1974.

15. Keough G. The need for nursing career development. J Cont Educ Nurs 1977; 8(3):5-6.

16. Hickman CR, Silva MA. Creating excellence. New York: New American Library, 1984.

17. NANR analyses nursing shortage (News). Am J Nurs 1980; 80(4):602.

Study questions

Chapter One

1. After studying these articles, reflect on your experiences as a nurse. Do you agree with the definition of nursing in the American Nurses' Association's *Social Policy Statement,* or do you support Orlando's argument, Schlotfeldt's, or another viewpoint?

2. Write your own definition of nursing. Why do you think the nursing profession is having so much difficulty developing a definition that all nurses can accept?

3. What is your opinion of Orlando's discussion of the dependent and independent paths of nursing? Do you agree with Lynaugh and Fagin that the health care system has been "built on the back of nurses"? What are the implications of this statement?

4. What is your opinion of Diers's definitions of nursing and professionalism? Is nursing caring? How can you help the nursing profession achieve the level of authority Diers describes?

Chapter Two

5. Do you think specialization could be included in associate-degree, baccalaureate-degree, or master's-degree education? Why? Do all nursing specialists have to be prepared at the master's-degree level, or should some specialists be prepared on the job or through continuing education?

6. How do you see nursing roles changing? Which roles do you see for yourself? Have you experienced the frustration of being floated to a nursing unit without prior orientation? How can you gain control of your own practice?

7. What is your opinion about certification? Describe why you think certification may or may not result in better patient care.

Chapter Three

8. Are all three levels of nursing education needed? Could client care be improved if nursing education began at the baccalaureate level?

9. Should two different licensing examinations be given, one for professional nurses and the other for technical nurses?

10. Why did you select the nursing program you are following? What are your plans for advancement? What is your opinion of Christman's proposal concerning the clinical doctorate degree for nurses? What do you and four classmates think of completing the doctorate by age 26?

Chapter Four

11. As you reflect on your clinical experience, which skills will you need to be considered competent when you graduate? What is your opinion of the clinical ladder concept?

12. Do you aspire to become a clinician who advances by clinical competence or a manager who advances by other skills? Why?

13. What is your opinion of the proposals to abandon centralized decision making for shared governance? Discuss the issue with your classmates. List the advantages and disadvantages of each system. In which system would you prefer to practice?

14. Do you believe that nurses should have autonomy and control in their clinical practice? On what do you base your belief?

15. Have you decided in which field of nursing you wish to practice? How do you plan to accomplish your goals? Where will you seek assistance in planning your career advancement?

Additional assignments

1. Write a paper addressing the following questions:
• What sets me apart from the other members of the health-care team?

• Am I a member of a profession? On what do I base my opinion?

• What does the term "nurse" mean to me?

• Can I define what "nursing" means to me? If not, why?

2. Establish a discussion group with your classmates and address the following questions:
• How does my role differ from those of other members of the health care team?

• Do I really understand where my functions start and end?

• Do I see myself as a generalist or a specialist? On what information do I base my decision?

3. Take some time to consider the following questions:
• Where do I see myself professionally in five years? Will I be in a clinical position or an administrative role? On what basis will I make my decisions?

• How will I contribute to the profession and to my own professional growth over the next five years?

UNIT TWO

Discipline issues: Nursing research, theory, and practice

DEVELOPING A KNOWLEDGE base for nursing — also referred to as developing the discipline of nursing — enables nursing to claim professional status. This is in contrast to activities such as collective bargaining and setting educational standards for registered nurses: These advance the profession of nursing but do not distinguish it as a discipline.

Fawcett (1980), a forceful advocate of developing a knowledge base for nursing, states her position succinctly and powerfully in "A Declaration of Nursing Independence: The Relation of Theory and Research to Nursing Practice":

> Traditionally, the primary determinants of nursing practice have been institutional policies and politics, largely influenced by economics and interprofessional turf wars. This situation has left nursing with an intuitive, trial and error practice that has become increasingly ritualistic. As a result, nurses are second class citizens in what is viewed by other professionals and the public as an ancillary occupation.
>
> Yet nurses have continuously strived for recognition as members of a separate discipline and independent profession. Their emergence as such can occur only when they iden-

tify a distinct body of knowledge about the individuals, groups, situations, and events of interest to nursing. The specification and explanation of these phenomena will provide the knowledge needed to move nursing practice to a reproducible process with predictable outcomes.

> The only way to generate, refine, or enlarge the knowledge base needed by nursing is through scientific research. Therefore, it is incumbent upon nurses to conduct investigations of nursing phenomena. However, unless this research is guided by theory and unless the theory is tested through research, both are in danger of being isolated and, therefore, trivial enterprises. Moreover, since the ultimate aim of all nursing theory and research is to improve the quality of client care, theory and research must have some bearing on nursing practice.

Most nurses agree with the need to develop the knowledge base for nursing as rapidly as possible, but debate continues about the characteristics of that knowledge base and the processes for developing new knowledge. Some hold that a knowledge base for nursing, similar to the knowledge bases of other disciplines, should contain a body of theoretical formulations derived from the generation and testing of research hypotheses. They feel that nursing knowledge derived in this way can be used in practice only after rigorous testing of the ideas under controlled conditions. In contrast, others view nursing practice as a primary source of nursing knowledge, the equal of research in importance. This debate (and others like it) will continue — a sign of the growing sophistication of the discipline.

Fortunately, we can expect acceleration in developing a knowledge base now that nursing research has its own agency, the National Center for Nursing Research, within the National Institutes of Health. Nursing leaders and researchers will be working to clarify such issues as the following:

1. What relationship exists between theory, research, and practice in a discipline such as nursing? For example, should all nursing practice be based on nursing research?

2. What criteria should be used to evaluate nursing research for its application in practice?

3. What is the role of the staff nurse in the development and use of new nursing knowledge?

Historical perspective on nursing research

Interestingly, Florence Nightingale viewed research as an essential component of nursing practice. She believed that nurses should collect and analyze data as a means of improving practice. For example, she used research to prove the value of nursing in England by collecting morbidity and mortality statistics both before and after nursing care was available. The dramatic improvement in the "after" statistics clearly supported the importance of nursing care.

Unfortunately, Nightingale's recognition of the relationship between research and practice was lost in the United States, where early training programs emphasized "learning by doing" together with behaving submissively toward physicians. In the late 19th century, nurses were not expected to evaluate the effectiveness of medical care, and it was not until the 1950s that U.S. nurses began to use the research process to address nursing practice problems.

By then, the federal government had declared nursing a profession, and nurses had realized that one of the criteria of a profession is that its members develop a knowledge base through research. Also by the 1950s, some nursing schools were located in academic settings where nursing faculty were expected to conduct research; graduate nursing programs were developing that emphasized advanced knowledge and specialization; and nurses pursuing doctoral degrees were receiving research training.

It was in this exciting era of nursing change and growth that Abdellah and Levine (1958) conducted the first national nursing study. Using a survey design, they collected data from various types of hospitals, then analyzed the data to find the relationship between hours of nursing care by type of nursing personnel (registered nurse, licensed practical nurse, and aide) and levels of patient satisfaction with nursing care. Abdellah and Levine concluded that hours of nursing care by registered nurses correlated with high levels of patient satisfaction, but that this did not hold true for the other categories of nursing personnel.

This landmark study demonstrated the value of the research process for nursing. At the same time, it raised questions about the use of research findings (research utilization). For example, some nurses thought the study solved the problem of how to obtain quality nursing care: Employ only registered nurses, they concluded, and the quality of care would be high. But other nurses challenged this view; they saw nursing research primarily as a means for generating and validating knowledge that could be translated directly into nursing practice. These nurses viewed the study by Abdellah and Levine more critically, recognizing that evaluating quality of care requires consideration of many other factors such as philosophy of care, work load, and nursing interventions.

During the 1950s, nursing research became firmly established within the profession. In the 1960s, much of the nursing research focused on the nurse and nursing education and was used to resolve problems within the profession. By the 1970s, it had shifted focus to the patient care setting and nursing interventions. Nursing research had also increased in quantity and quality. The 1980s saw the link between nursing theory and nursing research and a mushrooming of methods and settings for studying nursing phenomena. Today's nursing research generates and validates nursing knowledge.

The influence of the "logical empiricist" philosophy

Most nurse researchers of the 1950s, 1960s, and 1970s received their doctoral degrees and research training in disciplines such as sociology, education, and psychology, disciplines associated with a 20th century scientific philosophy labeled "logical empiricist" (also called "logical positivist"). According to this philosophy, science is a truth that describes aspects of the world, scientific theory can be formalized in the language of mathematics, theory is either true or false based upon empirical verification, and complex phenomena can be broken down into smaller units (the whole equals the sum of its parts).

In addition, the logical empiricist philosophy incorporates the concept of hierarchical importance of information: The basic sciences, such as physics and chemistry, are considered more important than the applied sciences, such as medicine and agriculture, that derive from them. The basic and applied scientists are considered a hierarchical elite in comparison to the practitioner and client, who use and benefit from the knowledge the scientists generate.

Nursing researchers with this educational background directly influenced the developing relationship between nursing research and nursing practice: They taught, conducted, and evaluated nursing research — and defined research use and the relationship between nursing research and practice — according to the logical empiricist philosophy.

Currently, the logical empiricist philosophy is under attack by clinicians and nurse researchers. Clinicians, eager for knowledge that can improve practice, have little interest in research whose value comes primarily from the methods used rather than the knowledge generated. Furthermore, increasing numbers of clinicians want to generate and test research ideas, rather than be passive recipients of research. Clinicians want research conducted under conditions that reflect complex reality rather than ones contrived to suit the researcher's purpose. Similarly, nurse researchers find the logical empiricist philosophy too restrictive.

Nursing theorists such as Watson (1983) argued that this view of science was inappropriate for interpreting the phenomena of nursing science. For example, Watson questioned how the reductionist view could be adequate to deal with the indivisible and central phenomenon of nursing: caring. Ellis (1982) noted that the logical empiricist philosophy emphasized the process of deduction and excluded creativity. Ellis advocated a view of science that valued both. Ketefian (1975) surveyed practicing nurses to determine the impact of research utilization; her data showed that research had minimal impact on practice. Newman (1982), another nurse-theorist, criticized the logical empiricist view for its emphasis on quantitative data and experimental design. She believes that some nursing phenomena are better explored through qualitative research methods.

Nursing is not the only discipline to challenge the logical empiricist view of science. Leaders in the fields of psychology (Schon, 1983), sociology (Bernstein, 1978), education (Reason & Rowan, 1981), medicine (Feinstein, 1983), and philosophy (Polkinghorne, 1983) are proposing alternate views of both the scientific process and the relationship between research and practice.

Historical perspective: The development of nursing theory

Florence Nightingale, the first nurse researcher, was also the first nurse theorist. Nightingale's theory emphasized the concept of environment as a force in healing. Most important for Nightingale, theory is not separate from practice because practice is theory in action.

In the 1950s in the United States, parallel to the pioneering investigations of nursing researchers, nursing educators began to articulate a theoretical view of nursing based on theory development and testing in disciplines such as education, sociology, and psychology. These educators assumed that by modeling the behavior of other disciplines, nursing would enhance its position within the academic community. They also assumed that nursing theory would benefit nursing practice, just as educational theory benefited classroom teaching.

Unfortunately, these educators tended to develop nursing theory from complex concepts unfamiliar to most nurses. For example, Rogers's theory of the Unitary Person (1970) described the human being as an energy field that is more than, and different from, the sum of the biologic, physical, social, and psychological parts. The environment is another energy field. Helicy (the diversity of the human and environmental field emerging from their interactions and manifesting nonrecurring rhythmicities); resonancy (ongoing change

from lower to higher frequency wave patterns in the human and environmental fields); and complementarity/integrality (continuous, mutual, and simultaneous interaction between human and environmental fields) are critical concepts in her theory.

The nursing literature describing the value, purpose, and nature of nursing theory also seemed ambiguous and complex. For practicing nurses, the knowledge used in practice is more than a "set of definitions, postulates, and deductions" or "invented or discovered reality." Researchers' efforts to differentiate theory from theoretical formulation, conceptual framework, model, paradigm, and empirical generalization further frustrated practitioners. The literature also described theory as general, grand, meta, middle-range, single-domain, explanatory, predictive, prescriptive, and grounded.

Yet, during the 1970s and 1980s, significant nursing theories emerged. (Today, some would argue that they are not theories but conceptual models.) In addition to Rogers's theory of the Unitary Person, significant theories include Levine's Conservation Theory (1973), Johnson's Behavioral Systems Theory (1980), Roy's Adaptation Theory (1980), and King's Open System Theory (1981).

Nurses have also applied theory from other disciplines to nursing problems. Once example is the use of the concepts of "internal and external locus of control" to study client response to health promotion interventions. Another example is included in the readings for Chapter Seven. Vicki Buchda, a clinical nurse specialist, describes her use of an existing theory of loneliness to deduce nursing interventions (in her case, 13 interventions for reducing loneliness).

Although nurses do not agree on a clear, succinct definition of nursing theory, and although members of the profession continue to debate the value of theory for nursing practice, nursing has continued to develop and test theory (including non-nursing theory) as a means of developing the discipline.

"Scholarly practice": Challenge for the future

As nurses challenge traditional views of research and theory, they are challenging traditional views of the relationships among theory, research, and practice. They are also challenging traditional views of the roles of theorist, researcher, and practitioner. In essence, nurses are proposing different paradigms (models) for developing the discipline. In some of these paradigms, the practitioner is both theorist and researcher.

Rosemary Ellis (1969), in addressing the topic "The Practitioner as Theorist," claims that the theorists in nursing are not the ivory tower thinkers; they are the nurses who work directly with patients.

Edgerton (1973), in the *Journal of Thought,* urges that the staff nurse be recognized as a theorist in nursing. She states that in the process of providing care, the staff nurse must conceptualize and reconceptualize the circumstances confronting her and conceptualize and reconceptualize available scientific theory. If necessary, the staff nurse must be able to create new theory. This, she says, requires imaginative reconstruction and the ability to identify and isolate significant phenomena. In this sense, the staff nurse is the real theorist and researcher in nursing.

In this view, the staff nurse is the scholarly practitioner who possesses the cognitive skills necessary to manipulate knowledge as it is being applied in practice. Knowledge does not take the form of a standard intervention. It cannot, because it changes with use. Theory, research, and knowledge from past practice are incorporated into the practitioner's knowledge base as dynamic facts, concepts, and theories.

Diers (1988) says this about the scholarly clinician:

Clinical scholars can be spotted in a half-hour's conversation. They talk about their exposure to people and events — the clinical work — with color, flavor, and texture. They describe patients or situations with acute observation, but always with what the observation produced as mental image or intellectual work. The repertoire of clinical scholar is not just a collection of empirical observations, for what makes the process into scholarly work is the constant analysis that pits today's events against accumulated learning, and makes the learning available to help understand the event. And it makes the scholar hunt for more explanations, more ideas, more theory, research, or study. And finally, what makes clinical scholarship is a hunger for understanding as regular as the sensations that make one eat breakfast.

What is most intriguing about the views of Ellis, Edgerton, and Diers is their tie to Nightingale's vision of nursing. Will we finally embrace her paradigm for the discipline?

The issues selected for review in Unit Two are significant to the development of the discipline. They pose critical "why," "how," and "who" questions.

REFERENCES

Abdellah, F.G., and Levine, E. (1958). *Effect of nursing staffing on satisfactions with nursing care.* (Hospital Monograph Series #4) Chicago: American Hospital Association.

Bernstein, R.J. (1978). *The restructuring of social and political theory.* Philadelphia: University of Pennsylvania Press.

Diers, D. (1988). On clinical scholarship (again). *Image, 20*(1), 2.

Drew, B.J. (1988). Devaluation of biological knowledge. *Image 20*(1), 25-27.

Edgerton, S. (1973). The technological imagination: A philosopher looks at nursing. *Journal of Thought, 8,* 57-65.

Ellis, R. (1969). The practitioner as theorist. *American Journal of Nursing, 69*(7), 1434-1438.

Ellis, R. (1982). Editorial, *Advances in Nursing Science, 4*, x-xi.

Fawcett, J. (1980, June). A declaration of nursing independence: The relation of theory and research to nursing practice. *The Journal of Nursing Administration, 10*(6), 36-39.

Feinstein, A.R. (1983). An additional basic science for clinical medicine: I. The constraining fundamental paradigms. *Annals of Internal Medicine, 99*(3), 393-397.

Johnson, D.E. (1980). The behavioral system model for nursing. In J.P. Riehl and C. Roy (Eds.): *Conceptual models for nursing practice* (2nd ed.). New York: Appleton-Century-Crofts.

Ketefian, S. (1975). Application of selected nursing research findings into nursing practice. *Nursing Research, 24*(2), 89-92.

King, I.M. (1981). A theory for nursing: Systems, concepts, process. New York: John Wiley and Sons.

Levine, M.E. (1973). *Introduction to clinical nursing* (2nd ed.). Philadelphia: F. A. Davis, Co.

Newman, M. (1982, July). Editorial. *Advances in Nursing Science, 4*(7).

Polkinghorne, D. (1983). *Methodology for the human sciences.* Albany, New York: State University of New York Press.

Reason, P., & Rowan, J. (1981). *Human inquiry: A sourcebook of new paradigm research.* New York: John Wiley and Sons.

Rogers, M.E. (1970). *The theoretical basis of nursing.* Philadelphia: F. A. Davis.

Roy, C. (1980). The Roy adaptation model. In J. P. Riehl and C. Roy (Eds.), *Conceptual models for nursing practice* (2nd ed.). New York: Appleton-Century-Crofts.

Schon, D.A. (1983). *The reflective practitioner*, New York: Basic Books.

Watson, J. (1983, October). Unpublished keynote presentation. University of Colorado School of Nursing.

CHAPTER FIVE

The relationship among theory, research, and practice

THE EDITORS OF BOTH *Advances in Nursing Science* and *Nursing Management* have chosen to address the issue of the controversy regarding the relationship among theory, research, and practice. In one sense, this is a controversy between knowing and doing: Chinn, in her editorial entitled "Knowing and Doing," discusses the gaps and dichotomies that have characterized our discipline and stimulates us to reflect on our personal views as well as on the collective views of our profession.

Can we use similar approaches to knowing and doing? Should we expect first to know and then to do, or the reverse?

We do not have that unity today. Many practicing nurses associate theory and research with the "ivory tower" mentality and not with the realities of day-by-day practice; they take great pride in being "doers," not just "thinkers." Other nurses, pointing to the failures in the health care system, take the most pride in being "thinkers" about how to make the system better. For their part, some theorists and researchers believe that their work has value apart from its capacity to improve nursing practice, and a few state frankly that they don't care whether their work can be used in the clinical setting.

Whereas Chinn calls for new thinking and doing, Curtin believes that time, patience, and tolerance will bring theory and practice together. In "Thought-full Nursing Practice," she attributes the dichotomies and misunderstandings to the fact that "nursing is a young discipline — vital and impatient."

Knowing and doing

PEGGY L. CHINN, PhD, FAAN

"Copper Woman warned Hai Nai Yu that the world would change and times might come when Knowing would not be the same as Doing. And she told her that Trying would always be very important."[1]

WE ARE ALL FAMILIAR with persistent voices decrying the various and sundry gaps that exist between the realms of theory and practice (also called, for us, the education *v.* practice gap). Indeed, those of us who have walked in both the worlds of academia and service have experienced very real and distressing senses of "other worldness" as we pass back and forth from one world to the other. Yet we continue to hear pleas for someone to bridge these gaps and wish for some magic formula that might make it possible for one world to better inform the other.

As nurses we are particularly vulnerable to an unrelenting sense of disparity between what we know and what we do. We know we would be stronger as a profession if we were unified with each other and with other health care providers, but we are not unified. We know we would be able to provide a high quality of care if we were free to practice nursing as we envision it to be, but we do not and cannot practice in these ways. We know we would better serve society if we focused our practice on health and developed greater knowledge about health, but we practice in an illness care system, not a health care system.

When we attempt to sort out the underlying issues and dynamics of these disparities, we experience clouded vision. We are confronted with circumstances and factors we would rather not see, that do not fit with our experience of ourselves and the world. We find contradictions, extremely complex situations, and a multitude of internal and external voices screaming dilemmas we already know too well. In the face of what seems to be an impossible challenge, I believe that there are brave steps that we can all take toward healing the perceived gaps. There is no single path, and some of the paths that we attempt may turn in a direction we would not intend. But it is vitally important that we begin to take the steps....

One step is to no longer accept the notion that we are doomed to experience fundamental gaps between what we know and what we do, and to begin to act and think in a way that reflects our desire to more fully express unity between our theory and our practice. We can begin to act in accord with our ideas about the way nursing should be, with firm conviction that what we think and what we do are vitally important. We can increase our conviction that what we think and what we experience *are* related, by thinking systematically about what we experience and consciously forming our experiences in light of our fundamental ideas about the world. We can give voice to our doubts and our questions about the ways that things are and listen attentively to the voices of others, especially those who are doubting, questioning, angry, or aggrieved. We can begin to discuss, with nurses from all walks of life, all areas of work, all levels of preparation, how we might move beyond our doubts and questions and anger, to create something that will make a difference. We can begin to believe, and act on the belief, that what we think and what we do can, indeed, make some difference in the structures that exert control over our lives.

Another step is to recognize that as we express unity in our knowing and doing, we will begin to enter dimensions of experience that have been previously unfamiliar. We will recognize paradoxes in our own thinking and in the thinking of other nurses that we wish did not exist. With recognition will emerge vision of how to move beyond the paradoxes. Bunch[2] has named one of these the "too hard/too easy" paradox. Some nurses assume that theory must be esoteric and far removed from daily life, if it is to be properly called theory. It must be too hard for most people to understand if it is to be taken seriously in the academic community. On the flip side, as Bunch notes, some of us want all theory to be easy—to have words that do not require a dictionary, to be able to be read rapidly and easily, if it is to be of any use. Both of these attitudes represent barriers to serious consideration of ways to move beyond the disparities between what we know and what we do. If we recognize that reading and writing theory is not easy but can be done, and theory can be comprehensible to all nurses, then we will begin to experience both theory and practice in ways that we cannot imagine in advance.

Healing what we experience as the theory-practice split in nursing cannot be left to someone else to do. As each of us, regardless of our work orientation, begins to heal the splits within our own thinking and in our own actions, we will begin to see movements toward unity that we all yearn for.

REFERENCES

1. Cameron A: *Daughters of Copper Woman*. Vancouver, British Columbia, Press Gang Publishers, 1981. Told from the stories of the native women of Vancouver Island.

2. Bunch C: *Passionate Politics: Feminist Theory in Action*. New York, St. Martin's Press, 1987.

Thought-full nursing practice

Leah L. Curtin, rn

Alfred north whitehead once remarked that "Intellect is to emotion as our clothes are to our bodies; we could not very well have a civilized life without clothes, but we would be in a poor way if we had only clothes without bodies." In like fashion, theory is to nursing practice as our clothes are to our bodies; we cannot very well teach or practice nursing without an underlying theory, but we are in a very poor way if we have only theory without practice.

The trouble with theorists

Theorists who isolate themselves from practice, who couch their work in inexplicable terms, and who claim that their theories need not be demonstrated in practice do no service for the profession. At best their efforts are a distraction. At worst, they serve as a justification for anti-intellectualism among nurses. And thus, nursing theorists who sacrifice relevance and utility to elegance and polish actually rob patients of the benefits of efficient, thought-full nursing care. Nursing is an art to be practiced, a science to be applied in an imperfect world. Theory adds perspective, not perfection.

The trouble with anti-intellectuals

Practicing nurses who despise "theory" are condemned to performing a series of tasks — either at the command of a physician or in response to routines and policies. Often, the purpose or goal of each task (if it was ever known) is lost. *You cannot maintain a purpose without a principle*. So...daily, nurses wash the old man with parchment dry skin; daily they measure his urine to fill-in the I & O sheet; and daily they tie him to his bed "to keep him safe." And no one exercises his body or his mind, and no one knows why he doesn't want to live anymore.

Following "orders" is the easy way out. It doesn't take as much time. Moreover, it helps us avoid responsibility. And administrators like us because we are "productive." And doctors like us because we don't ask questions. And no one can blame us when things go wrong: we've "gone by the book."

Leads to trouble for the public

But, in the long run, patients suffer because they do not receive personal care, nor do they benefit from nursing care's *unique* contribution to their recovery and/or well-being. Physicians become disgruntled about the nursing care (or, to be more accurate, the *lack* of it) — unquestioning obedience leads to accidents, errors and patient complaints. Hospitals actually run *less* efficiently: we now have proof that effective nursing practice reduces [length of stay] *and* recidivism.

To put the matter in as few words as possible, simplistic obedience (rote response to external structure) is no substitute for thought-full practice. Theory *internalizes* principles which increase adaptability and flexibility and enables one to transfer *experience* from one situation to the next. The problem is not with theory *per se,* not with practitioners, and not even with theorists.

But the real problem lies elsewhere...

The real problem is that nursing is a young discipline — vital and impatient. Eager to explain their experiences, nurses are engaging in research. Since there is not yet, in these early days, a coherent theoretical framework which encompasses the broad range of nursing phenomena, nursing theories proliferate. As the number of theories increase, nursing texts grow thicker rather than more discriminating and, more often than not, degenerate into a catalog. Authors apparently feel obliged to include as many theories as possible, thus sacrificing comprehension to comprehensiveness.

At the moment, the body of nursing knowledge is in some disarray: a situation which should *not* dismay nurses. Today's chemist probably would find the content of a "chemistry text" written at the same stage in the development of his discipline difficult to follow and mostly not worth learning. But they were necessary, even critical, steps to today's knowledge. Such is also the case in nursing.

Promoting growth

Patience and tolerance for ambiguity are essential. Far too often nurses' statements are impeccably dressed in precise (if somewhat *obscure*) terminology and shrouded discreetly in careful qualifications. Such precision and reticence may be commendable, but they do not stir debate or arouse passions. Rather, they leave the reader with that sense of ennui which is the natural partner to the bland notion that, on every theoretical issue, there is much to be said on both sides, and, in every content area, further research is needed. True, but boring.

One of the worst insults we throw at another nurse is to accuse her (or him) of *stating opinions*. God forbid that nurses ascribe expertise to a colleague, yet, "expert opinion" is eagerly sought in other disciplines! An emphatic statement made in *clear* language is remembered — and provokes discussion, reaction and debate. The danger of overstatement is preferable to the security of understatement. If

nursing is to progress, nurses, long conditioned by authoritarian structures, must learn that any theory *does not* deal in absolute truth, but only successive approximations to the truth. That precision in practice does not require rigidity in thought. That debate, dimension and opinion *are* the meat and bone of progress. That obscure language is the mark of the *over-schooled* and *under-educated*. That the purpose of theory is to give meaning and focus to practice.

Just as Whitehead's statement infers that emotion is superior to intellect (emotion represents the "body," intellect merely its clothes), so nursing practice — which consists of helping people change their lives, improve their lives, save their lives — is superior to the theories which describe it. So also, as intellect disciplines emotions — sharpens, directs and focuses it — theory guides practice.

...To promote human well-being

Some years ago, in an address to the California Institute of Technology, Albert Einstein said: "It is not enough that you should understand about applied science in order that your work may increase man's blessings. Concern for man himself and his fate *must always form the chief interest* of all technical endeavors, concern for the great unsolved problems of the organization of labor and the distribution of goods — in order that the creations of our mind shall be a blessing and not a curse to mankind. Never forget this in the midst of your diagrams and equations."

Nursing theory — the creations of our mind — [and] nursing care — its application in practice — create what we are as nurses as surely as we create our profession. And the profession *is* the promise to help...to bless.

CHAPTER SIX

Evaluating research in practice

IN THE ARTICLE "Evaluating Research for Use in Practice: Guidelines for the Clinician," Tanner argues that Ketefian's study of the procedures nurses use to take oral temperatures and Kirchoff's study of nurses' implementation of coronary care precautions show that practicing nurses are not making deliberate use of research findings. Why? According to Ingram (1988), one reason may be that little is known about how to disseminate nursing research effectively. For example, are organizational structures such as unit-based quality assurance committees effective in supporting innovation and change in nursing practice? In the next article, "Research in Practice: The Role of the Staff Nurse," Lindeman suggests that nurses view this problem from the perspective of *knowledge* use rather than *research* use; she claims that unless the knowledge view is adopted, the minimal use of research findings to improve nursing practice will continue.

Nursing leaders advocating use of research findings in nursing practice typically cite the research evaluation criteria developed by Haller et al. "Developing Research-Based In-novation Protocols: Process, Criteria, and Issues," describes these criteria, which are also referred to as the Conduct and Utilization of Research in Nursing (CURN) criteria, after the name of the project that facilitated their development and initial use.

Conduct and use of research in nursing

These criteria first assess the scientific merit of the research, then the significance and usefulness of the research to the practice setting, and finally the suitability of the findings for application to practice.

Tanner, however, offers an alternate set of criteria. She proposes consideration of research utilization as an aspect of clinical decision-making. According to this view, the criteria for evaluating research begin with an evaluation of the findings' clinical relevance; Tanner identifies decision points that reflect the process of clinical decision making.

REFERENCES

Ingram, M. (1988). Origins of nursing knowledge. *Image, 20*(4), 233.

Evaluating research for use in practice:
Guidelines for the clinician

CHRISTINE A. TANNER, RN, PhD, FAAN

FOR WELL OVER A DECADE, nursing leaders have expressed concern about the limited use of research in nursing practice. Ketefian's frequently cited study[1] points to the failure on the part of clinicians to take oral temperatures properly even though the procedure yielding the most accurate readings had been well documented in the literature. More recently, Kirchoff's study[2] revealed that nurses have continued to use coronary care precautions in spite of their knowledge of the research literature, which provided evidence that such practices were unnecessary.

In defense of practicing nurses, Downs[3] criticized Ketefian's conclusions, suggesting that by the time Ketefian had conducted her study, electronic thermometers were rapidly replacing the glass thermometers used in the research base, thereby making the knowledge somewhat obsolete. The nurses in Kirchoff's study[2] may have been making a wise choice in not eliminating coronary care precautions on the basis of the research literature. At least one study in the research base[4] was sharply criticized for its methodologic and conceptual inadequacies.[5-7] Moreover, the risk-benefit analysis suggested as part of the research utilization process[8] may well have favored continuation of coronary care precautions.

Despite these controversies in nursing, there is substantial evidence that the gap between knowledge production and knowledge utilization is on the order of several years. It is clear that knowledge utilization in general and research utilization in particular are complex processes. Indeed, a relatively new discipline, focusing specifically on the use of knowledge, is evolving.[9,10] In nursing, three large-scale projects have been conducted to investigate various approaches that may be used to foster the use of research.[11-13]

This article focuses on one aspect of utilization — the practicing nurse's evaluation of reports of research findings and the decision to use or not use the findings in practice. Guidelines for evaluating research are provided that emphasize (1) the potential utility in clinical practice, (2) the critical components of scientific merit, and (3) other factors that ought to influence the decision to use the research in practice, such as the feasibility of making a systematic evaluation and doing a risk-benefit analysis.

Utility in clinical practice

Three aspects of research utilization form the framework for the guidelines for evaluating the clinical relevance and utility of nursing research: the nature of research utilization, the scope of utilization, and the nature of clinical decision making in nursing.

Nature of research utilization. A basic assumption of researchers has been that research was "used" when it was implemented as part of a program or directly led to some decision — that is, that some specific action could be directly attributable to the use of research findings. However, current conceptions of research utilization recognize at least two general ways in which research might be used by individuals. Caplan and Rich[14] have used the terms "instrumental utilization" and "conceptual utilization." The former refers to cases in which the user can describe the specific way in which knowledge is being used for decision making. The latter term refers to the influence of one or more studies on a decision maker's thinking about an issue, without putting the information to any specific, documentable use. Weiss[15] suggested the term "enlightenment" to describe this type of utilization.

It is likely that both kinds of utilization figure prominently in decision making in nursing. For example, a nurse may be able to justify a decision to use a ventilator to hyperventilate a patient with an Fio_2 of 100% on the basis of one or more studies examining this approach to reducing hypoxemia. The nurse's action may be directly linked to his or her knowledge of the research literature. Alternatively the nurse may be aware of the various complications of endotracheal suctioning and may include this awareness as a part of deciding, for example, how long to apply suction or how many passes to make with the catheter. In the latter instance, the procedure employed is not that prescribed by the research literature but, rather, is one that the nurse adopts because of an awareness of the research and of several other factors related to the individual patient.

In instrumental utilization, it is possible that the research report can provide guidance for the practicing nurse in one or more of the following ways:

1. The findings and/or conclusions per se may be used to the extent that they provide evidence for a solution to a specific practice problem. For example, a number of studies have been conducted to identify ways to prevent diarrhea in tube-fed patients, hence providing a solution to a significant practice problem.[16]

2. The study has provided support for a theory that can guide practice. The specific intervention tested or the findings per se may not be useful, but the theory may serve to guide practice. For example, Johnson's series of studies[17] on sensory preparation before medi-

cal or surgical procedures has provided substantial support for the theory guiding this intervention.

3. Certain measures or tools used in the study might be helpful to a clinician to employ in practice. For example, a measure of risk for the development of pressure sores that has been tested and used in research[18] might be adopted as an assessment tool for use in practice.

Scope of research utilization. The scope of a research utilization endeavor may vary widely, from the individual nurse's decision to use research in a particular patient situation to institution-wide adoption of a research-based change in practice. Current conceptions of research utilization, both in general and in the nursing discipline, tend to focus on the broad-scale, organizational efforts needed to encourage research-based innovations.[9-11,19] Regardless of the scope of utilization, the critique of the research literature by nurses in practice for its utility, merit, and feasibility of implementation and the subsequent evaluation of the outcomes of the utilization effort are essential elements.

Nature of clinical decision making. The use of research in nursing practice is directed toward the goal of assisting nurses to make sound clinical decisions. This is true regardless of whether the way in which nurses use the research is instrumental or conceptual and regardless of the scope of the utilization effort.

Clinical decision making, like research utilization, is a tremendously complex process that requires the use of knowledge from several sources, as well as the use of both rational-analytic and intuitive judgment skills.[20-24] Clinical judgments by experienced nurses are apparently informed by (1) extensive practical knowledge, which derives from experience with similar (and dissimilar) cases over time,[23] and (2) scientific knowledge, derived from either application of basic science research or the use of nursing research. Investigations of the analytic approaches to clinical decision making[20-22] support the notion that nursing research may assist clinicians in making judgments in the following ways:

1. Deciding on appropriate observations to make in order to rule in or rule out particular diagnoses. For example, research on sensory deprivation has provided rich descriptions of its symptoms, providing guidance to nurses who suspect that a patient may be experiencing the consequences of sensory deprivation.

2. Identifying the extent to which patients may be at risk for certain problems or complications. For example, research on pressure sore formation conducted over the last two decades has provided clear indications as to which patients are at high risk for pressure sores and therefore require more aggressive preventive measures.

3. Deciding on the appropriate intervention most likely to produce the desired outcomes, reduce the probability of complications, or both. Research on numerous procedures, such as endotracheal suctioning, has provided assistance to nurses in performing the procedure in such a way that tracheal trauma and hypoxemia can be minimized.

The first part of the research critique is intended to provide for systematic and comprehensive assessment of the potential utility for clinical practice (Appendix I). The questions, which are adapted from several published critique guidelines,[8,11,25] assume that the goal of the reader is either to find a solution to a practice problem or to use the research literature as a way to initiate an innovation in practice. Some research is designed toward a goal other than immediate application in practice and is therefore not useful to the clinician. Other research is designed with utilization in mind but falls short of this goal because the research question is now viewed as salient by the reviewer. The questions probe for every possible use of research: to employ the findings, the theory tested, or the instruments; to use any aspect of the study conceptually or instrumentally; or to facilitate decision making. If no use for research in practice can be found through addressing these questions, then no further review is necessary.

Scientific merit

Once the research report has passed critical review for clinical relevance, then the evaluation of its scientific merit becomes salient. Three aspects of this evaluation are included in the guidelines: (1) the extent to which the conceptualization and/or justification for the study makes sense and thereby provides a sound basis for the remainder of the report (termed internal consistency) (Appendix II); (2) the degree to which there has been sufficient methodologic rigor for the reader to believe the results and conclusions (Appendix III); and (3) the representativeness of the sample and setting and the evidence of replication of the study, allowing for some confidence in the generalizability of the results (Appendix IV).

Conceptualization and internal consistency. The justification for study may be derived from the research or theory literature, from concerns in practice, or from both. Ideally, consideration of all these sources will be evident in the introductory portion of the report. The conceptualization ought to make sense to clinicians who wish to use the study in their practice, and it ought to provide the basis for the study design and reporting of findings. For example, if an investigator's interest is in the need for precautions in the care of patients with myocardial infarction, it would make sense to study such patients, assuming that the safety of such an investigation had been ensured through basic research with normal subjects. If the original problem was based on observations of patients' displaying obvious signs of distress while hospitalized in intensive care units, then an appropriate measure might be observation of these distress signs, rather than a paper-and-pencil trait anxiety scale. The results ought to be reported in a way that clearly addresses the research questions. In short, the report should make sense and hang together.

Believability of the results. If the report meets the criteria for conceptualization and internal consistency, then further critique of the methodologic rigor is in order. The first aspect to be considered is the internal validity of the results. The validity, or truthfulness, can be jeopardized by having a biased sample, resulting from convenience sampling without adequate attention to extraneous variables, or by not randomly assigning subjects to groups in an intervention type of study.

The types of measures used are also important in ensuring the validity of the study results. "Reliability of the measure" refers to the accuracy and stability of the instrument. For example, if an individual is weighed daily and a wide variation in weight is obtained, then there is considerable measurement error and the scale would be said to be unreliable. "Validity of the measures" refers to the extent to which the instrument measures what it is supposed to measure. For example, a measure of trait anxiety would not be a valid measure of distress experienced by hospitalized patients. Frequently a discussion of either the reliability or the validity of the instruments used in the study is omitted from the research report, making it extremely difficult for a reader to believe the results of the study unless he or she happens to be familiar with the instruments used.

The second aspect of the believability of the study is the conclusions drawn by the investigator. Here the reader must examine the explanations for the results offered by the in-

vestigator and attempt to generate alternative explanations. If the rival explanations seem equally plausible, based on the reader's knowledge and experience, then some caution is warranted in the decision to use the study results.

Generalizability of the results. Having ascertained that the results are believable, the reader must now assess the extent to which the research is applicable in his or her practice setting or with a particular patient. Questions about the sampling procedures used — and hence the presumed representativeness of the sample — are salient here. Because true random selection is rarely possible in clinical research (at least random selection from the target population of hospitalized patients in the United States), replication of the study takes on greater importance. If the total study has been replicated, a theory has been tested and supported in a variety of studies, or a measure has been evaluated with several different samples, then the reader can have greater confidence in the results — and in the possibility of achieving some degree of success in using the research in decision making with specific patients. Unfortunately, since replication is more often the exception than the rule in nursing research, other factors must be considered in the decision to use research in practice.

Other factors to consider in research utilization

The questions relating to this section are designed to balance the reader's judgment about utility and merit of the research with practical considerations (Appendix V). The consideration of these questions allows for the decision to use some research that may not meet all the criteria for scientific merit but that holds some promise of leading to beneficial outcomes.

The first question, that of the feasibility of making a systematic evaluation of the research-based practice, is critical regardless of the strengths of the research report and the degree of generalizability evident. As Barlow et al.[26] have pointed out, the individual clinician's decision to use research for an individual patient rests on the judgments (1) that the patient to which the clinician wishes to apply the new practice is like the average patient in the study who benefited from the practice and (2) that a clinically significant improvement will result from research-based practice when only statistically significant results have been reported. It would greatly advance the science of nursing if practicing nurses who attempt to use research-based practices would document the effectiveness (or ineffectiveness) of the practice with individual patients. Such documentation is the result of planning for systematic evaluation.

The remaining questions probe risk- and cost-benefit issues. Both the risk of changing practice based on the research and the risk of not changing practice should be explored. The reader may make a judgment that the latter risk is greater and hence decide to implement the practice even though other criteria have not been completely met. One may find that although benefits in patient outcomes might accrue from a change in practice, the benefits are not of sufficient magnitude to warrant the added cost. Each of these practical aspects must be considered before the decision is made to implement an institution-wide change in practice.

Summary

Research in nursing has the potential to contribute substantially to the quality of patient care. However, this potential can be realized only if the research base is critically evaluated and used appropriately as a basis for practice. At best, research will always be only a guide for practice. The astute clinician will combine his or her practical wisdom, derived from experience, with an understanding of the individual patient's situation and with knowledge derived from research to make a clinical judgment thought to be of benefit to the patient.

Appendix I. Criteria for evaluating a study for clinical relevance

Instructions

After reading the first sections of the article (through the methods section), respond to the following questions:

1. What was the problem that was studied? Does this study have the potential to help solve a problem that you currently face in your practice?

2. Does the study have the potential to help you with any of the following types of decisions?

a. Deciding on appropriate observations to make in order to rule in or rule out particular diagnoses.

b. Identifying the extent to which patients may be at risk for certain problems or complications.

c. Deciding on the intervention most likely to produce desired outcomes, reduce the probability of complications, or both.

3. Is a theory or proposition that might serve to guide practice tested by the study? What kinds of decisions might be guided by this theory?

4. Did the investigator test an intervention in this study? If yes, describe the intervention. Do you see the potential for using the intervention in your practice? Consider the following: (a) under nursing control and (b) feasible in your setting, given staffing patterns and cost constraints.

5. How did the investigator measure the dependent variables or outcomes? Do you see the potential for using any of these measures in your practice? Consider the following: (a) under nursing control, (b) would be of assistance to nurses in their assessment of patients or evaluation of outcomes, and (c) feasible in your setting, given staffing patterns and cost constraints.

Decision point

If the answer to any *one* of questions 1 to 5 is yes, then the study deserves further consideration. It has potential for use in practice. If you answered no to *all* the questions, then the study is probably not relevant to your practice and there is no need to evaluate it further (unless you are reviewing the study for other reasons).

Appendix II. Criteria for evaluation of scientific merit: Conceptualization and internal consistency

Instructions

Read the remainder of the study report and then respond to the following questions:

1. Overall, does the report hang together and make sense to you?

2. Does the underlying conceptualization make sense? Specifically:

a. Is there justification for the study?

b. Do the study questions relate to the justification?

3. Overall, do the methods fit with the conceptualization or justification for the study and with the study questions in the following areas: (a) subjects and setting, (b) sampling procedures, (c) instruments, (d) procedures, and (e) analysis?

4. Do the investigators answer the questions that they posed?

Decision point

If there are major conceptual problems (e.g., the underlying justification doesn't make sense) or if there is no internal consistency in the report (i.e., the methods do not fit with the conceptualization or the research questions are not adequately or properly addressed), then you have several possible options: (1) to continue with more detailed evaluation of the study, hoping that additional reading will clarify the confusing aspects of the report; (2) to seek consultation from a person with some of your questions; (3) to evaluate the report no

further, because it is sufficiently confusing that its usefulness in practice is jeopardized.

Appendix III. Criteria for evaluation of scientific merit: Believability of results

Instructions

For this section of the critique, the methods, results, discussion, and conclusion portions of the report should be reread with more attention to details. The questions that follow are screening questions and serve to alert the reader to major methodologic issues:

1. Are the methods used likely to lead to believable, internally valid results? Specifically:

a. What subjects were studied and how were they selected? If a convenience sample was used, did the investigator control for sample characteristics that might influence the results of the study?

b. If an intervention was tested with different treatment groups, were the subjects randomly assigned to these groups? If not, did the investigator control for possible initial differences between the groups?

c. Does the author discuss reliability of the measures: Is reliability satisfactory?

d. Does the author discuss validity of the measures? Are you confident of the instrument validity?

2. Are the conclusions drawn by the author based on the data presented and believable in light of the methods used? Specifically:

a. Does the author stay within the boundaries indicated by the subjects, the types of interventions attempted, and the measures used?

b. If there were statistically significant findings (e.g., a positive correlation between two variables, a difference between two treatment groups), does the author have a reasonable explanation? Based on your knowledge and experience, what other explanation might there be for these results?

c. If the findings were not as expected or

were not statistically significant, does the author provide a reasonable explanation? Could any of the following be possible explanations for these results: small sample size, invalid or insensitive measures, an unusually heterogeneous sample, or an insufficiently strong intervention?

Decision point
The set of questions in item 1, above, identify critical issues in methodology. If any one of these aspects is not adequately addressed in the research report, it *may* be grounds for the reader to decide on nonutilization — depending on the risk involved in using the results and depending on the availability of other studies that corroborate the results of this study.

If the methodologic issues in item 1 are adequately addressed, the reader then evaluates whether the conclusions drawn are appropriate. There frequently will be explanation or conclusions other than those which the author provides; negative review on this aspect is not sufficient by itself to decide on nonutilization. However, if results can be clearly attributed to factors other than those raised in the original research question, additional caution in using the study is warranted.

If both items 1 and 2 are adequately addressed in the study report, then the reader should proceed to the fourth component (see Appendix IV) of the critique.

Appendix IV. Scientific merit: Generalizability of the results
Instructions
The methods and conclusions sections, as well as the literature review, provided in this study are to be used as the basis for responding to these questions.

1. Is the sample and setting similar or dissimilar to the sample and setting to which you wish to generalize (target population)?

2. Have other studies been conducted that address the same problem, test the same intervention, evaluate the same measure, or test the same theory (replications)? Were the results similar to the results obtained in the present study?

Decision point
In the ideal situation, there will be considerable similarity between the study sample and the target population, *and* the study will have been replicated. The nurse can have confidence in the study findings and have more confidence in using the study in his or her practice. More frequently, one or both of the criteria are not met. If, however, the study has met other criteria, and if it is possible to systematically evaluate the use of the study in practice, then utilization is recommended. Failure to meet the criteria of generalizability, alone, is not sufficient justification for a nonutilization decision.

Appendix V. Other factors to consider in utilization
Instructions
The following questions can be addressed either from the standpoint of the individual nurse's making a judgment as to whether to use research in the care of a particular patient or from the standpoint of instituting a major change in practice throughout the institution. If the intended scope is the latter, then the reader will need to anticipate a major effort in planning, with involvement of multiple groups. [11] In either case, the following questions must be addressed before the research base is implemented in practice:

1. What is the feasibility of doing systematic evaluation of the research-based practice?

2. What is the risk of changing practice based on the research?

3. As important as the preceding considerations, what is the risk of maintaining current practice (i.e., not trying the practice suggested by the research)?

4. What is the cost of changing practice on the basis of this research?

5. What are the benefits of changing practice?

Decision point

If the benefits outweigh the costs, the risks are minimal, and it is feasible to systematically evaluate the outcomes, even with a single patient, then it is appropriate to proceed to use the research in clinical practice. This is true even if not all the criteria for scientific merit have been met. If costs or risks are high, and if some aspect of scientific merit is questionable, then additional research should be conducted before practice is changed on the basis of the research.

REFERENCES

1. Ketefian S. Application of selected nursing research findings into nursing practice: a pilot study. Nurs Res 1975;24:89-92.

2. Kirchoff K. A diffusion study of coronary precautions. Nurs Res 1982;31:96.

3. Downs FS. Clinical and theoretical research. In: Downs FS, Fleming JW, eds. Issues in nursing research. New York: Appleton-Century-Crofts, 1979.

4. McNeal G. Rectal temperatures in patients with acute MI. Image 1978;10(1):18.

5. Erickson R. Letter to editor. Image 1979;11(1):30.

6. Tanner C: Letter to editor. Image 1979;11(1):30.

7. Blainey CG: Letter to editor. Image 1979;11(1):31.

8. Haller KB, Reynolds MA, Horsley JA. Developing research-based protocols: process, criteria, and issues. Res Nurs Health 1979;2:45.

9. Stetler C. Research utilization: defining the concept. Image 1985;17:40.

10. Larsen J. Knowledge utilization: what is it? Knowledge: Creation, Diffusion, Utilization 1980;1:421.

11. Horsley JA, Crane J, Crabtree MK, Wood DJ. Using research to improve nursing practice: a guide. New York: Grune & Stratton, 1983.

12. King D, Barnard K, Hoehn R. Disseminating the results of nursing research. Nurs Outlook 1981;29:164.

13. Krueger J, Nelson A, Wolanin M. Nursing research: development, collaboration, and utilization. Rockville, Md.: Aspen. 1978.

14. Caplan N, Rich RF. The use of social science knowledge in policy decisions at the national level. Ann Arbor, Mich.: Institute for Social Research, University of Michigan, 1975.

15. Weiss C. Knowledge creep and decision accretion. Knowledge: Creation, Diffusion, Utilization 1980;1:381.

16. Horsley JA, Crane J, et al. Reducing diarrhea in tube-fed patients. New York: Grune & Stratton, 1981.

17. Johnson JE. Coping with elective surgery. Ann Rev Nurs Res 1984:2.

18. Goldstone LA. The Norton score: an early warning of pressure sores? J Adv Nurs 1982:419.

19. Horsley JA, Crane J, Bingle JD. Research utilization as an organizational process. J Nurs Adm 1978;8(7):4.

20. Putzier DJ, Padrick KP, Westfall UE, Tanner CA. Diagnostic reasoning in critical care nursing. Heart Lung 1985;14:430.

21. Westfall UE, Tanner CA, Putzier DJ, Padrick KP. Clinical inferences in nursing: a preliminary analysis of cognitive strategies. Res Nurs Health 1986;9:269.

22. Tanner CA, Padrick KP, Westfall UE, Putzier DJ. Diagnostic reasoning: an analysis of cognitive strategies used by nurses and nursing students. Nurs Res (in press).

23. Benner P: From novice to expert: power and excellence in clinical nursing practice. Palo Alto, Calif.: Addison-Wesley, 1984.

24. Benner P, Wrubel U. Skilled clinical knowledge: the value of perceptual awareness. Nurse Ed 1982;7(3):11.

25. Van Servellen GM, Stetler CB. Utilization of research: critiquing research for practice. In Lieske AM, ed. Clinical nursing research. Rockville, Md.: Aspen, 1986.

26. Barlow DH, Hayes SC, Nelson RO. The scientist practitioner: Research and accountability in clinical and educational settings. New York: Pergamon Press, 1984.

Research in practice: The role of the staff nurse

CAROL A. LINDEMAN, RN, PhD, FAAN

ALTHOUGH MOST NURSES agree that research should be applied in practice, there is little evidence that it is. We wonder what keeps nurses from using research. Yet nursing is not the only discipline concerned with the application of research in practice. Disciplines such as education, psychology, and sociology are raising questions similar to those raised in nursing. Why don't practitioners consciously apply research in practice? Is the research process suitable for generating the knowledge needed by practitioners? What is the best method for communicating research findings?

Central to any discussion of the application of research in practice is one's understanding of the relationship between research and practice, and the practitioner. In this article, two contrasting views of the relationship between research and practice, the role of the staff nurse, and the nature of nursing practice are described. The process of applying research in practice is illustrated using examples of research in preoperative teaching.

Traditional view

The traditional view of the relationship between research and practice is well stated by Fawcett (1980):

> The only way to generate, refine, or enlarge the knowledge needed by nursing is through scientific research. Therefore it is incumbent upon nurses to conduct investigations of nursing phenomena...since the ultimate aim of all nursing theory and research is to improve the quality of client care, theory and research must some bearing on nursing practice.

For the purposes of this article, the following characteristics of the traditional view of research are important to note: (a) The primary responsibility for developing knowledge belongs to the nurse-scientist; (b) neither the staff nurse nor the patient is an active participant in developing new knowledge; (c) the staff nurse applies knowledge in the real world; and (d) decisions about how new knowledge will be used are not a part of the research process.

According to this viewpoint, nursing interventions that had been tested under rigorous scientific conditions would be standardized and applied in practice. The staff nurse would then apply this standardized intervention as a problem solver, using standardized knowledge to solve problems presented by patients.

Disciplines such as psychology, education, and nursing are critical of the traditional view and have proposed new ways of viewing research and research application in practice (Schon, 1983). Within these new views, (a) the research subject is given an active role in the research process, (b) knowing "how" is viewed as equally important to knowing "that," (c) the scientist and practitioner are partners in research, and (d) research takes place in clinical practice settings.

Edgerton (1973) urges that the staff nurse be recognized as a theorist. She states that in the process of providing care, the staff nurse must comprehend and interpret the circumstances confronting her in order to apply or adapt available scientific theory. If necessary, the staff nurse must be able to create new theory. This requires imagination and the ability to identify and isolate significant events and facts.

In the emerging view, the staff nurse is knowledgeable, possessing the cognitive skills necessary to manipulate and apply research findings in clinical practice. Knowledge does not take the form of standard intervention, but it changes with use. Research becomes the foundation of the staff nurse's knowledge of facts, concepts, and theory.

Research in preoperative teaching

During the last 20 years, preoperative teaching has been a focus of nursing research. The effectiveness of teaching, teaching strategies, and timing of teaching has been investigated. It is clear from this literature that preoperative teaching does influence postoperative recovery. For the purposes of this article, the study "Nursing Intervention with the Pre-Surgical Patient: Phase I" (Lindeman, 1971) is summarized.

The purpose of the study was to determine the effects of preoperative teaching of deep breathing, coughing, and bed exercises. Reduction of postoperative respiratory and circulatory complications as a result of breathing, coughing, and bed exercises, known as the "stir-up routine," is discussed in the nursing literature as early as 1941 (Dripps, 1941). At that time only meager, inconclusive research was available to guide nurses.

The effects of systematic preoperative teaching were compared with unstructured preoperative teaching. Data were collected on ventilatory function, length of hospital stay, and number of postoperative analgesics. Subjects included patients, 15 years of age or older, admitted for elective surgery using a general anesthetic. The following principles for teaching a skill served as the basis for the structured preoperative teaching: (a) analyze the skill before attempting to guide the learner; (b) demonstrate the skill correctly; (c) guide the initial practice attempts verbally

and, if necessary, physically; (d) provide for practice; (e) encourage additional periodic practice; (f) assist the learner to evaluate his or her own performance so that he or she can be independent in performing the skill correctly.

A Sound-on-Slide Preoperative Teaching Program was developed. This program consisted of twenty-four 35-mm slides with a sound track.

Procedures for structured teaching included (a) distributing a patient-teaching pamphlet; (b) explaining the importance of the postoperative regimen; (c) showing the slides; (d) demonstrating and having the patient return the demonstrations for deep breathing, coughing, and bed exercises; (e) assisting the patient to evaluate each exercise; and (f) instructing the patient to practice.

The following conclusions were drawn from the study: (a) The ability of patients to deep-breathe and cough postoperatively was improved by the structured preoperative teaching; (b) the average length of hospital stay was reduced by the structured teaching method; and (c) the structured teaching plan had an effect upon the number of postoperative analgesics administered.

Application of research in practice

Traditional view. The staff nurse wishing to apply this research in practice would focus on the procedure for preoperative teaching. The lesson plan and perhaps even the Sound-on-Slide Program would become the standardized procedure. This standardized approach would be used with all patients having elective surgery and a general anesthetic. The staff nurse would assume responsibility and accountability for correct implementation of preoperative teaching and for evaluating patients' postoperative progress.

Emerging view. In the alternate approach to application of research in practice, the staff nurse gives more attention to the principles and less attention to the procedural components of the preoperative teaching research. The staff nurse will note that an important part of the preoperative teaching was supporting the patient in taking responsibility for his or her own care. The patient was less dependent on the nurse and was able to implement and evaluate activities on his own behalf. As staff nurses apply this knowledge in practice, they assess and evaluate each patient-situation to determine the most effective ways to implement the teaching principles. Depending on the nurses' assessments, families may or may not be involved in the teaching intervention. Depending on the patients' responses, the nurses may or may not add additional practice sessions. An anxious patient may be given additional printed material to minimize forgetting. Nurses evaluate the effectiveness of the teaching intervention by focusing on the patients' abilities to implement postoperative self-care behaviors. Over time, nurses will develop standardized ways of doing some aspects of preoperative teaching, but these will be altered to account for individual differences.

Summary

The nursing research literature contains numerous studies regarding the effectiveness of preoperative teaching of deep breathing, coughing, and bed exercises. The staff nurse can use this research base either to develop standardized procedures or to identify critical concepts that can be added to her existing knowledge base. By focusing on developing procedures, the staff nurse will promote the view of her role as problem solver who matches standardized interventions to standardized categories of patient problems. Alternatively, the nurse can focus on the critical concepts identified through research and base her practice on validated knowledge adapted to the specifics of individual patient situations.

Until the latter view of application is accepted, there will be limited evidence of the application of research in practice. The staff nurse knows the limitations of trial-and-error practice. The nurse, more than anyone (except perhaps the patient), wants a scientific base for practice. However, the staff nurse also knows that although all patients are similar in some respects, they are all unique in some respects. Research results will only be valued and applied in practice by staff nurses if the results clearly help enhance the care of individual patients with unique needs.

REFERENCES

Dripps, R.D., & Walters, R.M. (1941). Nursing care of surgical patients I: The stir-up. *American Journal of Nursing, 41*, 530-534.

Edgerton, S. (1973). The technological imagination: A philosopher looks at nursing. *Journal of Thought, 8*, 57-65.

Fawcett, J. (1980, June). A declaration of nursing independence: The relation of theory and research to nursing practice. *The Journal of Nursing Administration*, pp. 1036-1039.

Lindeman, C.A. (1971). Nursing intervention with the presurgical patient: Phase 1: The effects of structured and unstructured preoperative teaching. *Nursing Research, 20*, 319-332.

Schon, D. (1983). *The Reflective Practitioner*. New York City: Basic Books.

Developing research-based innovation protocols: Process, criteria, and issues

KAREN B. HALLER; MARGARET A. REYNOLDS; JO ANNE HORSLEY

THIS PAPER DEALS WITH the criteria and issues involved in a process of transferring research-based knowledge into innovation protocols for nursing practice. Content for the paper developed from work on a funded project titled the Conduct and Utilization of Research in Nursing (CURN). Now in its fourth year of activity, CURN is addressing a widespread and critical problem in the nursing profession. The amount of sound nursing research has been increasing steadily, but often this research has had little appreciable impact on nursing practice (Aydelotte, 1976; Ketefian, 1975; Krueger, 1978). Project staff are investigating ways in which scientific knowledge may be transferred to the practice of nursing and ways in which clinical practice might influence nursing research so that it more closely approximates the clinical setting's methods and goals.

Requisite to this work is the identification and evaluation of nursing research that is suitable for transfer to practice settings. This process has involved retrieving, reviewing, and organizing studies into areas of conceptually related research, followed by an evaluation of each area's potential for use. The final step in this sequence is the development of "innovation protocols" for nursing care interventions based on the identified research. Although specific criteria have guided the process of transforming clinical research into such protocols, several issues of concern have emerged. It is our intent in this paper to describe the process and the criteria used and to delineate the issues that have arisen.

Process

The project staff's experience with research utilization to date has demonstrated that considerable confusion exists among nurses regarding the differences between the conduct of research and the utilization of the knowledge resulting from such research. For example, when asked to describe how they might use research in their practice, nurses often cite a process of replication. It is important to differentiate the goals and, therefore, the people, knowledge, and context relevant for research conduct and research utilization, respectively. Research conduct is directed toward the production of knowledge that is generalizable beyond the population directly studied. The process of research utilization, on the other hand, is directed toward transferring specific research-based knowledge into actual practice. The conduct of research generally occurs in the academic context where people with specialized knowledge and skills in the methods of scientific inquiry can obtain the resources and control of conditions necessary. To be effective, however, research-based knowledge should be implemented and evaluated in a practice context where people with knowledge, skills, and experience in the methods of nursing practice can examine the relevance, means, and utility of new techniques (Horsley, Crane, & Bingle, 1978).

A key dimension on which the conduct of research varies from research utilization is methodology. The tenets of scientific methodology can be contrasted with those of the methodology of practice. Nurses in settings where research is conducted rely on scientific methodology that is systematic, controlled, and generally inflexible. Research methods are relatively rigorous and attempt to minimize personal bias. The researcher takes a logical approach and attempts to discover common patterns in a population. In nursing practice, however, skill is of paramount concern and methods are individualized. Clinical measures are relatively flexible, may rely on precedent, and call on clinical judgment. The clinician takes an intuitive approach and views each case as unique. These methodological differences are important because they affect the interactions that occur between the research and practice settings. Such differences have tended to preclude the use of research in practice as well as to inhibit the conduct of practice-relevant research. A process of methodological approximation, or a systematic effort to close the gap between research methods and practice methods, is essential to research utilization. Both researchers and clinicians need to assume responsibility for approximating one another's methods. The innovation protocol may be viewed as one step in a series of methodological approximations that are necessary for utilization. Later approximations can occur when nurses in a practice setting transform the protocol for their own particular needs and again when the change is implemented. The process used to develop innovation protocols will demonstrate this notion of methodological approximation.

The approach used to identify research-based knowledge with potential for use in nursing practice is based on the idea that there are areas of research in which studies can be related to one another by common variables and by relationships between those variables. Studies contributing to a particular area of research form the base from which nursing knowledge and nursing activities may be derived. When the activity suggested by the research base is different from traditional practice, that is, it either adds to practice in some way or calls for the extinction of a practice, it

is an "innovation." Innovations in nursing imply changes in practice that are new to those using them and that are intended to benefit clients. Once a potential practice innovation has been identified, an attempt is made to "package" the information into an "innovation protocol"; this represents a methodological approximation of research to practice. An effort is made to write the protocols in a form that will be useful to nurses interested in implementing research-based planned change in nursing practice. An innovation protocol, therefore, is research-based knowledge put in the form of a product: the product is nursing knowledge that has clearly definable parameters for use in practice.

The protocol

At this point it might be useful to describe the form and content of an innovation protocol. Each protocol begins with a section on the need for change, documenting the extent of the clinical problem and the relevance of the problem to nursing practice. The second section gives a description of the innovation, including information on the types of patients most likely to benefit from the innovation. The protocol then provides a summary of the research base and identifies "research-based principles" to guide the implementation of the innovation. Although the use of the term "principle" is not scientifically accurate, CURN Project staff have persisted in using the term because it was found to communicate the appropriate intent to nurses who use the protocols. It is more accurate, however, to say that what are extracted from the research bases are empirical generalizations.

The remainder of the protocol deals with implementation of the innovation and systematic evaluation of its effects. With regard to both of these processes, the protocol describes the materials that will be required, the personnel development that may be necessary to carry out the activities suggested, and the costs that are likely to be incurred. Finally, each protocol is summarized by a discussion of the benefits that can be expected to result from a successful trial of the innovation. Additional materials may be appended to the protocols as they are available or can be developed. These materials always include the primary sources of the research base. They may also include an annotated bibliography, an evaluation procedure designed by the author of the protocol, and any additional tools or resources that are available from the original researchers.

Ten research-based practice protocols have been developed by project personnel and are being field tested. These include:

1. Structure preoperative teaching
2. A lactose-free diet
3. Sensation information: distress reduction
4. Sensory information: recovery rate
5. Nonsterile intermittent urinary catheterization
6. Prevention of catheter-associated urinary tract infections
7. Intravenous cannula change regimen
8. Prevention of decubiti by means of small shifts of body weight
9. Mutual goal setting: goal attainment
10. Deliberative nursing: pain reduction

Criteria for utilization of research in nursing practice

When project staff began the search and retrieval process for research bases, a number of well-known nursing researchers were asked to identify areas of clinical research which they felt were sufficiently developed to merit use in practice. Responses indicated a wide range of opinion; for example, some felt that "anything may be utilized; the determination rests with those who want to incorporate the ideas in any given study into their clinical work." Others responded toward the opposite end of the continuum: "No area of clinical nursing research is currently adequate for utilization in prac-

tice." Clearly such a range of answers suggested that different processes, criteria, and issues were considered by the respondents. The nursing literature also offered little assistance in defining how or with what criteria one may determine the adequacy of clinical research bases. Therefore, CURN Project personnel established criteria for selecting the research that is used in the development of protocols and in the utilization efforts of the projects. The criteria were organized into three major categories: (a) criteria that pertain to evaluating and integrating studies that constitute a base, (b) criteria that address the issue of how relevant the base is for nursing practice, and (c) criteria related to the potential for evaluation in the clinical setting. Each of these will be discussed.

Evaluation and integration of studies

Replication. The first criterion for identifying studies that constitute a research base is replication. Ideally there is more than one study in a research base to provide greater assurance against committing a Type I error, thereby inferring an effect where none exists. Some researchers criticize this approach by noting that the Type II error can be just as costly in inferring a lack of effect when there actually is one. Certainly, postponing implementation of a valid study is of concern; however, the possibility of implementing an innovation based on a "false positive" has legal and ethical ramifications that project personnel were unwilling to risk. Therefore, when developing protocols in any given area of research, an effort is made to establish that the conceptual and constructive propositions have been confirmed in more than one study; this is a process of construct replication. According to Lykken (1968), construct replication tests the validity of the "relation between meaningful constructs, generalizable to some broad reference population, which the [original author] claimed to have established" (p. 156). Construct replication is achieved when a second investigator begins with a similar problem statement but formulates original methods of measurement and design to verify the first author's findings. The advantage of construct replication over literal or operational replication is that it validates previous work, extends the findings, and offers great utility because it builds knowledge efficiently.

In order to obtain a solid research base for an innovation, it has been necessary to organize studies according to the concepts tested and to actively seek instances of construct replication. For example, numerous investigators (Felton, Huss, Payne, & Srsic, 1976; Fortin & Kirouac, 1976; Johnson, Rice, & Endress, 1975; Lindeman & Van Aernam, 1971) studied structured preoperative teaching and its postoperative effects. At the time the literature search was done, it was clear that these studies did not directly replicate one another. Yet the studies did demonstrate — in varied settings, using different populations, and a number of methodologies — that structured preoperative teaching does have a positive postoperative effect on clients. In other instances such replication has not been found. For example, numerous investigators studied various treatment modalities for decubitus ulcers (for a review of the literature, see Berecek, 1975). In these studies, to date, the findings are not corroborated; therefore, in spite of the extensiveness of the research, no base is available from which to develop a particular nursing innovation for treating decubitus ulcers.

Scientific merit. The second criterion for studies constituting a research base is scientific merit. Each study with potential for contributing to the base is reviewed in terms of its design and methodology. Validity and reliability are key issues. The appropriateness of the sample for the clinical problem is also considered; generalizability is at issue here. At least one study in the research base must be con-

ducted in a practice setting. Finally, the study's assumptions, findings, and conclusions are examined. The value of a study to the conceptual base is not determined entirely by the statistical significance of the findings; rather, an attempt is made to understand the functional relationships between variables in a base. The conclusions and implications of each study are evaluated in terms of their power to corroborate, extend, or delineate the conceptual base.

In the process of evaluating individual studies and comparing each with other studies in the base, conflicting findings may be found. Attempts are made to resolve contradictory findings either through identification of methodological weaknesses or through a theoretical explanation for the discrepancy. It is also recognized that in a series of replications of the same study, a non-significant difference may be expected to occur a certain number of times on the basis of chance alone. For example, the research base underlying the regimen for changing intravenous cannula consists of some 20 studies (e.g., Collin, Collin, Constable, & Johnston, 1975; Thomas, Evers, & Racz, 1970). Collectively, these studies support the proposition that duration of cannulization is positively related to local venous infection and infusion phlebitis. The findings of one study (Crossley & Matsen, 1972), however, resulted in a departure from this generalization. Closer scrutiny revealed that only intravenous infusions of greater than 24 hours' duration were included in the calculations. In truncating the data at one end of the scale, the significant effect of time on the dependent variables of infection and phlebitis may have been lost. Theoretically, this suggested that the findings were not necessarily contradictory to the research base but that there was probably a maximum time beyond which duration of the intravenous infusion does not correlate significantly with complications. Further search and retrieval was indicated to confirm this suspicion and to define what the maximum time might be. The example demonstrates that each study in a conceptual area is evaluated on its own scientific merit as well as on its power to contribute to a research base for practice by corroboration or extension.

Risk. The third criterion used to identify clinical research bases is risk. The concept of risk is used to mediate the stringency with which the criteria of replication and scientific merit are applied. Where the risk to the client is small, a generalization is made more readily than in those instances where the risk is great. For instance, studies exist that can be grouped conceptually into an area; yet, considered together, these studies do not deal fully with the functional relationships among the variables. There may be some weaknesses in methodology; there may be conflicting findings; or perhaps the case for construct replication is not strong. If there is little potential harm to the client, the practice action suggested by the research base may be tentatively implemented *pending clinical evaluation.* Such is the case in the decubitus prevention protocol. The nursing innovation derived from the base calls for unscheduled small shifts of body weight in addition to routine, scheduled turning. Although this research base has some weaknesses, implementation of the innovation requires requires little time or training on the part of the staff and does not jeopardize the client in any way. In other protocols where risk to the client is greater, the criteria have been applied more stringently.

Relevance to practice

Once it has been established that a research base exists, the second major category of criteria needs to be considered; these criteria deal with the issue of practice relevance. When applied to an innovation, practice relevance means that the innovation derived from the base meets the demand of a nursing problem in a clinical setting. To state it another way, a research-based innovation that is practice relevant means that it has approximated the practice setting's goals and methods. The degree to which this approximation has occurred may be judged by four criteria: (a) degree of clinical merit, (b) extent of clinical control over the variables, (c) feasibility, and (d) cost.

Clinical merit. Clinical merit is the degree to which the research base addresses a problem of significance to the practice setting or the degree to which the suggested innovation will be potentially useful. Clinical merit represents an approximation of the research problem to the clinical goal.

Clinical control. A second consideration is clinical control. It is essential that nursing has, or is able to achieve, clinical control of the independent and dependent variables in the research base. If nurses are to use the research base, they must be in control of the events required for implementation and evaluation of the innovation. Control is problematic for two reasons: (a) the outcomes of nursing practice are often influenced by multiple factors external to the nurse-patient relationship; and (b) the instruments used to measure the effects of the innovation may not be available for use by nurses in the practice setting.

In the first instance, control over the outcomes of nursing practice is the concern. Occasionally, the variables in the research base fall clearly within the purview of nursing and control becomes almost automatic. An example of this occurs in the decubitus prevention protocol where the independent variable is small shifts of body weight and the dependent variable is occurrence of pressure sores. Clearly both variables are within the purview of nursing with minimal input from other professionals. In most of the protocols, however, clinical control of the variables must be achieved through the development of collaborative decision making with other practitioners. For instance, implementation of the non-sterile intermittent catheterization protocol requires cooperation with physicians. Input by physicians is necessary in making the decision to use nonsterile intermittent catheterization with individual patients, in prescribing drugs used in conjunction with the innovation, and in ordering laboratory studies to determine the effectiveness of the innovation. Clearly, securing the involvement of physicians is crucial to clinical control over implementation and evaluation of this innovation.

The second control problem relates to measurement. The protocols require the use of some of the dependent variables from the research base for evaluation of the innovation. Frequently, however, the methods that the researchers used to measure the dependent variables are not immediately available in the clinical setting. In some cases, an approximation to practice can be made by the substitution of valid clinical measures for the research instruments. In other cases, the clinical setting may approximate the researchers' methods by acquiring the new knowledge or skill needed to use the research tools. When the preoperative teaching protocol was implemented in two different Michigan hospitals, one setting chose to substitute tape measurement of chest expansion and auscultation for spirometry as measures of respiratory status. This particular substitution was adapted from work done by Horn and Swain (1977) and demonstrates an approximation to practice. The second setting chose to work with the respiratory therapy department to gain access to the knowledge and skills needed to do spirometry; in this case, a clinical approximation to research methodology was made.

Feasibility. Feasibility is the next factor that is considered in determining practice relevance. Given the constraints of the environments in which nurses practice, is it feasible to implement the innovation? Feasibility varies from institution to institution because it is related to the availability of resources (e.g., time, personnel, expertise, and equipment) and to the dominant feeling about change in the clinical setting. Each of these factors will vary in turn by the nature of the innovation, such as the degree of change it implies, the relative compatibility of the innovation with current nursing practice, the number of clients who will be affected, or the number of staff nurses to be involved.

Cost benefits. Closely related to feasibility but treated as a separate factor is cost. The financial cost of implementing and evaluating the innovation suggested by the research base is balanced against the potential benefit to clients. Since this type of analysis is rarely documented in the research literature, an estimate is made. Estimates most frequently balance the costs of materials, laboratory expenses, personnel development, and staff time against such benefits as reduced incidence of complications and patient or staff satisfaction.

Potential for clinical evaluation

Each research base must be reviewed in relation to its potential for permitting adequate clinical evaluation of the proposed practice change. A key distinction between research utilization and replication of research points to the importance of clinical evaluation. Utilization implies that the practitioner transforms the new knowledge for use in the practice setting. Even under ideal conditions of clinical control, utilization of research in the clinical setting constitutes a change in the independent variable. To assure that this change or transformation has not extended beyond the limits of the research base, it must be possible to evaluate clinically the effects of the innovation once the protocol has been implemented. More specifically, the criterion states that there must be one or more dependent variables in the original research base that can be reliably measured by clinicians in practice settings.

There are actually two components to this criterion: (a) the clinical knowledge and skills of the general nursing staff necessary to measure reliably the dependent variable and (b) the clinical control of the variable, which was discussed earlier. Using this criterion, project staff found that many of the dependent measures in the research base are not useful for clinical evaluation. Further, those measures that do meet the demands of the criterion are often the weakest in the research base in terms of validity and reliability.

Purposes of innovation evaluation. Evaluation of an innovation serves multiple purposes. Clinical evaluation moves practitioners to approximate research methodology more closely since such evaluation requires a systematic and controlled process involving measurement, data collection, and analysis. Evaluation can also be used to assess the extent to which research knowledge is applicable to practice settings. This information can then provide useful feedback to the original researchers. In addition, clinical evaluation questions whether the innovation is relevant to a practice problem, that is, whether or not it produces an outcome that justifies its use. The data base provided by clinical evaluation can serve to justify the new practice to others and is useful in meeting legal and ethical concerns related to accountability.

Characteristics of innovation evaluation. Initially, it was anticipated that the research base would identify the outcome variables and also assist in the development of appropriate measurement procedures for use in evaluation. This has not always been true, and as a result, greater flexibility has been required in the design of evaluation procedures to accompany the innovation. For instance, the original work on nonsterile intermittent catheterization was done by physicians. Some of the dependent variables, such as cystoscopy results, were not felt to be appropriate as nursing outcomes. On the other hand, some of the variables of keen interest to nursing were not accounted for in the research base: these included patient satisfaction, patient mobility, and degree of social interaction. Therefore, an evaluation procedure was devised that included variables from the research base and also drew on introspection about clinical practice.

Evaluation of the innovation is structured into a process component and an outcome component, providing a format that parallels current efforts in quality assurance. Independent variables from the research base are measured in terms of process to assure that the innovation has been implemented accurately and consistently; dependent variables are measured as outcomes. Once such an evaluation has been designed, it is easily placed into the ongoing quality assurance system.

To date, all evaluations use a pre- and postimplementation design. Baseline data and postimplementation data are usually summarized by frequency tables, ranges, rates, or means for purposes of comparison. Differences in the data are not tested for statistical significance. Again, a process of clinical evaluation rather than replication is advocated.

Conclusion

Development of research-based practice innovation protocols begins with a search for conceptually related studies that have potential for utilization in clinical nursing settings. Each potential practice area is then appraised according to the three major criteria that have been established by the CURN Project staff. If the area has an established research base, is practice relevant, and can be reliably evaluated by clinicians, it is judged sufficient for utilization in practice settings. An innovation protocol is subsequently developed, serving as a form of methodological approximation.

In many instances, potential practice innovations fail to meet the criteria and thus do not merit utilization in practice. Perhaps a replication of the original study is all that is necessary to permit its utilization, or it may be that a more valid and/or reliable tool is required in order to evaluate clinically the effects of the innovation. Through the process of subjecting each area to the demands of the criteria, missing links and deficiencies that preclude utilization become apparent. The identified deficiencies are of major importance, for they point to areas that need further research. Therefore, the process can also serve to guide future research efforts in nursing.

REFERENCES

Aydelotte, M.K. Nursing research in clinical settings: Problems and issues. *Sigma Theta Tau Reflections,* 1976, *2,* 3-6.

Berecek, K.H. Treatment of decubitus ulcers. *Nursing Clinics North America,* 1975, *10,* 171-210.

Collin, J., Collin, C., Constable, F.L., & Johnston, I.D.A. Infusion thrombophlebitis and infection with various cannulas. *Lancet,* 1975, *2,* 150-153.

Crossley, K., & Matsen, J.M. The scalp-vein needle: A prospective study of complications. *Journal of the American Medical Association,* 1972, *220,* 985-987.

Felton, G., Huss, K., Payne, E.A., & Srsic, K. Preoperative nursing intervention with the patient for surgery. Outcomes of three alternative approaches. *International Journal of Nursing Studies,* 1976, *1,* 83-96.

Fortin, F. A randomized controlled trial of preoperative patient education. *International Journal of Nursing Studies.* 1976, *13,* 11-24.

Horn, B., & Swain, M.A. *Development of criterion measures of nursing care.* Unpublished manuscript, School of Public Health, University of Michigan, 1977.

Horsley, J.A., Crane, J., & Bingle, J.D. Research utilization as an organizational process. *Journal of Nursing Administration,* 1978, *8*(7), 4-6.

Johnson, J.E., Rice, V.H., & Endress, M.P. Making psychological concepts concrete for medical education. *Proceedings of the 14th Annual Conference on Research in Medical Education.* Washington, D.C.: Association of American Medical Colleges, 1975, 125-130.

Ketefian, S. Application of selected nursing research findings into nursing practice. *Nursing Research,* 1975, *24,* 89-92.

Krueger, J.C. Utilization of nursing research: The planning process. *Journal of Nursing Administration,* 1978, *8*(1), 6-9.

Lindeman, C.A., & Van Aernam, B. Nursing intervention with the presurgical patient—The effects of structured and unstructured preoperative teaching. *Nursing Research,* 1971, *20,* 319-332.

Lykken, D.T. Statistical significance in psychological research. *Psychological Bulletin,* 1968, *70,* 151-159.

Thomas, E.T., Evers, W., & Racz, G.B. Postinfusion phlebitis. *Anesthesia and Analgesia,* 1970, *49,* 150-159.

CHAPTER SEVEN

The role of the clinician in development and use of knowledge

IN THE LOGICAL empiricist philosophy of science, the scientist uses a controlled-phenomena research process to uncover the laws of nature and thus find truth. According to this philosophy, truth cannot be found in practice settings because the practitioner cannot control events.

This philosophy of science predominated long into 20th century nursing, fostering a view of the staff nurse as a user of knowledge developed by the scientist, not as a developer of nursing knowledge. In this view, nurses were not expected to need time in their practice for doing research. For example, pressures within the clinical setting, such as cost containment, impeded nurses' implementation of roles that included research activities.

Since the 1960s, however, nurses in clinical settings have challenged this, believing that their involvement in research will increase both its relevance to their practice and its credibility. In the first article, "Loneliness in Critically Ill Adults," Buchda describes how theory from another discipline can be applied to nursing practice. In so doing, she also describes how nurses in the clinical setting can link theory and practice — thereby improving patient care.

Hathaway and Strong provide a concrete illustration of a clinical setting that incorporates theory and research into practice. Their experience, as described in "Theory, Practice, and Research in Transplant Nursing," shows the limitations of the logical empiricist philosophy to a practice discipline such as nursing. Their experience supports the view that the staff nurse is a theoretician and a researcher. The inquiring mind of the clinician is the key to bringing theory, practice, and research together.

In the final article, "Use of Research-Based Knowledge in Clinical Practice," Goode et al. implement the research guidelines developed as part of the Conduct and Utilization of Research in Nursing (CURN) project in a small, rural, 42-bed acute-care hospital. This approach does not conflict with the logical empiricist philosophy in that nurses in the clinical setting use knowledge developed by researchers. Based on their experience, they endorse research that is "user ready" for application in settings like theirs.

Loneliness in critically ill adults

VICKI L. BUCHDA, RN, MS, CCRN

LONELINESS IS A COMMONLY overlooked psychosocial problem in the critically ill patient, which can stem from both acute illness and hospitalization. One nursing study revealed that over 50% of adults hospitalized on medical and surgical units experience loneliness and 90% of those patients felt that the nurse might help relieve their loneliness.[1] Patients were able to identify measures nurses could take to help alleviate their loneliness. Social isolation and other components of loneliness have been cited as contributing factors in the development of ICU syndrome[2] and a sudden cardiac death.[3,4] Loneliness has also been linked to immunodepression.[5]

Nurses can diagnose and treat the problem of loneliness. Although loneliness is not itself an accepted nursing diagnosis, it may be the basis for several others, including anxiety, fear, social isolation, and sleep pattern disturbance. Prevention, early recognition, and prompt treatment of loneliness are important aspects of nursing care. The purpose of this article is to 1) explore the phenomenon of loneliness by comparing and contrasting types of loneliness and research findings; 2) discuss the manifestations of loneliness in the critically ill adult; and 3) identify potential nursing strategies to prevent and treat various types of loneliness.

The nature of loneliness

Although it is well-documented that loneliness occurs in hospitalized adults, nursing literature about the concept of loneliness is scarce and confusing. One factor which may explain the confusion is that there is no one definition or set of definitions of loneliness; a second factor concerns the lack of one specific nursing theory or theoretical framework which provides guidance for research and practice. Consequently the nurse must examine the theory and research from other disciplines and apply it from a nursing perspective. For a synopsis of four theories relevant to nursing care and research, see "Theories of Loneliness."

Definition of loneliness and related concepts. In using the loneliness concept to build assessment and intervention techniques, the nurse needs to distinguish between loneliness, aloneness, lonesomeness, and social isolation. Hildegarde Peplau was instrumental in first influencing nurses to examine the problem of loneliness and to incorporate the concept into nursing care.[6] In the psychodynamic tradition *loneliness* was viewed as pathological, rooted in life experiences, and resulting in a multitude of defense mechanisms. The lonely person did not choose to be lonely and was not aware of the loneliness or the defense mechanisms developed to avoid experiencing the pain of loneliness.

Peplau[6] contrasted loneliness with *lonesomeness,* which is described as a common, ordinary, normal experience resulting from being without others while wanting to be with others. The person recognizes that he is lonesome and takes steps to relieve the lonesomeness.

Aloneness is the chosen state of being alone for a purpose. Artists, scientists, and writers may choose to be alone by removing themselves from the social stream in order to improve concentration and limit interruptions. It is possible to be alone without being lonesome or lonely. In contrast to aloneness, loneliness is not a chosen state.

Peplau and Perlman[7] found three commonalities in a dozen definitions of loneliness offered by social scientists. The three commonalities include: 1) "Loneliness results from deficiencies in a person's social relationships."[7] 2) "Loneliness is a subjective experience; it is not synonymous with objective social isolation. People can be alone without being lonely, or lonely in a crowd."[7] 3) "The experience of loneliness is unpleasant and distressing."[7] Moustakas[8] and Weiss[9] both describe loneliness as extremely distressing and state that people will go to great lengths to avoid it, a supposition supported by other research as well. For example, Andren and Rosenquist[10] reported that people who used the emergency department repeatedly tended to be living alone and feeling lonely.

Social isolation has been addressed by nursing in the development of a nursing diagnosis titled "Social Isolation." In the nursing diagnosis context it is defined as "the state in which the individual experiences a need or desire for contact with others but is unable to make contact."[11] It is further described as "a negative state of aloneness...that exists whenever a person says it does and is perceived as imposed by others."[11] This definition of social isolation shares all three of the common elements that Peplau and Perlman[7] identified in their analysis of various definitions of loneliness. Mills[12] differentiated between social isolation and loneliness according to how it is perceived; social isolation is perceived as imposed by others, loneliness is not. Social isolation is an important nursing diagnosis because it is often a precursor of loneliness,[7] and can be thought of as a type of loneliness.[9] It is not, however, as inclusive as the diagnosis of loneliness, which has more emotional aspects than only social isolation. A patient may feel loneliness even in the presence of the numerous health care professionals common in critical care units.

Watson's[13] theory of nursing is an excellent vehicle for examining loneliness because it encompasses many of the concepts and approaches just examined, but emphasizes care of the person as a whole. Nursing is unique because the individual is viewed as a whole and the mind, body, and soul are seen as inseparable.[13]

Every human needs to be loved, cared for, and cared about, and seeks a union with another human. If a person feels separate and alone, there is incongruence and disharmony, resulting in illness.[13] Loneliness, then, contributes to illness and disease and is manifested in various ways.

Loneliness in the critically ill adult. Upon admission to the critical care unit, an individual experiences many changes that can precipitate feelings of loneliness. These feelings may be expressed as feeling empty, self-enclosed, awkward, restless, and bored.[14] The patient may appear quiet, withdrawn, or tearful, and may frequently have requests that bring the nurse into the room. Patients may also request to have their "own" nurse to care for them. The patient may experience existential loneliness or loneliness anxiety.

The critically ill person may experience *existential loneliness* related to the threat of the illness or to psychological and physiological pain.[15] An existential experience represents what is real for the individual and is unique because only that individual can know the experience; no one else can duplicate the exact feelings of that person. The threat of the illness or injury itself is real for the individual, who experiences the potential loss of organs, body parts, body function, and even life itself. This threat causes severe psychological pain, and the awareness of loneliness is embodied in that pain.

Another contributing factor to the psychological pain of loneliness is the separateness

Theories of loneliness

Psychodynamic approach

Zilboorg[19] published what was probably the first psychological analysis of loneliness. He differentiated between being lonesome and being lonely, and described lonesome as "normal" and "transient," usually related to missing a specific person, whereas loneliness was defined as "overwhelming," "persistent," and related to man's "narcissism." Lonesome people miss other people because they care about those people, whereas lonely people miss other people because there is no one to provide them with love. In typical Freudian tradition, Zilboorg linked the origins of loneliness to experiences in infancy and childhood. He contended that from birth the infant learns and expects that life is nothing else but being loved and admired and later this surfaces as self-centeredness, self-admiration, and loneliness.

Sullivan[20] and Fromm-Riechmann[21] built upon Zilboorg's views and supported the importance of childhood experiences in the development of loneliness. They also emphasized the inherent human needs for intimacy, and attributed the problem of loneliness to an inability to form relationships related to faulty interaction with parents[20] and "premature weaning from mothering tenderness."[21]

Loneliness was viewed as undesirable and pathological by all three of these theorists. Many of their ideas were based on observations and work in clinical settings, and they focused on the personal traits and conflicts which contribute to loneliness. Loneliness was thought to end in psychotic states.[7]

Existential approach

Existentialists view humans as ultimately alone; loneliness is considered a part of human existence. Although they share many of the same philosophical views, some existentialists vary in their differentiation of the types of loneliness.

Von Witzieben[22] divided loneliness into two types, primary and secondary. Primary loneliness is described as omnipresent, a universal human characteristic, and can be referred to as cosmic or existential loneliness.

It is the loneliness of "one's self, inborn in everyone, the feeling of being alone and helpless"[22] in the world. Secondary loneliness is the result of "temporary separation (as compared with permanent separation by death) from persons and things to whom one is closely attached".[23] Secondary loneliness was found to affect a large portion of hospitalized adults.[1]

Moustakas[8] considers the loneliness of modern life in two ways. Existential loneliness is viewed as an intrinsic condition of existence, the real loneliness of genuine experience. This true loneliness results from the knowledge that no one else can ever experience what one is feeling in exactly the same way. Moustakas contrasts existential loneliness, which is inevitable and a part of being, with loneliness anxiety, which he sees as being brought on by the conditions of modern life. Fear or anxiety occurs when a person is unable to experience a sense of relatedness to self, to others, and to nature. A person will seek the company of others and will participate in different relationships to try to deal with the anxiety.

Moustakas' views were influenced by Thomas Wolfe, who believed that as a result of existential loneliness a person develops deeper sensitivities and awareness, is strengthened, develops and maintains a true self-identity, and is more creative. Unlike Wolfe and Moustakas, most other authors do not consider this existential loneliness as an enriching positive experience.[7]

Interactionist view

Interactionists emphasize that loneliness is the interactive effect of both personality and situational factors; neither factor alone can explain what triggers loneliness.[24] Weiss[9] divided the loneliness experience into two parts, emotional isolation and social isolation. Emotional isolation is described as the loss or lack of a truly intimate tie, such as a spouse, parent, or child, while social isolation is the consequence of lacking a network of involvement with peers. Weiss focuses on current conditions as causes of loneliness and views loneliness as normal.[9] The problem of

---

Theories of loneliness (continued)

---

social isolation is addressed by nursing diagnosis, but is not seen as part of the loneliness experience.[12]

Cognitive approach
Peplau and Perlman[7] use the cognitive approach and view loneliness as occurring when the individual does not achieve the levels of social contact desired. Loneliness is

not based on an outsider's assessment, but on how the person perceives his or her own social relationships and whether or not they are characterized by the quality, intimacy, and quantity (or number of friends) desired. They have been influential in their work with loneliness, and their framework was used by Mahon in her nursing research regarding loneliness during adolescence.[14]

---

that the patient experiences upon admission to the critical care unit. The person is separated from familiar events, values, ideas, and significant others. Closed intensive care units with private rooms are conducive to a quiet environment with more privacy, but one study shows that patients in private rooms tended to feel more lonely and fearful of loss of love and support.[16] Feelings of relatedness to both the body and mind may be lost, conditions precipitated by dependence or perceived dependence on machines and equipment for life support, such as ventilators and hemodialysis. Physical pain can also cause existential loneliness because it is naturally interpreted as a threat to life.

Loneliness anxiety in the critically ill patient stems from the fear of being lonely in the critical care unit, and fear of the implications of the critical illness. A person who lacks a sense of relatedness to other people may feel like an object, a thing, or a commodity. This is accompanied by a loss of the sense of self and self-worth, and consequently the person may feel that life is meaningless. Moustakas[8] identifies the loneliness of a meaningless existence; the absence of values, convictions, and beliefs; and the fear of isolation as the most terrible kinds of loneliness anxiety.

There are, however, many ways in which the nurse can decrease loneliness and facilitate harmony within the critically ill adult.

Nursing techniques to reduce loneliness

Using Watson's theory, the nursing goal is to facilitate the individual's spiritual sense of relatedness to the body and mind, significant others, familiar events, values and beliefs, and to the nurse as a person. Increasing the patient's sense of relatedness to self and to others will decrease loneliness. Reduction of the causes of loneliness, both the threat of illness and pain (emotional and physical pain), will also decrease loneliness.

Nursing interventions need not be extremely time-consuming and can be incorporated into the nursing care already being provided. Interventions include:

1. Provide immediate and on-going patient teaching about the stages of healing and therapy. Reducing the fear of illness and treatment can decrease loneliness.

2. Include the family and significant others in teaching. The family can also experience loneliness. In his qualitative study, Speedling[17] found that patients and families often had grossly different perceptions of the severity of illness and its threats. The family often perceived the person to be much more ill than the ill person perceived himself or herself to be. Realistic understanding of the person, family, and significant others will decrease the threats of illness.

3. Increase relationships. Facilitation of the individual's sense of relatedness to his body, mind, significant others, familiar events, val-

ues, beliefs, and the nurse can reduce loneliness. The following techniques are specific ways to increase relationships and feeling of belonging for the critically ill patient.

4. Ask the person what name they would like to be called and always address the person by name. Calling a person honey, sweetie, or granny, etc., is demeaning, demoralizing, and can increase feelings of loneliness by decreasing a sense of relatedness to self.

5. Encourage patients and family members to participate in care when appropriate and to ask questions. Give them something to do which increases their interaction with the patient such as holding a hand, applying lotion, or assisting with feeding.

6. Touch the person when appropriate. Touch is often used to comfort and soothe those in pain, can enhance self-esteem and self-image, and increase awareness of another's presence.

7. Encourage verbalization of feelings about the illness, injury, accident, and/or pain to decrease the fright, which increases loneliness. Listen attentively and acknowledge these feelings as real (existential loneliness). Do not just quickly say "you will be fine"; instead listen to the patient's experience of loneliness, then offer realistic perspectives regarding cause of accident, quality of life, and potential duration of the pain. Mahon's[18] study of 209 subjects demonstrated that the more one disclosed oneself, the less lonely one tended to be.

8. Allow the patient to get to know you as a nurse and as a human being by sharing feelings and subjectivity. By not sharing oneself, the nurse is in effect refusing to acknowledge the other person's subjectivity. The result is that the person is reduced to an object deprived of any relationship with another, which will increase his or her sense of loneliness. This does not mean to "gripe" about short staffing, but instead to share your concern for the patient.

9. Offer psychological support by initiating short, frequent visits with the patient. Patients in Odell's study[1] indicated that they would like the nurse to "stop by to talk" and to come by "even when they don't have to do something to me." Do a care plan with the patient in the patient's room rather than at the desk and tell him or her you want to do the paperwork there because you "want to be with him."

10. Allow family members and significant others to be with the person as much as possible to facilitate close relationships. The quality of the visit is as important as the length in reducing loneliness, so work with family members on expressing caring. When family leave, have them tell the patient where they will be, repeat it to the patient later, and offer to call them with messages.

11. Ascertain from the person and/or family what kinds of routines the person prefers. Provide the person with familiar objects, such as a child's drawing or even a family picture. Ask the family what they can leave for the patient.

12. Frequently orient the person to time and inform them of the length of time between visits so that the patient can anticipate the next visit and focus on family visits more than loneliness. The critically ill person has perceptual distortions and may have a diminished sense of time. The time between visits can seem like an eternity to the ill, lonely person.

13. Always attempt to communicate with the individual. An inability to communicate precipitates frustration and anxiety, thus compounding a person's loneliness.

Loneliness is a real phenomenon and feeling for the critically ill patient. By applying the concept of loneliness, the critical care nurse can identify patients most likely to experience this problem and provide strategies within the normal nursing plan to prevent or reduce it for these patients.

REFERENCES

1. Odell SH. Someone is lonely. Issues in Mental Health Nursing 1981; 3(1-2):7-12.

2. Kleck HG, ICU syndrome: Onset, manifestations, treatment, stressors, and prevention. Critical Care Quarterly 1984; March: 21-28.

3. Lynch JJ, Convey WH. Loneliness, disease, and death: Alternative approaches. Psychosomatics 1979; 20(10): 702-708.

4. Ruberman W, Weinblatt E, Goldberg JD, Chaudhary BS. Psychosocial influences on mortality after myocardial infarction. N Engl J Med 1984; 311(9): 552-559.

5. Kiecolt-Glaser JK, Ricker D, George J, Messich G, Speicher CE, Garner W, Glaser R. Urinary cortisol levels, cellular immunocompetency, and loneliness in psychiatric patients. Psychosom Med 1984; 46(1): 15-23.

6. Peplau HE. Loneliness. Am J Nurs 1955;55(12): 1476-1479.

7. Peplau LA, Perlman D (Eds). Loneliness: A Sourcebook of Current Theory, Research, and Therapy. New York: John Wiley & Sons, 1982.

8. Moustakas CE. Loneliness. Englewood Cliffs, New Jersey: Prentice-Hall, Inc., 1961.

9. Weiss RS. Loneliness: The Experience of Emotional and Social Isolation. Cambridge, Massachusetts: MIT Press, 1973.

10. Andren KG, Rosenquist U. Heavy users of an emergency department: Psycho-social and medical characteristics, other health contacts and the effect of a hospital social worker intervention. Soc Sci Med 1985; 21(7): 761-770.

11. Carpenito LJ. Nursing Diagnosis: Application to Clinical Practice. Philadelphia: J.B. Lippincott Co., 1983.

12. Mills WC. Alienation: A basic concept underlying social isolation. In: Kim MJ, McFarland GK, McLane AM (Eds). Classification of Nursing Diagnosis: Proceedings of the Fifth National Conference. St. Louis: C.V. Mosby Co., 1984, pp. 343-351.

13. Watson J. Nursing: Human Science and Human Care. Norwalk, Connecticut: Appleton-Century-Crofts, 1985.

14. Mahon NE. Developmental changes and loneliness during adolescence. Topics in Clinical Nursing 1983; 5(1): 66-76.

15. Roberts SL. Behavioral problems in the critically ill patient. Critical Care Update 1979; June: 8-13.

16. Leigh H, Hofer MA, Cooper J, Reiser MF. A psychological comparison of patients in "open" and "closed" coronary care units. J Psychosom Res 1972; 16: 449-457.

17. Speedling EJ. Social structure and social behavior in an intensive care unit: Patient-family perspectives. Soc Work Health Care 1980; 6(2): 1-14.

18. Mahon NE. The relationship of self-disclosure, interpersonal dependency, and life changes to loneliness in young adults. Nurs Res 1982; 31(6): 343-347.

19. Zilboorg G. Loneliness. Atlantic Monthly 1938; 161:45-54.

20. Sullivan HS. The Interpersonal Theory of Psychiatry. New York: W.W. Norton, 1953.

21. Fromm-Reichmann F. Loneliness. Psychiatry 1959; 22:1-15.

22. von Witzleben HD. On loneliness. Psychiatry 1958; 21:37-43.

23. Francis GM. Loneliness: Measuring the abstract. Int J Nurs Stud 1976; 13(3): 153-160.

24. Weiss RS. Issues in the study of loneliness. In: Peplau LA, Perlman D (Eds). Loneliness: A Sourcebook of Current Theory, Research and Therapy. New York: John Wiley & Sons, 1982; 71-80.

Theory, practice, and research in transplant nursing

DONNA HATHAWAY, RN, PhD; MARGARET STRONG, RN, BSN, CNA

THE INTEGRATION OF theory, practice and research on one nursing unit is rare, even though the importance and relationship of these three activities have been addressed for decades (Dickoff, James, & Weidenbach, 1968a, 1968b; Jacobs & Huether, 1978). In this article, we will describe how our transplant unit was able to incorporate theory and research into practice. First, we will briefly clarify what the relationship is among theory, practice, and research and why the integration of the three components is important to the advancement of nursing. Following this introduction to the theory-practice-research (TPR) triad, we will describe our theoretical framework and how this relates to our practice and research.

The TPR triad

A theory is a set of testable relational statements that describes, explains, predicts, and controls given phenomena (Meleis, 1985; Walker & Avant, 1983). The phenomena referred to are events encountered during nursing practice. For example, the nurses on our transplant unit observed that transplant patients frequently displayed dependent behaviors. Chronic illness theories address this observation and provide a description and explanation for the dependent behaviors (Strauss, et al., 1984). The theories direct practice by providing statements that may be able to predict and control the phenomena with which nurses are concerned, serving as a basis for decision making.

In contrast, nursing practice often yields insights into phenomena and uncovers gaps in existing theories. In our case, the theories that address chronic illness were found to address

it as an ongoing, often degenerative state. In end stage renal disease (ESRD) treated with transplantation, this is not the case. Patients can be viewed as becoming more healthy and as having an entirely new set of health problems, a situation not fully addressed by chronic illness theories. In this way, nursing practice provides ideas, observations, and substance with which theorists can formulate relational statements that would comprise a new theory or build upon existing theories.

The research component of the TPR triad validates a theory's ability to describe, explain, predict, and control. Through research, nurses can determine if a theory is capable of these activities and therefore useful for decision making. This relationship is also reciprocal because research not only influences the development of theory, but the theory will also influence the design of research by determining what variables should be examined when studying a particular problem.

Finally, research and practice are related in the same reciprocal fashion. Questions raised during nursing practice frequently lead to the formulation of a research study, as did our nurses' observations. In this manner, research is directed by problems or observations encountered in practice. As research is conducted, findings generated through study are brought back to the practice setting for incorporation into practice.

This discussion clarifies the theory-practice-research relationship by explaining that all components are interrelated in a reciprocal fashion. This relationship is illustrated in Figure 1.

Each component influences the others

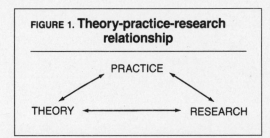

FIGURE 1. **Theory-practice-research relationship**

while at the same time is influenced by the others.

The impact that integration of theory and research into practice could have for nursing is profound. Historically, nursing has been based on intuition and tradition that has resulted in nursing being viewed as an art without a real scientific component. This view sees nursing as merely an adjunct to other health care disciplines with uncertainty even among ourselves regarding what is uniquely nursing. Achieving the status of a professional discipline that includes both art and science components is desirable if we want to assume autonomy and control over our practice. In order to achieve status as a discipline, we must clearly demonstrate that nursing has a unique body of knowledge; this is what the integration of theory and research into practice will provide.

The framework

The theoretical framework used on our unit as a basis for research and practice combines elements of chronic illness theory (Strauss, et al., 1984) and self-care theory (Orem, 1985). Chronic illness theory suggests that any illness can potentially cause multiple problems of daily living. These problems include: (a) preventing and managing medical crises; (b) controlling symptoms; (c) carrying out the prescribed regimens; (d) preventing social isolation; (e) adjusting to changes in the course of the disease; (f) normalizing interactions with others and lifestyle; (g) finding necessary money; and (h) confronting psychological,

marital, and family problems. Using this framework, the problems individuals with chronic illness face are not just the medical crises, symptoms, etc. Rather, the problems that directly relate to daily living become how the individuals will be able to undertake activities that will, for example, prevent and manage the medical crises and control the symptoms, etc.

In order to deal with multiple key problems, individuals must develop basic strategies that may call for the assistance of others. The basic strategies employed by the individual or those assisting will necessitate organizational or family arrangements. These arrangements may in turn have consequences for the individual and those assisting. This framework is illustrated in Figure 2.

The self-care component of our framework is being incorporated into our attempt to assist patients as they learn to deal with a new set of problems after transplantation. All the key problems identified by chronic illness theory are pertinent to our transplant patients, but adjustment to changes in the course of the disease is the major nursing concern.

Transplantation marks a dramatic change in the course of most ESRD patients' conditions, a change that influences all other problems. The change is generally one toward a more healthy life and one with a totally new set of health care problems. These changes not only influence all other key problems addressed by the chronic illness framework, but affect them differently than most other forms of chronic illness. Usually, chronic illness results in a progressive dependency on others to deal with multiple key problems. Following transplantation, patients are instead met with a totally new set of problems that can usually be dealt with independently.

Improvement in health status is welcomed by patients, although being chronically ill often has become routine. This routine frequently includes development of dependent

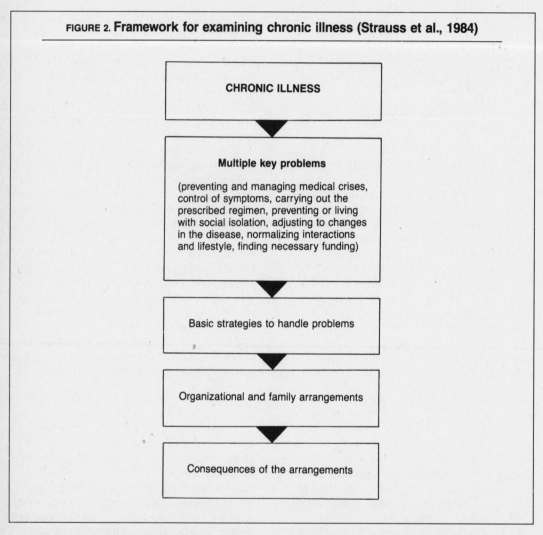

FIGURE 2. **Framework for examining chronic illness (Strauss et al., 1984)**

behaviors that require much assistance from others. It is changing this routine and taking a new approach to their problems that necessitate the incorporation of a self-care component into our framework. Through supportive-educative interventions during hospitalization, patients are encouraged to assume increasing responsibility for their own care. This enables patients to see a new set of problems and as-

sume greater responsibility for their own care.

This theoretical framework serves as a cornerstone of our TPR triad. To further illustrate how we have incorporated the theoretical framework into our research and practice, we will examine each component of the TPR triad and their relationships. Although we have separated the TPR components and relationships for the sake of simplicity and clarity, it must be stressed that in reality they cannot be viewed separately. The components and inter-relations are not separate but have a great deal of overlap with activities and conceptualizations occurring simultaneously.

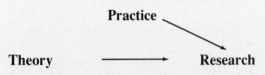

Theory ⟶ **Research**

A 10-bed transplant unit opened in May 1982 at the University of Tennessee, Memphis, William F. Bowld Hospital. Approximately 1 year after the transplant unit was opened, the staff identified the need to increase self-care abilities among among transplant recipients. Observations led the staff to believe patients were not attaining an optimal health care orientation, vocational rehabilitation or psychosocial status, deficiencies believed to be related to continued dependence on others for self-care needs. To establish baseline data prior to change in our practice, a research project was undertaken to document the observations made by practicing nurses. In this way, practice directed our research.

The theoretical frameworks proposed by Orem (1985) and Strauss et al. (1984) refer to others who assist a person with self-care needs as agents. Patients who have ESRD often are dependent on others to act for them as assisting agents. During critical phases of the disease, when individuals are totally unable to care for themselves, they require a wholly compensatory system of nursing care in order to meet their self-care demands. As the condition stabilizes, and the individual is able to assume some aspects of care, a partially compensatory system of care will need to be devised and the responsibilities of the assisting agent are diminished.

Immediately following transplantation, the patient is in a wholly compensatory state. As quickly as possible after the first 24 hours, the patient is moved through the partially compensatory system toward the supportive-educative system of care delivery. This system of care provides the patient with the support and education required in order for them to achieve self-care. During the transition from wholly compensatory to supportive-educative systems of care, the nurses function as assisting agents.

With this framework in mind, we designed a study to examine aspects of the patients' multiple key problems and their related self-care abilities. The Psychosocial Adjustment to Illness Scale (PAIS) has seven subscales that measure health care orientation, vocational environment, domestic environment, sexual relationships, extended family relationships, social environment, and psychosocial distress (Derogatis & Lopez, 1983). This instrument was chosen for our research because the subscales were consistent with our theoretical framework; the scale had established reliability and validity; and norms existed for dialysis patients. In this way, theory directed our research by guiding the choice of variables to study and the instruments used.

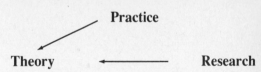

Theory ⟵ **Research**

During our study, 87 transplant recipients from the total clinic population participated by completing a demographic and PAIS questionnaire during a routine clinic appointment. The data were collected over a 4-month period and analyzed. At the conclusion of our research, the data analysis showed no significant differences in the transplant patients and the norms established for dialysis patients (Hathaway, Winsett, & Peters, 1987).

Observations made during practice are contradictory to those found during our research. Our patients are healthier and happier following transplantation, reporting a fuller life of a much higher quality. Yet, our research showed them to be no different than dialysis patients.

First, contemplation of our research findings and practice observations leads to several insights. Among them was the notion that after transplantation expectations of the patients and the staff probably influence each group's judgement of success. If the patient does not expect to gain independence, remaining in a partially compensatory system of care is not failure. Instead, success is measured only by being free of dialysis. On the other hand, staff expects patients to regain functional abilities and not rely on assisting agents to meet self-care needs. We believe these patient and staff differences are reflected in the instruments developed by providers for research, which are biased toward provider expectations and do not take into account the patient's perspective.

Second, practice and research discrepancies reflect the manner in which transplantation changes the course of a chronic disease. Although the theoretical framework attempts to deal with the usual remissions and exacerbations that occur in some chronic illnesses, the framework seems most appropriate for a progressive illness. Following transplantation, the patient's condition dramatically changes. ESRD is no longer a concern but organ rejection and the effects of immunosuppression are the concern. This is not merely a remission but rather is an entirely new condition, a phenomena not addressed by chronic illness theory.

These insights acquired through practice and research observations can direct theory formulation by identifying gaps in existing theory. Chronic illness theories need to address the unique circumstances surrounding transplantation, and nursing care systems need to be more attuned to discrepancies between provider and patient expectations.

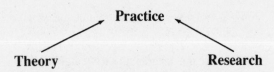

Current research with our transplant patients is designed to examine the expectations of the patients and staff, and problems encountered during the patients' first year following the transplantation. To accomplish this, interviews are being conducted with patients and staff during the acute hospitalization, and with patients at 6 months and 12 months after transplantation.

Our preliminary findings suggest that the patients have a lack of knowledge related to transplantation. To address that problem, the unit educator is preparing a group of learning modules for patients. These will include an outline with outcome objectives to guide staff in their patient teaching, an expected time frame for completion of the learning modules, teaching aids, and a checklist that patients and staff can use to monitor progress in acquiring essential knowledge and skills.

The learning modules address the new course the patient's disease has taken and are incorporated into a supportive-educative system of nursing care where patients are increasingly given more responsibility for their own care. In this manner, our research and theory have given direction to our practice.

Conclusion

Incorporating theory and research into a practice setting has been an evolutionary process, not something that we decided to do one day and incorporated the next. Theory, practice, and research became subtly ingrained on our unit without much fanfare as problems were observed, questions asked, and answers sought. Theory and research cannot become a part of nursing practice without staff who are unafraid to ask questions, seek answers, contemplate alternatives, and try new pathways. This is because at the heart of the TPR triad are inquiring minds. It was only in retrospect as we examined our work over the past several years that the impact of our endeavors became clear.

REFERENCES

Derogatis, L. & Lopez, M. (1983). *The psychosocial adjustment to illness scale: Administration, scoring & procedures manual—I.* Baltimore: Johns Hopkins University School of Medicine.

Dickoff, J., James, P., & Wiedenbach, E. (1968a). Theory in a practice discipline part I: Practice oriented theory. *Nursing Research, 17*(5), 415-435.

Dickoff, J., James, P., & Wiedenbach, E. (1968b). Theory in a practice discipline part II: Practice oriented research. *Nursing Research, 17*(6), 545-554.

Hathaway, Winsett, & Peters. (1987). Psychosocial assessment of renal transplant recipients. *Dialysis & Transplantation 16*(8), 442-444.

Jacobs, M., & Huether, S. (1978). Nursing science: The theory-practice linkage. *Advances in Nursing Science, 1*(1), 63-73.

Meleis, A. (1985). *Theoretical nursing: Development and progress.* St. Louis: J.B. Lippincott Company.

Orem, D. (1985). *Nursing: Concepts of practice* (3rd ed.). St. Louis: McGraw-Hill Book Company.

Strauss, A., Corbin, J., Fagerhaugh, S., Claser, B., Maines, D., Suczek, B., & Wiener, C. (1984). *Chronic illness and the quality of life* (2nd ed.). St. Louis: The C.V. Mosby Company.

Walker, L. & Avant, K. (1983). *Strategies for theory construction in nursing.* Norwalk, CT: Appleton-Century-Crofts.

Use of research-based knowledge in clinical practice

COLLEEN J. GOODE, RN, MS, CNAA; MARILYN K. LOVETT, RN, BSN; JO E. HAYES, RN, BSN; LORI A. BUTCHER, RN, BSN

THE PRESSURES FOR research-based practice are increasing. The literature speaks to the gap between research and clinical practice and to the fact that nurses who work directly with patients in the clinical setting are not using research findings.[1-6] Within the profession and from external sources, there are demands for nursing to demonstrate the scientific basis for its practice. Only two major research utilization projects have been reported which attempt to close the gap between research and practice.

The first research utilization project was the Western Interstate Commission for Higher Education (WICHE) Regional Program for Nursing Research Development,[7] started in 1971. Nurses from various clinical settings and agencies were taught methods relating to the change process and research utilization at a 3-day workshop. In this project the nurse participants identified a nursing care problem within their particular agency. Research that related to the problem was then critically reviewed, and a plan was developed for instituting a research based change and for evaluation of the change. The plan for change was then implemented in the participants' health care agency.

The second major effort, initiated in 1975, was the Conduct and Utilization of Research in Nursing (CURN) project,[8] carried out under the auspices of the Michigan Nurses Association. One of its primary goals was to translate research outcomes into clinical knowledge that could then be used in nursing practice. Another goal was to assist practicing nurses to use the knowledge in their patient care. The CURN project emphasized identifying current

research findings, using research methods in practice, learning the tasks involved in implementing research findings, and facilitating organizational changes necessary for effective research utilization.[8]

Using the CURN project guidelines, we will explain the phases of three research utilization projects and illustrate these phases with a systems theory model. The phases include: (1) preparing nurses to read, critique, and use research; and (2) conducting, implementing, and evaluating research utilization projects. The model for nursing research utilization was derived from our experience in developing and maintaining these projects.

Where to begin?

A major question we had to address was the feasibility of developing methods to use nursing research findings in clinical practice in a small, rural, 42-bed acute care hospital. There was no nurse researcher on staff to serve as resource person. Additionally, our staff nurses lacked preparation and experience in reading, critiquing, and using research. Two key ingredients were present however: (1) a nursing administrator with basic research knowledge and a keen interest in the research process and in using research, and (2) a group of professional nurses willing to take on the challenge of developing research utilization projects.

A research committee was established to act as change agents to engineer the research utilization process as recommended by the CURN guide; to review, discuss and evaluate findings from current research; and to make recommendations regarding use of research findings.[9] A committee already serving as an audit committee was selected by the nursing administrator to act as the nursing research committee. This group was selected because of its experience in reviewing practice while fulfilling its responsibilities for nursing audits and nursing quality assurance. The committee members had experience in identifying clinical problems, collecting data, interpreting data, and reporting findings. However, the committee also had some limitations. Most of the members did not have much experience in critically reviewing research articles. None had attended conferences at which nursing research was reported, and only two members had received research preparation in their basic nursing education. The committee was composed of five staff nurses, the education director, and the director of nursing; three members had BSN degrees; two had associate degrees; one a diploma; and one a master's degree. A month before the first research committee meeting, the nursing administrator assigned articles to be read. The articles were selected so that initial discussion would center around the importance of research to practice and how to use research findings. Each committee member was required to give a report on the articles she had read and to discuss the implications with the group. Also at the initial meeting, the goals for the committee were established. The goals were:

Main Goal: To use research based knowledge in clinical practice.

Supportive Goals:

1. To learn to read reports of research.

2. To review and discuss findings from current research.

3. To evaluate the research and make recommendations regarding its use.

At the second meeting, committee members were assigned articles on how to read research and were given a format for a research critique developed by Polit and Hungler.[10] Drawing heavily from the Polit and Hungler research text, the committee read many research studies as a group. This was not an easy task and required considerable support from the nursing administrator who chaired the committee. The remarkable dedication and interest of the committee members resulted in their spending many hours at home reading about the research process. Even with assurance that their skills would improve with experience, approximately 6 months passed before the committee members felt comfortable in reading and critiquing research.

As the committee learned more about research and research utilization, it became evident that specific criteria for determining what research should be used in practice were needed. The decision was made to consider changing nursing practice, policy, procedures, or teaching protocols when it was determined that the research studies had adequate sample size, and that there was consistency in findings from one research study to another. Because the Committee soon realized that all research has limitations, we adopted Haller, Reynolds and Horsley's [11] criteria in determining whether research is ready for use in practice. These criteria included: (1) the need for replication to provide greater confidence in the reliability and validity of findings as ideally there is more than one study in a research base; (2) examination of each study's scientific merit, especially concerning validity, reliability, generality, and statistical significance; and (3) determination of any potential risk to patients.

The process of research utilization is both orderly and deliberative. Translating research into practice, however, was neither easy nor quick. The Committee identified a complex set of activities involved in using research in practice, including:

1. Identification of problems occurring in the clinical area.

2. Gathering information from research studies that add knowledge regarding the problems.

3. Assuring that the nurses have adequate knowledge to read the research studies critically and understand their implications.

4. Determining if the research is relevant to the type of patients and clinical setting in which it was to be used.

5. Devising ways to transform knowledge so that it can be used in clinical practice.

6. Defining what patient outcomes are expected.

7. Providing education and training that is needed to get the practice change into the system.

8. Evaluating and adjusting or modifying the new practice protocol.

Selection of problems for study

Clinical practice problems for study were selected by staff nurses. Three examples follow of completed research utilization projects.

Temperature study. We wanted our first research utilization project to be an aspect of patient care to which all of our nurses could relate. Directed by hospital policy, temperature measurements were taken twice daily and were yielding many low readings. Electronic thermometers had just been purchased. There was some concern about the basis of the low readings, and this encouraged us to study our technique for temperature taking as the first project. As a result of review and evaluation of the research literature, we found substantial support for making the following changes in both policy and procedures:

1. Oral temperatures may be taken on all patients receiving oxygen by prongs. [12,13,14]

2. Rectal temperatures may be taken on the acute myocardial infarction (MI) patient if an oral temperature cannot be taken accurately. We learned that the repositioning technique is more critical in cardiac rate change than the stimulation of a rectal temperature probe.[15,16,17,18]

3. We now wait 15 minutes to take an oral temperature if the patient has just smoked or

had a hot or cold drink. If the patient has been chewing gum, we wait 3 minutes.[13] The time that our routine temperatures were taken was changed so that temperatures were not taken before oral care or food intake.

The committee learned from this project that just because "that is the way we've always done it" is not reason enough to explain our practice. Previous to this, we did not take oral temperatures on patients receiving oxygen, and we had a policy forbidding taking rectal temperatures on coronary care unit patients. Several weeks after implementation of the research findings for temperature taking, an audit of 25 charts revealed that we were indeed observing higher morning temperatures and probably more accurate readings. We continue to monitor both temperature readings by time of day.

Breastfeeding study. The need for a standardized teaching program on breastfeeding was perceived when, on follow-up visits, mothers expressed exasperation because "one nurse told me one thing; another nurse told me something else; and the doctor told me the exact opposite."

We had nurses who had breastfed their own babies and who had helpful ideas and good intentions, and we had physicians who tried their best to be of assistance but who were not always knowledgeable about current literature on breastfeeding. All staff needed assistance with a step-by-step program based on current research on breastfeeding.

To develop the teaching program (Figure 1), we used three textbooks, *The Womanly Art of Breastfeeding,*[19] *Nursing Your Baby,*[20] and *A Practical Guide to Breastfeeding*[21] to bring committee members up to date on current ideas regarding breastfeeding. A review of current research on breastfeeding was the next step. A bibliographic computer search was completed, and articles were selected and reviewed by the nursing administrator and one of the committee members who worked in the

FIGURE 1. **Excerpt from teaching protocol**

TEACHING CRITERIA	DATE & INITIAL	PATIENT UNDERSTANDING	EXPLANATION GIVEN TO PATIENT
Physiology of lactation			Milk is produced in response to baby's suckling, the more he suckles, the more milk you produce.
Let down reflex			Stimulated by sucking, felt as a light or strong tingling in breasts about a minute after baby starts sucking. It's caused by oxytocin hormone, causing milk ducts to contract and eject milk so it's available to baby. Milk may run from opposite breast. Initially, it may happen even between feedings or if you just think of your baby or hear him or another cry. It may take until you get home to become established. Occasionally mother never feels this let down but still can nurse successfully.
Colostrum			Present in last weeks of pregnancy. Very important for immunologic properties. 7% glucose solution—acts as a laxative to rid baby of initial meconium and bilirubin—lowering jaundice. Small quantity—great quality. Baby is born with water surplus and colostrum is sufficient until milk comes in.

obstetric unit and had knowledge about breastfeeding. Appropriate research articles were then distributed to committee members to read and critique. Through group discussion, information concerning breastfeeding was compiled and used to develop a standardized teaching program on breastfeeding.

Among the reports of research, Cohen[22] demonstrated the positive effect that a postpartum teaching session about breastfeeding can have on the subsequent use of milk supplements and duration of breastfeeding. In 1976, Johnson, in addition to identifying that successful breastfeeding at 1 hour of age was an important factor in overall success, also demonstrated the importance of the nurse's role in the breastfeeding experience.[23]

A frequent point of conflict has always been "how long should a breastfeed last?" A 1980 study by that title and six other studies on the subject led to the recommendation for unlimited suckling and illustrated the positive role frequent suckling plays in diminishing nipple soreness, diminishing incidence of engorgement, and decreased milk supply — all factors that contribute to unsuccessful breastfeeding experiences.[24-30]

Other problems frequently discussed by nursing and medical staff included those experienced by the working breastfeeding mother, and management of jaundice occurring in the breastfed infant. Recent studies in both areas, as well as studies on biologic benefits of human milk, suggested new approaches to management.[24,31-34]

By following the teaching program, all

breastfeeding mothers were given the same information by all obstetric nurses. Follow-up telephone interviews with patients have indicated that mothers who participated in the teaching program were knowledgeable about breastfeeding and that they perceived the teaching they received to be helpful.

Preoperative teaching study. In our hospital, preoperative teaching attained problem status when audits revealed that our preoperative teaching procedures were not uniformly carried out and were sometimes ineffective as regards to teaching coughing, deep breathing, and exercises. A bibliographic computer search found several studies on preoperative teaching were appropriate for our setting.

Felton et al.[35] compared three different nursing approaches to preoperative teaching and found that patients taught in a structured format using films and demonstrations had lower levels of anxiety and higher psychological well being. When an individualized teaching approach was used, Chapman found a 2-day shorter length of stay resulted,[36] a critically important criterion with the advent of prospective reimbursement.

When operation room (OR) nurses used an informative, supportive, and caring approach, Nolan found that patients had positive recall,[37] a finding that convinced us that a caring and supportive OR staff should be part of our teaching team. Fortin and Kirourac,[38] using a structured systematic patient education program, found their patient sample had higher scores on physical functioning at 2, 10, and 33 days postoperatively, increased patient comfort, shorter length of hospital stay, and returned to work sooner. Comparable findings had been reported by Lindeman and VanAernan.[39]

Finally, Johnson and co-workers demonstrated that sensory information increased rate of recovery both in hospital and after leaving hospital and that instructing patients in coping activities reduced the use of analgesics and increased patients' mobility.[40] Such consistency of research findings encouraged us to revise our teaching protocol and to re-educate our nursing staff on the importance of procedures for structured preoperative teaching.

In developing materials for our revised protocol, we modified an exercise check list devised by Rice and Johnson.[41] The check list gave specific instructions, a technique the investigators have found to improve the level of learning.

We feel we have increased the quality of our postoperative teaching program to an extent that will enhance patient well-being. A follow-up audit is planned to evaluate the outcomes of the new preoperative teaching plan.

A systems theory model for research utilizing

Based on our experience, systems theory assisted us in depicting the process we used in the knowledge-driven approach to nursing practice. Theorizing that all systems interact with their environment in the form of input, transformation, and feedback,[42] the model depicts an open system with interaction between the system and the environment. Parts of the system are always in the process of adjusting to the changes taking place as the system receives energy from the environment, transforms the energy into usable form, and discharges transformed energy back into the environment (Figure 2).

The model contains a number of concepts that need to be considered and clarified if an organization is planning to use research based knowledge in clinical practice.

Input. Six concepts were considered to be part of input: information, knowledge, involvement, planning, value, and consensus. Input information was supplied to the staff through a literature search that identified pertinent reports of research. Three new journals were added to the hospital periodical subscription

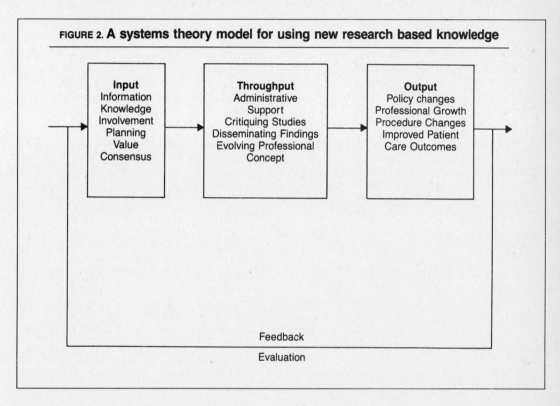

FIGURE 2. **A systems theory model for using new research based knowledge**

file: *Nursing Research, Research In Nursing and Health*, and *Advances in Nursing Science*. The staff already had available to them *The Journal of Nursing Administration, Nursing Management, Nursing Outlook, The American Journal of Nursing, Nursing Administration Quarterly, The American Journal of Maternal Child Nursing, Birth,* and *Critical Care Nurse.* Because there is no University Library available in our rural setting, by using the State Library of Iowa and interlibrary loan services, we were able to obtain most of the research reports we needed. Knowledge was gained through reading and discussion, a practice that produced more and more involvement from committee members. Mutual sentiments and beliefs about the need for a research utilization project began to emerge. Nurses often dis-

cussed the need to deliver "quality" care. Research utilization was seen as a key to quality in the practice of nursing. A consensus evolved that we were engaged in important worthwhile work. Planning was essential to insure success of the project. Through the planning process, committee members understood the group's purpose and objectives and the methods of obtaining them. Because the nurses placed high value on what they were doing, they were stimulated to work hard and to make the project successful. There was a belief among Committee members that research utilization would bring a degree of excellence to patient care and although a great deal of work was involved, it was worth striving for. *Throughput.* The concepts addressed at this stage of the model include: administrative support, critiquing studies, disseminating findings, and an evolving professional concept. Administrative support is essential. Research utilization takes time and staff must be provided time to find and read studies. It would be difficult if not impossible to have the project succeed if nursing management does not support development activities.

Because not *all* nursing research is good research and not all research findings are applicable to the small rural acute care hospital, critiquing reports of research is a major function of the research utilization committee. The committee is attuned to the fact that changes cannot be based on the results of one study, with one small sample. The committee reviews and discusses findings from current research and makes recommendations regarding the quality of the research and its use of the findings. The committee also encourages other staff members to bring research studied to the committee's attention. In our experience, new BSN graduates who have some research knowledge are the first to do just that.

A monthly staff inservice meeting is the channel through which research findings are disseminated and changes are planned and communicated. One committee member takes the responsibility for presenting each research utilization project at an in-service meeting. The committee member gives a summary and critique of each study used to support the utilization project. The inservice meeting is the method used to provide the education and training needed to get the practice change into the system. Another method used for communicating research is through a bulletin board on which studies are posted with segments of the study highlighted.

It is not surprising that through this process the professional self-concept of nurses improves. Conway speaks to such a change when nurses participate in research.[43] We believe that this also happens as nurses learn to under-

stand and use research findings. Nurses for whom research was previously irrelevant see its relevancy firsthand, and those who did not perceive themselves to be capable of reading, understanding, and using research soon learn that they can indeed do so. Perceptions of self as professionals are thus raised.

Output. Four concepts were addressed as an aspect of output: policy changes, professional growth, procedure changes, and improved patient outcomes. As research is replicated and findings validated, the scientific basis of practice emerges, obviating policies and procedures governing patients and delivery of nursing care based on tradition rather than on empirical evidence. As we learn more from research and use of research findings, we discover that tradition alone is not adequate to explain our practice. In some cases policies and procedures are changed. In other cases our range of interventions is increased or more finely defined. The research process thus becomes a method to obtain new knowledge or validate old knowledge. Evaluation to determine if patient care outcomes have improved involves both the process and outcome components. In term of process, the committee evaluates to ensure that the innovation has been implemented accurately. The outcome component involves collecting and analyzing data to determine if the predicted outcomes did in fact occur. In any event the quality of nursing care is improved. Nurses involved in research utilization grow professionally. The research skills of registered nurses are enhanced as they work on these projects. Staff nurses develop and maintain a seriousness about research and lose many of their fears. As critical reading and thinking skills develop, nurses are motivated to higher levels of thinking. Finally, involvement in research is considered an expectation of the practicing professional nurse.

Feedback. An ongoing process of evaluation is necessary to determine whether the policies and procedural changes improved patient care outcomes. Feedback from peers and colleagues is essential. Moreover, to assure that the change or transformation has not extended beyond the limits of the research base, we evaluate the effects of the innovation once a clinical protocol has been implemented [4] through audit studies and patient interviews.

Conclusion

The success of research utilization depends on organizational cooperation, as well as the skills and motivation of nursing staff members.[44] Nursing in clinical settings needs a practical systematic approach to the process of research utilization. Only then can we hope to effect research driven change to our practice.

In today's technological world, we talk about computers and programs that are "user friendly," meaning easy to use. We would like to see research that is "user ready," meaning already critiqued by experts and found to be "good" research and ready for use. As a committee, it would then be our responsibility to study the research, to understand its implications, and to determine if it fits our clinical setting. Perhaps more nurses would become involved in research utilization if this were accomplished.

As we carry out more research utilization projects, we acknowledge that we continue to increase our depth of knowledge. We are in our fifth year of work and the number of utilization projects are increasing. The audit/research committee has become a prestigious committee within our organization because of the important work of its members. Staff nurses volunteer to serve on this committee; however, we are reluctant to change the membership because of the amount of knowledge required of committee members and the amount of time it takes to acquire this knowledge.

We hope this article encourages nurses to begin research utilization projects. There is nothing more rewarding than instituting a protocol based upon research that improves patient outcomes.

REFERENCES

1. Crane J. Using research in practice-research utilization: theoretical perspectives. West J Nurs Res 1985;7(2):261-267.

2. Kirchhoff KT. Using research in practice: teaching research utilization. West J Nurs Res 1984;6(2):265-267.

3. Horsely J. Using research in practice: the current context. West J Nurs Res 1985;7(1):135-139.

4. Stetler CB. Research utilization: defining the concept. Image 1985;17(2):40-44.

5. Duffy ME. Research in practice: the time has come. Nursing and Health Care 1985;6(3):127.

6. Duffy ME. Research utilization: what's it all about. Nursing and Health Care 1985;6(9):474-475.

7. Krueger JC, Nelson AH. Wolanin MO. Nursing research: development, collaboration and utilization. Germantown, MD: Aspens Systems 1978.

8. Horsely J, Crane J. Using research to improve nursing practice: a guide. New York: Grune & Stratton, 1983.

9. Stokes JE. Utilization of research findings by staff nurses. In: Krampitz SD, Pavlovich N, eds. Readings for nursing research. St. Louis: CV Mosby, 1981.

10. Polit DF, Hungler BP. Nursing research: principles and methods. Philadelphia: JB Lippincott, 1978.

11. Haller KB, Reynolds MA, Horsley J. Developing research based innovation protocols: process, criteria, and issues. Res Nurs Health 1979;2245-51.

12. Grass S. Thermometer sites and oxygen. Am J Nurs 1974;74(10):1862-1864.

13. Levy F. The effect of oxygen inhalation on oral temperatures. Nurs Res 1982;31(3):150-152.

14. Nichols GA, Kucha DH. Oral measurements. Am J Nurs 1972;72(6):1091-1094.

15. Blainey CG. Site selection in taking body temperature. Am J Nurs 1974;74(10):1859-1861.

16. Gruber PA. Changes in cardiac rate associated with the use of the rectal thermometer in the patient with acute myocardial infarction. Heart and Lung 1974;3(2):288-292.

17. Mathewson M. Nursing rule: rectal temperatures should not be taken on a patient with coronary disease. Crit Care Nurse 1983;3(1):49.

18. McNeal GJ. Rectal temperatures in the patient with an acute myocardial infarction. Image 1978;10(1):18-23.

19. The womanly art of breastfeeding. Franklin Park, Illinois: LaLeche League International, 1981.

20. Pryor K. Nursing your baby. New York: Harper & Row, 1973.

21. Riordon J. A practical guide to breastfeeding. St. Louis: CV Mosby, 1983.

22. Cohen SA. Postpartum teaching and subsequent use of milk supplements. Birth and the Family Journal 1980;7(3):163-167.

23. Johnson NW. Breastfeeding at one hour of age. Am J Maternal Child Nurs 1976;1:12-16.

24. Carvalho M, Klaus MH, Merkatz RB. Frequency of breastfeeding and serum bilirubin concentration. Am J Dis Child 1982;136:737-738.

25. Carvalho M, Robertson S, Friedman A, Klaus M. Effect of frequent breastfeeding on early milk production and infant weight gain. Pediatrics 1983;72(3):307-311.

26. Cerutti ER. The management of breastfeeding. Birth and the Family Journal 1981;8(4):251-256.

27. Egli GE, Egli NS, Newton M. The influence of the number of breastfeedings on milk production. Pediatrics 1961;27:315-317.

28. Howie PW, Houston MS, Cook A, Smart L, McArdle T, McNeilly AS. How long should a breastfeed last? Early Human Development 1981;5:71-77.

29. L'Esperance CM, Pain or Pleasure: the dilemma of early breastfeeding. Birth and the Family Journal 1980;7(1):21-26.

30. Slaven S, Harvey D. Unlimited suckling time improves breastfeeding. Lancet 1981;1:392-393.

31. Carvalho M, Hall M, Harvey D. Effects of water supplementation on physiological jaundice in breastfed babies. Arch Dis Child 1981;56:568-569.

32. Maisels MJ. Breastfeeding and jaundice. Birth and the Family Journal 1981;8(4):245-249.

33. Auerbach KG. Employed breastfeeding mothers: problems they encounter. Birth 1984;11(1):17-20.

34. Mata L. Breastfeeding: main promoter of infant health. Am J Clin Nutr 31:2058-2065.

35. Felton G, Huss K, Payne EA, Srsic K. Preoperative nursing intervention with the patient for surgery: outcomes of three alternative approaches. International J Nurs Studies 1976;13:83-96.

36. Chapman JS. Effects of different nursing approaches upon selected postoperative responses of male herniorrhaphy patients. In: Downs F, Newman M, eds. A source book of nursing research. Philadelphia: FA Davis, 1977.

37. Nolan MR. Effects of nursing intervention in the operating room as recalled on the third postoperative day. In: Batey MV, ed. Communicating nursing research. Boulder, Colorado: Western Interstate Commission for Higher Education, 1977.

38. Fortin F, Kirouac S. A randomized controlled trial of preoperative patient education. Int J Nurs Studies 1976;13:11-24.

39. Lindeman CA, Aernam BV. Nursing intervention with the presurgical patient: the effects of structured and unstructured preoperative teaching. Nurs Res 1971;20:(4)319-332.

40. Johnson JE, Rice VH, Fuller SS, Endress MP. Sensory information, instruction in a coping strategy, and recovery from surgery. Res Nurs Health 1978;1:4-17.

41. Rice VH, Johnson JE. Preadmission self instruction booklets, postadmission exercise performances, and teaching time. Nurs Res 1984;33(3):147-151.

42. Richl JP, Roy C. Conceptual models for nursing practice. New York: Appleton-Century-Crofts, 1980.

43. Conway ME. Clinical research: instrument for change. J Nurs Adm 1978;8(12):27-32.

44. Krone KP, Loomis ME. Developing practice relevant research: a model that worked. J Nurs Adm 1982;12(4):38-41.

Study questions

Chapter Five

After reading the two editorials, reflect on your experiences in nursing.

1. Have you sensed a gap between what you study in the classroom and what you do in the clinical setting?

2. Do you detect a gap between the way students practice and the way the regular nursing staff practices?

3. Do the nursing practitioners in the clinical setting articulate the theory that guides their practice?

4. If you have experienced the gap that Chinn and Curtin describe, do you believe the resolution will occur through time and patience or by changing fundamental thought patterns of nurses?

5. If you haven't experienced the gap, identify the factors that contribute to the situation.

Chapter Six

After reading the articles, reflect on the issue of research utilization.

6. Compare the CURN criteria with those proposed by Tanner. In what ways are they similar? In what ways do they differ?

7. Should research of great clinical relevance but of marginal scientific merit be used in practice? Defend your position.

8. Is Lindeman splitting hairs by distinguishing between research (procedure) utilization and knowledge utilization? Why do you agree or disagree with her position?

9. What assistance should a nursing organization give to its staff to assist with the process of evaluating and using research? What is the responsibility of the individual nurse?

Chapter Seven

10. After reading the Buchda article, think about nursing practice. Try to identify theory from non-nursing disciplines that you have used. For example, some nurses use Maslow's Hierarchy of Needs as they develop care plans. When you use theory, do you think of yourself as a theorist or a practitioner? Why?

11. Contrast the approach to incorporating research and theory into practice described by Hathaway and Strong to the approach described by Goode et al. What are the strengths of each approach? What are the limitations of each approach? What are the responsibilities of the staff nurse in the two approaches?

12. After reading the three articles, develop your own position on the role of the clinician in *developing* and *using* knowledge.

UNIT   TWO

Additional assignments

1. In your curriculum, what is the underlying assumption regarding the relationship between knowing and doing? In your most recent clinical experience, what knowledge did you use as the basis for the care you provided? Based on that experience, how would you describe the relationship between knowing and doing? How would you describe the relationship among theory, research, and practice?

2. Select a nursing research article that interests you. Will you or have you used it in practice? How? Why? How do you think nurses will incorporate research into practice?

3. Select a nursing theory article that interests you. Will you or have you used it in practice? How? Why? How do you think nurses will incorporate theory into practice?

4. Organizational structure can enhance or detract from the use of nursing research in nursing practice. What nursing research is being conducted in your nursing organization? Where? Does the primary clinical agency used by your nursing school have a research committee? If so, what are its functions and effectiveness? If not, why and how is research applied?

U N I T   T H R E E

Health care delivery issues

ON APRIL 20, 1983, President Reagan signed into law H.R. 1900 (P.L. 98-21, the Social Security Amendments of 1983), and a new era in health care financing — and health care delivery — began. Throughout the 1960s and 1970s, hospital care had been financed through the cost-reimbursement system, a retrospective (and inflationary) system that put most of the financial risk on the payer. The new law implemented the Medicare prospective payment system (PPS), with incentives to hospitals to manage costs.

Under the Medicare PPS, a hospital is paid a preset price for each Medicare patient based on the patient's Diagnosis-Related Group (DRG). The introduction of prospective financing of hospital care for Medicare patients has had profound effects on health care delivery:

• The length of stay for hospitalized patients has decreased.

• As a result, the acuity of patients in hospitals and long-term care and home health care settings has increased.

• More cost-effective organizations for health care delivery have emerged.

• These changes have been assisted and accelerated by rapid advances in technology.

• A severe nursing shortage has developed.

With these sweeping changes still revamping our health care delivery system, the only principle we can be certain of is that the past is no longer an accurate predictor of the future. Rapid and ongoing change will continue to create challenges — and opportunities — for nursing.

Current nursing issues

The Medicare PPS has succeeded in slowing the increase in health care expenditures — but, ironically, at a price. With patient acuity higher in all care settings, the demand for the relatively fixed number of registered nurses is increasing, and the cost-effectiveness of other nursing personnel is decreasing. The resulting shortage of registered nurses has now become a national concern.

But prospective payment systems have created other health care delivery issues besides the nursing shortage:

1. How can nurses provide quality care under the economic restraints of prospective payment systems?

2. Changing demographics, disease patterns, and health care financing systems have altered the settings where care is delivered as well as the roles of health care providers. How can nurses make the most of these opportuni-

ties? Should nurses compete with physicians in the health care marketplace?

3. Tertiary care settings, such as acute care hospitals with intensive care units, show a trend toward using more and higher levels of technology. Nurses have rebelled, claiming they went into nursing to care for patients, not machines. Can nurses adhere to that attitude? How does technology affect nursing practice?

Financing of health care

Nurses, physicians, and hospital administrators traditionally differ in their opinions regarding the link, if any, between a patient's ability to pay for health care and his access to that care. Physicians and health care administrators tend to view ability to pay as a fair exchange for receipt of quality care; nurses tend to view a person's need for care as the only necessary criterion for receiving the best care the system can give. This dichotomy has always contributed to interprofessional friction among nurses, physicians, and health care administrators, but it is taking on new meaning today as the financing of health care undergoes significant and provocative changes.

With all the discussion about prospective payment plans and their effect on health care financing, we also need to consider the fact that nearly 40 million Americans do not have any health insurance — Medicare, Medicaid, or traditional private plans such as Blue Cross and health maintenance organizations. As a result, the base for financing health care in the United States is threatened with serious erosion.

This situation has not substantially changed nurses' position about ability to pay because their position is based on caring rather than billing. But the prospect of millions of uninsured patients has physicians and administrators arguing among themselves over who should control those patients' access to health care — and what quality of care they should receive.

The dropoff in health insurance coverage for Americans is a relatively new phenomenon. During the 1960s and 1970s, more and more Americans became covered by health insurance programs. As a result, health care expenditures increased, and the federal government and private industry assumed an increasing percentage of those expenditures. In 1965, Congress amended the Social Security Act to add provisions for Medicare and Medicaid. Medicare, a health insurance program for citizens age 65 and older, was amended in 1972 to make health care services available to selected disabled persons under age 65. The Medicaid program is a federally- and state-financed program to pay for health services for financially and medically needy persons in selected categories.

Although these government programs were intended to boost Americans' health status by making health care more widely available, for the most part they have not had the intended effect. The health of Americans has not generally improved, and the problems of the medically underserved, such as the elderly and the poor, have remained. Furthermore, the high cost of health insurance programs for employees drove personnel costs higher and higher, contributing to inflation. (For a time, Congress feared that Medicare payments would bankrupt the Social Security fund.)

In the late 1970s, the federal government attempted to control escalating health care costs by placing caps on various expenditures such as nurses' salaries. (This reflected the government's unwillingness to grapple with the high physician and hospital costs resulting from the cost-reimbursement payment systems then in use.) Yet costs continued to escalate until, in 1983, the federal government introduced the Medicare PPS, designed to achieve hospital cost control through built-in profit incentives.

Under this system, if the hospital spends

less than the government pays for patients in the various DRGs, the hospital makes a profit; if it spends more, it loses money. Hospital administrators, quick to see the advantage of tight cost controls under this new system, responded by rapidly reducing hospital staff, including registered nurses. (Since that initial response, the percentage of registered nurses has increased.) Hospitals also began implementing policies for reducing patients' length of stay, diverting to other hospitals patients who could not pay, and monitoring the consumption of hospital resources, particularly at the nursing unit level.

The ultimate impact of the PPS on access to care and quality of care is unknown at this time. What is known is that its apparent economic effects are encouraging the federal government to consider similar systems of reimbursement for other components of the health care system, such as nursing homes and home health care, as well as a fixed-fee system for providers.

And so, as reported in Chapter Eight, the controversy continues. We are certain to experience further changes in the health care delivery system as health care financing continues to undergo change. We are experiencing one such change already: the current shortage of registered nurses.

The nursing shortage

From the beginning of this century, issues regarding the number and distribution of nurses and nursing services, working conditions for nurses, and required education and skills for nurses have affected the nation's supply of nursing personnel. Interestingly, as reported in Chapter Nine, these same issues (exacerbated by the impact of prospective payment systems on the health care economy) characterize the nursing shortage of the late 1980s.

To help meet this shortage, economists such as Hornbrook (1988) are calling for new models of health care delivery, particularly a nurse-physician comanagement model that reconceptualizes every aspect of delivering health care. For Hornbrook, increasing salaries and improving working conditions for nurses without reconceptualizing the health care value system will not be adequate to relieve the current nursing shortage.

Unfortunately, the shortage of registered nurses as well as nurses with specialized knowledge and skills is continuing while various solutions are recommended and debated. The reader is urged to reflect on the similarities and differences in recommendations among the various studies described in Unit Eight.

Changing health care settings, new nursing opportunities

Among some health care professionals and legislators, awareness is growing that (1) the United States must have a system of health care that includes various settings and (2) the roles of traditional settings such as the hospital and the nursing home, and the roles of nurses, will change as this new system evolves.

Home health care is a rapidly growing component of our evolving health care system. Until recently, patient care was provided more efficiently and effectively in the hospital than in the patient's home; but with the advent of the Medicare PPS and the development of health care technology that can be transported and used in the patient's home, the home has again become a major setting in the health care system.

In fact, today's system of health care comprises many additional settings — nursing homes, schools, workplaces, hospices, ambulatory care settings, and day hospitals — where nurses (including public health nurses) are finding opportunities to assume new roles. Chapter Ten explores some of those opportunities and provides a glimpse into the future of nursing practice.

New technology, new nursing concerns

Rapid developments in health care technology have added to the costs of health care, increased the demand for nursing services, and increased the workplace frustrations of nursing personnel. Today's nurses must constantly update their skills in order to cope with a flood of new drugs, new instrumentation, new diagnostic and therapeutic radiologic devices, new metals and materials for joint replacement, and new computers for storing and retrieving information. Yet they often find that they are barely familiar with the "latest" piece of equipment when a new version is introduced, and the frustrating cycle begins again.

Perhaps this situation explains why data collected by such agencies as the Food and Drug Administration show that nurses are making a significant number of errors in applying patient care technology.

Do we really need all this new technology? Should nurses become involved at early stages in technology development so that equipment design takes their ease of use into account? Perhaps most important, what policies do we need for the ethical use of technology? These and other questions about the impact of technology on health care delivery are discussed in Chapter Eleven.

REFERENCES

Hornbrook, M.C. (1988). Economic models of nursing practice: Substitution, competition, and comanagement. In *Alternate conceptions of work and society: Implications for professional nursing.* (pp. 55-110). Washington, DC: American Association of Colleges of Nursing.

CHAPTER EIGHT

The financing of health care

FROM THE EARLY 1900s, financing of health care in the United States has reflected the social policy that all Americans should have equal access to quality health care. Today, however, that policy is threatened by changes in methods of payment for health care — changes that many health care professionals and Americans in general believe emphasize economic considerations over humane ones.

In 1980, Americans spent $75 billion on health care; by 1988, the yearly total had swelled to *$500 billion*. Furthermore, as a percentage of the gross national product, health care costs have increased from 7.4 cents on the dollar in 1970 to more than 11 cents on the dollar in 1988. Yet Americans' state of health is not demonstrably better than that of citizens in countries that spend less. For example, the United States ranks 17th in terms of infant mortality. Quality of care is under scrutiny, particularly in relation to steeply escalating health care costs.

Out of the exponential surge in health care spending by the federal government came the introduction of prospective payment systems, most importantly Medicare, for reimbursing hospital costs. This appears to be good economic policy. But is it good health care policy? How is it affecting patient care? How is it affecting nursing care and nursing practice?

The four articles in this chapter discuss these questions.

In "Nursing Megatrends Induced by Diagnosis-Related Groups," Wilson discusses the effects of prospective payment systems on a high-technology society such as ours. He is optimistic about their impact on nursing care. Joel, in "Reshaping Nursing Practice," sees prospective payment systems as an interim step toward total restructuring of health care. She identifies four challenging issues that nursing must address to survive in this new environment — for example, the issue of developing and implementing a philosophy of cost-effective nursing practice.

Kramer and Schmalenberg, in their two-part article "Magnet Hospitals Talk About the Impact of DRGs on Nursing Care," use data from interviews with nurses to detail the impacts of prospective payment systems. The nurses selected for interviews were employed at 16 magnet hospitals across the United States. (Magnet hospitals did not experience a nursing shortage in the early 1980s because they were attractive to nurses; indeed, they had waiting lists while other hospitals had shortages or full-time equivalent vacancies.) The interviews underscored the profound impact of prospective payment systems on nursing practice.

Nursing megatrends induced by diagnosis-related groups

THOMAS A. WILSON, RN, MS

"THINGS MAY BE getting better, but they are also getting different."[1] Such a statement by the former chairperson of Naisbitt Company is most appropriate in labeling today's health care system. In an ever-changing world comes the emergence of "megatrends" and the changes that these trends evoke. Something of a ripple effect is established because from the introduction of these changes come other changes necessary to meet the needs of the previous changes. The repercussions are vast and varied, especially in a high technological society such as ours.

Technology affects most aspects of our lives, including jobs, leisure time, economy, and, most important, health care. The medical profession's drive to discover, develop, and purchase the newest and best technological achievements and to cure, treat, and prevent illness and injury has caused a decrease in morbidity and mortality rates and an increase in life expectancy. Along with these achievements, however, has come an increase in health care costs and a limited allocation of resources.

Without some restructuring of our present health care payment system the same technology that preserves life would also be one of the contributing factors that plunges our society into debt — an indebtedness destined to shatter the sustenance of our economy. Such a restructuring was achieved in April 1983 with the passage of the Social Security Amendment, Public Law 241, and the emergence of the Diagnosis Related Grouping system.

Not since the development of Medicare, established by the Social Security Act, has a health care payment system made such a con-troversial impact on the health care industry. This new system has been greeted with much skepticism. It has been suggested that its implementation will not decrease the cost of health care but rather will decrease the services provided and the quality of care given. These accusations may be premature. If a high quality health care system, to which nursing contributes a large part, is to endure, it must be able to change with the times. It must identify the changes produced form present and future megatrends and act in an entrepreneurial manner. It is only by functioning in this manner that a high quality health care system, and by extension nursing, will continue.

Because of the impact of this new system, it is important for nurses to understand DRGs and to forecast the potential impact on their profession and the health care system.

Development

Along with the many benefits created from high technology come many disadvantages. Although technology, with its improved tools for the delivery of health care, has increased life expectancy, the surviving patients caused an increase in the consumption of human and material resources. In some instances this increased consumption has been found to cause excessive use of technology where unwarranted, unwanted, or both.[2] In addition, it has increased competition among hospitals to acquire expensive technology whether needed or not, encouraged the development and use of ancillary services, led to wastefulness caused by insufficiently skilled managerial staffs, supported the practice of defensive medicine with its excessive testing and diagnosing and further enlarged the exorbitant profit-taking by suppliers and users of medical products. Health care costs, already elevated, were pushed even higher because of these practices. These costs were then passed on to Medicare.

Until recently, hospital costs were paid by third-party reimbursement or patients as billed. In 1982, Medicare patients accounted for 30% of all hospital admissions. Consequently, 36 cents of every dollar spent on hospital admissions came from Medicare.[3] The Department of Health and Human Services (DHHS), which administers Medicare, had the third largest budget in the world.[4] With the continual surge of health care technology, its associated expenses, and the continual demand for the resources produced by its know-how, our present payment system would have become insolvent by the year 1988.[4] With the considerable rise in health care costs (17.5% annually), implementation of a prospective payment system was required by the federal government to deter these costs from further escalation until a new and more effective approach for reimbursement of health care costs was developed. This amendment depicts a major change in the policies that have governed the Medicare payment system during the past decade.

The prospective payment system was developed in the late 1960s and mid-1970s at the Yale University Center for Health Studies and the Yale–New Haven Hospital. Its purpose was to define expected lengths of patient stays for the quality-of-care services provided and for the utilization review of activities. Today its primary purpose is to construct definitions of case types, each of which is expected to receive similar services. Its main determinants are patient diagnosis, treatment, age, sex, and discharge status. Information obtained from these determinants is channeled into one of 23 major diagnostic categories, for example, diseases of the respiratory system. Once a category is defined it is further divided into 467 subgroupings based on elements contributing

to resource use, such as age, performance of surgical procedure, and complications or comorbidity.

The information produced by these classifications determines the average length of stay for patients with similar circumstances and data. A fixed fee, based on these tabulated norms, is then paid by Medicare. If the patient's stay is longer than the established norm, the hospital must absorb the extra expenses; in contrast, if the patient is discharged before the fixed norm, the hospital will profit. In the long run, shorter hospital stays should offset longer, more costly ones. However, if a hospital's cost per case (e.g., a complicated cholecystectomy) exceeds the defined limit, it will incur a loss for this case regardless of its departmental cost-to-charge ratio (e.g., 24-hour nursing care for 3 days). The government and the consumer stand to benefit, while the hospital sustains the cost of longer stays and increased usage of services. This system can also be adjusted to provide additional reimbursements for situations that turn out to be more expensive than anticipated, such as patients who remain acutely ill for unusually long periods of time or those patients who are awaiting placement in a skilled nursing home. These cases are called "outliers" and are compensated for approximately 60% of the initially assigned DRG rate per day.

Prospective pricing, therefore, is a method of holding down inflation. It is also a means of regulating the buyer's economy, making it no longer a seller's market. Such a system has many financial advantages. It can reduce expenditures to the Medicare Trust Fund by dispersing the costs of health care evenly throughout the system; the "haves" pay the same as the "have nots" of health insurance. It will not generate revenue but it will curtail costs to the trust fund. According to McMahon,[5] in the last quarter of 1982 hospital expenses increased at a rate of 14.5%; in contrast, in 1983 with the introduction of this new system hospital expenses were reduced by 6.7% for the same period. Thus, hospitals wavering on the brink of bankruptcy could be spared by these decreased costs and expenditures.

Impact on hospitals

Although many hospitals may benefit from this new system, the hospitals that once prospered at the expense of the government may now feel the financial pinch. The prospective payment system is designed to benefit the Medicare payment system. The American Hospital Association predicts that 20% (one out of five) of all existing hospitals could be forced to close under this system.[4] Those institutions that are able to maintain occupancy, control expenses, and operate efficiently will be in the best position to survive, those that cannot may falter.

The new system jeopardizes hospitals unless they control the type of patients admitted, the type of treatment provided, and the use of routine and ancillary services. No longer can hospitals admit patients for observation, no longer will physicians be permitted to conduct numerous diagnostic tests to prepare a patient's work-up while simultaneously ruling out other unrelated disorders.

Hospitals may also lose funds on transfer admissions and intensive care patients. Those that are unable to provide their patients with the highly technological care that they need (such as intensive care) will be compelled to transfer them to those institutions that can. Although the prospective payment system allows for these transferred outliers, it reimburses the transferring hospital only 60% of the initial admitting DRG; however, the receiving institution will acquire a full DRG payment based on the newly determined admitting DRG. Therefore, institutions that frequently transfer patients to other hospitals may suffer financially because the delicate balance between

early discharge and transfers may not even out financially.

Hospitals will be forced to firmly control their resource usage. Such control might minimize tests and procedures performed, cause the development of faster and more efficient billing systems, minimize risks to patients that might cause longer recoveries, and result in the use of the DRG system as a management tool to provide valuable information.

The implementation of the prospective payment system is altering the outlook for hospitals. Many changes in the hospital system are now being seen with many more soon to materialize. Health care is becoming increasingly competitive. An example of this rivalry is the recent growth of hospital advertising. Such competition, in theory, should advance the level of patient care by providing a high quality of care in the most economically efficient manner. Only institutions that can compete subject to these standards will endure.

Alternatives to hospital care are evolving. A drive is underway to provide care for the patient at home where it may be more economical and in keeping with the patient's own lifestyle. Because of this, hospitals are developing and opening affiliated home care agencies, alternative care clinics, free-standing emergency centers, and specialized hospitals to meet the new demands for care to counterbalance revenue lost by traditional hospital care. In addition, multihospital systems will also expand in number because of their ability to realize economies of scale and access capital.

Impact on nursing

Just as the DRGs will have an impact on hospitals, they will also influence those who provide patient care, especially nurses. Because nursing expenditures account for a substantial share of hospital personnel budgets, nurses are prime candidates for close examination and budget cuts. These reductions could be critical. Hospitals no doubt will attempt budget-cutting strategies that will directly affect nurses and the nursing profession. Hospitals may try to substitute licensed practical nurses, technicians, and other ancillary personnel for registered nurses. Cuts may be made in traditional nursing programs, such as staff development and patient education, because of their expense and involvement of the nurses' time. To further reduce costs, nurses might also be pressured into performing tasks of ancillary personnel, such as the transporting of patients and housekeeping chores.

Although these approaches might be attempted, nursing can endure and prosper from the implementation of DRGs. Nursing is faced with a challenge. Nurses must take a stand, meet this challenge, and labor to overcome it. If they do not, the consequences could be a fragmentation of patient care and a compromise in the quality of care rendered.

Nurses have a history of delivering a high quality care at a low price. In the past, however, they have had difficulty quantifying and substantiating this claim. Because of the impact of the DRG system, nurses are being compelled to justify this claim by conducting research to define what they do, and how the care that they provide makes a difference. According to Coleman et al.,[2] nurses have a commitment to improving patient care and have a well-developed ability to think analytically. Although it may be asserted that technicians and licensed practical nurses can provide less costly care, their usage also tends to fragment care and thus might shortchange the patient and society by delivering a suboptimal level of care in a health care industry that is ever increasing in its complexity. The professional nurse alone is equipped with the expertise and competencies that are essential to meet the critical changes produced by a technology-driven society. Shaffer[6] claims that, although hospitals might attempt to cut costs through the use of mixed staffing, this practice might actually lengthen patient stay because ancil-

lary personnel are often deficient in advanced nursing assessment skills and thus cannot identify actual or potential problems and initiate the nursing process in a timely manner. The implementation of this process can be provided solely by the professional nurse. The provision of high quality care by the registered nurse ensures a competitive edge over the technician. To keep this edge, nurses must pursue research to document their effect on patient care.

Not only can nursing endure under the DRG system, but it also has the potential to prosper. As the system evolves, so too may nursing if it progresses in an entrepreneurial manner and is willing to take necessary risks to guarantee its advance. DRGs will cause nurses to specialize, provide opportunities in alternate settings, provide opportunities for role expansion, and help secure nursing's "turf" from other entrepreneurs.

As hospitals become specialized so too must the nurse. With the rapid influx of technology it is impossible for a nurse to know everything about all areas of nursing. Any endeavor to do so would inspire the nurse to stretch his or her knowledge base thin and might conceivably cause a disservice to the patient. In addition, training staff members to be proficient in several services is expensive and will not be tolerated in the new cost-conscious health care system.

Opportunities for nurses to practice in alternate settings are opening and will continue to grow in the future. The biggest growth area is in the home care setting. Community health care nursing has always been a domain for nursing practice; however, with DRGs causing earlier discharges from hospitals the number of patients at home requiring competent professional care will enlarge considerably.

Other areas of opportunities for nursing practice are emergency centers and hospice care. Again, with the fixed rates attached to the DRG system and its estimated days of care, chronically ill patients will not spend the last days of their lives in cold sterile hospital surroundings. They will choose to die in the privacy of their own homes or in specialty centers, surrounded by familiar objects and comforted by their loved ones. Emergency centers will also thrive. Such centers will serve as ambulatory clinics within their communities and as feeders for their parent institutions. Opportunities for nurses in these areas of specialization will be increasing.

Under the new system, the nurse's professional role will broaden. Patients are becoming more informed consumers. They prefer economical, thorough, and individualized care. Nurse practitioners are educated to provide such care and might compete with physicians for patients because they frequently provide similar services such as health teaching and follow-up care at a lower cost. In addition, nurses are inclined to deliver a more personalized care providing the warmth, concern and caring attitudes that the consumer desires.

The demand for the clinical nurse specialist (CNS) may also grow. As hospitals, other health care agencies, and nursing itself become more concerned with reducing costs without lowering the quality of care provided, it is the nurse specialist who may offer alternatives. The role of the CNS converges on consultation, research, and education. Such a role is essential because it is through research and consultation that standards for delivery of improved care are investigated to emphasize the development of more efficient and effective practice of patient care. Improved patient care will lessen patient hospitalization time, thereby proving profitable for hospitals to hire the CNS. The bottom line, however, should remain the provision of better patient care. Documentation will obviously reveal that nursing does make a difference.

During the last decade or two, we have witnessed the diversification of the health care system and the out-growth of many "new kids on the block." These new kids were, among

others, the physician's assistant and the respiratory therapist. With the growth in technology the health care system became complex. Consequently, responsibilities once assumed by nurses became delegated to other ancillary personnel "for the good of the patient." Nurses, relieved of those additional tasks, became used to their new-found freedom. They reasoned that they now had additional time and stamina to provide more thorough patient care. The problem with this premise was that they kept delegating the responsibilities once unique to nursing. This action weakened their professional status and bargaining power while the influence of the new ancillary groups evolved because they could be reimbursed more easily and more readily.

Under the new prospective payment system there is a call for curtailment of services that are not essential or cost-effective. The ancillary personnel providing these services are prime candidates for reduction or elimination. Because nurses delegated those tasks initially, nurses may be designated to consolidate them back into a more homogeneous portrayal of primary nursing. Such an image would elevate the status of nursing and provide a more coordinated and cost-effective patient care system. Failure of nursing to capitalize on these opportunities might force the nurse to become a co-ordinator of care rather than a primary care provider. The very subsistence of nursing as we know it is endangered. Nurses must reclarify their roles. The DRG system may very well provide the drive toward such an opportunity.

Nursing management

John Naisbitt in his book *Megatrends*[7] expresses the belief that our society is moving from a centralized form of management to one of decentralized decision-making. This change is becoming visible in nursing, and the implementation of the DRG system will have an impact on managerial decision. Because nurse managers and head nurses control the allocation of nurse resources and expenditures, they are becoming more influential under this new system. It is vital that they, as middle managers, develop a knowledge of managerial skills focused on organization theory, computers, and data processing.

Administrative skills are necessary to maximize productivity, as well as to market nursing favorably. Nurse managers must identify the nature and extent of nursing resources that DRGs address, indicate the influence that these resources have on costs, and assert equitable claim for their reimbursement. A compatible system must be developed by which patient conditions determine daily consumption of nursing resources and functional needs.

The implementation of such a system is a significant step forward for nursing. It justifies the hiring of registered professional nurses in the health care setting by substantiating, via statistical correlations, their direct influence on patient care. [Currently] under the new DRG system, this interrelation does not exist, because nursing care costs are lumped under general hospital costs such as room and board. The costs are not specific. DRGs, coupled with a specific nursing costs tool, will associate nursing care and financial data simultaneously for the first time. Such a system would enable nursing to determine the actual care that each patient requires and should receive each day on the basis of the DRG classification. By converting nursing functions to time consumption, budgeting needs can be decided on the basis of productivity. This will allow nursing to be viewed as revenue producing rather than as an expenditure. The conversion of nursing care to time consumption and then to cost figures allows nursing to substantiate its professional existence because it provides an appropriate source of verifiable information. This is significant because information in our society today is a source of power. Such power is influential if nurses are to negotiate for control of procedures, pay, and policies that govern their

specific contributions to the hospital's economy and prosperity.

Impact on critical care setting

No other area within the health care system has seen such dramatic use of technology as the critical care setting. Over the last 25 years intensive care beds and technological expenditures for them have soared. There was a rush to purchase and apply whatever new technology became obtainable, regardless of cost. Within an increasingly cost-conscious environment, however, the need for such equipment will be more closely reviewed.

Clearly, DRGs will have an influence on hospitals and considerably affect their intensive care units. Because increased numbers of patients will be discharged earlier, patients left within the locale of the hospital will be most acutely ill. Hospitals will, therefore, become enormous critical care facilities. Large university hospitals will become referral centers for the acutely ill, and smaller community hospitals will provide treatment for the less acutely ill and limit services to those that are revenue producing. Because of this change, more intensive care and intermediate care units will expand within these megastructures. In addition, the patients within these units generally require more complex care and are more likely to have complications. On the basis of this assumption, it is safe to speculate that hospital stays will also be longer for critically ill patients than for patients who are not critically ill.

Alternative sites of critical care delivery will also emerge. Among these will be emergency centers and the home. As methods to cut the length of the hospital stay unfold, considerable growth will occur in the number of acutely ill patients cared for at home. To care for these enlarged numbers of critically ill, intensive care nurses will be needed outside the setting of the intensive care unit.

For the entrepreneurial-minded critical care nurse this is the burgeoning area of practice on which to focus. It represents a young and unstructured setting where standards of care must be developed and implemented. Such occasions present the critical care nurse a challenge and permit him or her to perform those independent nursing functions with more autonomy, outside the direct influence of the hospital bureaucracy and the physician. Consequently, the independent practitioner is totally cognizant of the direct cause and effect of his or her actions. Extreme satisfaction, as well as ample power, can be acquired because the effect of the nurse's care on the patient's condition is not obscured by the actions of others.

The critical care nurse must be able to meet the constant bombardment of patient data derived from the high technological equipment. This is crucial in a system of care that frequently produces more information than can be used therapeutically. Equipment is only as good as the interpretation of the data it creates. Because nurses are the ones most frequently working with the data, they will be relied on foremost to translate the data to other health care providers. In fact, such interpreting skills delineate a significant opportunity for nurses to attain greater influence and input into decision-making because "information equals power."

Conclusion

We are living in the time of the parenthesis, the time between eras....We are clinging to the known past in fear of the unknown future.... Those who are willing to handle the ambiguity of this in-between period and to anticipate the new era will be a quantum leap ahead of those who will hold on to the past. The time of the parenthesis is a time of change and questioning....Although the time between eras is uncertain, it is a great and yeasty time, filled with opportunity. If we can learn to make uncertainty our friend, we can achieve much more

in stable eras. We will have extraordinary leverage and influence — individually, professionally, and institutionally — if we can only get a clear sense, a clear conception, a clear vision, of the road ahead. [7]

The impact of high technology on the health care system has created enormous challenges to the nursing profession. Nursing should perceive the advent of the new prospective payment system as a challenge that ought to be met in an entrepreneurial manner. Nursing can no longer maintain its accepted practice of maintaining the status quo by "not rocking the boat." A lackadaisical position would further diminish the professional status of nurses, as well as endanger their posterity. Instead, by acting as entrepreneurs, nurses can welcome these new challenges eagerly and open-mindedly. Nursing can reclaim some of its status lost in the past and safeguard its future. It can also recognize the evolving changes in the health care system and thus broaden its horizons. Acceptance of the DRG system as a potential friend, rather than an enemy, is an attitude that will ensure the future of nursing within a complex changing world — a world filled with evolving megatrends.

REFERENCES

1. Hallet J. The challenge of looking at tomorrow through today's eyes. American Nurses' Association Fifth Convention. New Orleans, Louisiana, June 23, 1984.

2. Coleman J, Dayani E, Simms E. Reorganization of health service delivery: emerging systems. In: Curtin L, Zurlage C. eds. DRGs: the reorganization of health. Chicago: S-N Publications, 1984.

3. Plomann MP, Shaffer FA. DRGs as one of nine approaches to case mix in transition. Nurs Health Care 1983; 4:438-43.

4. Sanford S. Prospective payment: get out your baseball mitt! Heart Lung 1984; 13(5):24A-7A.

5. McMahon JA. Letter to the editor. New York Times 1984 April 12:A26.

6. Shaffer F. Prospective pricing: impact on the hospital team. In: Curtin L, Zurlage C, eds. DRGs: The reorganization of health. Chicago: S-N Publications, 1984.

7. Naisbitt J. Megatrends. New York: Warner Books, 1984.

Reshaping nursing practice

LUCILLE A. JOEL, RN, EdD, FAAN

THE 1980s FIND US confronted with the social mandate to control escalating health care costs. Our conviction that health care is a right does not change the fact that resources in both public and private sectors are restricted. A shrinking tax base and competing demands have curtailed money for health care.

The Medicare system of prospective pricing — the now infamous Diagnosis-Related Groups (DRGs) — is only an interim step toward more dramatic economic restructuring of health care. As our ability to use data for predicting the cost of illness improves, the DRG case-specific calculations for hospitalizations will progress to a capitation system that will pay for the total cost of an episode of illness regardless of where service is delivered or by whom.

Even greater efficiency in predicting costs could divorce health care coverage from the episode-of-illness concept and lead to a system of paying a capitated amount for a time period, perhaps even as great as a lifetime. Case mixing every service and the services of every provider is only one step toward more inclusive measures of resource use that will break down artificial barriers between levels of care and care providers.

Higher-acuity nursing

Hospitals that remain fiscally sound under DRGs develop a profile of increased volume and occupancy rates, decreased length of stay, and complex case mix. Each change holds serious implications for nursing intensity.

Increased volume means more admissions. Anyone who has nursed can attest to the fact that new admissions demand significantly more nursing time and energy in order to establish a data base and coordinate the initial plan of care.

In the 1980s, medicine can diagnose, prescribe, and stabilize the treatment regimen very expeditiously in the community. In fact, physicians experience less economic constraint and can practice with the least intrusion if patients are treated on an ambulatory basis. Patients who come for major surgery need intensified nursing.

Even patients with "brittle" conditions or in medical crisis are hospitalized for the biophysical and psychosocial surveillance that nurses provide. If patients don't overtly come for nursing, the fact that they stay for nursing is apparent. While a physician may be the appropriate admitting provider, a nurse may be more qualified to assess readiness for discharge.

In fact, excessive nursing intensity in patients who exceed the usual length of stay was documented in New Jersey through experimentation with the Relative Intensity Measures (RIMs) methodology to calculate case-specific nursing resource use.

Decreased length of stay creates additional nursing intensity. Patients, whether their needs are complex or simple and relatively inexpensive, will be treated so as to shorten their length of stay. Discharge planning, as we are now beginning to see, must begin before admission.

Fast on the heels of intensity issues come the economic dilemmas. As hospital finances become more constrained, all departments have been expected to accept cutbacks. Even if nursing departments have not been asked to absorb any more than their proportionate share, that request is likely to be inequitable in view of the emerging clinical and utilization patterns. While the use of pharmacy, X-ray, laboratory, and other services can be trimmed, nursing services have actually intensified.

Foolish cuts or caps

Faced with patients who are less functionally able and more acutely ill, the fool's answer to economic constraints is to dilute staffing; the foolish will sacrifice two professional positions to hire three ancillary workers. This reasoning proves disastrous. In other situations, nursing positions are frozen as they are vacated through attrition, or salaries are capped. As a labor-intensive department, nursing becomes a moving target for cost cutting. Staffing has an elastic quality that invites abuse.

Our inability to document nursing intensity has put us in a compromising situation economically. Collective bargaining problems surface here. New Jersey nurses, for example, suffered an 84-day strike when management held firmly to the position that the hospital was unable to offer any increase in a wage and benefit package because of controlled increases in hospital rates.[1] In a second case, labor was asked to reconsider guaranteed increases in an existing contract because of DRG-related economic pressures.

Controlled rate increases create other unique problems. Adjustments in the DRG rate are calculated on an economic factor consisting of two elements: the rate of inflation capped at a designated limit and a labor index. The labor index is a statistic computed for each of many federally designated and geographically defined labor areas. Averages are established for salary increases within these geographic areas.

When nurses have had greater salary gains than other occupational groups, a labor-area average puts nurses at a disadvantage. This is because labor-area calculations are not sensitive to the history of wage inequity for nurses in acute care nor to the relationship between these economic situations and rate setting.

The relevance of geographically defined labor areas is also in question. Rate-setting constraints in one state bordered by states that have a higher economic factor and consequently higher salaries may create a serious drain on the supply of nurses. Within reason, nurses will seek employment where compensation is most attractive. No provisions have been made to allow bordering areas to keep pace with one another. Such situations build a case for adherence to a national economic standard, as long as calculations are based on an appropriate index.

Improving cost efficiency

The survival of nursing under DRGs is contingent on attention to four areas:

• carrying out a philosophy of cost efficiency at the bedside

• fine-tuning unit routine, personnel utilization, and clinical programs to maximize the use of increasingly limited resources

• creating and managing internal data to document the change in nursing intensity and nursing's contribution to hospital fiscal solvency

• costing out nursing resource consumption case by case.

Discussion of creating new efficiencies cannot proceed without admitting that our history includes significant inefficiencies. Per diem anonymity has allowed nursing to avoid any painful precision in manpower deployment, or to scrutinize the efficacy of care, or to define with conviction our autonomous areas of clinical decision making.

We have paid the price of being victimized by a tradition of cross-subsidization and down-substitution: nurses used for nonnursing duties and at inappropriate skill levels. Studies in New Jersey show 38 percent of hospital nursing resources were used in nonnursing areas.[2] Using nurses to their best advantage requires both an administration that values nursing as an essential clinical resource and nurses who recognize the value of their service. The first and most critical step, one that is often ignored, is the need to enlist the support of nurses at the bedside by helping them develop a healthy respect for the expanse of hospital care and for themselves as providers of a costly service that, if rendered properly, can have a major economic impact.

Sophisticated clinical nursing promises to create a competitive financial edge for hospitals. Hospitals can survive and even thrive economically where there is no cost-conscious use of resources and clinical responsiveness to patients.

Nurses have the potential to speed discharge, avoid complications or reduce their severity, fine-tune the unit routine to see that the diagnostic and treatment regimen is accomplished expeditiously, reduce the use of costly supplies, and make clinical recommendations about the use of special care for individual patients.

RNs are the logical choice for providing timely, comprehensive, and therapeutic care. They can make independent practice decisions under the aegis of their own licenses. They have the knowledge and skill to generate clinically sophisticated document ation, so interdisciplinary respect can grow. Primary nursing with 24-hour responsibility for patients and access to the "state-of-the-art" abilities of clinical specialists should be an economically viable and desirable model in this DRG era, and beyond.

Since patient acuity is the common basis for day-to-day staffing adjustments, we most profile a hospital's usual case mix and the average number of hours of nursing care provided to patients. This creates an acuity baseline from which we are then able to observe change.

Tracking nursing dollars

Identify those DRGs that are most frequent, most costly, and most nursing intensive. Characteristically, 50 percent of hospital resources are consumed by 30 DRGs. Carefully track changes in acuity that build a case for more nursing hours. Through data management it becomes possible to dig into budgets of other departments that have not experienced a similar increase in intensity and demonstrate where nursing has reduced cost or generated revenue.

Analyze role activities common to nurses. How do nurses use their time? What patterns exist related to downtime, turnover, and job satisfaction? Loss of a seasoned employee and recruitment of a person who needs to be oriented, groomed, and socialized anew should be computed in terms of the full direct and indirect costs.

Finally, the need for a practice framework with a structure, process, and outcome elements should not be overlooked. Does a standard of care exist with a complementary structure, such as clinical guidelines, to enable compliance? Have the components of a data base for clinical practice been identified and formalized? Does the quality and nature of documentation validate the nursing resources invested in teaching or counseling? Is patient nonresponsiveness to care documented? DRG survival requires a fully conceptualized plan based on the answers to questions like these.

Nursing cannot continue in economic anonymity. Even though nursing is indistinct in DRG calculations, patient-specific billing for nursing services consumed is justified and critical. The literature is rich with proposals for how to do this.[3,5] Enough billing experience could generate a credible standard for use in case-mix calculation of nursing for rate setting.

Two-thirds of all registered nurses are salaried professionals working in hospitals. Any set of circumstances that allows us to demonstrate our contribution to hospital solvency is welcome.

DRGs are an opportunity, not an obstacle — an opportunity to establish the power of specialty practice and a new pride for nurses in the work they do. It is essential to recognize that adjustments in our traditional view of nursing education also are necessary. These times are only an interlude in a process of even greater health care delivery.

REFERENCES

1. 84-day strike ends: major issues resolved. *NJ Nurse* 14:1, July-Aug. 1984.

2. Joel, L.A. DRGs: The state of the art of reimbursement for nursing services. *Nurs. Health Care*. 4:560-563, Dec. 1983.

3. Curtin, L. Determining costs of nursing services per DRG. *Nurs. Manage*. 14:16-20, Apr. 1983.

4. Trofino, J.A. Reality based system for pricing nursing service. *Nurs. Manage*. 17:19-24, Jan. 1986.

5. Patients pay for nursing services under hospital's new billing plan. *Am. J. Nurs*. 82:1333-1361, Sept. 1982.

Magnet hospitals talk about the impact of DRGs on nursing care — Part I

MARLENE KRAMER, RN, PhD; CLAUDIA SCHMALENBERG, RN, MSN

"DRGs CREATED AND sanctioned a business mind about health-care." This major effect, noted by one of the Associate Directors of Nursing interviewed in this study, was echoed by hospital nursing staff at all levels. It is this "business mind" which has led to a shift in emphasis for many nursing departments — a shift from a goal-driven concept of nursing services to a resource-driven model; a shift from "quality at all costs" to "How much quality can be given with the resources available?" Whether the prospective payment system of the future will be a continuation of DRGs or a shift to a total capitation system, the revolutionary changes brought about by prospective cost payment demand that we assess the effects of Prospective Payment Systems (PPS) on nursing care and nursing delivery systems *now*. To what extent are nurses at all levels feeling the impact of Prospective Payment Systems? To what extent are they making the shift to a "business mind"?

Only three studies could be found in the literature related to the impact of PPS on nurses and nursing care. In 1984 *Nursing Life* reported the results of a magazine poll of 200 nurses and a New Jersey mail survey of 166 nurses.[1] Contrasting the two groups (the New Jersey nurses had been working under DRGs since 1980), they found that nurses are indeed "worrying" about patient care, increased workloads, and job security. Generally reactions appeared to be strongest where DRGs were newest, but more definitive and serious where DRGs had been operative for a longer period of time. The New Jersey nurses: 1) were more uncomfortable about decreased quality of nursing care; 2) recommended hiring more nurses as a way to making nursing departments more effective and 3) had higher percentages who felt patients were being discharged too early. Reporting on a survey of 118 nurse administrators after DRGs, Hartley found: 1) a shift toward all-RN staff; 2) reduced census and fewer budgeted positions; 3) shorter lengths of patient stay and 4) increased emphasis on discharge planning, medical records, productivity, and nursing cost.[2] Newman, reporting on a case study of the Twin Cities, Minnesota area in which 37 people in three hospitals were interviewed, found that the most apparent factors influencing delivery of nursing care within the current PPS are the increased acuity of patients' conditions and decreased length of hospitalization. This leads to an increased density and intensity of workload for the nurse.[3] While the above studies are important beginnings, they they do not go far enough. The first was a limited poll of a nonrepresentative sample; the second was limited to the views of only top level nurse administrators; the third did not go beyond the initial impact of increased density and intensity to what this means for the practicing nurse.

This article, based on interviews with more than 1,000 nurses at varying levels within the nursing departments of sixteen Magnet Hospitals, will begin with a brief description of the legislation leading to prospective payment. The methodology for the collection of the data and the qualitative descriptions of the impact of DRGs on nursing in hospitals will then be presented. The article will conclude with a discussion of what might be done to foster the

practice of nursing in a prospective cost environment.

Prospective payment legislation

The Tax Equity and Fiscal Responsibility Act
and the Omnibus Reconciliation Act of 1982
were the beginnings of sweeping changes in
the health care field. While TEFRA provided
for specific cost-cutting measures in Medicare
and Medicaid, perhaps the single most significant change was the mandate for the development of a prospective payment proposal. By
1983 the mandate was realized, with the selection of DRGs as the prospective payment
methodology, and the amending of the Social
Security Act to provide for prospective payment for Medicare inpatient service.

PPS went into effect as of October 1, 1983.
The system provided for:

1. Transition to propective payment with
"blended" rates for the first three years, with
the fourth year being 100 percent, based on a
national DRG rate. Regional wage adjustments, urban-rural designation, and teaching
versus non-teaching institutions would account
for variation in the national rate.

2. DRG rates applied to Medicare patients
only, with no copayment or deductibles
charged beyond what was permitted by law.
Cost and length of stay outliers would be reviewed for reimbursement.

3. Capital costs to be reimbursed on a reasonable cost basis for the first three years with
prospective payment beginning October 1,
1986.

4. Direct and indirect teaching costs excluded from prospective payments related to
DRGs and separate arrangements provided for
handling these costs.

5. Hospitals are required to contract with a
Professional Review Organization (PRO) for
the review of quality of care, appropriateness
of admission and appropriateness of care to
designated outliers.

6. Psychiatric, long-term care, children's
and rehabilitation hospitals (and distinct units)
were excluded from DRG payment and will
continue on a cost system.

7. Provisions for limiting the reimbursement of hospital-based physicians were
applied.[4,5,6] It was predicted that these 1982-83
legislated changes would have profound effects on hospitals, nursing and health care
within a very short period of time. The effects
were expected to alter both financial and practice aspects of care. For many hospitals, the
PPS changes and corresponding effects would
occur before hospitals had recovered from the
economic conditions of 1981, during which
occupancy rates had plummeted. For other
hospitals, notably those in the "oil company"
states, the compounding effects of PPS and
economic recession would be delayed until
1984-86. To understand better the impact of
PPS on nursing and health care, it is wise to
examine the DRG system for classification of
patients, which is the basis for PPS.

Diagnostic Related Groups (DRGs) is a
classification system with 23 major diagnostic
categories and 467 subdiagnoses. The system
organizes patients into groups based on homo-
geneity of resource consumption. The major
factor underlying the use of resources in this
system is length of stay of the patient. Each
patient is assigned a DRG upon discharge
from the hospital. The discharge summary
serves as the basis for classifying patients according to the following major variables: use
of the operating room; discharge diagnosis;
age; existence of complications or significant
comorbidities; and length of stay. Once the
DRG is assigned, the hospital receives the reimbursement set for that DRG. If a patient exceeds the expected length of stay or is within
the length of stay but exceeds cost, he becomes defined as an outlier and is reviewed by
the PRO for reimbursement.

PPS is expected to provide positive incentive to hospitals to cut costs. With this system,
if patients are discharged with a decreased

length of stay (when compared to means established through DRG data), the hospital profits. However, if patients have long stays and over-utilize services and resources, the hospital is expected to absorb the losses. With most services included under DRG payment, the system is expected to decrease the use of unnecessary tests and services to patients, thus decreasing overall costs.

While DRGs initially applied only to Medicare, it has been stated that "We want to prospectively price not only Medicare services but eventually Medicaid and all personal health care services regardless of provider or setting."[3] It is expected that eventually the DRG system of PPS will directly or indirectly affect all medical and health care practices.

Various studies have been done to ascertain whether DRG reimbursement rates reflect nursing costs.[7-12] Findings indicate that for some DRGs, the patient's DRG classification is *not* an adequate measure for determining, assigning, or allocating nursing costs within the institution. The literature warns that hospitals that do not track actual nursing costs risk unanticipated cost overruns. New Jersey led the way in the development and testing of Relative Intensity Measures (RIMs), a method designed to incorporate a sensitivity to nursing resource use in the DRG payment mechanism. RIMs, however, have been roundly criticized for methodological failures and for the assumption that care delivered equals care required.[13,14] While the jury is still out on these two major approaches, virtually all hospital nursing departments have or are instituting some method of classification or acuity system to determine nursing costs and to describe and/or predict utilization of nursing resources.

Predicted effects of DRGs and PPS

What effects were anticipated as a result of the movement to prospective payment? There were many, and they included the following:

1. There was immediate concern about the financial viability of hospitals which cared for large percentages of the Medicare and Medicaid populations.

2. Hospitals were expected to examine their programs and admission policies and to shift to those patients and programs which spelled greater profitability.

3. Since length of stay would be the major consideration in profit and loss, there was concern about patients being discharged before they were ready.

4. Since hospitals would attempt to shorten length of patient stay, the volume and complexity of case-mix would increase, not only in hospitals but in home health agencies and extended care facilities as well.

5. The necessary of decreasing operating costs would force examination of supply and manpower expenditures. Quality of care was viewed with anxiety! As hospitals cut costs, labor-intensive departments such as nursing would suffer massive reductions in staff.

6. There would be increased emphasis on outpatient treatment and teaching programs.

7. Increase in competition between hospitals for the "profitable" patient would occur.

8. While DRGs were questioned as the appropriate method for the PPS by many, nursing administrators doubted the ability of DRGs to predict the intensity of nursing care.

9. Everyone, especially third party payors, expressed concern about massive cost shifting. As a result of cost shifting, the end result of DRGs would be to increase health care costs for everyone else. Ultimately this would result in having more individuals who could not afford or could not gain access to care.

10. Changes in the character of the nursing work force were predicted, with two quite different pictures emerging. One scenario called for the demise of primary nursing because of the high cost of a complete or high ratio RN staff. There would be an increased use of ancillary workers, thus further eroding quality

care. Retention and recruitment of professional nurse staff would become difficult, due to decreased satisfaction in the work place. The other scenario called for marked shifts to an all RN staff, thus augmenting the practice of primary nursing. There would be a corresponding decreased utilization of nonprofessional staff (LVN and nurse aide) because of increasing "down" time with more acutely ill patients. Registered nurse job satisfaction would increase because of more direct nurse involvement in patient care and less time spent supervising nonprofessional workers.

11. There was much concern as to the adequacy of the recording and coding systems, since accurate documentation and accurate assigning of DRGs to case would be absolutely essential. Overall, the atmosphere of the health care would became charged with insecurity and anxiety.

Have the predicted effects of the new health care legislation come true? Which of these concerns materialized? And to what extent have practicing hospital nurses adopted a "business mind" or resource-driven models to accommodate to these revolutionary changes in health care economics?

Study methodology

In 1982, a nationwide survey was conducted by the American Academy of Nursing to locate those hospitals which had been particularly successful in attracting and retaining qualified nurse staff.[15] Forty-one hospitals were located and accorded the appelation, "Magnet Hospitals." These hospitals had certain characteristics in common: 1) they had 85 percent of all budgeted RN positions filled on an annual basis; 2) they had a predominantly professional nursing staff; 3) they had high occupancy rates; and 4) they had well-educated nursing leadership.

The published study received nationwide attention. Although not studied or measured directly, the conclusion was that a high level

of performance by registered nurses is inseparable from high quality patient care. The inference throughout this study is that because the Magnet Hospitals were "good places to work," there was high job satisfaction and high quality of nursing care given. Since the data upon which the Magnet Hospital study was based occurred prior to the implementation of DRGs and PPS, and since, by general acclaim, these are generally considered to be among the "best" hospitals in the country, the Magnet Hospitals serve as an appropriate group of hospitals and nurses from which to ascertain answers to questions regarding the impact of DRGs on hospital nursing care.

In the Fall of 1985, an in-depth follow-up study of one-third (n=16) of the 41 Magnet Hospitals was begun. The hospitals were chosen proportionately by region of the country. In some regions (e.g., the Southern region, where there were fewer than three Magnet Hospitals identified), a 50 percent sample was obtained. Both quantitative and qualitative studies were done to ascertain answers to several research questions. This report is based primarily on the qualitative data related to PPS and DRGs as obtained through: 1) interviews with individual staff nurses; 2) group interviews with head nurses, clinical nurse specialists, staff development nurses, assistant and associate clinical directors and 3) an individual interview with the Chief Nursing Executive. Each of the group interviews lasted about 90 minutes; the same questions were asked of each group: What impact, if any, have PPS and DRGs had on you as a nurse? on your nursing practice? on the Department of Nursing?" Short, informal interviews were conducted with more than 800 staff nurses before and after the testing sessions, and in conference rooms on the patient care units. In addition to the interviews, quantitative data were collected on a 25 percent random sample of the staff nurse population in each of the 16 hospitals. A total of 1634 staff nurses participated in the study. Utilizing the same questionnaire used in the 1982 study, quantitative data relative to hospital and nursing department department characteristics were obtained at the same time as the interviews. All data collection and interviews were conducted by one of the authors during a personal visit to each hospital lasting from two to five days, depending upon the size of the hospital.

Quantitative data relative to the impact of PPS on nursing care are difficult to obtain. Even more difficult is the goal of attributing causation. In this study, no attempt was made to differentiate between or differentially to attribute causation to DRGs or to the economic conditions such as high unemployment, unless specifically noted by the nurses.

Results

Whether attributable to DRGs or to economic conditions, or to both, there is no question that there has been a reduction in the number of operating beds (i.e., licensed beds that are staffed on a regular and routine basis) in the 16 Magnet Hospitals studied. In 1982, the 16 hospitals had a total of 6,454 licensed and operating beds. In 1985, while the number of licensed beds remained about the same, the number of operating beds had declined to 5,542. Although some of this reduction was due to refurbishing and renovating of patient care units to accommodate new services, the large majority was due to closure of patient care units because of low census.

The qualitative data obtained will be organized and presented relative to three outcomes; the outcomes relative to the patients, the outcomes relative to the nurses and the outcomes relative to the department of nursing as a whole. Patient outcomes are covered in this article; the remainder will be in Part II.

Effects on patients

The impact related to patients coincides with the predicted effects of DRGs as described

earlier. In 15 of the 16 Magnet Hospitals, the reported level of occupancy for inpatients *decreased* over the past four years. In 1982 occupancy rates ranged from 72 to 98 percent with a median of 84 percent. In 1986, occupancy rates ranged from 40 to 92 percent, with a median of 78 percent. The hospital with the occupancy rate of 40 percent appeared different from the other 15 Magnet Hospitals. If this hospital is excluded from the sample, the range was 56 percent to 92 percent.

While the actual percent of occupancy decreased, the number of patients increased. In some hospitals, nurses reported that as many as three patients occupied the same bed in the course of a 24-hour period. Thus the decrease in occupancy rate is a direct result of an overall decreased length of patient stay. Nurses report a very high level of activity in caring for patients. In addition to the shortened length of stay, without exception, the nurses indicate that the patients are at a higher level of acuity. Thus the "sicker and quicker" phenomenon discussed in the literature is felt keenly and reported universally by all nurses.

While the staff nurses interviewed did not report and did not seem cognizant of the predicted shifts in the paying status of patients, the head nurse and Clinical Director groups were very knowledgeable about the percentage breakdown by paying versus non-paying patients, how many Medicare patients, etc. They could not say whether there was a substantial change in one composition over the past four years because as one nurse put it: "I never paid any attention to that before. It wasn't important. But now when they tell me that my cost center is a loser for the hospital, I know what that means. If my unit is filled with non-paying patients, or has many 'outliers,' then the difference has to be made up somewhere else."

Although the nurses interviewed did not report any particular shift in the kinds of medical conditions for which patients were hospitalized, they validated repeatedly the prediction of a shift to more outpatient care and treatment. Comments indicated that patients who normally have been admitted to the hospital for a procedure or surgery were now in day care surgery or coming in as outpatients for diagnostic tests. While the nurses generally were in favor of outpatient treatment, there was a prevailing sense that there were patients for whom outpatient care was not really safe. Nurses noted that patients having some complication due to day care surgery, who would have been admitted a year ago, were now being sent home. These patients, as well as hospitalized patients whom the nurses felt were discharged too early, constituted the *single greatest concern* for all groups of nurses interviewed. "The pressure to discharge patients early, in fragile condition, to an uncertain environment, is the biggest problem I face in nursing today." This included ethical, moral, and legal considerations.

Interestingly, while nurses generally reported increased dissatisfaction with the quality of care that they were providing to patients, in 12 of the 16 hospitals studied, the nurses reported that Patient Satisfaction Questionnaires indicated the same or higher levels of satisfaction than they had over the last five years — and all indicated that patients were highly satisfied with their care. Despite no changes in Patient Satisfaction Questionnaires, staff nurses did not utilize this information to mitigate (or adjust, or assuage) their level of satisfaction with the level of care they were giving. Head nurses, on the other hand, did connect these two facts and stated that they were trying

to use these facts to help their staff become more satisfied with the level of nursing care they were delivering.

REFERENCES

1. *Nursing Life* Special Poll Report: "How Many Staff Cuts Ahead?," *Nursing Life*, 4(6):21-25, 1984.

2. Hartley, Susan, "Effects of Prospective Pricing on Nursing," *Nursing Economics*, Jan. 4(1):16-18, 1986.

3. Newman, Margaret and Sharon Autio, *Nursing in a Prospective Payment System Health Care Environment*, (University of Minnesota: School of Nursing, 1986).

4. Grimaldi, Paul L., "Regulations Proposed for Second PPS Year," *Nursing Management*, 15(9):60-62, 1984.

5. Maraldo, Pamela J., "The Challenge: Health Care in Crisis," in Shaffer, Franklin A. (Ed.), *DRGs: Changes and Challenges*. (New York: National League for Nursing, 1984), pp. 9-14.

6. Shaffer, Franklin A., "DRGs: History and Overview," in Shaffer, Franklin A. (Ed.), *DRGs: Changes and Challenges*, (New York: National League for Nursing, 1984), pp. 15-34.

7. Franz, Julie, "Challenge for Nursing: Hiking Productivity without Lowering Quality of Care," *Modern Health Care*, September 1984, pp. 60-64.

8. Mowry, Mychelle and Ralph Kropman, "Do DRG Reimbursement Rates Reflect Nursing Costs?," *JONA*, 15(7,8):29-35.

9. Piper, L.R., "Accounting for Nursing Functions in DRGs," *Nursing Management*, 14:46-48, 1983.

10. Reschak, Gary *et al.*, "Accounting for Nursing Costs by DRG," *JONA*, 15(9):15-20, 1985.

11. Schaefers, Vicki, "A Cost Allocation Method for Nursing," in Shaffer, Franklin A. (Ed.), *Costing Out Nursing: Pricing Our Product*, (New York: National League for Nursing, 1985), pp. 69-84.

12. Urosevich, Patti, "How Nurses are Learning to Live with DRGs," *Nursing Life*, 4(2):64-66, 1984.

13. Grimaldi, Paul L. and Julie A. Micheletti, "A Defense of the RIMs Critique — RIMs Reliability and Value," *Nursing Management*, (14):40-41, 1982.

14. Grimaldi, Paul L. and Julie A. Micheletti, "RIMs and the Cost of Nursing Care," *Nursing Management*, 13:12-22, 1982.

15. McClure, Margaret *et al., Magnet Hospitals,* (Kansas City, Missouri: American Nurses' Association, 1983).

Magnet hospitals talk about the impact of DRGs on nursing care — Part II

MARLENE KRAMER, RN, PhD; CLAUDIA SCHMALENBERG, RN, MSN

SINCE 1983, Diagnosis Related Groups (DRGs) have caused a shift in emphasis in many nursing departments — a shift from a goal-driven concept of nursing services to a resource-driven model. Very little has appeared in the literature relative to the impact of Prospective Payment Systems (PPS) on nurses and nursing care. This study reports the results of interviews with over 1000 nurses in 16 Magnet Hospitals throughout the country. In Part I the effects on patients were reported. This article discusses the impact of DRGs on nurses and on nursing departments.

Effects on nurses

Before reporting on the results of the interview data, a composite picture of the nursing staff in the 16 Magnet Hospitals is in order. In the 1982 study,[1] it was reported that the nursing staff in Magnet Hospitals were largely professional nurses, with an overall ratio of 1.1 nurses per occupied patient bed, and a 10:1 RN to LPN ratio. In the present study (1986), the ratio of RNs to occupied patient bed ranged from 1.0 to 2.0 with a median of 1.4. The median RN to LPN ratio increased slightly in four years from 10:1 to 11:1, with one hospital reporting no LPNs on staff. The RN to nursing aide ratio dropped from 12:1 in 1982 to 8:1 in 1986.

The Magnet Hospitals continue to demonstrate their ability to attract and retain professional nurses. In 1982 it was reported that almost all of the Magnet Hospitals reported having at least 85 percent of their budgeted registered nurse positions filled on an annual basis. In 1986, the 16 Magnet Hospitals in this study reported that the monthly average budgeted registered nurse positions filled ranged from 75 to 99 percent, with a median of 97 percent. Resignation rates were not reported in the 1982 study. In the current study, yearly RN resignation rates (total No./total RN FTE [full-time equivalents]) ranged from 6.76 percent to 45.69 percent, with a median of 18.06 percent. (If the one hospital that was an outlier is omitted, the range is 6.76 percent to 29.38 percent, with a median of 14.51 percent.)

One of the most immediate effects of DRGs noted by large numbers of staff at all levels was increased cost consciousness. One of the staff nurses commented: "It seems like overnight we woke up to the fact that there was not an unlimited amount of money out there to pay for nursing services, which are a very valuable commodity. Equipment, tests, supplies, as well as the nurses time cost money, and it has to be rationed, in sense. It is not limitless."

One example of increased cost consciousness was the staff nurses' involvement in the explanation of costs to patients. In the past, this role was assumed entirely by the business office. Now nurses reported that they often discuss costs in relationship to early discharge, as well as explaining costs for the varying alternative treatments. Several of the Magnet Hospitals reported that they provided staff nurses with specific classes on how to do this effectively with patients and families. While the nurses interviewed did not generally object to this role, they did report that they were not yet comfortable with it, mainly due to inexperience.

Another factor raising the cost conscious-ness of the nurses is the increased emphasis on documentation. The constant theme is the need for clear, concise and complete documentation of the patient's condition, the treatment pro-vided and the patient's response to that treat-ment. Not unlike previously heard cries, staff nurses reported that they were so tied up with paperwork that there was not enough time for patient care.

One of the areas of planning and documen-tation that was the most vulnerable and most frequently mentioned was written nursing care plans. "I hate them; I hate them; I hate them. They really take time away from my patients." "At the same time that I realize they are im-portant and very necessary for documentation, I despise having to do them." The nurses inter-viewed did not object to planning nursing care. They did not object to communicating this plan of care verbally from one nurse to the other. As a group, they objected vehemently to the "drudgery, repetition, and time-consuming writing out of a plan of care." "No other pro-fessional group has to write out in such detail what they plan to do; why do nurses have to do so?" In only three of the 16 Magnet Hospi-tals visited were the nurses, on the whole, not angrily and vocally opposed to the writing out of nursing care plans. In the other two hospi-tals, nursing care plans were on line in the computer system.

This cost consciousness did not just happen; in many instances, the nurses detailed specific factors that brought it about. The staff in virtu-ally all 16 hospitals indicated that they had participated in educational sessions to learn about PPS and DRGs and about their role in using cost-saving measures. Additionally, the staff stated that they noticed a change in the quantity, quality, and availability of supplies. The inventory of supplies kept on the units de-creased markedly. In one hospital, nurses re-ported that they became acutely aware of costs

when they discovered (in doing an inventory) that much costly patient care equipment was scattered throughout the hospital in patient care rooms. In some instances, decreased unit inventories meant delays in getting supplies needed for patient care. In addition, nurses re-ported reduced quality in general supplies, such as kitchen stock. It was reported that the plastic eating utensils often break and that it is not uncommon to have styrofoam cups leak, due to the lower quality of materials being purchased. While the staff finds the lack of medical supplies extremely frustrating, the poor quality of kitchen supplies was viewed with a remarkable degree of humor.

One of the indirect effects of DRGs on nursing care is increased specialization. Many hospitals have organized their units around like patients to a greater degree than ever be-fore. As a result of the growing acuity and the inability of a nurse to know everything about everything, there has been increased educa-tional emphasis. Many hospitals provide pro-grams for certification of nurses in their new specialty. Nurses report increased feelings of self-worth as a result of the in-depth knowl-edge and increased ability to provide compre-hensive care for the specialty patient. With the increased knowledge has come increased au-tonomy for decision making in regard to the care of the patient. Of course, the flip side of this coin is that there was tremendous hesi-tancy and resistance when a nurse was asked to float out of her specialty area, and increased concern over incompetence in caring for other types of patients. In general in the 16 hospitals studied, nurses were not obliged to float out of their cluster or service. Nurses reported that they have found new confidence and respect for one another as specialization has grown.

Another effect of DRGs on nurses has been increased job dissatisfaction because of the perceived quality of nursing care given to pa-tients. "It scares me to death how fast we dis-charge patients who are still really so sick, and who need nursing care; I shudder to think of the legal liabilities if something should happen to them." "Oftentimes we are teaching the patient and his family as the patient goes out the door. It's not right! We know how to give good care and we know what this patient really needs to know, but they aren't here long enough to give it to them." "I've given up teaching the patient; you have to concentrate on the family. The patient simply isn't conscious long enough or ready to learn while he is here."

The perceived increase in overall acuity level of patients also contributes to job dissatisfaction. But the real issue is that noted in the literature; it is not necessarily that the patients are sicker than ever before but rather that patients are cared for in the hospital only while they are at their highest level of acuity. When the lower acuity ends of an illness are cared for outside the acute care setting, the end result is an increase in the averages.[2] Nevertheless, to the staff nurse, it definitely feels like the patients are "sicker."

In combination with the "quicker" aspect of care, the workload seems to be increasing exponentially. There is increased activity associated with the acuity as well as increased admission and discharge of patients, with almost all patients being urgent or emergency admissions. All of this has led to decreased satisfaction with the very act of nursing care. Nurses don't see patients getting better or getting well. They always see the patient at his worst; they miss the satisfaction derived from helping someone and seeing that their actions made a difference.

In conjunction with the increased acuity and shorter length of stay is an increased emphasis on teaching and discharge planning. The value of preparing a patient for discharge at the time of admission is truly in operation now. However, the nurses find themselves engaging in a highly satisfying role behavior

(teaching) which leads to decreased job satisfaction (trying to teach someone who is so sick, unconscious, or is in so much pain that he is not ready or able to learn). Nearly half of all preoperative patients are now admitted the morning of surgery, making it difficult to prepare them properly. This leads to a perception of less positive postoperative results. For other patients, the length of stay is so short that there is insufficient time to do all the teaching that is necessary. Patients are sometimes discharged without adequate skill to take care of themselves at home. This has increased the use of community resources, but in some instances the community resources are not yet developed enough to handle the needs. The positive side of this is that patients are being discharged to recover at home, which is where they really want to be, and what nurses have been taught is optimal. The discomfort of the staff in dealing with this constant "unfinished" feeling is increasing with time. Some of the Magnet Hospitals have introduced programs specifically designed to handle this problem with both nurses and patients.[3]

As mentioned at the outset of this report, the decrease in occupancy rates has led to the closing of some units in most of the 16 hospitals. Reduction in staff was generally accomplished in one of four ways. First, in 13 of the 16 hospitals, initial reduction was done through termination or reassignment of the NA and LPN work force. A second mode was reduction in or eradication of one of the supervisory or staff layers in the organization, with subsequent reallocation of responsibilities. The dominant groups that were affected were evening and night supervisors and Assistant or Clinical Directors. In two of the 16 Magnet Hospitals studied, the staff development department was terminated, although some portion has been reestablished in both hospitals. The third way of reducing the work force was through non-replacement when positions become open. Although this was perceived generally as being superior to the fourth method — layoffs — it is not without hazards. Resignations do not occur on a planned or equal basis, so the work force is out of balance while waiting for attrition to occur. On the other hand, some of the staff viewed layoffs as being done by the hospital to decrease benefits and also to save money by hiring new nurses at lower salaries. Actual layoffs of Registered Nurse staff occurred in only two of the 16 Magnet Hospitals studied. The numbers were very small, and in some instances, the nurses were rehired within a short time.

The end result of any of the above methods is the breaking up of long-time work groups. As nurses are moved to other units to concentrate occupied beds or to redistribute staff following normal attrition, naturally established working teams are split up. For many of the staff, this was almost as difficult, if not more so, than layoffs. Both activities led to marked feelings of job insecurity defined in one of two ways: 1) fear of losing one's job completely or 2) fear of losing a particular job on a particular unit. Both were classified as "job insecurity." In 10 of the hospitals, the nurses reported feeling very secure about their jobs (8 or higher on a 10-point scale). In four of the remaining six hospitals, the nurses reported moderate job insecurity, while not at all sure they would have a job tomorrow or next week.

In only one area was there a marked difference between the staff nurses and nurse management relative to the effects of DRGs. Nurse managers were much more inclined to see DRGs as an opportunity for collaboration with the physicians and for ascription of increasing importance to the role of the nurse on the health team. The staff nurses were much more inclined to see DRGs as a resurrection of the "policing of medical practice" role. With the advent of primary nursing and change in the role of the nurse, the staff had felt that much

progress had been made in getting the nurse out of the "medical police" business. DRGs have definitely brought an unwanted return to this role.

Nurse managers also were much more inclined to report increased competition between hospital departments since the advent of PPS. Who will provide services in overlapping situations between departments such as physical therapy or social work? Who will pick up and provide the services neglected when personnel are laid off from support departments? Again, from the perspective of all nurses, this is an unwanted dinosaur from the past.

The nursing department

For the majority of the nursing departments, the need to decrease and control costs has led to increasing decentralization of the department. In 10 of the 16 hospitals, the supervisory or assistant director level had been eliminated; the head nurse had been elevated either officially or by default to the level of department head. One of the smaller Magnet Hospitals had accomplished this major undertaking almost three years earlier when the whole idea of cost containment was still in its embryonic stages. Stimulated by its charismatic leader and an article in the literature, this nursing department executed this change in an unbelievably smooth manner.[4] Such adherence to and implementation of planned change seems to be a major characteristic of these Magnet Hospitals.

Elimination of layers in the organization and decentralization of responsibility and decision making was not seen as completely desirable. A frequently heard quip was, "When you've cut direct care as far as you can cut it, there is only one place left to look." In general, at all levels, decentralization was viewed positively. Autonomy and decision making focused at the bedside for patient care was perceived as having positive results, although some head nurses had mixed reactions. They are caught in the squeeze between managing and giving care. Although organizational expectations varied, head nurses reported a range from "no direct care responsibilities" to 80 percent of their time giving direct care. The usual dissatisfactions from not being able to give patient care yet wanting to do so, and wanting to manage but having insufficient time to do so were present in this group. However, unlike a few years ago when the role of the head nurse first started to change and the staff objected to this new manager role, the staff nurses in this study reported that, first and foremost, they wanted their head nurses to be good managers.[5] Once again the "head nurse as caregiver/manager" dilemma must be faced.

Another change for most nursing departments involves staffing patterns. There has been a decrease in occupancy, accompanied by wider ranging variations in census than ever before. Most of the hospitals were staffed for between 60 percent to 70 percent occupancy. Whereas one used to expand from 87 percent to 105 percent occupancy, now one expands from 65 percent to 95 percent occupancy. The latter range of expansion is much more difficult. To cope with the degree of flexibility required, most hospitals either increased the number of part-time staff, increased the number of inhouse float nurses, or both. These options are fraught with the usual problems. The one most frequently mentioned by the staff nurses in these Magnet Hospitals is that they objected to the loss of work group cohesiveness that these measures introduced — so much so that in one Magnet Hospital, the staff made it a common practice to "adopt" certain float nurses for specific units — which practice was sanctioned by Nursing Administration. To handle what was termed the "biggest management problem of today"— fluctuating census — virtually all hospitals utilized some kind of mandatory and/or voluntary furlough. In the 16 hospitals, the range was from zero to 40 FTEs in a given week for time off without pay because of low census.

• *Desirable staff mix:* Definite movement toward all-RN staffing was noted in the 16 Magnet Hospitals studied despite (or because of) the need to cut costs and regardless of literature statements concerning staff mix.[6-9,20] The percentage of RNs on staff ranged from 67 percent to 97 percent, with a median of 78 percent. Newman found that the RN complement in the Twin Cities ranged from 69 to 88 percent in three hospitals she studied.[10] National trends indicated by a survey of 23 cities showed that the RN ratio of nursing staff increased from 59 percent to 69 percent over the past four years, with the highest complement of RNs being 87 percent in Seattle. The Nursing Life study indicated that the New Jersey nurses who had been working with DRGs longer perceived a greater need for an RN staff than did the comparison nationwide group.[11] Comparable data for the Magnet Hospitals in 1982 are not available, so it is not known whether the figures above represent an increased proportion of RN staffing. However, all CNEs [chief nurse executives] interviewed indicated that they had increased their RN complement since 1982.

In spite of an increase in RN staffing, the unsettled question of desirable staff mix is reflected in the wide range of ratios of RN to LPNs found in these Magnet Hospitals. In five of the 16, a very clear decision to go toward a predominantly RN staff has been made. RN to LPN ratios were 1:299; 1:128; 1:106; 1:66, 1:38. In five other hospitals where the ratio was 1:4, clearly the opposite decision had been made. In the remaining six hospitals, five reported that they were increasing the ratio of RN to LPN through natural attrition, upgrading of vacated positions, reassignment to other departments, or by setting deadlines stating when LPNs have to have earned their RN licenses. In two of the Magnet Hospitals, specific educational programs were in process to get all LPNs back to school to study for an RN.

• *Nursing care delivery system:* Perhaps the greatest impact for DRGs and PPS on the nursing department was in the delivery system for nursing care. The 1982 Magnet Hospital study reported that Primary Nursing was the dominant delivery system operative in Magnet Hospitals. In this 1986 study, it was found that the dominant delivery system was either eight-hour Total Patient Care or something variously labeled "district," "modified primary" or "modified team" approach; this meant that an RN, usually assisted by an LPN or NA, cared for a group of patients who were housed in a given geographical area.

During the interviews, the nurses were presented with five primary tenets of Primary Nursing, namely: 1) 24-hour accountability; 2) case method of assignment; 3) caregiver to caregiver report; 4) decentralized decision making; and 5) nurse/patient continuity. They were asked the extent to which these five were operative on the nursing units of that hospital. In only two of the 16 hospitals were all five generally operative. The two factors most commonly in place in all 16 hospitals were decentralized decision making and [the] case method of assignment. Only one hospital did not use the case method of assignment; two did not have centralized decision making. All but four of the hospitals utilized a system with caregiver to caregiver report. The factor least present was 24-hour accountability; only two of the 16 hospitals reported that their system includes this. Nurse/patient continuity is questionable and is raising serious concerns as to the viability of primary nursing to today's health care environment.

Both in the literature and in this study, nurses questioned this viability.[7,10] There was no question as to the desirability of the RN giving comprehensive, direct patient care, planning of care, and continuity of care between hospital and discharge. There was no question about their not wanting to return to a "functional" nursing system. But disrupted continuity — of both patient and staff — was identified continually as a deterrent to primary nursing. The shortened length of stay, increased use of part-time staff, and voluntary or mandatory low census days were cited frequently as the major inhibitors. When neither patient nor nurse is present for several continuous days, nurses felt that it was next to impossible to practice Primary Nursing. One of the hospitals in which Primary Nursing was superbly practiced had an almost all RN-BSN, full-time salaried staff.

• *Classification systems:* Various schemes have been used to cost out nursing services, to estimate nurse resource utilization, or to serve as a basis for measuring nursing workload or projecting staff needs and mix. Classification systems — either of the patient, time expended, or nursing resources — form the bases for these. Probably the most extensively studied have been DRGs and Relative Intensity Measures (RIMs): both have been found wanting.[6,9,12,13] It has been shown that for some very common DRGs, nursing resource consumption varies within the DRG; this can result in significant unanticipated cost overruns.[14] RIMs have been criticized for methodological failures and for the assumption that care delivered equals care required.[13,14]

The Magnet Hospitals are a microcosm of the health care system with respect to the status of classification systems and their relationship to consumption of nursing resources. Only one has an operative system for costing out nursing services and billing by patient acuity.[15] Several had published or described their own patient classification systems in the literature.[16,17] All of them were involved in some way in classifying nurse resource consumption. The specific purpose of the activity was not always clear.[18] From the perspective of the staff nurses interviewed, the purpose of all patient classification activity was "to justify an increase in staffing."

Unclear or diverse purposes for patient classification or acuity systems can lead to major problems for the institution. Several CNEs reported that there is no way that they can afford to staff by what the acuity picture says is needed. Some believe that hospitals are probably getting as much of the health care dollar as they are going to get. Putting nurses through the exercise of classification and acuity rituals when nothing can come of it is not only a distraction from nursing care but also the source of anger and frustration.

While there was some expression of interest and concern about the costing out of nursing care, it had not led to rapid movement in this direction. In general, there was some consensus that such costing out may not be helpful and may not be effective unless one's professional nurse staff was salaried. There were some expressions that it may, in fact, be detrimental to the nursing department.

Conclusions and discussion

This follow-up of the 1982 Magnet Hospital study was designed to get an answer to the question, "What impacts have PPS and DRGs had on hospital nurses and nursing care?" Magnet Hospitals were chosen to obtain the answer because they are perceived generally as being among the leading hospital nursing departments in the country, and because some comparative data prior to PPS were available. With or without the coexisting economic conditions, PPS seems to have had its greatest impact in the following areas:

1. While nursing and patient care may still be of the very highest quality (and Patient Satisfaction questionnaires would seem to validate that this is so), nurses don't *feel* as good about the quality of care that they are giving

now because they don't *see* patients getting well.

Undoubtedly, this is a problem that is not going to go away and must be dealt with. Many nurses expressed the concern that it was all right if *they* did not actually nurse the patient back to a higher level of wellness, but they wanted to be assured that someone who was competent did so. Three of the Magnet Hospitals studied had in operation programs specifically aimed at dealing with this problem. One had instituted a decentralized home care program in which the staff nurse, in the role of Case Manager, worked directly with the hospital employed home care nurses in seeing to it that the patient continued with the home care needed. Another hospital had a separate department of Continuity of Care whose Clinical Nurse Specialists worked with the primary nurses on the unit in planning and delivering care to patients in their homes. The third hospital had a highly effective and operative primary nursing system wherein the primary nurses directly planned and made arrangements for the continued postdischarge care of their patients. Alleviating the anxiety of nurses for their patients after discharge is something that would do a great deal to reestablish for a nurse the job satisfaction that comes from seeing and knowing that her patient is doing well. This tremendous concern of nurses today for the welfare of the patient after discharge is reflected also in some of the excellent research being done currently on this problem, such as that of Brooten.[19]

2. Nurses at all levels in the organization are becoming more cost conscious. They definitely have begun to develop a "business mind."

While nurses generally saw the necessity of developing a business mind, they were quite resentful of physicians (and to a lesser degree, other department personnel) who were not made to play by the same rules. In a few instances where nursing and hospital administration insisted that the medical staff work with nurses in cost containment, a much more collaborative relationship between nurse and physician was established. For the most part, nurses are looking forward anxiously to the day when medical price tags will be regulated; they believe that this will encourage physicians to cooperate more with cost containment measures.

3. There is evidence that, if available, more and more acute care hospitals are moving toward all-RN staffing. Whether this is possible or desirable is beyond the scope of this article. But there is no question that staff nurses, head nurses, and nurse administrators are strong in their conviction that with the increased acuity level, the most educated nurse is the one best able to provide the needed care, and that, with the low "down" time for the RN, it is the most cost effective. The use of nursing assistants, who assist the nurses rather than giving direct care to patients, seems to be an established practice that is continuing.

4. With the "sicker, quicker, and early discharge" phenomenon, some established nursing care practices, such as primary nursing, and written, detailed nursing care plans, may need to be altered somewhat, without losing sight of the desired goal.

In all likelihood, staff nurses themselves will work out the delivery system that works best for them. Many are very clear about principles and about the type of care they wish to achieve — continuous, planned, comprehensive, and non-fragmented. Also, they are very flexible in adapting daily to the system of care that best fits the resources available for that day. The kind of help needed will be assistance in holding on to the principles, while working within a resource-driven model, to effect the best delivery system possible.

Written, individualized nursing care plans were developed by nurse educators for the education of the student. For this purpose they

work quite well. They have never been embraced enthusiastically by the majority of nurses at the bedside. Part of this is because many nurses do not see the NEED for them; part is because they are not USED by other nurses; part is because in many instances they are not part of the permanent record; part may be because some nurses are not comfortable in doing them. But perhaps the biggest impediment to the written, detailed nursing care plan is a negative cost-benefit analysis. In a resource-driven market, the nurse practitioner has to decide: "Given the limited amount of time and the many patient care needs, what are the most important things for me to do with the time available?" The documentation aspect of nursing care planning is understood clearly and strongly ascribed to: it is the advanced writing out of the plan that brings resistance. It was quite evident in the present study that computerization of nursing care plans greatly overcomes resistance; in fully activated systems, care planning and documentation can be done simultaneously.

5. The PPS may change over time, but clearly the dollars for inpatient health care will continue to be restricted. Clinical research is needed to determine which treatment modalities are most beneficial, from a cost-benefit perspective.

Through the years, nurses have developed a variety of different treatment modalities for nursing problems such as decubiti or incontinence. As yet, there has been minimal research done to determine which methods produce the best results — let alone which methods produce the best results at the lowest cost. Scientific studies to look at nursing treatments are needed. Studying the treatments does not necessarily mean that just because a treatment is costly, it will be abandoned. However, where possible, the most effective treatment for the least cost should be our aim.

6. Some positive features emanating from PPS are recognized: increased specialization

has led to increased pride, self-esteem, and respect from others for many nurses. Early patient discharge has fostered increased taking of responsibility for health care by the patient and his family. More and more families are learning to provide health and illness care in the home. What is learned in one illness episode can be utilized by the family in caring for family members in subsequent episodes.

Because of the crucial role the nurse plays in getting the patient ready for discharge, the nurse role has become more powerful in the inpatient setting. The opportunities and necessities for collaboration with medicine and other members of the health care team have increased. There can be no summary better than that expressed by one of the staff nurses interviewed. "Sure, since DRGs, the nursing role has changed somewhat. I've certainly become more conscious of cost and length of stay, and outliers. But the nurse role has become more powerful and more important also. The most important thing for me to do now is to develop the confidence to respond with independent thought to the interdependent relationships in which I find myself."

REFERENCES

1. McClure, Margaret, et al., *Magnet Hospitals* (Kansas City, MO: American Nurses' Association), 1983.

2. Schaefers, Vick, "A Cost Allocation Method for Nursing," in Shaffer, Franklin A. (Ed.), *Costing Out Nursing: Pricing Our Product* (New York: National League for Nursing, 1985), pp. 69-84.

3. Rusch, Sue, "Continuity of Care: From Hospital Unit Into Home," *Nursing Management,* 17(12):38-41, 1986.

4. Fanning, Jane A. and Ruth Busch Lovett, "Decentralization Reduces Nursing Administration Budget," *JONA,* 15(5):19-24, 1985.

5. Taylor, Dori and Marlene Kramer, "The Head Nurse: Manager? Clinician? or Both?" in McCloskey, J. and Helen Grace (Eds.), *Current Issues in Nursing,* Second Edition (Boston, MA: Blackwell Scientific Publications), Chapter 30, pp. 405-424.

6. McKibbin, Richard, *et al.*, "Nursing Costs and DRG Payments,"*AJN*, December, 85(12):1353-1356, 1985.

7. Marram van Servellen, Gwen and Mychelle Mowry, "DRGs and Primary Nursing: Are They Compatible?," *JONA,* 15(4): 32-36, 1985.

8. Minyard, Karen, *et al.*, "RNs May Cost Less Than You Think," *JONA,* 15(4):32-36,1985.

9. Wolf, Gail A., Linda Lesic, and Allison Leak, "Primary Nursing: The Impact on Nursing Costs Within DRGs," *JONA,* 16(3):9-11, 1986.

10. Newman, Margaret and Sharon Autio, *Nursing in a Prospective Payment System Health Care Environment*, (University of Minnesota: School of Nursing, 1986).

11. Nursing Life Special Poll Report: "How Many Staff Cuts Ahead?," *Nursing Life,* 4(6):21-25, 1984.

12. Reschak, Gary, *et al.*, "Accounting for Nursing Costs by DRG," *JONA,* 15(9):15-20, 1985.

13. Grimaldi, P.L. and J.A. Micheletti, "RIMs and the Cost of Nursing Care," *Nursing Management*, 13:12-22, 1982.

14. Mowry, Mychelle and Ralph Korpman, "Do DRG Reimbursement Rates Reflect Nursing Costs?," *JONA,* 15(7,8):29-35, 1985.

15. Ethridge, Phyllis, "The Case for Billing by Patient Acuity," *Nursing Management*, 16(8):38-41, 1985.

16. Urosevich, Patti, "How Nurses are Learning to Live with DRGs," *Nursing Life,* 4(2):64-66, 1984.

17. Nyberg, Jan and Nora Wolff, "DRG Panic," *JONA,* 14(4):17-21, 1984.

18. Giovannetti, Phyllis, "DRGs and Nursing Workload Measures," *Computers in Nursing,* 3(2):88-91.

19. Brooten, Dorothy, *et al.*, "A Randomized Clinical Trial of Early Hospital Discharge and Home Follow-up of Very-Low-Birth-Weight Infants," *New England Journal of Medicine*, (315):934-939, 1986.

20. Adams, Rella and Brenda Johnson, "Acuity and Staffing Under Prospective Payment," *JONA,* 16(10):21-25, 1986.

The nursing shortage

ECONOMISTS DEFINE *demand* as the amount of a service people will purchase at a particular price. Viewed in this way, the demand for nurses equals the number of nurses that employers will hire at a particular price. A shortage exists when demand exceeds supply — that is, when employers wish to employ more workers with certain qualifications, at certain salaries, than are available.

The nursing shortage of today, however, reflects a far more complex set of circumstances. It appears to result not from a contraction of the supply of registered nurses but from a dramatic increase in demand for their services — from 80.8 RN full-time equivalents (FTEs) per 100 patients in community hospitals in 1983 to 97.8 RN FTEs in 1987. According to those statistics, at the same time that hospitals were reducing their numbers of beds, they were hiring more nurses. And at the same time that hospitals were terminating many hospital workers, including licensed practical nurses, they were hiring more registered nurses.

Currently, unemployment rates for registered nurses are at an all-time low, and work force participation rates (the percentage of eligible persons actually working) for registered nurses are very high. Furthermore, because of the impact of prospective payment systems, the acuity of hospital patients continues to increase, and hospitals predict an even higher demand for registered nurses. Of course, unless dramatic solutions for the nursing shortage are found, higher demand will only make it worse.

The readings in this chapter focus on (1) the extent and nature of the nursing shortage and (2) immediate and long-term strategies for responding to the shortage.

The first article, "Secretary's Commission on Nursing: Final Report, Volume I, December 1988," by the Department of Health and Human Service's Commission on Nursing, concludes that the reported shortage is of "significant magnitude" and "primarily a result of an increase in demand as opposed to a contraction in supply." The commission has formulated 16 recommendations and 81 strategies designed to alleviate the current shortage and ensure an adequate supply of nurses in the future.

Aiken and Mullinix, in their article "The Nurse Shortage: Myth or Reality," also believe the current nursing shortage results from increased demand, but in their article they cite compelling data that underscore the low economic rewards of nursing and the reluctance of hospital management to implement necessary changes in the work environment. These authors, who point to the versatility of nurses and their relatively low pay as the major reason demand has increased, have evolved a relative-wage theory that deserves careful reading and reflection.

The third article, "CNA Sets Forth Shortage Solutions," is a position statement of the California Nurses Association (CNA). Believing that the current nursing shortage is the result of increased demand for nursing services, the CNA has proposed a process and plan to solve the shortage over the long term. Their plan includes strategies for the practice environment as well as for job structure, compensation, career development, image, and recruitment into the profession.

The fourth article, "A Look Ahead: What the Future Holds for Nursing," differs from the preceding ones in that it does not present a consensus opinion. The editors of *RN* sought the views of six influential nurses on nursing shortage issues and the future of nursing. Their views are not entirely positive: Five of the six panelists do not predict a resolution of the entry into practice issue discussed in Unit I by the year 2000 — or even 3000.

The American Medical Association (AMA) has proposed a new category of health care worker to alleviate the nursing shortage: This non-nurse, bedside care technician, called a *registered care technologist,* is the subject of this chapter's fifth article, "American Medical Association's Proposal on Introduction of Registered Care Technologists (RCTs)," by Shurbet, et al.

The next three articles are intended to be read as a set and to stimulate discussion of nurse-physician relationships and solutions to the nursing shortage, including the AMA's proposal for RCTs.

In the article "Coming to Terms with the Nursing Shortage — Asserting the Role and Initiatives of Academic Health Center, Kassebaum states that nursing education is at fault: "The shortage arises because of attrition and because the graduate models of various educational programs do not align with patient-care needs."

Pounds, a physician and former nurse, puts the blame for the problems of nursing on nurse educators and their failure to use the apprenticeship model as it is used in medical education. In "Beyond Florence Nightingale: The General Professional Education of the Nurse," she proposes a longer basic education program for the registered nurse, a smaller nursing work force, and the use of an increased number of nursing assistants.

In her article entitled "Nursing Education and Practice," Lindeman is critical of the RCT proposal and the process used to develop it. Calling for a very different set of strategies for responding to the nursing shortage, she puts the responsibility on physicians, health care administrators, the public — and nurses.

Final report, volume I, December 1988

DEPARTMENT OF HEALTH AND HUMAN SERVICES SECRETARY'S COMMISSION ON NURSING

Executive summary

IN LATE DECEMBER 1987, in response to reports of widespread difficulties recruiting and retaining registered nurses (RNs), Health and Human Services' Secretary Otis R. Bowen, M.D. established the Secretary's Commission on Nursing. The charge given to this 25-member, public advisory panel was to: 1) advise the Secretary on problems related to the recruitment and retention of RNs; and 2) develop recommendations on how the public and private sectors can work together to address these problems and implement immediate and long-range solutions for enhancing the adequacy of the supply of RNs. The Commission was given the calendar year 1988 to accomplish these tasks. The first five months of the commission's tenure were devoted to an assessment of the magnitude, causes, consequences, and future implications of the nurse shortage. The results of this assessment were presented in the Commission's *Interim Report*, presented to the Secretary in July 1988. Based on this assessment, the Commission concluded:

• The reported shortage of RNs is real, widespread, and of significant magnitude. There is evidence to support the conclusion that the current shortage cuts across all health care delivery settings and all nursing practice areas. The shortage is most acute in urban hospitals, critical care and medical/surgical units, and nursing homes.

• The current shortage of RNs is primarily the result of an increase in demand as opposed to a contraction of supply. Although RN supply continues to grow, the number of new RN graduates has declined, and there are strong indications that RN supply has not kept pace with increased demand.

• The shortage is contributing to the deterioration of RNs' work environment and may also be having a negative impact on quality of patient care and access to health services.

• Projections for the future are not encouraging. In the short term, the quantity of care provided by the existing pool of RNs will be difficult to increase without significant intervention. In the long term, there is considerable evidence to suggest that the demand for RNs will continue to increase, and a continued imbalance with supply is anticipated.

Working from this assessment, the Commission then turned its attention to the task of developing action-oriented recommendations designed to alleviate the current shortage and assure a healthy nurse labor market in the future. Recommendation development was an iterative process that spanned five public meetings of the Commission and that led not only to the drafting of recommendations but also to the construction of a series of companion strategies designed to secure the successful implementation of each recommendation....

The Commission advances 16 specific recommendations and 81 directed strategies to achieve them. These are presented in groups, as they address the following issues:
• utilization of nursing resources
• nurse compensation
• health care financing
• nurse decision making
• development of nursing resources
• maintenance of nursing resources.

The specific recommendations are listed below, along with a brief statement explaining the rationale which supports each set of recommendations. Section 3 of this report contains all of the recommendations, more detailed rationales, and specific implementation strategies. These strategies provide guidance regarding the Commission's assessment of viable actions that can be undertaken to realize the objectives stated in the recommendations. Although not listed here in the Executive Summary, these implementation strategies are an integral component of the recommendation package and should be given careful consideration by all readers interested in the Commission's work.

Utilization of nursing resources. As stated earlier, the Commission has concluded that the current nurse shortage is primarily the result of a rapidly-increasing demand for RNs. Some of this increased demand for RNs is arising because health care delivery organizations are compensating for reductions in non-nursing staff — both clinical and non-clinical — as well as in other categories of nursing personnel. The four recommendations advanced in this area are intended to encourage nurse employers to use scarce RN resources in an efficient and effective manner, thereby enhancing the adequacy of the existing RN supply. These recommendations call for the provision of adequate support services for nurses, utilization of the most appropriate mix of nursing personnel, adoption of automated information and other labor-saving technologies in order to increase RNs' productivity, and improvement in the internal management of nurse resources within health care delivery organizations. The specific recommendations are as follows:

1. Health care delivery organizations should preserve the time of the nurse for the direct care of patients and families by providing adequate staffing levels for clinical and non-clinical support services.

2. Health care delivery organizations should adopt innovative nurse staffing patterns that recognize and appropriately utilize the differ-

ent levels of education, competence and experience among registered nurses, as well as between registered nurses and other nursing personnel responsible to registered nurses, such as licensed practical nurses and ancillary nursing personnel.

3. The federal government should sponsor further research and encourage health care delivery organizations to develop and use automated information systems and other new labor-saving technologies as a means of better supporting nurses and other health professionals. Health care delivery organizations should work with researchers and manufacturers to ensure the applicability and cost-effectiveness of such information systems and technologies across all practice settings.

4. Health care delivery organizations, nursing associations, and government and private health insurers should develop and implement methods for costing, budgeting, reporting and tracking nursing resource utilization, both to enhance the management of nursing services and to assess their economic contribution to their employing organization.

Nurse compensation. Evidence analyzed by the Commission indicates that nurse compensation is inadequate and that the severe wage compression over the span of a nurse's career is of particular concern. The Commission believes that inadequate compensation is one of the roots of the current nurse shortage. On the demand side, low RN compensation levels relative to those of other personnel for which RNs can substitute encourage employers' inappropriate utilization of RNs in carrying out non-RN functions. On the supply side, compensation levels lower than those of other professions requiring comparable educational preparation may encourage existing nurses to leave the profession, thus exacerbating the current shortage. In the longer run, inadequate compensation is also likely to discourage potential nurses from entering the profession, contributing to a continuation of the shortage.

The following compensation recommendation is advanced to address these concerns.

5. Health care delivery organizations should increase RN compensation and improve RN long-term career orientation by providing a one-time adjustment to increase RN relative wages targeted to geographic, institutional and career differences. Additionally, they should pursue the development and implementation of innovative compensation options for nurses and expand pay ranges based on experience, performance, education and demonstrated leadership.

Health care financing. The Commission recognizes that many employers of nurses, especially those in the nursing home and home health sectors, may not have sufficient financial resources to support the compensation enhancement advocated in the preceding recommendation. Thus, the health care financing recommendation listed below and its accompanying implementation strategies given in Section 3 are put forth in the hopes of ensuring that the reimbursement levels and procedures do not constrain the efforts of efficiently-organized health care delivery organizations to offer competitive compensation packages.

6. Government should reimburse at levels that are sufficient to allow efficiently-organized health care delivery organizations to recruit and retain the number and mix of nurses necessary to provide adequate patient care.

Nurse decision making. The Commission believes that failure on the part of the health care delivery organizations, physicians, and health policy making bodies to fully recognize the decision making abilities of RNs has contributed to problems in recruiting and retaining nurses, hindered the development of a career orientation in professional nursing, and limited the efficiency and effectiveness of patient care delivery. With improved representation on policy-making, regulatory, and accreditation bodies, nurses can make unique, critical, and effective contributions to the health care delivery system. Furthermore, the technological, ethical, and managerial challenges facing health care delivery organizations dictate more collaboration among members of the health care team. The recommendations below address the active involvement of nurses in decision making at all levels.

7. Policy-making, regulatory, and accreditation bodies that have an impact on health care at the national, state, and local levels should foster greater representation and active participation of the nursing profession in their decision-making activities.

8. Employers of nurses should ensure active nurse participation in the [organization's] governance, administration, and management.

9. Employers of nurses, as well as the medical profession, should recognize the appropriate clinical decision making authority of nurses in relationship to other health care professionals, foster communication and collaboration among health care team, and ensure that the appropriate provider delivers the necessary care. Close cooperation and mutual respect between nursing and medicine is essential.

Development of nursing resources. While nearly all evidence indicates that the current nurse shortage is demand-driven, the recent downturn in nursing school enrollments is cause for serious concern that the shortage will grow worse in the future. Additionally, the distribution of RNs across specialties and employment settings is currently problematic, and there is evidence that the formal education received by many new nurses leaves them inadequately prepared for the rigors of clinical practice in today's complex health care environment. Finally, the Commission believes that increased public awareness regarding the image of nursing can contribute to a reversal or recent enrollment trends. The recommendations contained within the development of nursing resources category are aimed at facilitating the education of nurses, and thereby increasing the supply of qualified RNs, through increased targeted financial support and improved program accessibility, updating the relevancy of nursing curricula, and promoting nursing as a career.

10. Financial assistance to undergraduate and graduate nursing students must be increased. The burden of providing this assistance should be equitably shared among the federal and state governments, employers of nurses, philanthropic and voluntary organizations. The preferred method of providing this support is the use of service-payback loans as well as funding for those in financial need.

11. State governments, nursing organizations, schools of nursing and employers of nurses should work to minimize non-financial barriers to nursing education for individuals desiring to enter the profession as well as for nurses wishing to upgrade their education.

12. Schools of nursing, state boards of nursing, and employers of nurses should work together to ensure that the curricula are relevant to contemporary and future nursing practice, prepare nurses for employment in a variety of practice settings, and provide the foundation for continued professional development.

13. The nursing profession should take primary responsibility for providing immediate and sustained attention to the promotion of positive and accurate images of the profession and the work of nurses.

Maintenance of nursing resources. Although certain in their assessment of the current status of the nurse labor market, and confident that the recommendations put forth in this report embody the best approaches to resolving the current nurse shortage, the Commission believes that the federal government should spearhead a sustained effort devoted to: monitoring the nurse labor market; collecting improved data and conducting further research on the demand for nurses, as well as the supply and nursing practice; and following through on the implementation of the recommendations and strategies outlined in this re-

port. The recommendations that follow are designed to accomplish these goals.

14. The Department of Health and Human Services should create a commission having a duration of at least five years that will monitor the implementation of the recommendations in this report as well as the development and maintenance of nursing resources. This commission should be constituted as an advisory body reporting directly to the Secretary.

15. The Department of Health and Human Services, private foundations, and employers of nurses should support and carry out research and demonstrations on the effects of nurse compensation, staffing patterns, decision-making authority, and career development on nurse supply and demand as well as health care cost and quality. Research should be sponsored on the relationship of health care financing and nursing practice.

16. The federal government should develop data sources needed to assess nursing resources as they relate to health planning and manpower. The Commission does not view the development of these recommendations as the final step in addressing the nurse shortage. Rather, the more important and challenging task still lies ahead. The Commission strongly encourages the organizations addressed in this report to examine carefully the Commission's diagnosis of the problem, to assess honestly and carefully the relevance of each issue to their own particular organization, and to implement without hesitation the appropriate recommendations. The Commission recognizes that some of the identified problems transcend the interests of one particular organization and expects that, in these cases, the relevant institutions, organizations, associations, and individuals make a good faith effort to collaborate in the implementation of the recommended solutions to the problem. *It is the sincere belief of the Commission that the health of this nation will be at risk if the changes suggested in these recommendations do not occur.*

The nurse shortage: Myth or reality?

LINDA H. AIKEN, RN, PhD; CONNIE FLYNT MULLINIX, RN, MPH, MBA

THE PROPORTION OF vacant positions for registered nurses in hospitals doubled between September 1985 and December 1986,[1] reaching the levels of the last national nursing shortage of 1979. Current reports of vacancies are perplexing in the light of the size of the nation's supply of nurses. The output of nurses has doubled over the past 30 years, greatly exceeding the population growth, and licensed registered nurses now number 2.1 million. Between 1977 and 1984 alone, the number of employed nurses increased by 55 percent, as compared with an 8 percent growth in population.[2] Intuitively, it would seem that an increased number of nurses would be the solution, but the problem persists nevertheless.

The reported shortage of hospital nurses exists in the midst of a substantial reduction in hospital inpatient capacity nationally. The demand for acute inpatient care in general hospitals has fallen, resulting in 50 million fewer inpatient days in 1986 than in 1981. Since 1983, hospitals have closed more than 40,000 beds and average hospital occupancy rates dropped to 63.4 percent in 1986.[3] Enrollments in nursing schools have also decreased markedly, raising the possibility that fewer nurses than anticipated will be available in the future.

There is now a contentious debate about whether a shortage of hospital nurses truly exists and about its causes. In 1981, the Institute of Medicine was commissioned by Congress to reconcile the evidence of an increased supply of nurses with continued reported shortages. The study concluded that the national supply of generalist nurses was adequate for the present and short-term future.[4] Cyclical vacancies in positions for hospital nurses were attributed primarily to local labor-market conditions, although a shortage of nurses in certain specialties was noted. Recommendations were made to the hospital industry on the need to restructure nursing roles and develop improved financial rewards and opportunities for career advancement in clinical care.[5] The National Commission on Nursing made remarkably similar recommendations in 1983.[6] But in 1986, the American Hospital Association was again reporting that high vacancy rates in positions for nurses were disrupting hospital care,[1] whereas the U.S. Department of Health and Human Services again concluded that the national supply of nurses was in balance with the demand.[7]

Employment patterns of nurses

The shortage of nurses is measured by the hospital industry as vacant budgeted full-time-equivalent positions for registered nurses. Vacancy rates, however, are not an objective measure of the need for bedside nurses. Moreover, the number of factors, including budget constraints as well as local wage rates. Despite these limitations, we have chosen to analyze vacancy rates because they are used by the industry to reflect the changing supply of nurses.

There are several commonly held but erroneous beliefs about nurses' work patterns. One misconception is that nurses have left nursing in large numbers and are either inactive or working at jobs outside health care. In contrast, nurses have one of the highest rates of participation in the labor force among workers in predominantly female occupations. Almost 80 percent of registered nurses are actively employed[2] either full-time or part-time, as compared with 54 percent of all American women. Not much is known about those who do not renew their licenses and, therefore, are not counted in the population of registered nurses. But less than 6 percent of registered nurses are employed in other occupations and are not seeking a position in nursing.[2] Given the responsibilities of women for child rearing and other domestic concerns, an employment rate of 80 percent may be almost as high as can be expected. Thus, it is unlikely that un-employed nurses represent a large potential re-source for hospital employment. However, nursing is somewhat unusual in that 27 percent of the total pool of registered nurses work part-time. Clearly, a change in the number of hours worked by more than 500,000 part-time registered nurses could substantially affect the supply of full-time-equivalent nurses.

Some observers have suggested that the shortage of nurses in hospitals may be due to the increased demand for nurses in ambulatory settings and new administrative positions in health care. However, hospitals' share of the ever-growing pool of nurses has not changed substantially since 1960. Sixty-eight percent of all employed nurses work in hospitals.[2] Hospi-tals have dramatically increased the number of nurses they employ in the aggregate and in re-lation to numbers of patients, even when the recent increase in out-patient visits is taken into account. In fact, hospitals are employing more registered nurses than ever before and are even replacing non-nurses with nurses — just the opposite of what would be expected during actual shortage of nurses.

In response to reduced numbers of inpa-tients, hospitals employed 133,376 fewer full-time-equivalent workers in 1986 than in 1983.[3] In contrast, the number of full-time equivalent nurses increased by 37,500 during the same period.[8,9] A substantial increase in the ratio of nurses to patients resulted. In 1972, hospitals employed 50 nurses per 100 patients (average adjusted daily census); by 1986, the figure had increased to 91 nurses per 100 — an 82 per-cent expansion (Fig. 1). Aides and licensed practical nurses were replaced by registered nurses. In 1968, registered nurses accounted for only 33 percent of hospitals' total nursing-service personnel; by 1986, registered nurses accounted for 58 percent.

The changing demand for nurses

The rapidity with which the current shortage developed suggests that increased vacancy rates must be due to a changing demand for nurses, not to a declining supply. There are three primary explanations for recent increase in the demand for hospital nurses. First, hospi-talized patients are sicker and require more care than in years past, on average, because of the reduction in discretionary admissions and the shorter average length of stay. However, there is no basis to suggest that the average condition of hospitalized patients changed dra-matically enough between 1982 and 1986 to require a 26 percent increase in the ratio of registered nurses to patients. Although the changing case mix may provide a partial ex-planation for the increased demand for nurses, it cannot be the only explanation.

A second explanation for the recent in-crease in vacancy rates is related to changing budget constraints in hospitals. When vacancy rates were at an all-time low of 3.7 percent in 1984, the Medicare Prospective Payment Sys-tem was just being implemented and fears of severe hospital-budget limits were widespread. As a result, some budgeted positions were eliminated. Unexpectedly high operating mar-gins, however, provided the opportunity for hospitals to budget for more nursing positions.

A third explanation is related to changes in nurses' relative wages. In most labor short-ages, wages are adjusted and other incentives are developed to attract additional workers. These market adjustments fail to occur in

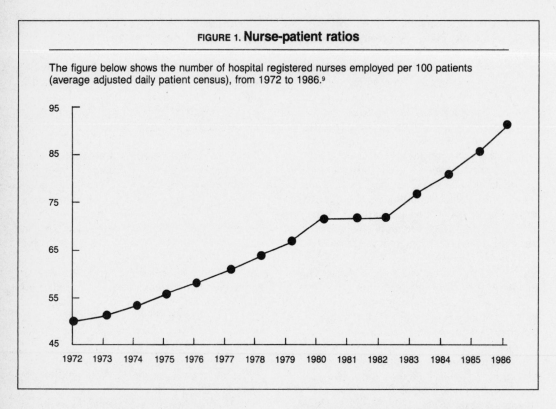

FIGURE 1. **Nurse-patient ratios**

The figure below shows the number of hospital registered nurses employed per 100 patients (average adjusted daily patient census), from 1972 to 1986.[9]

nursing with the rapidity or magnitude seen in other labor markets. Labor economists have described nursing as a "captured" labor market.[10,11] In any given community, a small number of hospitals employ most of the local nurses — a phenomenon known as oligopsony in labor economics. Employers offering nurses jobs with weekday hours usually have no trouble employing nurses and thus do not compete with other employers on the basis of salary. There is no demand for nurses outside the health care field that is sufficient to create competitive pressures on the hospital industry, as there is, for example, for computer programmers. Moreover, hospital administrators tend to assume that there is a finite number of nurses in any given community and that wage

competition among hospitals will be costly and will not resolve community shortages. The majority of nurses, if they want to work, must accept the terms offered by hospitals.

Registered nurses are versatile employees in a hospital context.[12,13] They can provide all the services for which hospitals sometimes employ nurses' aides and licensed practical nurses, and they can also often perform a wide range of other functions, including those assigned at other times to secretarial and clerical personnel, laboratory technicians, pharmacists, physical therapists, and social workers. Nurses substitute for physicians under some circumstances, and commonly assume hospital management roles after regular work hours. Thus, when nurses' relative wages are low as compared with other workers', it is advantageous

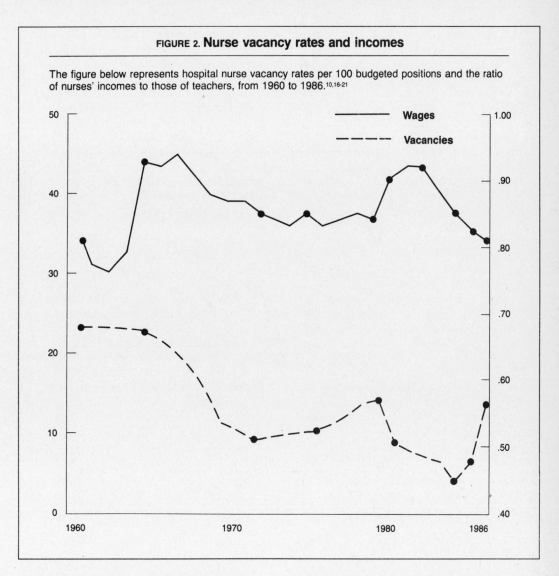

FIGURE 2. **Nurse vacancy rates and incomes**

The figure below represents hospital nurse vacancy rates per 100 budgeted positions and the ratio of nurses' incomes to those of teachers, from 1960 to 1986.[10,16-21]

for hospitals to employ them in greater numbers and in lieu of other kinds of workers. Even if nurses' wages are 20 to 30 percent higher than those of licensed practical nurses or secretaries, it may still be more economical to hire nurses, because they require little supervision and can assume responsibility for a wide range of duties. The increased demand for nurses created by low relative wages can lead to shortages in some geographic locations, in specialty units, and on undesirable evening, night, and weekend hours.

The relative-wage theory is supported by data spanning several decades[14,15] (Fig. 2).

From 1946 to 1966, for example, the increase in nurses' wages lagged behind those in comparable women's occupations. Nurses' wages over the period increased by 53 percent, whereas teachers' salaries increased by 100 percent and female professional and technical workers' salaries increased by 73 percent. In the early 1960s, more than one in five budgeted positions for nurses were vacant. There was great concern at the time that the increased demand for hospital care accompanying the introduction of Medicare and Medicaid would exacerbate the shortage of nurses. But these new programs were accompanied by substantial wage increases for nurses. Employment rates among nurses increased substantially after these wage increases, as did enrollments in nursing schools. The proportion of vacant budgeted positions for nurses in hospitals dropped from 23 percent in 1961 to 9 percent by 1971 and after hospital wage and price controls in 1971 and state rate setting and the voluntary hospital cost-containment effort a few years later, nurses' wages declined relative to other groups' and the proportion of vacant positions for nurses in hospitals increased again, leading to the shortage of 1979. There was a wage response to the 1979 shortage; nurses' wages rose an average of 13 percent annually in both 1980 and 1981. By 1984, the proportion of vacancies had reached a low of 3.7 percent.

The substantial wage increases received by nurses in 1980 and 1981 did not continue subsequently, and by the time the new Medicare prospective payment system was implemented, nurses' wages had been eroded. Hospital nurses have received only modest wage increases sine 1982. By 1985, average salaries for teachers were 19 percent higher than those for nurses, and average salaries for all female professional and technical workers were 10 percent higher. Despite all the publicity about the shortage of hospital nurses, nurses' wages increased only 4 percent in 1986.[18]

Declining nursing school enrollments

Since 1983, enrollments in nursing schools have dropped by 20 percent[22] (and National League for Nursing: unpublished data). The number of new nurses graduating annually is predicted to fall from a high of 82,700 in 1985 to 68,700 or lower by 1995.[7] All types of nursing programs have had declining enrollments; associate-degree programs have had a decline of 19 percent, and baccalaureate programs 12 percent (National League for Nursing: unpublished data). Enrollments in three-year hospital diploma programs have been declining for more than two decades and now account for only 14 percent of graduates annually (Fig. 3).

The country's demographic profile is partly responsible for declining enrollments because of the smaller size of 18-year-old cohorts in recent years. However, interest in nursing as a career has fallen precipitously among college freshmen in both community colleges and four-year institutions. The University of California, Los Angeles, national survey of first-time college freshmen indicated a 50 percent decline since 1974 in the proportion of full-time women students planning to pursue nursing career. In contrast to an almost threefold increase in the proportion interested in careers in business[23] (Fig. 4). Moreover, the College Board recently released data indicating that the SAT scores of high-school students interested in nursing careers were well below the national average for college-bound students, and that the SAT gap between prospective nurses and non-nurses was widening over time.[24]

There are many reasons for the declining interest in nursing. Whereas starting salaries of nurses are now comparable to those of other college graduates, the average maximum salary for nurses is only $7,000 higher than the average starting salary.[18] Since more women are choosing to work continuously in the labor force, the low raises discourage them from choosing a career in nursing. Moreover, em-

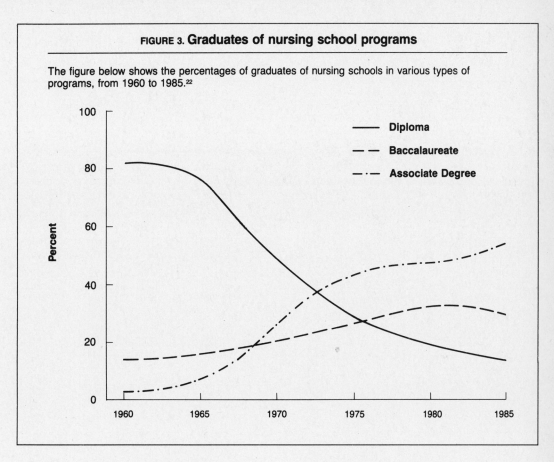

FIGURE 3. **Graduates of nursing school programs**

The figure below shows the percentages of graduates of nursing schools in various types of programs, from 1960 to 1985.[22]

ployers do not offer substantial differences in salary in return for advanced education in nursing. Thus, the economic return on a baccalaureate degree in nursing is poor as compared with the return in alternative fields. Women today have many more career options than they had in years past. Most other careers offer comparable or higher economic rewards and do not require night and weekend work — a notable disadvantage of nursing.

Recommendations for change

A number of issues deserve careful reconsideration and experimentation. First, public-policy makers must recognize that hospital rate

setting can induce labor shortages by artificially depressing wages in occupations like nursing, in which hospitals are the dominant employers. In the short term, depressed wages will increase the demand for nurses, because they can substitute for other personnel, and result in acute spot shortages and high vacancy rates. Over the long term, recruitment to nursing will be seriously eroded by the absence of an adequate salary range that rewards skill and experience.

Second, one of the most unattractive aspects of nursing is the requirement of night and weekend work. With sicker patients, hospitals now need many more nurses on these

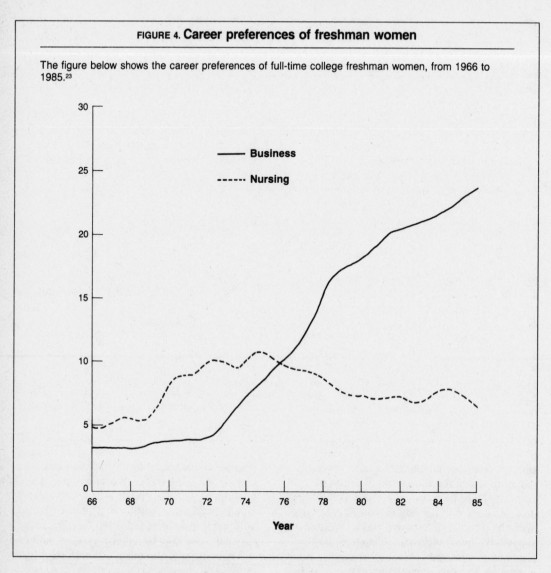

FIGURE 4. **Career preferences of freshman women**

The figure below shows the career preferences of full-time college freshman women, from 1966 to 1985.[23]

unpopular shifts than they needed in the past, when it was not unusual to have a single nurse covering a unit at night. Most women want to work regular daytime hours and will even choose less interesting, less skilled, and worse-paying jobs to accomplish this. Preference for day work explains why vacancy rates are low in ambulatory care despite lower average salaries. Other industries that operate on a 24-hour basis offer substantial difference in wages for evening, night, and weekend work in order to attract sufficient voluntary staff coverage.

Hospitals offer only small differences and try to make shift rotation a requirement of employment. Curiously, most of the innovations hospitals have adopted to reduce vacancies during unpopular shifts actually encourage nurses to work fewer hours. For example, some hospitals pay nurses a full-time salary to work two 12-hour weekend shifts (24 hours per week) but will not pay full-time nurses equivalent hourly rates for unpopular shifts. In view of all the expenses associated with continued high vacancy rates, increasing marginal wage rates to fill vacancies on unpopular assignments might not be as costly as is commonly assumed.

Third, the work requirements of nurses and other personnel in hospitals should be restructured. The ratio of support personnel to professionals is substantially lower in the hospital industry than in other industries. Given the complexities of operating busy hospital inpatient units there is an astounding absence of secretaries, administrative assistants, and mid-level non-nurse managers. Moreover, the computerization of hospitals has lagged for behind that of other industries. Nurses are currently performing many nonclinical, administrative, and management functions in hospitals. Fewer better-paid and better-educated nurses in combination with an improved nonclinical support staff might yield better care without substantial increases in operating costs.

Fourth, hospital management should introduce incentives to encourage experienced nurses to remain in clinical care. A differentiated wage structure that recognizes experience and advanced education is critical. Employment benefits such as pension, tuition support, and sabbaticals could be used much more effectively to develop "loyalty" and thus reduce costly staff turnover.

Fifth, physicians should take leadership roles in the development of more effective collaborative models of practice with nurses in hospitals. Much of the dissatisfaction of nurses with hospital practice is related to the absence of satisfying professional relationships with physicians. Many nurses choose administration over clinical practice in an effort to obtain greater status in their interactions with physicians. More effective nurse-physician collaboration in clinical care activities would improve the professional satisfaction of both groups and contribute to improved patient outcomes as well.[25]

Conclusions

The evidence suggests that under current market conditions in many local communities, the demand for nurses is greater than the supply. Regardless of the reasons for this imbalance, there is only a limited number of possible solutions. Expansion of nursing-school enrollments to increase the national supply of nurses might eventually solve the vacancy problem but is unlikely to occur, given demographic trends and the declining interest of young people in nursing careers. Recruiting inactive nurses into the work force is also not a promising solution because employment rates are already high among nurses and may have reached a ceiling. Expanding the number of nurses trained abroad is an expedient option but one that might create more problems, in terms of quality of care, than it would solve. The development of incentives to induce part-time nurses to work more hours is a promising option that should be pursued. Finally, if all the above methods to increase the supply of nurses still do not eliminate disruptive vacancies, restructuring hospitals to make more appropriate use of the special expertise of nurses is a difficult but obvious alternative.

None of these recommendations are new; they have been advocated consistently by every panel studying nursing shortages. Implementation, in contrast, has been slow, despite encouraging evidence from the few hospitals that are making the suggested changes.[26] The fact is that nursing shortages are a consequence of complacent management and the reluctance of administrators to re-examine traditional practices. In the light of the attitudes of young women and their changing aspirations, what is now an artificially created shortage may become a critical problem in the future. Nurses are an essential resource for hospitals and the nation's health. Addressing their needs and aspirations realistically and examining their work conditions meaningfully are prerequisites for high-quality patient care now and in the future.

REFERENCES

1. Curran CR. Minnick A. Moss J. Who needs nurses? Am J Nurs 1987: 87:444-7.

2. Department of Health and Human Services. The registered nurse population. 1984. Springfield, VA: National Technical Information Service, 1986. (DHHS publication no. (HRP) 0906938.)

3. Economic trends. Vol 3 No. 1. Chicago: American Hospital Association, 1987.

4. Institute of Medicine. National Research Council. Nursing and nursing education: public policies and private actions. Washington, DC: National Academy Press, 1983.

5. Aiken LH. Nursing's future: public policies, private actions. Am J Nurs 1983: 83:1440-4.

6. National Commission on Nursing. Summary report and recommendations. Chicago: Hospital Research and Educational Trust, 1983.

7. Department of Health and Human Services. Fifth report to the president and congress on the status of health personnel: report on nursing. Springfield, VA: National Technical Information Services, 1986. (DHHS publication no. (HRP) 0906804.)

8. Hospital statistics. Chicago: American Hospital Association, 1983.

9. Hospital statistics. Chicago: American Hospital Association, 1986.

10. Yett DE. An economic analysis of the nurse shortage. Lexington, MA: Lexington Books, 1975.

11. Feldstein PJ. Health care economics. New York: John Wiley, 1979.

12. Aiken LH. Nursing priorities for the 1980's: hospitals and nursing homes. Am J Nurs 1981: 81:324-30.

13. Mechanic D, Aiken LH. A cooperative agenda for medicine and nursing. N Engl J Med 1982: 307:747-50.

14. Aiken LH, Blendon RJ, Rogers DE. The shortage of hospital nurses: a new perspective. Ann Intern Med 1981: 95:365-73.

15. Aiken LH. The nurse labor market. Health Aff (Millwood) 1982: 1:30-40.

16. Mullner R, Byre CS, Whitehead S. Hospital vacancies. Am J Nurs 1982: 82:592-4.

17. Report of the 1986 Hospital Nursing Supply Survey. Chicago: American Hospital Association, 1986.

18. National Survey of Hospital and Medical School Salaries. Galveston, TX: University of Texas Medical Branch at Galveston, 1987.

19. Money, Income, and Poverty Status of Families and Persons in the U.S.: 1979-1986: Current Population Reports. Washington, DC: Bureau of the Census. (Series P-60.)

20. National Center for Education Statistics: Digest of education statistics, 1979-1987. Washington, DC: Department of Education, 1987.

21. American Hospital Association. Nurse vacancy rates: analysis from the 1982-1985 annual survey. Chicago: American Hospital Association, 1986.

22. Nursing data review 1985-1986. New York: National League for Nursing, 1986.

23. Astin AW, Green KC, Korn WS. The American freshman: twenty year trends, 1966-1985. Los Angeles: American Council on Education, UCLA, 1986.

24. Feinberg L. Area nursing schools seek cure for decreasing enrollment. Washington Post, August 11, 1986.

25. Knaus WA, Draper EA, Wagner DP, Zimmerman JE. An evaluation of outcome from intensive care in major medical centers. Ann Intern Med 1986: 104:410-8.

26. Magnet hospitals: attraction and retention of professional nurses. Kansas City, MO: American Academy of Nursing, 1983.

CNA sets forth shortage solutions

CALIFORNIA NURSES ASSOCIATION

The plan

SOLUTIONS TO THE increased demand for nursing services require a comprehensive, totally integrated approach. Piecemeal solutions are inadequate and ineffective in the long term. Implementation of the following solutions by health care facilities will result in increased retention and recruitment of registered nurses.

The plan should be developed using the following steps:

1. Assessment of current internal and external nursing environment unique to the setting.

2. Analysis of the future vision of nursing in the specific setting.

3. Development and implementation of a transition plan to achieve the future vision in the specific setting.

The plan to address the demand for nursing services must address these six areas:

1. The Practice Environment
2. The Structure of the Job
3. Compensation
4. Career Development
5. Image
6. Recruitment into the Profession

The practice environment

Nurses work best in an environment that encourages autonomy and respect. Facilities should provide staff development, good facility design, and efficient documentation systems.

The practice environment should foster:

• A philosophy of nursing that recognizes that clinical nursing is the essential patient care service.

• Formation of Nurse-Physician Forums to enhance communication, respect and mutual understanding.

• Formation of staff nurse-administration forums or Professional Performance Committees to identify specific problems and discuss solutions to these problems.

• Development and implementation of models of clinical practice that improve and provide increased autonomy and control of practice, such as shared governance and case management.

• Provision of sufficient education time before equipment or programs are initiated to ensure ongoing staff education to master new equipment and technology.

• Implementation of a thorough educational program for first-line managers.

• Knowledge of financial picture of the organization, including reimbursement methods, capital improvements and portion attributed to nursing care, in order to negotiate responsibility for nursing dollars.

• Facility design which maximizes efficient provision of patient care.

• Provision of patient care management and documentation systems which facilitate comprehensive and efficient documentation of care provided.

• Institutional support for preceptorship and mentorship during the orientation process and beyond.

The structure of the job

Nurses need control over their own practice, authority to supervise, and physicians who want to work collaboratively. Nurses want to take responsibility and be accountable.

• Effective and efficient utilization of registered nurses' skills, knowledge, and experience.

• Efficient use of support personnel under the control of nursing.

• Elimination of non-nursing tasks from registered nurses' responsibilities by efficient use of traditional support personnel, such as transportation escorts, housekeeping, and clericals.

• Utilization of a system of accountability for ancillary and support services to ensure complete and efficient performance as it relates to direct patient care.

• Avoidance of situations where critical care units use new graduates as the only registered nurses on the shift.

• Utilization of a patient classification system that is relevant, includes nurse input, and is useful for staffing.

• Education of nurses on rules and regulations governing nursing practice and licensing of agencies, such as Title 22 licensing regulations.

• Satisfiers built into the job, such as opportunities to develop expertise, job diversity and cross-training, contact with patients over an entire illness episode.

• Development and utilization of nursing research on models of delivering care that are cost-effective and improve the quality of care.

• Documentation of unsafe patient care assignments using Assignment Despite Objection forms, and incident/notification reports.

• Maximum flexibility in scheduling of work hours such as short shifts, job sharing, part-time positions, and input hours.

Compensation

To attract the best and brightest, nurses need compensation and benefit packages commensurate with their education, experience, and responsibility.

• Implementation of compensation and benefits packages designed to deal with issue of salary compression so as to attract and retain the best and the brightest women *and men* to nursing.

• Compensation commensurate with levels of responsibility, preparation, and experience.

• Recognition for certification by ANA and speciality organizations.

• Career ladders to reward nurses who have mastered clinical skills to keep excellent nurses at the bedside.

• Negotiation with facilities for payment of affordable child care, preferably on the premises.

• Promotions related to evaluation of competence, performance, and seniority using objective standards.

• Pay differentials for difficult-to-fill shifts and weekends.

• Pay increase for years of experience or tenure with the hospital.

• Recognition of previous experience and benefits when transferring from setting to setting.

Career development

To encourage the best nurses to remain in patient care, opportunities for advancement based on experience and expertise should be built into nursing jobs.

• Incentives and recognition for clinical practice and direct patient care providers.

• Development of clinical ladders in hospital and agency settings.

• Institutional support for educational advancement of nurses, such as financial support, leaves/sabbaticals, release time, and opportunities to utilize new knowledge.

• Institutional support for professional development such as conferences and participation in professional organizational activities.

• Staff nurse involvement in agency committees and policy development.

• Improved articulation among various nursing education programs.

• Encouragement of staff nurses who obtain more education to remain in the clinical setting.

Image

Nursing suffers from an inaccurate and outdated image. Nurses provide the most comprehensive, preventive, and cost-effective health care. The wide variety of nursing services should be emphasized in public relations efforts.

• Emphasis on the positive, rewarding aspects of the profession.

• Programs to educate junior and senior high school counselors and other career advisors about the nursing profession.

• Development of a public relations effort within institutions to market nurses and their services to other health care personnel.

• Development of a long-term public relations campaign about the advantages of nursing as a professional career.

• Utilization of minorities and men in public relations campaign.

Recruitment into the profession

To ensure continued delivery of health care, legislation, scholarship/loan programs, and efforts by health care employers should focus on recruiting more people into nursing.

• Development of cooperative efforts between nursing service and education to enhance educational programs.

• Legislation to increase availability of financial assistance to prospective students.

• Sponsorship by health care employers and institutions of scholarship/loan programs and other innovative financial incentives that support nursing education.

• Development of innovative recruitment efforts using a variety of media formats targeted to elementary and junior high school students, minorities, and individuals seeking alternative careers, and those returning to nursing.

• Encouragement of flexible hours for educational programs to enable students to work while enrolled in school.

A look ahead: What the future holds for nursing

THOUGH THIS ANNIVERSARY issue celebrates the past, it seems fitting also to take a look ahead.

• How bad will the nursing shortage get, and how long will it last?

• How will the shortage affect nursing pay?

• What will hospitals do to attract more qualified nurses — and what *should* they do?

• When and how will the debate over one versus two levels of practice be resolved?

To answer these and other questions about the shape of things to come, we sought the views of six well-informed and influential nurses — a national cross-section of nursing expertise and opinion. From their vantage points in education, management, law, and consulting, not to mention staff nursing and private practice, they told us what they thought would happen to nursing by the year 2000.

The group included:

Connie Curran, RN, EdD, FAAN, is a vice president of the American Hospital Association in Chicago. She has held teaching positions at Loyola University in Chicago, the University of San Francisco, and the Medical College of Wisconsin. She has also served as corporate chairman of nursing at Montefiore Medical Center in New York City.

Marie C. Infante, RN, JD, MS, MBA, is a lobbyist — her title is Director of Legal Affairs — for the American Health Care Association in Washington, D.C. Trained in Maryland as an orthopedic nurse, she once served on the board of directors of the National Association of Orthopaedic Nurses.

Jean Mueller, RN,C, MSN, an instructor at Bellin College of Nursing in Green Bay, Wis., has worked as a psych nurse at a mental health center and as a staff nurse at two community hospitals in Wisconsin. At one hospital she also served as inservice director. She is a member of the *RN* Editorial Board.

Carolyn Robertson, RN, MSN, CS, enjoys a dual career. Not only is she a nurse specialist at the New York University School of Medicine in New York City, but she's also a private practitioner, specializing in the care of diabetic patients.

Rachel Rotkovitch, RN, MS, is Vice President for Nursing at Yale–New Haven Hospital in New Haven, Conn., a post she's held since 1979. Her varied nursing career has spanned the globe. After starting out in Lebanon, she has worked in Washington, D.C., New York, Egypt, and Israel.

Donna Ojanen Thomas, RN, MS, CEN, a frequent contributor to *RN*, is Director of the Emergency Department at Primary Children's Medical Center in Salt Lake City, where she has worked since 1975. She, too, is a member of the *RN* Editorial Board.

They met with our staff on May 27 for a provocative, wide-ranging look at what the future holds for nursing....

How long will we face a nursing shortage?

None of the six panelists sees an early end to the current nursing shortage. Most feel that this shortage will be with us for a very long time — certainly through the 1990s and maybe even into the next century. That forecast suggests that, generally, nurses should have little trouble finding jobs, even though hospitals may decline in number and shrink in size.

The discussion included this illuminating exchange:

Rotkovitch: There's no doubt about it. The nursing shortage will not go away; it will be with us for the next five, 10, or 15 years. That means competent nurses will not have any problem finding hospital jobs.

Curran: I agree. Surveys made by the American Hospital Association show that hospitals are already moving toward a nursing vacancy rate of 15%. In the future, that percentage may climb even higher.

Will the shortage of nurses lead to better pay?

Yes — but that's a Yes with certain qualifications. Since nurses make up such a large part of the hospital labor force, their wages account for a correspondingly large part of a hospital's costs. That's why hospitals hate to pay nurses any more than they absolutely have to. In years past, they managed to ride out shortages without raising nursing salaries too much. They'll undoubtedly try to do that again, but their long free ride may be over.

Here's what two of the panelists say about nursing pay:

Rotkovitch: In my opinion, a beginning nurse should earn $40,000.

Curran: I agree that nurses deserve a bigger piece of the economic pie, and I think they're going to get it. Remember, though, that the nursing shortage is a two-edged sword. When this kind of shortage arises, does that mean hospitals should increase salaries? Or does it encourage them to hire other types of workers to do nursing jobs?

Who will hospitals hire to replace nurses?

Patients will see a lot more white uniforms at bedside, but all of that white won't be worn by nurses. That's because hospitals may try to offset the nursing shortage by bringing in or training less qualified employees — aides and technicians, or the like — for some nursing tasks. Dangerous? You bet, say our panelists, but not at all unlikely.

Thomas: I won't be surprised if hospitals try to substitute technicians for nurses. If a patient is hooked up to a machine, all the technician has to do is operate the on-off button. You can teach anyone to do that, but it's no way to provide good patient care.

Rotkovitch: Hospitals could just look for an extra pair of hands, as they did after World War II, when a lot of aides were brought in.

Curran: Hospitals will try to save money by hiring nurses from foreign countries. They're already recruiting in Canada, Ireland, the Philippines, and England — and I'm sure overseas recruiting will continue. But I worry about hiring foreign-trained nurses. They've been educated in a different culture, and that could produce real liability problems. There's no doubt in my mind that hospitals need nurses trained in the United States.

Will nurses even want to work in hospitals?

Not if they can help it! The panelists predict that hospitals may soon start to pay a price for their failure to get their act together insofar as nurses are concerned. By the year 2000, fewer and fewer nurses will be providing inpatient care in hospitals, while more and more will work in outpatient settings and other alternative delivery systems. Indeed, Marie Infante estimates that no more than four or five nurses out of 10 will be employed in hospitals by the end of the century. Fully six nurses out of 10 work in hospitals today.

Other comments:

Rotkovitch: Many nurses will be able to find 9-to-5 jobs in HMOs and corporations. That helps explain why so many of them will opt for employment outside the hospital.

Infante: There'll also be new opportunities for nurses in nursing homes and extended-care facilities. This country's long-term care system is going to be federalized, so someone will have to manage the payment system in each facility — a case manager type of job. That's a role that can be — and should be — filled by nurses.

Thomas: There's no doubt that more nurses than ever will hold down managerial jobs in nursing homes. They'll continue to go into home health care, too. Insurance companies will hire a lot of nurses, and so will law firms, which can use nurses to review charts involved in malpractice suits. All in all, nurses will be getting out of the hospital unless hospitals start treating them better.

Curran: Nurses won't hesitate to shun hospital jobs because, so often, hospitals are not pleasant places to work.

What should hospitals do to attract nurses?

Nurses want better treatment — bigger paychecks, greater autonomy, and more respect. By zeroing in on what nurses really want, hospitals can improve retention as well as recruitment.

The panelists offer these specific suggestions:

Infante: Pay big bucks.

Rotkovitch: Provide refresher courses for nurses who are currently out of the job market.

Mueller: Money and education are important, but the intangibles may be even more important. If nurses don't get the respect they deserve, hospitals can pay them $40,000 a year and they still won't stay. Right now there are a million RNs who aren't working as nurses. Autonomy and respect would help bring them back. At Johns Hopkins there is a program that allows nurses to set their own hours and fill in their own schedules. That's the kind of thing nurses want.

Curran: If hospitals gave nurses money, plus autonomy, prestige, and self-determination, that would go a long way toward overcoming the nursing shortage.

Infante: We have to match nursing training with people who don't have jobs. What about reaching out to unemployed workers in areas where plants have closed? There may be billions of government dollars available for retraining such people, and some of them — even steel workers! — might well be potentially fine nurses.

What changes will nurses see in hospital jobs?

Nurses may become an endangered species as far as hospitals are concerned. Patients will need more complicated care — the type of care that only RNs can give. With fewer and fewer nurses to go around, hospitals will have to make better use of their energies. Primary nursing may disappear, Carolyn Robertson says, because nurses won't have enough time to spend at the bedside. Instead, many more RNs will be employed as case managers — assessing problems and directing care. That means the return of team nursing with, the panelists hope, the kinks untangled.

Rotkovitch: The first time we tried team nursing, the RN was a team leader who did nothing but give out medications; the actual bedside care was in the hands of people who weren't competent to make judgments. I don't know how many patients died, but I can assure you that a lot of them did.

Robertson: If we expect team nursing to make a comeback, we'll need better nurses as team leaders. Part of the failure in the past was due to the lack of educational and administrative support for team leaders. If hospitals are smart, they won't let that happen again.

Rotkovitch: By the year 2000, we'll see teams made up of a professional nurse and associate nurses, many of them upgraded LPNs.

Only one level of nursing by 2000? Or two levels?

The debate over one level of nursing practice versus two levels has gone on for so long that many nurses have given up hope of seeing it resolved in their lifetimes. Still, Rachel Rotkovitch believes that two levels of nursing may become a reality by the end of the century. Other panelists feel that prognosis is not very realistic.

Mueller: In at least 40 states, there are moves underway to make the BSN the basic requirements for entry into nursing practice. If those states act affirmatively, we will have two categories of nurses — professional nurses with BSN degrees and associate nurses with AD degrees — but I don't see that happening as early as the year 2000.

Rotkovitch: On the contrary, LPNs will be grandfathered into the associate role in the majority of states by the year 2000, and diploma and AD grads will be grandfathered into professional roles. From that point on, the BSN will become the basic requirement for professional nursing, just as a college degree is for every other profession.

Curran: I don't think many hospitals will prepare themselves for two levels of nursing or even go along with it. Hospitals don't believe there's a difference between BSN and AD nurses, and as a result, they're definitely not going to encour age two levels. That's why I really can't predict when we'll have two levels of practice.

Thomas: The way things are going now, we won't see two levels of nursing before the year 3000.

What changes are in the offing for nursing schools?

Survival will be hard for many nursing schools unless they try harder to attract students. Otherwise, capable students who would have gone into nursing in an earlier era will go into other professions. Career choices for women are wider now than they used to be, and they will inevitably continue to widen. To compete for students, nursing schools have got to market themselves, just as businesses do. If they do it right, Ms. Rotkovitch avers, "we will have a new influx of students into the schools of nursing."

Other comments:

Mueller: We can expect to see more advertising and promotion by nursing schools. These schools, moreover, need to get high school guidance counselors on their side. Right now, counselors are not encouraging students to go to nursing school.

Infante: Advertising alone is not enough. Nursing schools need to foster the kind of atmosphere you find in other professional schools. They tell their students: "You'll be decision makers." Nursing schools don't send that message.

Curran: Quite the opposite, in fact. Nurses are not taught to view themselves as decision-making professionals. In fact, a study shows that the one characteristic a person must have to remain in nursing is the willingness to accept authority.

Robertson: That is really too bad. By the year 2000, I hope nursing schools will teach nurses how to take risks and how to do strategic planning. Right now, nurses are rewarded for being passive rather than for being assertive. Nurses must begin to learn how to be more autonomous. In the future, after all, many of them will be working in independent settings.

Will nurses and physicians wage turf wars?

One traditional view of the future is that doctors and nurses will "stand shoulder to shoulder." But several panelists disagree. They predict that strains between doctors and nurses will worsen, exacerbated on at least in part by a growing glut of physicians.

Curran: I don't think nurses and doctors will stand shoulder to shoulder. Instead of welcoming autonomy for nurses, doctors could view nurses as competitors. I think we're in for a tough time for at least the next 10 years.

Thomas: It looks that way to me, too. The more the glut of physicians grows, the less autonomy nurses will enjoy. In our ER right now, nurses have to fight if they want to start IVs.

Robertson: When I started out in private practice, doctors looked upon me as an "extra gem" and were glad to refer patients to me. But when I started getting referrals from patients, a number of physicians got angry and began hinting that I was practicing medicine without a license. The truth is, doctors really don't want a more equal relationship with nurses.

Rotkovitch: Whatever happens, I'd like to think that by the year 2000, nurses will get what they're looking for — to be able to decide for themselves what nursing practice is, and to have the freedom to implement nursing judgments at the bedside, not subservient to but in collaboration with other members of the health-care team.

How will nurses get the clout they need?

Clout comes from unity, and nurses need a stronger and more responsive nursing leadership. Right now, nurses are splintered into diverse specialty groups, with only about 15% of them belonging to the ANA. One way of bringing nurses together would be to form an umbrella organization for specialty groups.

Rotkovitch: We need to get the specialty groups together so that they can speak with one voice for all nurses. This is a force we haven't mobilized.

Infante: Another approach, perhaps, would be specialty groups to have greater participation within the structure of the ANA.

Mueller: Nurses can also get stronger by working to improve their public image, particularly in the media. Let's put an end to those airhead blondes in the afternoon soap operas — the ones who have nothing to do but give a doctor his messages.

Robertson: We need unity. We can only achieve it by working together.

American Medical Association's proposal on introduction of registered care technologists (RCTs)

AT ITS FEBRUARY 1988 meeting, the American Medical Association (AMA) Board of Trustees approved a proposal to develop a nonnurse, bedside care technician, to be called a registered care technologist. The goal of the proposed registered care technologists (RCT) program is to contribute an innovative solution to the shortage of bedside personnel that will be timely, cost-effective, and efficient. The purpose of the plan is to provide a dependable supply of technically oriented bedside caregivers that will improve access of patients to needed medical care in hospitals. It is also the intention of the proposal to: 1) provide support services for nurses at the bedside and a recruitment pool for higher education in the health professions, 2) coordinate the fragmented education of certain hospital-based technicians, and 3) organize and implement accredited hospital-based apprenticeship programs and hospital-based inservice programs to teach technical skills to RCTs.

Background
At the interim meeting 1987, Report CC, "Nursing Education and the Supply of Nursing Personnel in the United States," was adopted by the House of Delegates. The recommendations supported the efforts of nursing to facilitate the recruitment, retention, and education of nurses to provide care at the bedside. In response to the growing shortage of bedside caregivers, the report also recommended support for hospital based programs to promote the education of nonnurse caregivers for acute and long term facilities. The report recommended that the AMA cooperate with other organizations to develop and accredit programs to increase the availability of caregivers at the bedside in order to meet the medical needs of the public.

Initiatives of organized nursing to solve the shortage of nurses at the bedside
Organized nursing has promoted several initiatives to solve the problems of bedside nursing shortage. These include the solicitation of funds from Congress to support higher education of nurses. Funds have been acquired for demonstration projects to differentiate practice between the two levels of entry into practice, the 2-year Associate Degree (ADN) for the "technical" nurse, and the 4-year Bachelor of Science in Nursing degree (BSN) for the "professional" nurse. It is the goal of nursing to promote the technical nurse as the bedside caregiver in long-term care facilities, to replace LPNs, and to place professional nurses in hospitals as case managers and providers of comprehensive care at the bedside. This strategy is consistent with the goals of the nursing profession to upgrade education for nurses. Organized nursing has also convened several conferences on the nursing shortage and has been the major influence in promoting Secretary Bowen's Commission on the Nursing Shortage. The Commission is charged to offer solutions for the registered nurse shortage by the end of 1988. An AMA representative sits on the the Commission.

In response to the shortage of nurses, the nation's hospitals have adopted various measures to maintain access to medical care. Substantial increases in nurses' salaries occurred. Nurse registries have provided bedside care on a temporary basis in places where the need is urgent. On-the-job training of technicians in various hospital units is taking place. Many hospitals engaged recruitment firms to sponsor nurses to come to the United States from the Far East and Europe. The House of Delegates adopted Resolution 121 (I-87) supporting efforts of members of the health-care field to extend H-1 visas of nurses actively practicing clinical nursing. While all these are necessary responses, a new approach is required to provide safe, effective, quality care for the basic and technical needs of patients at the bedside in the immediate and long-term future.

The proposal for a program to prepare registered care technologists (RCTs)

The RCT program is designed to meet the variable needs of patients for bedside care during the current shortage and beyond. The RCTs would work with nursing personnel and assist with bedside care at nonmanagerial levels. These technologists, however, will be oriented to the highly technical environment of modern medicine. The RCT would be part of a medical support system that will be of assistance to nursing in hospitals.

There are several kinds of technicians who already deliver direct patient care in hospitals and provide a safe environment and support for physicians and the health-care team. Surgical technologists, respiratory therapy technicians, and emergency medical technicians, among others, have programs that are accredited by the Committee on Allied Health Education Accreditation (CAHEA). Many technician roles at the bedside are not accredited by CAHEA, such as cardiopulmonary and dialysis technicians. In some hospitals where bed closures impede access to medical care, physicians report the training and supervision of technicians to monitor medical services in critical care and other highly technical units. The RCT program will offer a mechanism to

coordinate and extend the current training of technicians delivering direct patient services and assure consistent standards of education necessary for quality care.

RCTs will form a recruitment pool of experienced, skillful bedside care technologists who may consider advancement in the health field through higher education as part of their future career plans. At the same time, RCT training could provide a potential source of revenue for technologists seeking to defray the costs of higher education in the health disciplines of their choice. The RCT will maintain a special role, oriented to bedside care and assure access to needed medical care in an increasingly technological environment that requires highly personalized services.

Scope of practice of RCTs. The RCTs' scope of practice would be to continuously monitor and implement physicians' orders at the bedside in order to support and promote the welfare of patients in institutions. Three levels of competence would be included in the program: 1) assistant, 2) basic, and 3) advanced levels. The RCT is a resource for nurses but not a direct substitute for nurses in long-term care institutions and in acute care hospitals.

Functions of the three levels of competence of RCTs. The assistant to the RCT would be able to function as a bedside aide equal to assistants now required by the new federal law (PL 100-203 Omnibus reconciliation Act, 1987) for long-term care facilities. The basic RCT would subsidize work now performed at the level of licensed practical nurses. Licensure as an RCT would be available to LPNs who desire to monitor and implement bedside medical care, administer routine, nonintravenous medications with supervision. Advanced RCTs would require an additional 9 months of experience in several hospital intensive care units. RNs and hospital technicians already experienced in the delivery of direct patient care would be eligible to complete this course, which will be sufficiently rigorous to serve as a practical orientation program for new graduates from schools of nursing.

Structure of educational program for RCTs. Education for registered care technologists would be offered at a post–high school level and provide instruction for three contiguous levels of competence: Assistant, basic, and advanced registered care technologist. An assistant RCT would require 2 months of training; the basic level would be completed after an additional 7 months, after which the RCT would be eligible for licensure. An additional 9 months of highly technical education would provide certification as an advanced RCT. The total program could be completed in 18 months. The program is stringent but flexible and can be accessed at any level at the discretion of the student, or the RCT could be recruited for service by the hospital on completion of any stage of preparation.

Accountability. The registered care technologist would require licensure to assure minimal standards of practice and protect the public good. To avoid a multiplicity of licensure boards, the RCT would be licensed under an arm of the state medical boards. To assure quality of education, accreditation through a national body such as the Committee on Allied Health Education Accreditation (CAHEA) would be essential. Liability insurance would be under the auspices of the hospital employer, which would also be responsible for assigning technicians and relevant resources to the appropriate departments. The RCT would be accountable for physician orders for patient care in accordance with the scope of practice and would report to the head of the unit where they are assigned.

Recruitment. The program would be marketed to high school students, with emphasis on low income groups. The program may also attract male and female students who are uncertain about their choice of health-care careers. LPNs and many kinds of technicians with experience in the delivery of direct patient care may also be recruited for advanced training as RCTs. The program would be offered in hospitals in cooperation with local vocational schools or community colleges. Apprenticeship programs ordinarily pay partial salaries during the period of education. Current costs of hospital in-service education might be appropriately applied against salaries.

Coming to terms with the nursing shortage: Asserting the role and initiatives of academic health centers

DONALD G. KASSEBAUM, MD

MANY TEACHING HOSPITALS are suffering from the shortage of nurses that pervades the country. The unavailability of critical care nurses frequently causes emergency rooms to divert ambulance traffic, confusing the emergency care system and cutting down on the case material available for teaching. Clinical clerkships and electives, already victims of shorter patient stays, distorted case mixes, and greater patient acuity, are further compromised, because the number of admissions is limited more by the availability of nurses than by bed capacity.

Almost as appalling as the nursing shortage itself are the disagreement and empiricism marking the national dialogue about its causes and correction. The solution is beyond the power of any single agent. It will require the integrated commitments and resources of nursing educators, nursing service administrators, hospital directors, physicians, and the medical education establishment. The stewards of patient care and clinical education in academic health centers — the deans of medicine and nursing, hospital directors, and health center vice-presidents — have the opportunity, if not the obligation, to make the common cause and show how the problem can be rectified.

In theory, if not always in practice, academic health centers are adapted to integrate education, practice, and the organization or care into effective and durable models of professional partnership. The insights obtained in these more coherent and controlled settings can be synthesized and reflected for external application. The technically complex settings of the academic medical center have proved the mettle of nurses as partners in critical care and in numerous nurse specialist and practitioner roles that carry significant independent authority. Nurses have assumed increasing responsibility for the testing and introduction of new procedures of care and for quality assurance across a broad scale. Nurses' capacity to make clinical judgments and to combine patient assessment and education with care-giving has confirmed the superiority of primary nursing over task-oriented models. Hospitals that have adopted career-development ladders for nurses, with graduated responsibilities and pay for higher levels of achievement of skills, have tended to experience less staff attrition. When graduating nursing students are asked where they intend to work after licensure, they commonly identify hospitals where they have had satisfying clinical experiences during the third and fourth years of nursing school.

One would think it possible to cull some tactical approaches to the nursing shortage from these fairly well-known facts and observations: (1) Partnership between nurses and physicians has been proof-tested and should be accepted as normative. Argument about "medical" versus "nursing" models ought to be unnecessary when trust is the common coinage and the partners adopt appropriate ways to be supportive and reinforcing to their patients and to each other. (2) When a hospital involves nurses in matters of policy and assessment and encourages nurses to advance their professional careers and incomes over time, retention will be enhanced. (3) One of the best recruiting strategies to gain new nursing graduates is to nurture career choices in their formative years.

The world, or course, is neither this rosy nor this simple. But this does not negate the fact that these are highly important factors affecting the supply of nurses in hospitals. If we cannot come to terms with the fundamentals, working on other angles or inventing new species of nurses is likely to achieve only halfway remedies.

The output of nurses is increasing. The shortage arises because of attrition and because the graduate models of various educational programs do not align with patient-care needs. Nursing schools in academic health centers have differentiated increasingly into programs conferring master's degrees and doctorates for administrators, educators, and scientists. The baccalaureate-degree graduate tends to be of generic brand, albeit better prepared behaviorally and scientifically for a greater role in patient assessment and education. However, technical specialists are needed desperately in emergency rooms and critical care units; and existing shortage of nurses in major hospitals is exacerbated when few critical care nurses can be hired ready-made and most have to be impressed and trained from the general-duty ranks.

The academic health center is united around a set of common academic purposes and values. There is no comparable common ground or better chance to test the partnership of interests that will resolve the nursing shortage. We need to foster medical students' and nursing students' learning together in interdisciplinary settings if we are to overcome disabling prejudices and sensitivities. Hospital nursing administrators and deans of nursing must work together, the former welcoming nursing faculty practitioners and students, and the latter differentiating educational program lines more congruent with hospital needs.

Nursing schools would do well to diversify their clinical products, as medical schools have done, if their stewardship of nursing is to remain unchallenged. Nursing internships might also be employed on a broader scale to facilitate the transition to hospital practice. No less importantly, medical school deans consciously and publicly supportive of nursing roles and innovations if the tension between the two professions is to be overcome.

Assuring a supply of competent nurses at the bedside will take more than greater medicine-nursing collegiality, better coordination between nursing education and service, and improved involvement, career opportunities, and compensation for nurses. It also will require a considerable investment by hospitals to capitalize alternative personnel and automated systems to relieve nurses of the administrative duties that consume more than half their time. Nurses must be liberated from constructing staffing plans, ordering laboratory tests and taking reports, scheduling procedures, performing housekeeping and dietary service, giving physical therapy, performing phlebotomies and starting IVs, and handling the mass of paper work required by quality assurance programs.

Some academic health centers have established effective and durable nursing models, and these should be given greater national prominence. Others ought to test the transferability of these models to their own environments or invent and publicize workable alternatives. The common ground between medicine, nursing, and the teaching hospital in academic health centers affords an ideal opportunity to integrate the thoughts and efforts of the stakeholders. Now is the time to put these ingredients to work and rectify a national dilemma.

Beyond Florence Nightingale: The general professional education of the nurse

LOIS A. POUNDS, MD

I VIVIDLY RECALL, when I was a collegiate nursing student in the 1950s, an influential faculty member's spending an hour presenting the arguments for nursing to be regarded as a profession, not a trade. Seven years later I asked the dean for admissions at a medical school whether I would be considered as a candidate. His response was that medical schools did not take trade school graduates. When I entered medical school, I found that medical education in the 1960s was much like nursing education in the 1950s, a combination of classroom and laboratory science with apprenticeship education on the wards. By the time I was in medical school, nursing education had made what I consider to have been a disastrous decision to distance itself from this form and to shift its emphasis from the natural sciences to the social sciences. Since that time I have had many occasions to reflect on the never-ending murmurs of distress from my friends in nursing and the insensitivity of my colleagues in medicine.

History of nursing education

In the nineteenth century, Florence Nightingale lifted nursing from its scullery maid status to that of a service by gentlewomen. This was accomplished by a new training program that had a brief classroom component and a long period of apprenticeship. The model of nursing training promoted by Miss Nightingale spread rapidly and by the early twentieth century was the standard form of nursing education in this country. What had started as an elite program for a select few became a way off the farm and out of the factory or household service for generations of young women. Until the late 1920s, hospitals were largely staffed by the student nurses and the faculty members of their nursing schools. Graduates became private duty nurses in the homes of the middle and upper class and for well-off patients who had to be hospitalized. Nursing care was the largest part of what physicians could offer for most illnesses, and nurses were placed in their positions by physicians or hospital registries, establishing firmly who controlled whom. This state of affairs began to change with the advent of new drugs and surgical techniques in the 1930s as it became an advantage to hospitalize patients, and the depression ended the luxury of private nursing homes for most illnesses. World War II created a heavy demand for nurses in the military services and, in an interesting parallel to Florence Nightingale's Crimean War experience, changed nursing dramatically. Nurses went to war as officers, commanding staffs of corpsmen, doing procedures previously reserved for doctors, being strong members of the team and often running it. These nurses returned with a new view of what nursing was and could be.

From late in the nineteenth century to the present day, the leadership of nursing has been concerned more with the status of nursing and with establishing an educational elite than with the potential for developing a broadly based service career. During the 1940s, a series of maneuvers to move the education of nurses from the hospital schools to the college, that is, to the professional level, was begun. It was successful, but the process took 30 years, which may have led the leadership to wonder whether they were leading a wave or pushing a rock. In fact, the greatest resistance to this movement came from within nursing itself, although physicians were also opponents. The final straw that led to the demise of hospital schools was the cost of running educational programs, which eventually became too much for hospitals. The leaders in nursing early in this century did not want the proliferation of "trained nurses" but labored and argued for an elite cadre of hospital schools and graduates. After World War II, with a commitment to have nurses educated in colleges, leaders wanted these graduates called "professional" nurses, and hospital-trained nurses called "technical" or "hospital" nurses. In the drive to achieve professionalism the intention was never to upgrade all nurses but rather develop a layer of professionals on top of the existing nurses. It is small wonder that the rank and file were so resistant to the vocal nursing leadership. Today, the obsession with professional status continues. The latest initiative is to have nurses with master's degrees at all head-nurse and supervisory levels. This comes in the face of declining interest in entering the field of nursing and an apparent shortage of nurses to staff our enormous health care system.

Status of nurses

Nursing education leaders blame the lack of interest in nursing on low status and low pay and contend that physicians are responsible for the former and hospitals for the latter. I suggest that the heart of the problem lies in nursing itself. It must be granted that the practice of nursing in hospitals, beside nursing, is a dead-end career. In the drive to achieve professional status, nurses have made the decision to attract bright young people to competitive colleges and give them a baccalaureate degree. Then the graduates accept positions that require around-the-clock staffing. After five years of this work, the nurses would like to have the reward of steady hours, less weekend work time, and a rising pay scale, but to do this they are forced to leave the bedside. Nursing services are very reluctant to have a bedside nurse work 9-5, five days a week, let alone to have a beside nurse make as much money as their supervisors. The nursing solution is that nurses must get more education and advance into positions away from the bedside. I have observed that in every hospital, older nurses are found in the clinics, the employee health service, and material management, or in the ranks of nursing service administration. They are working, but not at nursing.

The best and the brightest leave nursing altogether. Some conform to nursing educators' dicta and earn master's degrees and doctorates, and only a fraction of these ever give nursing care to a sick patient again. The skills of nursing at the bedside are not learned except at the bedside, but nursing education has shunned apprenticeship education as task-oriented and not professional. What attracts young people to nursing is caring for the sick and being involved in the excitement of modern health care. Nursing means taking care of the sick at the bedside, making careful scientific observations, performing technical procedures of evaluation or treatment, and making judgments of the moment-to-moment changes in a patient's condition. It is also comforting, teaching and maintaining therapeutic interpersonal relationships with patients and their families. It is demanding, interesting, satisfying, and fun.

Proposal

Nursing education should parallel medical education. If there is a reason for medicine to have a scientific basis on which to build the art of medicine, there is a reason for nurses to be prepared in the sciences as well. I believe that to provide upward mobility the educational structure could provide a basic framework that could be built upon throughout a nursing career and allow career shifts within the health care system. The entering college freshman should take required and elective preprofessional course work, including modern biology, general and organic chemistry, psychology, and sociology. The junior student majoring in nursing should enter nursing school, and the curriculum should have a rigorous basic science component including biochemistry, physiology, anatomy, pharmacology, pathophysiology, and microbiology. Clinical courses and nursing skills would complete the major. The baccalaureate degree would then be followed by a one-year paid rotating internship in a hospital, where skills would be honed under [the] supervision of the nursing faculty and hospital staff. At the conclusion of the internship, the nurse would sit for a board examination, prepared to move to any position as a staff nurse. This model of nursing education would surely be limited and could never supply the needs of modern hospitals for nurses. This nurse could be a staff nurse, moving from bedside care and supervision of her assistants to charge nurse status or to nursing supervisor, based on her talents and skills.

If after this the nurse still wanted to expand her education and remain in direct patient care, she should have that choice: the nursing schools should offer nurse practitioner and clinical nurse specialist education at the master's degree level. This educational step should also be available through experience and continuing education. Once a nurse decided to get a master's or doctorate in psychology or sociology or physiology or biochemistry, she would become a psychologist or sociologist or a biochemist. She would no longer be a nurse. The nurses who chose to leave nursing to get M.B.A. or Ph.D. or M.D. degrees would be able to build on their strong preprofessional baccalaureate education to become hospital administrators, faculty members in schools of nursing or liberal arts programs or physicians.

These well-educated former nurses would be able to fill the ranks of the nursing schools with faculty members who would have a strong base in either the social or the natural sciences and who could establish themselves as academic investigators and teachers. This would be a strong incentive to colleges to offer baccalaureate programs in nursing, since current nursing school faculties are seldom able to attract the research dollars to support themselves and their academic programs.

Such an educational progression with the possibilities outlined would make nursing a very attractive career choice. Nurses today should have the opportunity to further their careers through experience or continuing education rather than being required to leave work to return to colleges or universities, which unfortunately has been the method of reform promulgated by the nursing leadership in the past.

The void in nursing care left by the reduction in the number of highly qualified nurses should be filled by an army of assistants to the nurse. Nursing assistants should be staffing the wards and clinics and even high-tech areas to relieve nurses of those responsibilities that are the residual of nursing practices at the same time of Miss Nightingale. Nursing educators should welcome the opportunity to provide leadership in planning for tiered levels of nursing care that would put the nurse at the top, responsible for a professional level of supervision and management. Instead, we in teaching hospitals find nurses all too eager to eliminate the nurse's aide and the licensed practical nurse as unprofessional and incapable. These nursing assistants should be educated by nurses in technical schools and community colleges with lower academic requirements and more apprenticeship training. The assistants should be able, with earning power and experience, to consider moving up to the college level and becoming nurses. In its collegiate mode, nursing has been inaccessible to disadvantaged and minority young people, who cannot afford the cost. If nursing would provide this entry to the health care industry with the dignity and the upward mobility it deserves, there should be an enthusiastic response. Nursing has never contained broad representation of our society, and there is no reason why it should not.

It is clear that the teaching hospital will face a patient care problem, to say nothing of a fiscal problem, if graduate medical education becomes less of an apprenticeship in style through reduction in working hours. Capable and well-educated nurses, nurse practitioners, and clinical nurse specialists can easily do much that residents do in day-to-day care of hospitalized patients. Clinical nurse specialists are already functioning in this manner in many intensive care nurseries. Both medicine and nursing need to be collegial in caring for patients, not drawing sharp lines over which the other may not step.

It is time for the parties involved in this crisis — nurses, physicians, and hospitals — to share in its resolution. Nursing education must take the responsibility to build an educational program that allows easy access to advancement. Nursing services managers and physicians must admit that Florence Nightingale is long dead and that the dedicated, fevered-brow–cooling, back-rubbing, capped, cloaked young woman of quality who does everything from cleaning to complex therapeutic and monitoring procedures did not survive the Second World War. Hospitals must accept that their work force is largely female and thus requires appropriate management, including flexible work hours, day care programs, and recognition of experience and quality of work with appropriate financial rewards. Physicians must work to establish a professional alliance with their nursing colleagues to meet the goal of both: quality patient care.

Nursing education and practice

CAROL A. LINDEMAN, RN, PhD

Q: What does everyone and yet no one know?
A: The definition of nurse/nursing!

Q: What profession has doubled its graduates in the last 20 years and yet can't keep up with demand?
A: Nursing.

Q: What profession or occupation has the smallest salary range, that is, potential for growth in salary?
A: "Bedside" nursing: direct patient care.

These simplistic questions and answers provide a glimpse of the quandaries surrounding the education of nurses and their practice. The many types of nursing education programs and the diversity of settings in which nurses practice add to the complexity of issues related to the supply and demand of nursing personnel.

In this essay, I discuss three issues that directly influence nurse-physician relationships and the supply of registered nurses — the nature of nursing practice, the education of registered nurses, and the American Medical Association (AMA) proposal for registered care technologists.

The nature of nursing

In the United States, nursing has been recognized as a full profession since the 1940s, when the federal government agreed to confer officer status on nurses entering military service. Nursing, then, like other professions, exists to serve the interests of the society of which it is a part. The relationship between a society and its professions has been expressed as follows:

A profession acquires recognition, relevance, and even meaning in terms of its relationship to that society, its culture and institutions, and its other members. Professions acquire recognition and relevance primarily in terms of needs, conditions, and traditions of particular societies and their members. It is societies (and often vested interests within them) that determine, in accord with their different technological and economic levels of development and their socioeconomic, political and cultural conditions and values, what professional skills and knowledges they most need and desire. By various financial means, institutions will then emerge to train interested individuals to supply those needs.

There is a social contract between society and the professions. Under its terms, society grants the professions authority over functions vital to itself and permits them considerable autonomy in the conduct of their own affairs. In return, the professions are expected to act responsibly, always mindful of the public trust. Self-regulation to assure quality in performance is at the heart of this relationship. It is the authentic hallmark of a mature profession.[1]

Because nurses view themselves as full professionals, they define their practice in terms of societal needs, that is, the needs of their patients. To the extent that expectations of medicine and health care administrations are consistent with the patient's or societal needs, nurses will fulfill them. When the nurse senses conflict or differences in priorities, the nurse's primary duty is to the patient. Obviously, this duty can create disagreement among nurses, physicians, and health care administrators.

It is also obvious that conflicting opinions about nursing practice existed before the current nursing shortage. For example, in 1970 Taylor[2] described conflicts between administration, medicine, and nursing regarding care of patients. One such conflict concerned admitting persons on the basis of their ability to pay, which Taylor described in this scenario.

> The administrator is responsible among other things, for keeping the hospital out of debt. He is delighted when patients can pay their hospital bills, and he is tempted to order "red carpet" treatment those patients who might donate money to the hospital in addition to paying their bills.
>
> The physician has inherited the tradition of allowing the "rich" patient to contribute to the care of the "poor" patient. Special consideration for the patients who are in a position to make substantial donations to the hospital, or for medical research, does not seem unreasonable to the physician.
>
> The nurse's reactions to the patient's pay category are more complicated than the reactions of the administrator or the physician. Like the administrator and the physician, the nurse believes that any sick person who needs care should receive care whether or not he can afford to pay for it. In addition, the nurse tends to resent the notion of "red carpet" treatment as a suggestion that she would give superior care to a patient merely because he could afford to pay for it.

Taylor then described how nurses ignore the priorities of the administrator and physician and create their own priorities based on nursing care needs.

Mingled with this view of the nurse's accountability is the issue of the nature of nursing practice. Many health professionals and members of the lay public see health professionals as existing in a hierarchy. They think of the tasks that are performed and arrange them in some order of complexity: the least complex tasks can be safely done by an unlicensed professional, while the more complex tasks require differing amounts of education and different types of certification.

Most nurses disagree with this hierarchical view of health professionals and with the substitution concept of practice. In general, could a physician replace a nurse on any nursing unit in an acute care hospital, make a home visit, or provide care and supervision in a nursing home? The nurses and health care administrations that I have talked to say "No!" Doctors and nurses provide different services — they are not substitutes for each other but offer services that are complementary. There is some overlap but there are significant differences.

Dr. Mitchell Rabkin, president of Boston's Beth Israel Hospital, in an essay regarding modern nursing practice,[3] described the differences in the origins of nursing and medicine and then stated:

> The public is little aware of that growing and sophisticated knowledge base, for example, which the Beth Israel primary nurse can bring to bear, or of the nurse's capacity to integrate the many specialized inputs — medical and otherwise — into a coherent whole. Combined with the insights the nurse develops into the patient while providing the hands-on nurturing, her or his knowledgeability leads to sophisticated evaluation and management of the patient's psychology and psyche. That new integrating role of the nurse, more so than mere handling of the sophisticated technology of modern medicine, has become of critical importance for care of the highest caliber. The nurse is fully accountable for these professional responsibilities, and the nursing role is thus vital to the hospital, patient and physician.

There will be little agreement between physicians and nurses on any question about the supply of nurses if there is disagreement regarding the most basic issue of all, the nature of nursing practice and its relationship to medical practice. Nurses are committed to the fullest development of nursing as an independent profession. The creation of the National Center for Nursing Research within the National Institutes of Health is evidence of the status of the profession. We in nursing hope that our physician colleagues will support the continued development of the profession of nursing. We hope they will share our vision of quality health care provided by physicians and nurses working as colleagues.

Nursing education

Although nursing personnel include three occupational groups — registered nurses, licensed practical nurses, and nursing aides — to me the title nurse refers to those individuals who have successfully completed the examination for licensure as registered nurses.

One may become eligible for the licensure examination for registered nurse through three educational routes: the hospital school of nursing, the community college, and the four-year college or university. At one point in time these programs differed in length and curriculum, but over the years all the programs have become more similar than dissimilar, probably because all graduates take the same licensure examination. Evidence of this in Oregon comes from comparing "true" requirements for admission to and graduation from associate degree and baccalaureate nursing programs. An associate degree nursing program just a few miles from our university nursing program requires 176 quarter credits for graduation. Our baccalaureate nursing program requires 186 quarter credits. This situation is true in many states. If there are differences in programs, they are likely to be in the areas of public-community health nursing, manage-

ment-leadership skills, and research. Students in baccalaureate programs are likely to have learning experiences in these areas, while other students are not.

In one sense, the differences in the three educational routes to the licensure examination for registered nurses are the differences in the philosophies and objectives of the parent institutions. Hospitals exist to provide services to the sick; they are not by definition educational institutions. An educational program funded by a hospital is, in keeping with its mission, designed to produce well-qualified people to serve in it, and most of the clinical experiences provided are in that particular hospital. Community college programs define themselves in terms of vocational or technical education, producing skilled people ready for technology roles in the work force. At the baccalaureate level, four-year colleges and universities are committed to a basic education in the liberal arts, to an attitude of inquiry and life-long learning, and to a beginning level of proficiency in a chosen field. Increasingly, nursing leaders in clinical settings emphasize that baccalaureate preparation is the desirable preparation for "bedside" nursing. This statement reflects the expected evolution of a nurse's practice over time, not merely entry-level performance. The professional nurse's background in the arts and sciences is associated with the ability of the practitioner to fulfill nursing's full contract with society.

According to the National League for Nursing, in 1986 there were 1,471 nursing education programs preparing students for registered nurse licensure. Of these, 16% (238) were diploma programs; 53% (774) were associate degree programs; and 31% (459) were baccalaureate programs. Although enrollments in schools of nursing have declined since 1984-85, the size of the nursing work force will increase, because the number of nurses added to the work force is greater than the number leaving the work force. This should be the case for the rest of the country.

Organized nursing continues to clarify the job expectations of graduates from baccalaureate and associate degree programs. This work, funded by the Kellogg Foundation, is being conducted as part of the National Commission on Nursing Implementation project.

I would like to see associate degree programs target their objectives to a particular setting and to preparing an excellent technologist. For example, one associate degree program might focus on preparing its graduates for jobs in home health care, another for jobs in long-term care, and another for jobs in acute care. Job expectations differ across settings and, in my opinion, a two-year program is stretched to cover more than one setting. Furthermore, technology is a major aspect of health care and nursing practice. The philosophy of the community college makes it an ideal setting for developing nursing personnel skilled in applying technology to patient care.

My observations suggest that the marketplace and student demand will continue to shape nursing education. I doubt that edicts from nurse educators will bring reason and rationality to nursing education — job opportunities and salaries commensurate with educational preparation and competence will.

Registered care technologist

Probably nothing in the history of medicine and nursing has so divided the two professions as has the AMA proposal for a new category of health care worker called the registered care technologist (RCT). Nursing has found the proposal itself divisive and the process for developing it inflammatory.

It is difficult to critique the proposal for the registered care technologist, as it continues to change. Will RCTs be licensed health care workers? If so, under which applicable practice act and licensure authority will they function? At the time the AMA reported to the

Secretary's Commission on Nursing, the issue of licensure had not been resolved by the AMA.

How can a person with a maximum of 18 months of training safely carry out physicians' medical orders in an acute care hospital? Ordinarily, a nurse exercises extensive judgment in implementing medical orders, beginning by evaluating treatment in terms of the fluctuating status of the individual patient. As most practicing physicians know, sound nursing judgment and input are necessary for an effective, efficient plan of medical care.

Patients are concerned about the dehumanizing aspects of health care. They often express the feeling of being known not by their names or persons, but by their diseases and room numbers, and they are concerned about the fragmentation of care and the feeling that there is no *one* person to turn to for understanding and reassurance about the total plan of care. In response to these concerns, the nursing profession developed an approach for delivering care known as primary nursing. On admission, patients are assigned a primary nurse who assumes responsibility and accountability for the patient's care through discharge. In the most successful primary nursing settings, the nurse and the physician share the authority for care.

In light of the advances made in decreasing the fragmented, dehumanizing aspects of health care, the nursing profession is opposed to the introduction of another health care worker who has a very limited scope of practice and requires extensive supervision. According to proponents of the RCT, there would be, in addition to the nursing aide and licensed practical nurse, three levels of RCTs on a given nursing unit. All five of these workers would have different job descriptions and functions. The creation of five slightly different health care workers is a piecework, assembly-line approach to health care. Research

from the 1960s and 1970s showed how inefficient and ineffective this model of care was
with only three categories of health care workers (RN, LPN, and aide).

Nurses also are skeptical that the RCT programs would attract the number of applicants
the AMA has proposed. The reasons cited for
why minorities would be attracted to the program reflect negative stereotypes, and the program would keep them in dead-end jobs. Nursing rejects this approach to increasing numbers
of minorities in health care.

Suggestions

To many, the problems posed by the current
nursing shortage and the conflicts over the
RCT proposal appear resolvable. In the past
year many columnists have discussed the nursing shortage and the RCT proposal. In general,
they have spoken of the need to provide nurses
the financial and professional recognition their
work deserves. The sentiment is to improve
the working conditions for nurses rather than
to add a new and ill-defined category of
worker.

Most doctors and nurses have their own pet
solutions. Here are some of mine.

1. Retain more nurses in the work force by
improving working conditions. For example,
nurses need to have job security and predictability. In the years just preceding the current
shortage, many nurses did not know from day
to day whether the census would be high
enough to assure them work. They might be
able to work only if they "floated" to an unfamiliar clinical area. Other days they would
find they had to work a double shift because of
an unexpected influx of patients. Every professional can accept some of this job insecurity
and unpredictability, but certainly it should not
need to be tolerated as a routine part of one's
job.

The work environment for nurses also is
characterized by high levels of verbal abuse:
everyone lets off steam by yelling at the nurse.

Certainly, this could be appropriately challenged.

Adequate salaries, recognition in the organization, and authority commensurate with
responsibility are clearly necessary.

The changes needed in the working environment for nurses are so fundamental they
need no discussion. It is time to do what is
clearly right to do. Nurses must be willing to
promote these changes. Physicians and medical boards must lend their support.

2. Increase the productivity of nurses by using technology to reduce the time allocated to
indirect patient care activities. Current estimates are that a staff nurse spends 50-60% of
working time charting or filling out forms. For
the most part, this is done by the nurse's writing on a record, writing on a care plan, or writing information on a form. The same piece of
information is entered by hand on numerous
forms designed for various aspects of (health
care) hospital administration. The technology
of the 1950s is still being used. Consider the
cost savings that could accrue if "nurse-
friendly" information-processing systems were
developed and were available on nursing units.

It is important to remember that some technology — the technology of a neonatal care
unit, for example — will increase requirements for nursing personnel. The technology
that would reduce requirements for nursing
personnel is not often available. I dream of a
voice-activated information processing system
housed in a robot that functions as a nurse assistant. The robot could retrieve necessary supplies but also it would be the entry point for
data that would appear on the clinical record
and the financial record. Each nurse would
have a personal robot as an assistant.

3. Destroy the myths that physicians love to
repeat regarding nursing education and nurses
with graduate preparation. Only this week I
again heard that the elite in nursing were responsible for the nursing shortage by empha-

sizing the baccalaureate degree for entry into the profession. The fact is that the shortage results from an increase in demand and not a decrease in supply. The American Nurses' Association's position on entry-level requirements has not caused the shortage. Another myth is that "nursing" caused the closure of diploma programs and stopped the supply of the only really good nurses. The facts are that hospital economics and societal trends led to the closing of hospital-based nursing programs, and educational institutions became the logical sites for nursing education. Doctors are as unhappy with new medical school graduates as with new nursing school graduates: none of these graduates fits the myth of what the past generation was able to do in relation to the increased knowledge and skill required.

4. Restructure health care organizations so that doctors and nurses serve together with equal voices on committees and boards. Let's re-examine the idea of community-based joint practice committees composed of physicians and nurses. Let's explore the use of these groups to formulate creative short- and long-term solutions to the many health care problems facing our nation. The country needs to see us function as leaders together.

5. Support the efforts of organized nursing to create a rational system of nursing education designed to prepare an adequate number of nurses appropriately to deliver quality health care in our complex health care system.

The current system is duplicative and inefficient, and it needs reform. There is support within nursing for a revised system that includes two types of programs: a technical nurse program and a professional nurse program.

At institutions across the country, short-term solutions to the nursing shortage are already being implemented. Salaries are increasing, nurses are assuming larger leadership and management roles at an institutional level, and recruitment activities are moving forward. Longer-term solutions are being developed by the U.S. Health and Human Services Secretary's Commission on Nursing, other national advisory councils, and national nursing organizations. Implementing these solutions will require a team effort of health professionals and the financiers of health care. The health needs of the public and not the vested interests of any one health profession must be the guiding force for these decisions. Our focus must be on the future, not the past. Nursing, the public, and physicians would benefit from the AMA's support for these solutions.

REFERENCES

1. American Nurses' Association. *Nursing: A Social Policy Statement.* Kansas City, Missouri: American Nurses' Association, 1980, pp. 3, 7.

2. Taylor, C. *In Horizontal Orbit: Hospitals and the Cult of Efficiency.* New York: Holt, Rinehart and Winston, 1970.

3. Rabkin, Mitchell T. The New Professionals. *Wellbeing.* Beth Israel Hospital, Boston. October 1982, p. 2.

CHAPTER TEN

New practice opportunities for nurses

CHANGES IN THE HEALTH CARE SYSTEM as well as in demographics, patterns of illness, health care financing, and technology are creating new practice opportunities for nurses. Some place the nurse into competition with the physician; others unite nurse and physician as comanagers of health care. For nurses with the specialized skills called for in today's health care marketplace, the career possibilities are practically endless.

The first article in this chapter, "Case Managers: Guiding the Elderly Through the Health Care Maze" by Parker and Secord, discusses the role of case manager for elderly patients, a role made necessary by the complex and fragmented nature of our health care system. Comparing and contrasting private case managers with case managers associated with clinical agencies, the authors forecast cautiously for the future but urge nurses to consider the case manager role.

The article by Floyd and Buckle, "Nursing Care of the Elderly: The DRG Influence," discusses the role of the home care nurse in a model of case management associated with an institution. The authors describe this role in respect to the special needs of frail elderly patients, but it is also applicable to other patient groups.

In "Nursing 2020: A Study of Nursing's Future," Sullivan et al. used panels of experts and the Delphi survey technique to forecast new nursing roles (such as the space health scientist) as well as major expansions of existing roles, such as occupational health nurse. The scenario projected for the year 2020 contains significant changes in the roles and functions of nurses.

In the final article, "A Case Study Involving Prospective Payment Legislation, DRGs, and Certified Registered Nurse Anesthetists," Garde discusses the impact of prospective payment systems on certified registered nurse anesthetists. Garde also describes ways health professionals and Congress can interact to create health care policy encouraging expanded roles for nurses, such as nurse anesthetist, nurse midwife, and nurse practitioner.

Case managers: Guiding the elderly through the health care maze

Marcie Parker, ma, mpa; Laura J. Secord

Private geriatric case managers exist for many reasons: to help elderly patients and their families break into and negotiate the complex and fragmented health care system; to serve those not served by public programs either because income or geography renders them ineligible or because they can't cope with the stigma attached to the public welfare system. Another reason is that clients often prefer a long-term relationship with a case manager who will be available to them any time, day or night.

Typically nurses, social workers, or psychotherapists, private geriatric case managers usually "hang out a shingle" because they too want long-term relationships with clients and families. Often public sector "dropouts" tired of spending almost half their time untangling the red tape of public agencies, they enjoy developing and implementing creative, cost-effective plans for their clients. For many, the flexibility and autonomy that go along with independent professional practice are just so much icing on the cake.

Is the movement toward private case management gathering momentum? Who are these managers? What services do they offer? What do they charge? Who pays? Where do they get their referrals? What share of the market do they hold? How do they relate to other case management providers? InterStudy, a private not-for-profit research and policy studies firm based in Excelsior, Minnesota, sought to find out.

Getting the scoop

InterStudy recently completed a one-year national study, funded by the Retirement Re-

search Foundation, of private geriatric case management services. For the study, they defined case management as "a systematic process of assessment, planning, service coordination and/or referral, and monitoring through which the multiple-service needs of clients are met." And they included only *private* providers of case management — those whose services are not usually paid for by Medicare, Medicaid, or other public programs and who bill for case management as a separate service.

InterStudy collected its data through literature review, telephone interviews with case managers and experts on case management, and a national mail survey to which 117 private case management firms responded. They limited their data to the case management of elderly clients paying privately for the separate and distinct service of case management.

Here, in a nutshell, is what they found:

Organization. Most private case-management firms have been in business no longer than four years. Seventy percent of the 117 private case-management firms that responded indicated that they are independent and self-managed.

Of the 117, 65 percent operate for profit; 75 percent of the remaining not-for-profit providers are affiliated with other organizations, predominantly hospitals, social service agencies, and nursing homes.

Staffing. More than 65 percent of the responding firms employ one or two managers who typically handle 1 to 20 cases per month. Less than half (just over 45%) employ administrative or secretarial support staff.

Most managers have postgraduate degrees, usually in either nursing or social work. Very

What else do private managers provide?		
SERVICE	NO. OF FIRMS PROVIDING*	PERCENT
Family/caregiver counseling	80	68.4
Client counseling	78	66.7
Nursing home placement	62	53.0
Housing placement	42	35.9
Psychotherapy	40	34.2
Retirement planning	35	29.9
Support groups	34	29.1
Financial counseling	31	26.5
Companion services	22	18.8
24-hour hotline	21	17.9
Guardian/conservatorship	20	17.1
Homemaker services (cleaning, cooking)	19	16.2
Transportation	19	16.2
Home health aide (personal care)	17	14.5
Respite care	16	13.7
Chore services (lawn care, home repair)	13	11.1
Estate management	12	10.3
Home health care (nursing care)	11	9.4

*Total number of firms responding to survey: 117

few federal or state regulations apply to private case managers. Of course, if theirs is a licensed profession, they must meet their state's requirements for licensure.

Services. The direct services most often provided by private case managers are family and caregiver counseling, client counseling, and nursing home or housing placement. Case managers also may include a range of functional, social, and financial assessments; ongoing patient monitoring and evaluation for community-based care or institutional placement; planning, referral, and coordination of services; help in completing forms; and hiring and monitoring staff from other agencies. Many firms provide direct home care services. Few firms provide transportation, help with chores, or respite care.

Because the managers have relatively small caseloads, they personalize their services, tailoring them for the client's unique problems and needs. This may involve any number of additional services, such as those listed here.

Firms that employ baccalaureate-prepared RNs tend more often to provide the services of a home health aide or companion than do those who employ, for example, managers with MSWs [master's degrees in social work]. Case managers with MSWs, on the other hand, tend to provide psychotherapy and related services.

Referrals. According to 77 percent of the respondents, referrals come primarily from physicians and from other clients. More than 50 percent also listed social workers, relatives and friends of clients, hospital staff, attorneys, and the clients themselves as other sources.

The services the case managers most often referred their clients to include home health aides, homemakers services, home health care, legal services, in-home meals, transportation, adult day care, respite care, companion services, senior centers, and nursing homes.

Fees and payment. Most firms charge an

hourly rate for services (either alone or along with a sliding fee scale) or a set rate per session (usually for an initial assessment or consultation). Firms that employ at least one RN more often reported using a set rate for package or services than did other firms.

Hourly rates range from $13 to $100 per hour. Slightly more than half (51.5)% of the firms charge between $41 and $60, and the bulk of these (53%) charge $50 per hour. The next most frequently reported range was $21 to $40 per hour. Only six respondents, all not-for-profit firms, reported fees of $20 or less per hour; and only seven firms, five of which are for profit, reported fees higher than $60 per hour. Several firms do pro bono work.

Eighty percent of the case management firms affiliated with hospitals charge $41 to $60 per hour. Unaffiliated firms reported hourly fees of $41 to $60 more often than the did any other range.

A third of the firms using sliding fee scales charge a maximum of $45 to $50 per hour; 69 percent charge $50 or less. Thirty respondents use set rates for services beyond those covered by the hourly rate or sliding scale. For example, monitoring might cost $300 a month or perhaps $75 a week; travel expenses might cost $70 an hour or maybe $0.25 a mile.

Eleven respondents offer package rates, typically covering assessment, establishment of a care plan, consultations, referrals, and monitoring. Rates rage from $4.52 to $400, with six firms reporting rates of $100 or more.

Most private case mangers are paid out of pocket by the client or family: almost 45 percent receive more than half of their payments and 44 percent receive all of their payments out of pocket.

Drawbacks. The managers described in some detail the tremendous investment of time their work involves. Not only are they available to their clients around the clock, seven days a week, but they are on their own with the business end of the operation as well. Many of the participants noted that private practice takes personal sacrifice and commitment. Finances and job security are risky at best, and without support from colleagues (as they may have had in more traditional settings), burn-out is always a risk. Having to establish and maintain a strong referral network is yet another stressor. *Rewards.* Most private case managers feel, however, that the rewards of private practice offset the drawbacks. They enjoy the satisfaction of seeing their clients progress and maintaining a long-term relationship. And their fee-for-service payment structure makes it possible for them to provide their clients many more service options than are generally available through public programs.

Case management bandwagon

The future of private cast management may depend considerably on the quality and accessibility of future public programs. If public programs add fee-for-service case management to their service packages, private managers will have to compete with them for clients, just as some now compete among themselves. Of course, the market for customized case management will always exist; it's just likely to grow somewhat less rapidly if public providers get into the act.

With diversification the buzzword at many hospitals, nursing homes, health care agencies, health maintenance organizations (HMOs), as well as insurance companies, private case management is coming under close scrutiny. Some of the managed care systems (HMOs, for example) are already convinced that private case management is the way of the future and are including it in their service packages.

More and more nurses are going into private case management (not to mention social workers and gerontologists). At the third annual meeting of the National Association of Private Geriatric Care Managers, held [in

1987] in Boston, 20 of the 150 attendees were RNs either interested in providing this service or already doing so.

Employers are beginning to recognize the need for case management services for employees caring for elderly family members. Private managers are already establishing contracts for providing employee assistance programs at the corporate level.

Undoubtedly the number of case management providers of all kinds is growing; whether the expansion is really due to unmet service needs is not so clear. Because the elderly are an especially vulnerable population, we need to keep a close watch on whether the services provided them by private managers are truly in their best interests. One clear way for nurses to do this is to provide the essential services themselves.

Nursing care of the elderly: The DRG influence

JEANNE FLOYD, RN,C, MS; JUNE BUCKLE, RN, MSN

WE LIVE IN A TIME of transition. Societal changes, specifically those triggered by fiscal constraints, are influencing the traditional system of healthcare delivery in the United States. Virtually all levels of healthcare providers are being forced to assess the degree of effectiveness and efficiency associated with their function within the system. For example, the traditional models of providing nursing care are being challenged to respond to the present needs of society.

Two specific changes are linked to the current demands on nursing. First, the changing nature of the age structure in the United States has increased the number of patients who are over the age of 65. Many of these patients claim at least one chronic illness.[1] Second, the Medicare prospective payment system (PPS) has decreased the length of inpatient hospitalization days and released patients into the community who often require complex nursing care.

Problem statement and purpose

Nursing is forced to address the following questions:

1. Will traditional models of delivering nursing care to the frail elderly or persons over the age of 75 meet the present and future needs of society?

2. Should nursing models differ in the acute and home care settings?

3. If different nursing models are proposed in each setting, can a bridge be developed between the settings to ensure continuity of patient care?

These questions are posed by nurses at The Johns Hopkins Medical Institutions (JHMI)

who deliver inpatient care to the frail elderly in the Department of Medicine and in the home care program known as the Post-Hospital Support Study. These departments communicate with each other as patients move between the acute care facility and the home setting.

This article focuses on the response of nursing to these demands by:

1. Presenting an overview with potential outcomes of the societal changes associated with the prospective payment system;

2. Discussing the elderly population at JHMI in relationship to special nursing needs;

3. Reviewing the traditional nursing models of delivering care in the JHMI acute and home care practice settings and stating some of the nursing practice problems that have surfaced within these models; and

4. Proposing recommendations for planning changes in the nursing models that will assist nursing to meet present and future demands successfully.

Overview

Blum[2] states that the major reason for planning is to obtain improvements in circumstances. Those who plan must understand the realities of the present. This includes the present and future age structure and the potential outcomes of the PPS.

Under the PPS, the federal government stipulates in advance how much it will pay for the treatment of a given episode of an illness. Basically, the new PPS classifies all patients in one of 470 diagnosis-related groups (DRG), with the exception of a small number of "outlier" patients. The hospital would receive a fixed payment per DRG regardless of treatment and length of stay. Those hospitals incurring lower costs than the fixed payment are allowed to keep the savings. The opposite is also true. Those hospitals spending more than allowed under the DRG would be required to absorb the costs.

The DRG program provides an incentive to manage hospital operations and deliver services to Medicare beneficiaries in a more efficient and cost-effective manner. With the incentive to reduce the length of stay, more emphasis is being placed on outpatient services, preadmission testing, same-day surgery, and care after discharge. Those who criticize the system are concerned that patients formerly treated in outpatient departments may be admitted to inpatient services, and some patients, particularly the frail elderly, may be discharged prematurely.[3]

Potential outcomes

Under the PPS, changes in clinical practice will be necessary as a result of the reduced length of stay. There will be less time to develop and implement discharge plans. More stress will be placed on healthcare providers as patients are discharged with more complicated plans of care.[4] There is growing consensus that elderly discharge planning is a requisite for survival under the PPS. Although most managers support discharge planning from the time of admission,[5,6] some advocate discharge planning before the patient is admitted.[4] Many are concerned about the adverse effects of PPS on patient care. There certainly will not be "as many frills or fringes as in the past."[7]

Although it is believed that this type of incentive program will decrease total healthcare costs, it is feared that the frail elderly population is at risk for compromised quality of care along with difficulty in accessing care. The reason for this fear is that hospitals stand to lose money by caring for those over the age of 70. The new prospective payment plan does not take into account that the average length of hospital stay increases with age, a factor that influences increased cost. In addition, the PPS does not recognize multiple clinical problems or severity of illness. Since the elderly often exhibit serious, multiple medical problems, hospital administrators may view the elderly as undesirable revenue losers. Hospital management could conceivably select against the high-cost elderly patient in favor of short-stay patients.[8]

Nursing administrators recently surveyed in New Jersey have evaluated some of the effects of PPS.[5] The new system has forced a strong commitment on the part of hospital employees to provide effective and efficient patient care. The survey revealed that personnel emphasized the value of patient care planning, patient classification systems, and discharge planning. This would not have been true prior to the implementation of the PPS.

Changes were also noted in the clinical area. There was an increase in the nursing care hours per patient and in the number of aged patients admitted. Patients who could receive care in alternative community-based services were not admitted to the hospital. Those hospitalized patients for whom home health services could be arranged were discharged early. As a result, an increase in referrals to home health agencies was noted. Some patients were deemed by the agencies to be too ill for solely daytime coverage. Such cases are being considered for evening home care coverage.[5]

The elderly population at JHMI

Changes in the age structure of the patients admitted to the Department of Medicine have been noted over the past several years.[9] In 1982, of the 7,504 patients admitted to the Department of Medicine, 30%, or 2,243 patients, were 65 years old or older. These individuals accounted for 35% of the total inpatient hospital days. In 1983 there was an increase in the number of patients 65 or older who were admitted for care; that is, 32% of all patients were over 65. This elderly population accounted for 36% of all patient days. These trends are projected to continue.

According to Metcalf,[9] the nursing staff has identified special care needs in the aged cohort. Many of these individuals, for instance, suffer auditory and visual deficits that result in communication problems. As many as half of those treated are thought to be cognitively impaired. Discharge planning and follow-up care must be reflective of these serious impairments. Patient teaching and discharge planning can be extremely difficult goals to implement with patients who lack the abilities to speak, hear, and process information.

Discharge plans are also affected by patient health decrements such as unsteady gait and decreased mobility. These conditions are often exacerbated by complete bed rest during hospitalization. In such cases, the independent functional ability of the patient must be measured prior to discharge, and physical therapy is instituted for rehabilitation, as indicated.

Malnutrition is also a major health problem. Some of the factors that contribute to compromised nutritional states include the inability of patients to adhere to recommended diets, functional limitations, cognitive deficits, and lack of knowledge about proper nutrition.[9]

Patients and their families may need assistance with planning for home care of health and nutrition problems. Additional care problems include urinary and fecal incontinence. Those with compromised nutritional states may require tube feedings. Patients may become depressed as a result of physical insult and environmental factors. These factors include the loss of independence that occurs with hospitalization, loss of familiar surroundings, and social isolation. Depression can impede immediate recovery and compromise the potential gains that contribute to successful re-

cuperation over time. In summary, Metcalf has proposed that the frail elderly experience physical decrements that require increased nursing contact hours and complex discharge planning.

Nursing practice at JHMI

Primary nursing is the model of delivering comprehensive nursing care within the Department of Medicine. Autonomy, accountability, advocacy, collaboration, coordination, and communication are among the key elements needed to operationalize the concept of primary nursing.[10] The primary nurse is the nursing representative to the patient during his or her contact with the hospital. The primary nurse plans for total patient care form admission to discharge for a select group of patients and their families.

The patient is the central focus for planning, implementing, and evaluating care. Aspects of the individual's physical, emotion, spiritual, and social well-being are considered. The primary nurse assumes 24-hour accountability for the patient care being delivered. He or she collaborates and communicates with other members of the healthcare team about the status of the patient and the plan of care. As the patient's advocate, the nurse addresses problems that the patient or the patient's family are experiencing within the healthcare system.[10]

The primary nurse begins discharge planning at the time of the patient's admission. The care of all patients is reviewed weekly at interdisciplinary rounds, which are attended by nurses, physicians, social workers, a pharmacist, occupational therapists, and physical therapists. A liaison nurse or social worker from home care services, such as the Post-Hospital Support Study, often attends rounds and accepts patients who would benefit from home services.

As a means of preparing registered nurses for the role of primary nurse, a variety of workshops are offered. These educational programs include content on the roles of charge nurse and primary nurse, methods of patient education, and theory on adult learning. Within this framework nurses learn principles of assertiveness and patient advocacy.

The frail elderly home care project known as the Post-Hospital Support Study delivers nursing care through the case management model. According to Bell,[11] this form of community or public health nursing cuts across professional boundaries and is responsible for identifying, securing, and coordinating all the resources necessary for the patient's life in the community. Direct physical care is delivered by the nurse case manager. After an assessment process, the manager is responsible for providing a 24-hour plan that coordinates the activities and services of those involved, which includes the quality of service and the patient response to the plan. The case manager also functions as an advocate, intervening on the patient's behalf when necessary.

Wiles[12] addresses collaboration as an integral part of home care nursing. Without effective collaboration there would be no continuity of care provided and the client's understanding of the home care program would be fragmented. Each client has an individualized care plan even though the client may have problems similar to others in a specific disease category classification. Wiles states that in home care, interdisciplinary services are documented. This requirement allows for accountability of each professional and fosters continuity of care. Wiles explains that in home care, as in other healthcare settings, professionals experience stress associated with changing roles and overlapping boundaries. In collaborating, health providers in the home should carefully analyze one another's roles to determine if overlapping occurs.

In addition to the communication skills required in the collaborative process, the case manager assumes broadly focused responsibilities. Arbeiter[13] states that the community or public health nurse must put a premium on self-reliance, flexibility, knowledge of systems, cooperation, and teaching. The author summarizes, "You have to learn to play the hand you're dealt." To do this, Wiles recommends that the case manager understand:

1. Application of the group process to achieve group goals;
2. Problem-solving process;
3. Role theory;
4. What other professionals do and how they see their roles; and
5. The conceptual differences between home care, practice, and institutional care practices.

In comparing the case manager role and the role of primary nurse, Bell[11] determines that both have accountability and responsibility for a 24-hour plan of care that includes implementation and evaluation. The roles are also similar in that it is easier for the patient to organize requests for assistance around one person, rather than negotiate individual requests with a variety of persons. In contrast with the primary nursing role, Bell states that the case manager role is also concerned with the development of a social network, which is an area of responsibility typically associated with the social worker. A nurse fulfilling this function can enlarge the scope of the 24-hour plan to include interventions that meet nursing and healthcare needs as well.

Nursing practice problems

In the acute care setting, the following problems have surfaced. First, there is an increasing sense of frustration experienced by the nurse in implementing complex care plans for the frail elderly. A significant number of patients in this population bear the potential for serious, multisystem physical problems. The related care plans and patient teaching needs are commensurately complex and labor-intensive. Often, as a result of the reduction in the length of stay, there is not enough time to carry out the plan of care or to meet the individual's teaching and learning needs. Therefore, planning must begin at admission and be continued after discharge. The present system does not allow for a smooth transition of the plan of care for the frail elderly from the hospital to the home.

Second, although gerontology has developed as a major science during the 20th century, knowledge about the care of the elderly is still missing in the academic and healthcare practice settings. Reflective of this deficit, the nurse is not educationally prepared to meet the special care needs of the frail elderly. Knowledge of the aging process and the potential iatrogenic consequences of medical therapies is lacking. No formal continuing education program is offered to or required of the nurse who cares for such a large, chronically ill population. Educational programs with content specific to age-related health changes, communication styles, and teaching-learning skills are essential. Nurses could then design complex plans of care. An important step in filling these educational needs has been taken. Several staff members within the department have developed written standards for delivering care to elderly patients.

In the course of developing the role of the nurse case manager in the home setting, problems in delivery of service to the frail elderly have also been identified. The profile of problems is as follows.

First, the home care nurse is seldom given adequate information by the acute care nurse to ensure that the care plan is immediately modified for the home setting. This lack of coordination makes for duplication of efforts and lost time, and negates the position of advocacy that the acute care nurse assumed on behalf of the patient. The home care nurse often faces a set of home needs that require immediate attention and are overwhelming for a single nurse.

Second, the home care nurse is inexperienced in the practice of community health nursing as previously defined by Bell. No formal continuing education plan has been designed to assist the nurse in gaining the necessary knowledge and skills. Some informal teaching has been conducted by the program director, who is an adult nurse practitioner, and the psychogeriatric nurse consultant, who is a community health specialist. These teaching sessions have occurred when the home care nurse has identified barriers to the delivery of care that are associated with inexperience or lack of knowledge.

Third, the home care nurse is assigned a patient and family to follow in tandem with a social worker, who is educated to assume the responsibilities of case management. The outcome is a shared form of case management with blurred lines of responsibility and accountability. Without guidelines or clear expectations, role ambiguity and role conflict have developed. The indistinct division of roles has been a source of major stress for both members of the care giving dyad.

The literature on planning for health care delivery in the 1980s addresses such problems. Blum[2] states that the problems themselves are sources of never-ending pressure for improvement. An awareness of possibilities for improvement come from several directions. The author explains that pressures for planning come particularly from our never-ending desire to create a better future, the distress created by current problems, and our increasing awareness that we need a new kind of understanding to rationalize our actions. Blum believes that as problems recur they become recognizable and involve more and more persons; problems then take on sizeable dimensions as forces for change. These remarks on the impetus for change apply to the delivery of nursing care to the frail elderly. As predicted, societal changes are influencing the current models of acute and home care nursing at JHMI.

Nursing model recommendations

The Post-Hospital Support Study may be viewed as a "project organization" that is operating within the functional, hierarchical structure of JHMI.[14] This combination is known as a "matrix organization." Cleland and King[15] claim that one of the advantages of a matrix organization is a better balance among time, cost, and performance. This balance occurs through a system of built-in checks and balances that are based on deliberate conflict and continuous negotiations between the project and functional organization.

In this open system, conflict is necessary to promote dynamic activity and growth. The statement on nursing practice problems can be interpreted as the necessary conflict that will promote developmental change within the matrix system. Two problems that have been empirically identified are the areas of unmet professional education needs and barriers to communication. The following recommendations are designed to alleviate these problems.

Education. Blum and Stein[16] advise that the first task of planning is to conduct a needs assessment. Support is required by the nurse managers in the acute and home care settings. Recognizing educational deficits, the management of inpatient nursing has set up a program to meet educational needs. For example, workshops are offered on the concepts associated with primary nursing. Nurses involved in case management might similarly be offered instruction specific to that portion of the delivery system. Content might include theory on case management, families, values, and change; communication with the multidisciplinary team in the community setting; and means of accessing community resources and services.

Development of an educational bridge is recommended to link both nursing groups in a shared workshop on the special care needs of the frail elderly. In response to the group needs in gerontological nursing, the content of the bridged program might include topics such as age-related physical and normative psychosocial changes, cognitive impairment, drug toxicities, advanced assessment skills, communication with the elderly, and rehabilitation concepts. In effect, this educational package could be designed to assist the nursing staff in meeting the requisites of the American Nurses' Association certification exams.

Nursing management can draw on the pool of experienced practitioners who are formally educated to deliver an advanced level of care within the hospital system. Costs can be contained by enlisting the aid of this network of available resources on a time-limited, brief basis. Library reference material should be updated so that the staff can review the literature as an expected step in solving complex practice problems. There are many creative, cost-effective educational possibilities.

Communication. As the educational bridge raises the group consciousness, communication between the nurses in the two segments of the delivery system is likely to develop. The bridge demonstrates that each group acts as an advocate for the patient within a network. Communications between interdisciplinary team members is likely to expand as nursing clarifies its practice position through an increased knowledge base and greater degree of accountability. Members of the team must learn to plan together and to recognize that blurred lines of involvement do not necessarily lead to a territorial dispute. The patient benefits if the team members join forces.

Management must be willing to give direction in assisting the providers in clarifying overlapping roles throughout the system. As an example of positive management intervention, the director of social work at JHMI offers supervisory assistance to the social work providers in both settings. Similarly, the director of the Post-Hospital Support Study assists the nursing and social work staff to increase communication skills and establish care-giving priorities. The psychogeriatric clinical nurse specialist offers consultation and instruction to management and staff about communication skills, group facilitation, and patient-related problems. The staff reports that these measures to facilitate communication are helpful.

Documentation. With staff assistance, managers can develop an improved documentation format. After reaching agreement on the necessary data base, documentation can be formalized and applied to the acute and home care settings. For example, a standardized patient problem list and medication calendar could be developed to serve as a patient assessment and evaluation tool over time. The list leads to a nursing diagnosis that is applicable in both care settings. This means that two nurses could conduct a rapid patient assessment in the same objective manner. At the time of patient transfer in either direction within the system, the accompanying information would ensure immediate and continuing interventions.

Enhanced continuity of care is likely to occur if the patient were responsible for safeguarding a copy of this document and for presenting it to professional providers each time the system is accessed.

Military personnel, for instance, carry documentation of blood type, immunization history, and health records as they transfer from one duty station to another. Costs to redesign the existing data base and discharge planning forms would involve minimal staff time and printing expenses.

Research. There is a need to conduct descriptive research. Such investigation would establish the pathway for future research treatments based on an experimental design. Certainly,

there is a growing need to explore the following research questions:

1. Is it possible to describe the relationship between age structure, prospective reimbursement, severity of illness, and traditional models of delivering nursing care?

2. Is there a measurable change in quality of care delivered to the frail elderly before and after the intervention of staff education?

3. Does the cost involved in a changing models of care make a difference in patient outcome as potentially measured by patient readmission rate, compliance to the plan of care, and morbidity-mortality rates?

Summary

The purpose of this article has been to present an overview of the potential relationship between the growing number of elderly patients with special healthcare needs and the traditional models of delivering nursing care. Nursing problems are barriers to communication and deficits in professional education.

Such problems provide an organization with the impetus to change and provide a more efficient and effective healthcare delivery system. Recommendations address the role that management might take to investigate these observations and to facilitate communication and the education process. Costs can be contained through use within the matrix organization.

Growth-promoting change can be the outcome of the questions that force nursing to address the problems faced in daily practice.

This is a time of transition for healthcare delivery systems. The role of nursing is an integral one in contributing to the advances that organizations are likely to make in the care of the frail elderly.

REFERENCES

1. American Association of Retired Persons: *A Profile of Older Americans.* Washington, DC.: AARP, 1984.

2. Blum H: The nature of the task, in Blum H (ed): *Planning for Health: Generics for the Eighties.* ed. 2. New York: Human Sciences Press Inc, 1981.

3. Urosevich, P: How nurses are learning to live with DRGs. *Nursing Life* 1984; 4(2):64-65.

4. Rosen S: Adapting discharge planning to prospective pricing. *Hospitals* 1984; 58(5):71-76.

5. Feldman J, Goldhaber F: Living with DRGs. *J Nurs Adm* 1984; 14(5):19-27.

6. Rutkowski B: DRGs: Now all eyes are on you. *Nursing Life* 1985; 5(2):26-29.

7. Editorial: Prospective plan needs public awareness. *Hospitals* 1983; 57(24) (October):19.

8. Berenson R, Paulson G: The medical prospective payment system and the care of the frail elderly. *J Am Geriatr Soc* 1984; 32(10):843-848.

9. Metcalf A: Geriatric consultation service: Nursing implications. Paper presented at the meeting of the Assistant Directors' Forum, Johns Hopkins Hospital, Baltimore, Md. October, 1984.

10. Zander K: *Primary Nursing: Development and Management,* Germantown, Md.: Aspen Systems Corp., 1980.

11. Bell R: Care of the chronically mentally ill patient, in Stuart G, Sundeen S (eds): *Principles and Practice of Psychiatric Nursing.* St. Louis, Mo: C.V. Mosby Co, 1983.

12. Wiles E: Home health care nursing, in Stanhope M, Lancaster J (eds): *Community Health Nursing: Process and Practice for Promoting Health.* St. Louis, Mo: C.V. Mosby Co, 1984.

13. Arbeiter J: The big shift to home health nursing. *RN* 1984; 47(11):38-45.

14. Rakich J, Longest B, O'Donovan T: *Managing Health Care Organizations.* Philadelphia: W.B. Saunders Co, 1977.

15. Cleland D, King W: *System Analysis and Project Management.* New York: McGraw-Hill Book Co, 1968.

16. Blum H, Stein S: Assessment: Measurement of where we are, where we are likely to be, and where we want to be, in Blum H (ed): *Planning for Health: Generics for the Eighties,* ed 2. New York: Human Sciences Press Inc, 1981.

Nursing 2020: A study of nursing's future

Toni J. Sullivan, RN, EdD; Jan L. Lee, RNC, MN; Myrna L. Warnick, RN, MSN; Lois Green, MHSA; Julena Lind, RN, MN; Deborah S. Smith, RN, MN; Patricia Underwood, RN, DNSc

The year is 2020. Space Health Scientist Carol Kole, RN, is one of 12 professional nurses assigned to the United States Space Exploration Team (USSET). As part of a multidisciplinary team of space health scientists, Dr. Kole or one of her nurse colleagues accompanies each manned space launch. Recognized by USSET as the most health-focused members of the team, these nurse scientists have the responsibility of diagnosing and treating alterations in the responses of the astronauts to such realities of space life as weightlessness, limited personal space, and altered sensory input. Nurse space health scientists also initiate and implement ongoing nursing research projects in space. For example, Dr. Kole is studying the relationship of locus of control and previous life experiences to the inclination to anthropomorphize the voice control panel. Research findings have included an ethnography of the tendency to anthropomorphize computer controls and their influence on personal and group behavior in space.

Science fiction? Far-fetched? A pipe dream? No! This is a possible future scenario. Will it come to be? That depends on the decisions that nurses make today and in the near and far future and on the strategic actions they take to achieve the preferred future.

How can the profession create a future that will demand a Carol Kole in space — and on earth? How does the profession get from here to there? Currently, nursing is existing in a dynamic and uncertain present (including an aging society, a better informed and more participatory clientele, a cost-conscious citizenry, and the opening of other career options for

women) and moving into an uncertain future. In the face of such uncertainty, the profession must reprogram and reposition itself for the future.

But which future? Which are the more probable futures? Which of the futures do we prefer? Which of the futures will we be prepared for? Futures research methods offer a way for the profession to engage in long-range strategic planning for the purpose of creating an intentional future and being prepared for it. Nursing 2020, a future research study, polled nursing experts' opinions to fashion alternative scenarios of nursing's future. Once scenarios are developed, nursing can employ them to guide the strategic planning process.

A national invitational conference of 40 nursing experts laid the groundwork for the project. From the raw data generated at the conference, 20 forecast statements were developed. Thirty-five nursing experts, including 7 clinical nurse specialists, 13 nursing service administrators, and 15 nurse educators, completed two rounds of a Delphi study over a six-month period. Panelists rated each forecast statement for both the probability and desirability of occurrence in the years 2000 and 2020. In addition, panelists were asked to rate the sufficiency of information available to them in making their judgments. Thus, in each round of the Delphi survey, panelists made five judgments for each of the 20 items for a total of 100 responses. On the second round of the Delphi, results of round one were shared and panelists' written comments were solicited. Data were then analyzed both qualitatively and quantitatively.

Results of the study

Forecast data about the future of nursing proved very provocative and revealing. An interrelation of the items with a high probability of occurrence (70% or above) and the items with a low probability of occurrence (30% or below) yielded three major themes of concern and change for the nursing profession: shifting nursing's level of autonomy in society and health care, strengthening of patients' rights in health care, and increasing the interrelationship of high technology with humanistic caring by nurses.

Predictions for the year 2000 showed little change from the present, but predictions for the year 2020 showed great change. It seems that this group of experts considered the year 2000 a near future — too near for noticeable change. Given the present rapidly changing health care system and nursing's need to position itself favorably within it, this slow rate of projected change is a cause for some concern. An interrelation of predictability scores with desirability ratings demonstrated that in the areas of upgrading nursing education and increasing nursing autonomy in practice, minimal change is predicted, although substantial change is desirable. This finding seems to indicate feelings of powerlessness in these key areas....See how your judgments compare to the judgments of the expert panel.

Scenario

In the year 2020, nursing is still in transition from occupational to professional status. Since the 1980s, substantial progress toward autonomy for nursing has been made in practice, research, and in the policy arenas of public health and welfare. However, the profession has not yet achieved a high standard of education for all entrants into practice. Consequently, the status and authority positions of nursing in health care delivery in relation to the other health sciences, particularly medicine, remain unchanged from the relative positions occupied in the 1980s. What is perceptible, however, is an intensified and widespread resolve within the profession to achieve full authority over nursing practice and education. Those familiar with nursing history recognize these tensions as yet another chapter in nursing's long and tortuous route to professional stature. But there are also differences, because nursing and nurses have played influential and visible roles in formulation of health care policy and provision of health care delivery in the past 35 years. The factors needed for success in standardizing and upgrading nursing education appear to be in place — societal support and internal demand. Nursing appears on the threshold of completing the journey to professionalism begun over 100 years ago.

In the year 2020, health care delivery continues to be highly regulated by state governing boards, despite the efforts of alterative providers to weaken state regulations and open health care to more freedom of choice by consumers. In collaboration with medicine on this issue, nursing has participated in limiting the scope and authority of alternative provider groups. The strong nursing support for continued state regulation has been effective; in most states, nurses can admit patients directly to nursing homes, home health agencies, and community nursing centers. This ability has increased nursing's internal cooperation; nurses are now able to refer patients to colleague nurses across these various health care settings. Nursing, a major provider group in occupational settings, is conducting much of the primary health promotion and secondary prevention activities that have become a major component of health care delivery in the United States. Occupational health nurses, particularly in urban settings, are often patients' first contact with the health care delivery system and often refer patients to other health care services.

This limited gatekeeping authority, denied

to nurses for so long, is viewed by nursing leaders as evidence of nursing's increasing power and influence in health care. The assumption by the profession of gatekeeping functions in health promotion and health maintenance settings is a triumph in research and public policy. Two major studies in the 1990s, one in nursing home care and one in occupational health in the auto industry, demonstrated that nursing care made a significant difference in the health status of patients and saved the federal government and the auto industry billions of dollars in health care costs. This created a favorable climate for improving nursing's authority in these settings, which the profession wisely recognized. Adopting a unified posture, nursing was able to achieve Medicare and Medicaid reforms at the Federal level that allowed nursing to assume more decision-making authority in long-term care and community settings. Nursing then quietly worked with major industries, most of which were self-insured, to increase nursing's authority to diagnose and treat health problems in occupational settings. At the state level, the profession was modestly successful in expanding nurse practice acts — or their interpretation — to increase nursing's authority and responsibility in community and long-term care.

Opposition by organized medicine was pervasive, but was for the most part viewed as self-serving by a public eager for widely available, cost-efficient health promotion and health maintenance care. Unfortunately, organized medicine, surprised by nursing's success in the 1990s, has been vigilant ever since. The nursing profession, in turn, has had to marshal its considerable resources periodically to prevent loss of gains made at both the state and the federal level.

Nursing, once concerned about its future in in-patient hospital care, has proven itself indispensable to the highly technological hospital. Nurses are humanistic knowledge workers in this setting, serving as a bridge between the technological environment and acutely ill patients and their families. New technologies in health care no longer enjoy instant demand and acceptance. Instead, the rightful focus has moved to technology assessment and ultimately to the ethical application of technologies, old and new alike.

Although neither community-based nor hospital-based nurses are authorized to admit directly to hospitals, nurses are playing an increasingly important role in case management. Case histories from nurses in community settings are often viewed as indispensable tools for care planning and care management in hospitals. Hospital-based nursing has contributed significantly to the development of nursing science. A large body of literature exists on clinical decision making. A standard nursing diagnosis nomenclature, agreed on by the profession, has expanded rapidly and is in use in hospitals and community-based settings in the nation's major metropolitan areas. In fact, several state nurse practice acts have mandated its use.

A growing societal movement toward humanizing health care, begun in the 1990s, has increased the financial support for nursing research that focuses on human responses to health and illness problems. Fortunately, the National Center for Nursing Research in NIH was already in place at that time and has been able to capitalize on this movement. At the federal level, about 30 percent of all biomedical research sponsored is now in nursing science.

Nursing, in 2020, is also in the forefront of the patients' rights movement. All hospitals and communities are required by federal mandate to have active humanistic impact study groups to assess the impact of biomedical technology/genetic engineering on patients' rights to freedom of choice and to death with dignity. Nurses, required by law to sit on these committees, have proven to be patients' rights advocates and have gained widespread recognition as such through several highly publicized cases.

Nursing's role in patient advocacy, in general, has become highly visible and widely recognized. This acceptance of an advocacy role for nursing within the profession and society is based on nursing's persistent efforts to ensure that both individuals and the public at large have access to quality health care regardless of ability to pay, and have a voice in health care decisions that affect the quality of life and the allocation of scarce resources. Nursing roles in advocacy also include consumer education, patient counseling regarding alternative treatment options, and nursing support for dying patients who choose to forego heroic lifesaving measures.

Overall, in the health care delivery system in 2020, patients' rights and humanistic values are alive and well. There is societal focus on health promotion, disease prevention, and the ethical aspects of health care decisions. Nursing is recognized — and recognizes itself — as being in the forefront of these movements. The unfinished business for the nursing profession includes elevating and standardizing its curricula for entry into practice and advanced practice roles. Articles appearing in the national press and television commentaries have recently addressed this topic. It appears that the stage is set for nursing to finally accomplish educational sanity. Will the profession finally repair its Achilles' heel?

A case study involving prospective payment legislation, DRGs, and certified registered nurse anesthetists

John F. Garde, MS, CRNA

THE SHIFT FROM a cost-plus payment system to a prospectively determined, fixed-price system for hospital care for Medicare patients in 1983 had and continues to have major effects on health providers, both institutional and individual. Whereas a variety of efforts previously had been undertaken to contain rising Medicare costs, none had been sufficiently successful to achieve desired outcomes. It became obvious to many health care planners, economists, industrial and business leaders, state and federal legislators, and administration officials that changes were needed, both in the health care delivery system and in reimbursement incentives if significant headway was going to be made to contain costs while not significantly affecting access to health care.

The reimbursement mechanisms utilized for paying for health care services often have been cited as the basis for the escalation of health care costs, along with increasing costs associated with major advances in science and technology. Health clients were blamed for the increased cost because they had been shielded from the actual cost of care through the third-party payment system that had evolved in the public and private sectors. The third-party payers came under criticism because they often restricted reimbursement to higher-cost care systems, like the hospital, rather than reimbursing ambulatory or outpatient services, creating the incentives to increase hospital admissions. Services aimed at health screening or maintenance were usually not reimbursed under health insurance plans, except within the few health maintenance organizations that had come into existence during and following World War II, particularly along the West

Coast. And physicians' organizations, believing that any health care system that interfered with the relationship between individual patients and their physician was inherently bad, also insisted that the fee-for-service payment system was essential for maintaining such relationships.

Unfortunately, the health care system is a very human system, subject to all human attributes, not merely altruistic ones. As such, perhaps everyone was at fault for the escalating costs, providers, patients, and payers alike. Most of us look upon health care as a right, rather than a privilege, and desire that all within our society have equal access to health services. But that remains a goal, rather than a reality, with little opportunity to actualize it without major changes in both the health care delivery and reimbursement systems.

It has been said that major change cannot be effected suddenly in large, bureaucratic organizations or systems but must be done incrementally. The Prospective Payment System (PPS) legislation, enacted into law in 1983, was true to this axiom in that it covered only Part A Medicare (hospital payments). Payments for physician services, under Part B Medicare, were not affected, though the ways physicians would practice, under PPS, had the potential to be greatly affected. Furthermore, hospital care consumed the highest portions of money spent by Medicare, and perhaps was a logical point to begin incremental change.

Basic characteristics of the PPS system
The economic theory underlying PPS had previously been tested in several states and was

believed to hold promise for containing Medicare costs. This theory, in its most simplistic terms, was that systems paid on a cost-plus basis had no real reimbursement incentives for providing cost-effective services. Thus it was felt that hospitals would provide cost-effective care only when their profits depended on their ability to do so. Moreover, it was felt that if hospital profits also depended on changes in physician behavior relating to hospital resource consumption, hospitals would be more apt to implement strategies for changing physician behavior related to resource consumption as opposed to those systems where hospital profits increased with increased resource consumption by physicians. Because these incentives were directed at the macro level of a major component of the health delivery system, though affecting every micro element of the system, little consideration was given to individual-type services and providers. The little attention that was directed at the micro level related to a prohibition within the legislation against unbundling of services and the shifting of costs from Part A to Part B Medicare, that is, shifting services, costs, and their reimbursement from the hospital to physicians. However, the time frame for implementing PPS permitted unbundling, and the reimbursement incentives underlying PPS fostered it.

The essential elements of the PPS legislation are important in understanding PPS's effect on certified registered nurse anesthetists (CRNAs) and the subsequent actions taken to minimize their adverse effects. Essentially, PPS legislation mandated that a fixed rate for hospital care, covering all Part A services, be paid to hospitals based on a Medicare patient's diagnostic-related classification (group), or DRG, that is, one of some 356 diagnostic groups (at last count). This fixed rate was to cover all costs associated with the hospital admission, including all services provided by nonphysician health providers, whether hospital employees or not. The rate of reimburse-

ment for the diagnostic categories was calculated on data from the cost-plus system and was to be regionally adjusted. It was to be implemented over a time frame of 4 years, with hospital payments being determined as a mix between the cost-plus and DRG rates, utilizing a decreasing cost-plus, increasing DRG formula until at the end of the fourth year all hospitals (not exempted from PPS, like mental health, children, and rehabilitation hospitals and units) would be 100 percent reimbursed on the basis of DRG payments. Although it was perhaps best, as well as easier, to pass legislation that affected only one major component of the system, it is obvious that the most difficult changes to be made in the system relate to physician (Part B) payment because of the political power of physicians and their organizations.

Essentially, under PPS, there is a health care reimbursement system in which pressure is applied to cap escalating costs on one side, without an equal and opposing pressure being applied to the other side. Thus, physical principles applied to this open health care system would indicate a tendency to shift some of the effects of that pressure into the noncapped sector, or Part B Medicare, rather than truly containing costs. In such a system, although hospital costs might be contained, costs for Part B could increase. Furthermore, whereas hospitals are mandated to accept Medicare payment over and above any patient-required annual deductible, physicians are not mandated to accept such assignment. Therefore, if some hospital services could shift to Part B, then the cost of those services would not have to come from the DRG payment. If physician payments were capped, physicians still could pass along increases in their charges to Medicare beneficiaries, and total health care costs would not necessarily be contained. The federal government would contain its costs, but beneficiaries would pay more, thus increasing total costs.

This, of course, was the basis for the prohibition against unbundling in PPS, a provision that would be difficult in some instances to enforce.

In addition, those hospitals that utilized large amounts of nonphysician services, rather than physician services, where substitutability between providers is possible, as in anesthesia, may have been affording cost savings to the Medicare system in the past. However, these hospitals stood to be hurt the most by the DRG payment. They would have to pay the nonphysician health professionals' salaries and benefits from the DRG payment. Hospitals, utilizing more physicians for such services, did not need to take such costs from the DRG because physician services were reimbursed from Part B and could still be reimbursed as before. Thus there was a potential for the latter hospitals to reap a so-called "windfall profit" for utilizing more costly providers, and a strong incentive for hospitals to shift such services to physicians and attain additional revenue over expenditures prior to, or early in, the implementation of the legislation that prohibited unbundling. Because the DRG payment was a mean figure based on an aggregate of all hospital costs at the time of its determination, no one was able to determine just what portion of that cost related to anesthesia or any other service, or whether it would be adequate to cover such costs.

Concerns were also high among private insurers that hospital costs for Medicare patients would be shifted to private patients. Industrial leaders, recognizing the potential for their costs associated with health care benefits for employees and other beneficiaries to climb, began to take measures to control the escalation they expected.

Reimbursement and anesthesia services
The cost of anesthesia services comprises three principal components: (1) professional service fees or costs, (2) drug and equipment charges, and (3) capital costs associated with facilities and capital equipment utilization and replacement factors. (Some hospitals put all these costs into one basic fee schedule. Also buried within either drug and equipment charges or capital costs are those administrative and logistic costs of a hospital that are passed along in such charges.) Historically anesthesia services have been one of the major profit centers of hospitals. Because nurse anesthetists have consistently provided a major portion of the anesthesia care within hospitals, hospitals have made significant profits from their services.

Many anesthesiologists were also hospital-employed prior to World War II. With increasing numbers of physicians entering the field, with increasing access to both private and public third party payment, and with medical societies, including the American Society of Anesthesiologists (ASA), discouraging hospital employment or salaried positions or physicians in their Ethical Codes, radiologists, pathologists, and anesthesiologists left such hospital positions in droves and took some of the hospitals' profits with them, forcing hospitals, in many instances, to increase charges associated with these and other services.

Impact of PPS on CRNAS
The American Association of Nurse Anesthetists (AANA) recognized early that the PPS legislation, as passed, would have an adverse impact on nurse anesthetists. It was enacted into legislation rapidly, without the usual time delays, thus eliminating opportunity to present testimony and point out deficiencies within the legislation, or to raise significant opposition to it. Under Medicare Part A, CRNA salaries and benefits, and charges by CRNA private contractors, had been fully reimbursed under the cost-plus reimbursement mechanism for hospitals. Now, such reimbursement would come from the DRG payment. Furthermore, if anes-

thesiologists could not charge for the services of their employed CRNAs under PPS, because all nonphysician services were to be paid from the hospital DRG, they would have to negotiate with the hospital in an attempt to recoup their perceived losses related to the CRNA salaries and benefits they paid for their employees. They also could begin providing these services themselves, which in all probability would significantly reduce their earnings.

Recognizing these and other problems with PPS, AANA formed a group to perform a definitive analysis of the legislation. Furthermore, the group was charged to develop a plan to try to control the damage to CRNAs and their practice. In addition, the membership was requested to keep the AANA informed about the effects of PPS being felt at the hospital level.

CRNA practice patterns

The extent to which CRNAs could be affected by this legislation is reflected in their three predominant practice patterns. At the time of passage of the legislation, approximately 44 per cent worked as hospital employees, 37 per cent worked as physician employees (predominantly employed by anesthesiologist groups), and about 11 per cent were self-employed and worked as private contractors.[1] From 1981 data from hospitals that provided services requiring an anesthesia capability, 16.9 per cent were serviced solely by anesthesiologists, 42.3 per cent were serviced by both CRNAs and anesthesiologists, 33.5 per cent were serviced solely by CRNAs, and 3.7 per cent got their anesthesia from other types of providers.[2] Thus about 17 per cent of hospitals could reap additional profits from the DRG, whereas for 75 per cent of the hospitals, CRNAs would constitute costs somewhat beyond that accounted for in the DRG. Furthermore, hospital costs could be lowered by utilizing more anesthesiologist services that had access to Part B Medicare.

This situation must also be viewed from the context of the times and the increasing number of physicians entering the marketplace, including the increased numbers of American-educated physicians entering anesthesiology. Moreover, when comparing incomes between anesthesiologists and CRNAs, the cost of anesthesia care to Medicare beneficiaries could be expected to escalate because anesthesiologists constituted one of the groups among the medical specialists with the lowest percent participation in Medicare assignment.

AANA plan of action and its results

Rather than taking a paranoid attitude toward Congress regarding this legislation, it was AANA's position that Congress had inadvertently created reimbursement disincentives to the utilization of CRNAs while bolstering such incentives for utilization of anesthesiologists. Also, much talk by Congress and the administration was centered on building competition in health care in an attempt to contain costs. Unfortunately, most of such discussions involved competition between physicians or between institutional health providers. The AANA recognized that competition could also be built into the system between selected physicians and nurses or other nonphysician providers. However, from studying reimbursement and reimbursement access, AANA also concluded that to be able to compete in this latter subsystem, equal access to reimbursement mechanisms (not necessarily equal reimbursement rates) had to be available to afford maximum opportunity for substituting nonphysician services for physician services. Having data to demonstrate that no significant differences existed in the outcomes of care provided by CRNAs and anesthesiologists, and evidence, though secondary, of the cost-effectiveness of CRNA utilization within the health care system in general, and Medicare specifically, the AANA devised a three-point program to overcome the adverse impact of PPS on CRNAs.

The AANA plan, devised by its Government Relations Committee and consultants, and adopted by its Board Of Directors, involved three components, all of which were pursued simultaneously. It required working with and lobbying both the administration, particularly the Health Care Financing Administration (HCFA), and Congress. It also took massive efforts for educating and motivating as many CRNAs as possible to become effective lobbyists.

The first two components of the plan related to short-term corrections to alleviate the inherent reimbursement disincentives for utilizing CRNAs. It consisted of requesting exception to the unbundling provision of PPS for physician-employed CRNAs and a temporary pass-through provision for costs of hospital-employed CRNAs and private practice CRNA contractors. The third component of the plan related to assuring that reimbursement access in the future did not create inadvertent disincentives for the utilization of CRNA services by assuring that services by either CRNAs or anesthesiologists be paid from the same part of Medicare, either Part A or Part B. It was felt by those who had analyzed the Medicare legislation that if both CRNA and anesthesiologist services were reimbursed under the same Medicare payment component (that is, Part A or Part B), competition could be enhanced and the chance for inadvertent reimbursement disincentives would be minimized.

In fact, it was felt by some individuals studying this matter that if Congress wanted to maximize competition in anesthesia care and/or implement a system that had the potential to be most effective at containing anesthesia costs, they would enact legislation for paying all anesthesia services under Part A, and give the money to the hospital administrator to buy anesthesia services. However, it was highly unlikely that Congress would do this for one medical provider and not for others. And if they did, undoubtedly a lawsuit would have been filed to test the constitutionality of the legislation. Thus, following these considerations, the AANA sought congressional support for direct reimbursement for CRNAs as a long-term solution, agreeing to support congressional efforts in the future that might change reimbursement for anesthesia services, so long as both anesthesiologists and CRNAs were being paid from the same so-called "pot."

With considerable discussions with, and an avalanche of letters to, HCFA, including a conference with Caroline Davis, its administrator, HCFA regulations were written authorizing an exception to the unbundling provision for a 3-year period for physician-employed CRNAs as a part of the regulations implementing PPS. Although AANA had made the major effort to obtain this, it also was supported by anesthesiologists who employed CRNAs, though without significant support from the ASA. (Many of the leaders of ASA saw this legislation as an opportunity to significantly decrease the utilization of CRNAs and thus their potential to compete with anesthesiologists for anesthesia services. This was consistent with the long-held position of many past and current leaders of ASA, that anesthesiology is a medical specialty and one into which nurses should not be admitted. This position is almost incomprehensible when it is recognized that the nursing specialty in this country evolved prior to the medical specialty and that today, nurses provide anesthesia, or are otherwise involved as an anesthetist in 70 per cent of the anesthetics administered in this country.) Although HCFA stated they had the regulatory authority to make the exception to the unbundling provision for physician-employed CRNAs, they did not believe they had authority to authorize a pass-through of costs for hospital-employed CRNAs and private contractors, thus necessitating an amendment to Medicare legislation to accomplish this goal.

It was necessary to sell the pass-through legislation to selected members of the appropriate congressional committees to get such a technical amendment introduced in both the House of Representatives and the Senate. Active lobbying, laying out AANA's total legislative agenda for CRNAs under PPS, drew the necessary support for the technical amendment. The amendment agreed on by the House and Senate conferees and signed into law by the President in 1984 put a time limit on the pass-through of 3 fiscal years and included the mandate for a study of "possible methods of reimbursement which would not discourage the use of CRNAs by hospitals." It is of interest that whereas some hospital administrators supported AANA in this particular effort, the American Hospital Association lent no support to this amendment. In discussions between AANA and AHA representatives, it appeared that because this pass-through had to be budget-neutral and its costs required a slight downward adjustment of the DRG, AHA saw it as a loss of control over a portion of DRG funding. They further felt it would delay the necessity for hospitals to be responsible for how all Part A Medicare funds were spent. The ASA did not take a public position either for or against this amendment.

The AANA recognized that selling direct reimbursement under Part B of Medicare would be the most difficult job of its three-part plan and that such a proposal would be opposed by not only the ASA but Medicine in general. Furthermore, many members of Congress believed, and continue to believe, that fee-for-service health care is not only a basis for escalating health care costs, but that it provides incentives to increase the number of services patients or health clients receive, whether they are actually needed or not. Thus most Congress members were not supportive of opening up fee-for-service Part B reim-

bursement to additional health providers.

The job of AANA was to convince Congress that CRNAs were concerned about health care costs as well as equitable reimbursement for their services for salaries from their employers. AANA also pointed out that other providers determined the need for anesthesia services, not CRNAs. As such, CRNAs were in no position to escalate the number of anesthesia services they provided merely to increase their earnings. The AANA also pointed out that something would have to be done if CRNAs were to remain a viable force in affording cost-effective anesthesia services at the time the exception regulation and the pass-through amendment were scheduled to expire. AANA agreed that if it would be helpful to gain passage, CRNAs would accept a clause mandating Medicare assignment, a condition still not imposed on physicians.

Direct reimbursement legislation for CRNAs was introduced in the Senate in August 1983 by Senators Matsunaga (D-Hawaii), Inouye (D-Hawaii), Sasser (D-Tennessee), and Pell (D-Rhode Island) and in the House in January 1984 by Barney Frank, Democrat from Massachusetts. Although it was Democrats on both the House and Senate side that made the introductions, support was gained for the legislation from a variety of Congress members of both parties. The legislation did not make it through the 98th Congress.

With the convening of the 99th Congress, this legislation was reintroduced in both the Senate and House. Sponsors for introduction in the Senate included Matsunaga, Inouye, and Pell, who had signed on in the previous Congress, with the following additional senators: Pressler (R-South Dakota), Humphrey (R-New Hampshire), Sarbanes (D-Maryland), Melcher (D-Montana), Burdick (D-North Dakota), and Leahy (D-Vermont). Representative Barney Frank again introduced the House bill. Additional representatives and senators signed on as cosponsors during the period following introduction, and others expressed willingness to support the bill after it was explained to them by CRNAs from their congressional districts. This legislation was passed as a part of the Omnibus Budget Reconciliation Act of 1986 and was signed into law on October 21, 1986. The effective date for direct reimbursement for CRNAs was set in the bill as January 1, 1989, with the unbundling and pass-through provisions achieved earlier being extended to cover the interim period.

The direct reimbursement legislation affects all CRNAs regardless of their practice setting. It permits CRNA employees to sign over their billing rights to their employer. All CRNA services are subject to Medicare assignment. An additional provision in the bill requires that the new system for reimbursement of CRNAs be budget-neutral.

After 4 1/2 years of intensive effort and expenditure of funds on the part of AANA, its members, staff, and consultants, a nursing specialty was finally recognized for direct reimbursement under Medicare legislation. Although not the first nonphysician group to achieve such status under Medicare, AANA was the first professional nursing organization to achieve such a goal for its members. Support for this endeavor came from some other nursing organizations, some hospital administrators, and a variety of other sources. Richard Verville, AANA's Washington attorney, and other congressional consultants (Debbie Hardy, former congressional aide to the late representative from Illinois, George O'Brien, and now a partner in Capitol Associates; and Jay Constantine, formerly chief staff member for the Senate Finance Committee) provided the continuous, on-scene Washington support for this endeavor. The AANA conducted yearly Government Relations Workshops during this process in Washington, D.C., and its

members roamed the halls of Congress visiting and talking with their representatives and senators; this communication continued when the members returned to their home states. In addition, at the AANA annual meeting in Washington, in 1986, the AANA held a major legislative reception, attracting one of the largest crowds of congressional members, staff, and constituents that many experienced staffers could remember.

The study mandated by Congress in 1984 was awarded to the Center for Health Economics Research and has recently been completed. The study provides interesting primary data to support AANA's contention that CRNAs are involved in all types of anesthesia care from the simple to the highly complex, and provides such services in all types of hospital settings. It is felt the implications of this study with regard to human resources will show that there is an even greater need to increase the total number of CRNAs in this country. The CHER data also imply that the services provided by CRNAs are essentially substitutable for physician anesthesia services. If HCFA translates these facts into new payment methodology reforms, Medicare would take the first step in reducing excessive overpayments.

AANA has proposed that the mechanism for direct reimbursement be based on a relative value scale as is utilized for reimbursement of anesthesiologists. Conversion factors could be specifically set for CRNAs. Unfortunately, HCFA is resisting such a proposal and is proposing utilization of a time unit for the actual anesthesia time, which does not take into consideration many aspects of the care provided by CRNAs. Such a payment rate may be particularly hurtful to rural hospitals and the CRNAs who service them. Thus AANA was not able to enjoy a lengthy respite from intensive federal government activities but rather must continue its activities to ensure a satisfactory mechanism for reimbursing CRNA services, one that will not create new disincentives to the utilization of CRNAs. For this purpose, AANA has engaged the services of Health Policy Alternatives, Inc.; Touche Ross; and Wexler, Reynolds, Harrison, and Schule, Inc. to assist us in bringing this matter to a successful conclusion. It was the expressed intent of Congress in the passage of AANA's pass-through amendment to correct problems in PPS legislation creating disincentives to the utilization of CRNAs. It may require AANA to pursue additional technical amendments to Medicare legislation to ensure that HCFA is not permitted to inadvertently create such disincentives this year through its regulations.

In the meantime, AANA continues to monitor activity related to possible changes in physician reimbursement under Part B of Medicare, and is prepared to continue to work with Congress to effect further refinements in legislation that have the potential to contain health care costs in a cost-effective health environment. Our experience has taught us that government, although perhaps well-meaning, is not all-wise. It has demonstrated to us that when people and Congress agree on goals, they can work together to bring about better solutions to the problems we face, so long as government intervention is indicated. It has also demonstrated to us that small lobbies, when those interests and those of the public are congruent, can achieve success even when larger lobbies with more financial resources oppose them for perceived or real self-interest reasons.

Conclusions

If nurses would unite on essential and relevant health care issues that we all can support, rather than allowing those issues on which we are divided to consume so much of our energies, we might all be surprised at the changes we could make in this nation's health policies, as well as its health care delivery system. And change must come if health care access is to be ensured for all who need it, and at a cost this nation can afford. It is the AANA's contention that although it will not be easy, nurses are essential to the achievement of such a goal, and in fact, if it is to be achieved, nurses must make it happen. For when the interests of the public and nurses are congruent, as they would be in such circumstances, required legislative support can be acquired regardless of the opponents. This has been the major lesson that AANA has learned from the PPS legislative activity — not to fear taking on giants when your members are united in a worthy cause.

REFERENCES

1. AANA Membership Survey, 1982.

2. Orkin FK, et al: Committee on Manpower Study, "The Distribution of Anesthesia Care Providers in the United States," American Society of Anesthesiologists, August 1983.

CHAPTER ELEVEN

Technology: Friend or foe?

RECOGNIZED AS HAVING the most technologically sophisticated system of medical care in the world, the United States nevertheless falls far below other countries in some measures of health status (see Chapter Eight). One reason for this is that the development of new social policies for using the new technology has lagged far behind its implementation. Since World War II, the federal government and the private sector have invested billions of dollars in biomedical research, generating a huge array of innovative diagnostic and treatment technologies. These advances, for the most part, were greeted with strong public support and enthusiasm. But about 10 years ago, a negative reaction began to set in with the recognition that such technology might do harm as well as good — for example, might prolong the life of a terminally ill person without consideration for the quality of that life.

In response to these concerns, investigators such as Daniel Callahan of the Hastings Institute have suggested slowing or halting research on new biomedical technology until the related ethical issues have been identified and considered (see Unit Five for a discussion of ethical issues). Yet academic medical centers continue teaming up with industry to ensure rapid development and dissemination of medical technologies.

Public concern has also arisen over the control physicians have in using new technologies, as expressed in the form of medical orders. Many persons concerned about the ethical and economic issues implied in this situation would prefer that other health professionals and knowledgeable lay people took part in this decision-making process.

The two articles included in this chapter deal thoughtfully with these important issues. The first, "The Potential of Expert Systems in Nursing" by Schank, et al., deals with expert systems in nursing — technology systems for increasing the effectiveness and efficiency of the way nurses' work is done. For example, the bar codes now common on food packaging are being evaluated in hospitals for inventory control and even patient charges. At this time, many clinical facilities are using computers for staffing decisions, charting, medical orders, and word processing, but only a few are exploring the development of expert systems for nursing. After answering the question, "What are expert systems?," the authors discuss these systems' uses in nursing practice.

The second article, "Technological Imperative and Decision Support" by Heaney, discusses the technological imperative "We can; therefore, we must," which appears to drive both physician behavior and the health care system. He provides examples of why this approach is not in the best interests of society and suggests some solutions for regulating the use of technology, including implementation of the care manager role. Heaney concludes his provocative article by suggesting why nurses are the most likely professionals to fill this role.

The potential of expert systems in nursing

MARY JANE SCHANK, RN, PhD; LLOYD D. DONEY, PhD, CDP, CNE; JANET SEIZYK, RN, MS

THE PHENOMENAL GROWTH in the availability of personal computers, and the attendant proliferation of general-purpose microcomputer software have made available to nursing professionals a substantial array of impressive, powerful, and easy-to-use computer capabilities. These tools offer nurses the potential of increasing personal productivity, contributing to increased organizational efficiency and effectiveness, and providing improved service to clients. Three of these tools, word processing, data base management systems, and electronic spreadsheet capabilities, are already being used by nursing practitioners, administrators, researchers, and educators. But a newly emerging tool, expert systems, places an even more provocative and potentially powerful computing capability at their disposal.

In this article, the authors examine expert systems and their potential as "intelligent assistants" for nursing professionals. The following questions are considered and discussed:
• What are expert systems?
• Where are expert systems being used?
• Are expert systems possible in nursing?
• Are expert systems economically feasible in nursing?
• What are the benefits of using an expert system?
• What are the limitations of expert systems?
• What is the future of expert systems?

What are expert systems?
Since the early 1950s computer scientists have been experimenting with computer programs for endowing computers with capabilities that previously had been considered inherently human. These efforts have come to be known as the field of artificial intelligence. The field of artificial intelligence generally is taken to include activities in the following areas: (1) natural language processing; (2) speech recognition; (3) pattern-matching; (4) robotics; (5) machine learning; and (6) expert systems. Of these six areas, the field of expert systems has produced some of the most successful and commercially viable results to date.

There is no single, universally acceptable definition of an expert system. However, some possibilities include:

> Expert systems are computer programs exhibiting behavior characteristic of experts, e.g., a medical expert diagnosing infectious diseases.[1]

> Expert systems are interactive consulting systems which provide users with expert conclusions about specialized knowledge domains.[2]

> [Expert systems involve] the creation of computer software that emulates the way people solve problems. Like a human expert, an expert system gives advice by drawing upon its own store of knowledge, and by requesting information specific to the problem at hand.[3]

> Expert systems are sophisticated computer programs that manipulate knowledge to solve problems efficiently and effectively in a narrow problem area. Like human edxperts, these systems use symbolic logic and heuristics — rules of thumb — to find solutions.[4]

These definitions may be summarized by saying that an expert system is a computerized capability in which the expertise of an expert or a panel of experts, in a relatively narrow area of knowledge, has been modeled and stored in a manner that allows this expert knowledge to be accessed and used by others to assist in making decisions and solving problems.

Expert systems are built by knowledge engineers who extract knowledge from experts and translate this knowledge to computers through one of the several expert system development tools available. The system usually consists of two parts, the knowledge base and the inference engine. The knowledge base contains the facts, empirical knowledge, formulas, statistical probabilities, and rules that use this information as a basis for solving a problem. The inference engine is separate from the knowledge base. It combines knowledge in the knowledge base with information supplied by the user to arrive at a decision or a solution. Though there are other ways to represent the knowledge in an expert system, the most frequently used scheme is a rule-based design, involving strategies expressed as: IF (premise), THEN (conclusion), or IF (condition), THEN (action) structures.

Expert systems differ from other computerized tools in that they manipulate knowledge rather than data. Both data base management systems and spreadsheet capabilities focus on the processing of data through the application of user-defined processing algorithms (sequences). Expert systems, in contrast, focus on the representation and use of knowledge through the application of heuristics (rules-of-thumb), using inferential (logical) processes. While expert systems may use the search capabilities of data base management systems and the computational features of spreadsheets, these activities are incidental to the more powerful capabilities of the system which use symbols to present the problem concepts and apply various strategies to search and manipulate those concepts.

Where are expert systems being used?

In spite of the fact that expert systems capabilities are a relative computing newcomer, the list of expert systems in use is impressive. Even more impressive are the considerable efforts that are underway to develop more workable systems and new software capabilities directed to facilitating the design, development, and use of future expert systems.

The earliest expert systems were developed in medicine, the sciences, and engineering. More expert systems have been developed for medicine than for any other problem area. Several expert systems are in use for assisting the physician in the diagnosis and treatment of specific diseases. Other medical expert systems assist the physician in determining the proper drug dosage for patients. Chemists are using expert systems to aid in the discovery and creation of new chemical structures. In engineering, an expert system is available to help nuclear power plant operators determine the cause of some abnormal event; in computer science, to assist in configuring a computer system to customer requirements; and in geology, to serve as a consultant to geologists searching for mineral deposits.

More recently, expert systems have been developed in law to help lawyers reason about civil cases and to assist in the out-of-court settlement of product liability cases; in auditing, to measure a client's potential for defaulting on a loan, and to plan the necessary audit activities for an audit client; in tax practice, to assist in tax and estate planning for clients; and, in education, to assist students in deciding what courses to take.[5]

Some expert systems activity in nursing is reported in the nursing literature at the time of this writing. A substantial nursing practice–based knowledge system at Creighton University is described by Ryan.[6] Cybernurse, a hybrid knowledge and data base management system in nursing developed by Cybernetic Health Systems of Ann Arbor, Michigan, is mentioned but not described by Schultz.[7] Ernst describes a system that is under development to assist in the planning and controlling of nursing staff.[2] Laborde proposes expert systems development for nursing diagnosis, patient care planning, and nursing theory.[8] Bloom and co-workers examine the development of an expert system prototype to generate nursing care plans based on nursing diagnoses.[9] Finally, Ozbolt and others propose an expert system approach to the organizing and codifying of existing nursing knowledge.[10] The diversity of knowledge domains which have served as the basis for the development and use of expert systems, and the activity that has been reported in nursing, suggest that there is the potential for the further development and use of expert systems in nursing practice, administration, research, and education.

Are expert systems possible in nursing?

Artificial intelligence scientists and knowledge engineers are reluctant to prescribe the general characteristics that make a problem appropriate for the development of an expert system. Nevertheless, some guidelines may be found. Waterman suggests seven criteria [4]:

- Task requires only cognitive skills.
- Experts can articulate their methods.
- Genuine experts exist.
- Experts agree on solutions.
- Task is not too difficult.
- Task is not poorly understood.
- Task does not require common sense.

Cognitive skills refer to abilities related to knowledge, comprehension, application, analysis, synthesis, and psychomotor (physical) skills and affective skills, which are related to morals, attitudes, beliefs, and values. While matters related to the affective and psychomotor domains are pertinent to some aspects of nursing, the majority of problem-solving and decision-making skills required lie in the cognitive domain.

Although the availability of experts is a necessary prerequisite to the development of an expert system, they must also be able to articulate and explain the methods they use to solve problems or make decisions. Further, in those instances where experts disagree, it is necessary that they come to a consensus so that the expert system's performance can be validated. The availability and participation of experts is a critical aspect of developing an expert system in any area of knowledge, but there do not appear to be any special or insurmountable problems related to those who practice in the various areas of nursing expertise.

On first analysis, many tasks appear to be too large for the successful development of an expert system. A large task can, however, be broken down into smaller, shorter, and relatively independent tasks for which expert systems can be developed. One of the basis features of expert systems is their inherent modular (building-block) design that facilitates both changes and additions to the knowledge base. Whereas an expert system to assist the nursing administrator of a large hospital in developing the nursing services budget might be too large, a system to assist the director of outpatient services in budget development may be of manageable size.

In addition to size, the level of the development and organization of knowledge in a particular area is relevant to whether the development of an expert system is possible. Most of the early successes in the development and use of expert systems were in areas of knowledge rooted in the physical or the biological sciences. These successes were due in part to the fact that the knowledge involved was precise, well-organized, and well-understood. In areas where the knowledge is new or poorly understood, it is difficult to create the required knowledge base. Since many segments of nursing knowledge derive from the physical and the biological sciences, it seems reasonable to expect that successful expert systems are capable of being developed and implemented in nursing.

Finally, if a task requires a lot of common sense, an expert system is likely to fail. The body of knowledge which comprises those skills referred to as common sense is simply too large to be computerized. For example, a human expert would recognize that a patient is not likely to weigh 15 pounds if the patient is 16 years old. But unless the knowledge base of the expert system included a table of probable ages and weights, the system would not recognize the apparent error (perhaps a zero was omitted in the weight) and seek to continue to generate a suitable recommendation or solution.

Expert systems appear to be possible in a number of areas of nursing problem-solving and decision-making, if the projects are carefully selected and not overly ambitious. Activities which are rooted in knowledge that is precise, well-organized, and well-understood are the best candidates for expert systems applications.

Are expert systems economically feasible in nursing?

Expert system development is costly and time-consuming. PROSPECTOR, an expert system that aids geologists in the exploration for minerals, took more than 30 person-years to produce. The accounting firm of Coopers and Lybrand reported that ExperTAX, an expert system that runs through more than 3000 rules to identify a client's best tax options, costs more than $1 million and took more than 7000 hours to develop.[11] Costs in six- or seven-figure amounts are not uncommon in those instances where development costs have been reported.

Given the likelihood of substantial development costs, some of the circumstances which can contribute to a correspondingly high payoff include a recurring need for the expertise, a scarcity of human experts, and the loss of human expertise. The potential payoff of an expert system increases directly in proportion to the number of times that the expertise is needed. Few computerized capabilities have been developed to solved onetime problems. The payoff in any commercial computer application comes with repeated use. Generation of nursing care plans, staff scheduling, quality assurance, patient classification, and staff continuing education are nursing activities where there may be a sufficient and repetitive need for expertise to justify expert system development.

The development and retention of nursing professionals is also costly, requiring a suitable combination of education and experience. Retention frequently requires increasingly larger rewards in the form of salary and benefits. An expert system is an alternative to developing additional nursing experts when such expertise is scarce, when the organization needs the expertise in a number of locations, or when the organization is losing expertise due to retirements, illness, or resignations.

What are the benefits of using an expert system?

The benefits which derive from developing and using expert systems include: providing consistency of performance; increasing productivity; preserving expertise; expanding expertise; gaining a better understanding of problems; and providing staff development.

Providing consistency of performance. A human expert at different times or human experts at different locations may reach conflicting conclusions about a particular situation for a variety of reasons. An expert system will always provide the same conclusion for the same problem. In addition, expert systems eliminate the occasional inadvertent omissions or errors that befall even the most careful of human experts.

Increasing productivity. Expert systems have the capacity for increasing organization productivity through expanding the available expertise within an organization and through relieving experts and other staff of some of the more routine tasks which are a necessary part of the problem. The development and use of expert systems by physicians have occurred primarily because they minimize many of the routine activities which are a necessary part of practice.

Preserving expertise. Where expertise is scarce or declining, expert systems are a way to preserve an organization's available expertise. The preservation of expertise may be continued, even as the number of experts in an organization decreases, by updating the knowledge base as circumstances change or as new expertise is developed. The development and use of expert systems technology in clinical areas may provide nursing administrators with a means of alleviating the staffing problems arising from the recent and recurring wide cyclical shifts in the availability of clinical nursing staff.

Expanding expertise. Expert systems are portable. It is therefore possible to expand expertise to all locations where the expertise is required. this aspect of expert systems has also been attractive to physicians because many of the same procedures and techniques are required by patients at several different locations.

Gaining a better understanding of problems. The efforts and analysis required to develop an expert system often lead to a better understanding of problems, and sometimes even to a recognition that expertise may be improved with respect to certain aspects of the problem. The necessary interaction between the expert and the knowledge engineer may lead to a refinement or improvement in the expert's approach. This effort may also reveal some of the limits of existing knowledge, and provide the impetus for further research efforts to expand that knowledge. Ozbolt and others confirm this benefit that expert systems development may bring to the organization and codification of existing nursing knowledge.[10] Laborde suggests that expert systems development effort may contribute to the further development of nursing theory.[8] The emerging concept of case management could lead to a combined nursing and physician knowledge base, to be used in the management of patient care.

Providing staff development. Expert systems provide a good learning tool for those who are seeking to develop as experts. Newcomers to the profession may use expert systems in case-type situations to either support or contradict their solution to a problem. Depending on the expert system development tool used, the system may allow the user to "track," step-by-step, the analysis leading to the problem solution or recommended decision. Many systems provide WHY and BECAUSE capabilities that enable the user to compare each facet of their own reasoning with that of the expert.

In addition to developing new experts, expert systems appear to be most effective in the training and development of employees in areas requiring technical knowledge and skills. They hold promise for reducing training costs and ensuring consistency in the presentation of skill-building programs to those who assist the professional nurse.

What are the limitations of expert systems?

The following factors currently limit efforts to develop and use expert systems: development costs; narrow scope of knowledge; user acceptance; incorrect or inconsistent knowledge base; and difficulty of representing certain kinds of knowledge.

Development costs. While development costs currently may preclude efforts to create and use expert systems in some areas, costs are falling and will continue to decline. Future users of expert systems will benefit from both the declining costs of the hardware and software necessary to implement expert systems. They also will benefit from the knowledge gained by those who are pioneering efforts in the field. It is the responsibility of nursing administrators to set priorities and to articulate the needs of nursing to information services and throughout the organization.

Narrow scope of knowledge. Current capabilities limit the size and scope of the knowledge base. There will always be some limitation, but improvements in systems development software and hardware will make it possible to enlarge knowledge bases under consideration.

User acceptance. The successful development and use of expert systems is dependent upon the willingness of those who are affected to participate. Moreover, expert systems are most successful when the impetus for their use comes from both the top and the bottom of the organization. Nurses and computers, however, are strangers, because nurses have been using computers for a number of tasks and problems for many years.

Incorrect or inconsistent knowledge base. Expert systems have difficulty with erroneous or inconsistent knowledge. They are not able to recognize such knowledge and are likely to produce incorrect results or advice when inconsistencies and/or incorrect knowledge are incorporated into the knowledge base.

Difficulty of representing certain kinds of knowledge. Currently, the tools for building expert systems are not as flexible and general as one would wish. Temporary and spatial knowledge are difficult to represent, and different types of knowledge representation schemes cannot be handled easily with the same expert system building tool. There also needs to be a greater ability of expert systems languages to interface with other software, particularly data base management systems and spreadsheet packages.

What is the future of expert systems?

In spite of some of the problems, the development and use of expert systems is growing rapidly. In a recent survey by the accounting firm of Coopers and Lybrand, 40% of the responding organizations reported that they were currently using some form of expert system technology. Another 12% said they were in the process of developing it. The sample included a wide range of manufacturing and service organizations.[12]

Efforts in the sciences will continue to dominate the field. In the past few years, however, there have been a number of new software companies exploring opportunities where the main activity of the organization is professional judgment. While there is sufficient evidence to suggest that the field is growing rapidly, it is somewhat difficult to measure precisely the extent of the application and use of expert systems. There is some suspicion that many expert systems are working so well that some organizations are reluctant to discuss or to publicize their use.

Expert systems will continue to occupy a central place in the evolution of computing capabilities to facilitate the efforts of those in the "think" professions. Competitive pressures and public efforts to contain health care costs will motivate health care providers to seek greater productivity in the knowledge professions. Expert systems will not replace nursing decision-makers and problem-solvers, but they do promise to serve them as effective "intelligent assistants," relieving them of many of the more routine and repetitive tasks which consume much of their time.

It is ultimately the task of nursing administrators to judge whether it is possible and economically feasible to develop and use expert systems in specific areas of practice, administration, and education. This brief examination of expert systems is intended to provide nursing administrators with some of the essential aspects of expert systems development that must be considered. Some of the knowledge bases which underlie the activities of the professional nurse appear to meet the necessary criteria which have been discussed, but nursing administrators will have to assume the leadership role in advocating and facilitating exploration of promising applications. Indeed, given the rapid pace of expert system development and use, it is quite possible that a number of nursing administrators are currently involved in such efforts.

REFERENCES

1. Borthick AF, West OD. Expert systems: a new tool for the professional. Accounting Horizons March 1987;9.

2. Ernst CJ. A relational expert system for nursing management control. Human Systems Management 1984;4(4):286.

3. Moose A. Shafer D. V-P Expert rule-based expert system development tool. Berkley: Paperback Software International, 1987;ix.

4. Waterman DA. A guide to expert systems. Reading, MA: Addison-Wesley, 1986;xvii.

5. Bell HA. Applied artificial intelligence: The Marquette University automated advising system (MARACAS). Milwaukee: Marquette University College of Business Administration, 1987.

6. Ryan SA. An expert system for nursing practice. J Med Syst 1985;9(1/2):29-41.

7. Schultz SI. Languages, DBMSs, and expert systems: software for nurse decision making. J Nurs Adm 1984;14(12);15-24.

8. Laborde JM. Expert systems for nursing? Comput Nurs 1984;2(4):130-135.

9. Bloom KC, Leitner JE, Solano JL. Development of an expert system prototype to generate nursing care plans based upon nursing diagnoses. Comput Nurs 1987;5(4):140-145.

10. Ozbolt JG, et al. A proposed expert system for nursing practice: a springboard to nursing science. J Med Syst 1985;9(1/2):57-68.

11. Coopers and Lybrand. C&L chairman discusses information management. Executive Briefing May 1987. (ExperTAX is a registered service mark of Coopers and Lybrand.)

12. Coopers and Lybrand. Survey on using expert systems in business. Executive Briefing November 1986.

Technological imperative and decision support

ROBERT P. HEANEY, MD, FACP

Introduction

I WANT TO SHARE with you some thoughts about what I see to be the major problem confronting our Health Care System today. Virtually everyone in the health professions has his or her own view about what is wrong, and undoubtedly the issues are complex. A typical list would include high cost, commercialism, malpractice liability, scandalous neglect of the indigent, government and third party interference — among a host of others. But, in my view, the principal problem is not any of these. Rather it is the very technology upon which the system is now based. For despite a literal explosion in our capacity to intervene effectively in the course of human illness, we have developed essentially no means to help us decide when we shall do so, or in whom, or to what extent, or with what means, or finally, for what purpose.

Technological imperative

The result is that our expanded technology has become essentially self-directed. What has evolved is what economist Victor Fuchs called, 20 years ago, the technological imperative.[1] Expressed in simplest terms, the technological imperative translates to "We can; therefore we must." And from the patient's point of view that often can be paraphrased as "The physician can; therefore I must let him." In both cases — for physician and for patient — choices are effectively proscribed. I, as physician, must do everything possible to you or for you; and you, as patient, must let me do it. No one seems to be free. Both patient and physician are equally captives. Can it

be true that no one has a choice? Are there no rational alternatives? I believe there are. The question can be refocused, therefore, to how can good decisions — real decision — be made in this kind of climate?

Human illness is almost never a trivial situation, even when the character of the illness is objectively minor. It is anxiety-provoking, it creates dependency, and it inevitably impairs judgment. It changes who I am: I become a *patient,* an *unwhole* person. It involves what Pellegrino calls the "wounded humanity" of the patient.[2] These impairments are worsened in the face of truly serious disorders. Then a deep sense of responsibility descends upon both provider and patient — a responsibility for the provider to spare no effort — leave no stone unturned — in order to do what is best for the patient, and the responsibility of the afflicted patient to do what is expected or prudent. The result too often is that the provider does all that is possible. Then this course almost invariably gets defined as giving the best possible care.

And yet we know from experience that "everything possible" simply cannot be synonymous with best. We have countless examples of the havoc wrought by excessive or inappropriate medical interventions. Every one of us is all too familiar with the many heroic interventions that occur at the end of life, ranging from the initiation of renal dialysis in permanently comatose patients, multiple cardiovascular resuscitations in the final week of life of people dying of multiple myeloma — the examples are too numerous and too painful to recount. Such unrestrained use of technology produces almost uniformly bad results —

increased suffering for all and huge costs that strain the health care financing system.

If one reads what is written by the people who do these things, one gets a clear sense of why Fuchs was right when he referred to what is happening as an "imperative." For they literally feel that they must. Robert J. White, a neurosurgeon at Case Western, in an article in *America* magazine entitled "Bioethical Shock,"[3] described four cases that he handled in a single week, each of which was incurably damaged or ill, and each of which he snatched from the jaws of death, at what he himself conceded was enormous financial, personal and psychological cost to all concerned. In no one of the four did he improve health status. And yet he seemed convinced that he was doing the right thing. He concluded his article with a statement of his own personal belief: "I have always struggled personally with this issue by simply offering and counseling that every single thing be done for each and every patient who comes into my area of responsibility." A textual analysis of his article reveals the operation of the technological imperative in his very choice of words —"need," "must," "requirement," "urgently needed," "had to"— over and over.

We see the technological imperative operative in other situations, as well. One example — but only one of many — is what happens when an otherwise ostensibly well person gets a label, particularly a label of some dread disease, most often "cancer." In addition to all the usual stages of reaction to loss that occur in such situations, there is finally one of fear and submission. As a result patients too often let things be done to them for which there is no good medical basis, which succeed only occasionally, and even then, often at unacceptable costs. They are, literally, desperation measures. Confronted then with a predictably bad outcome, one often hears "But, what choice did he have?" The

clear fact that there so often seems to be no choice underscores both why the problem is called an "imperative" and why there so badly needs to be good decision support mechanisms for patients and families facing such problems.

But the technological imperative is operative whenever there is an opportunity to intervene, either diagnostically or therapeutically, not just when life is threatened. There is the pervasive need to know, to find a cause, to make a diagnosis, and to try to fix what is broken.

Problem

Why is that a problem? Why is doing everything possible not the same thing as providing the best possible care? While we all recognize the excesses to which I have alluded, we somehow curiously interpret them as exceptions. Something unintended went wrong, something that couldn't have been predicted. We believe it probably won't happen next time. But that very attitude illustrates the pervasiveness of the technological imperative, the seductiveness of its power, and the extraordinary faith that we have placed in the ability of technology to intervene effectively in the course of our lives. The sober truth is that problems such as I have alluded to are not, in fact, exceptions. Rather, they are inherent in the nature of the medical interventions available to us, and they beset all such intervention.

Virtually all of our medical interventions have both good and bad effects, and both are probabilistic, in the sense that we cannot predict them with accuracy in any given case, though we often can do so, on average, in a large number of cases. There is both a chance of helping and a chance of hurting. There is nothing much new about that insight. It is the familiar relationship between risks and benefits, a relationship we have examined in far more detail in the context of the ethics of human investigation. Curiously we seem to believe that the principle is somehow less applicable in the context of illness intervention. I suspect we are too often trapped in an intention ethic which allows us to neglect the bad outcomes simply because they are not intended. The fact that we are trying to help the patient seems to justify exposing him or her to almost any risk. That, unfortunately, is a classic example of denial. The fact is: We directly cause those bad outcomes when we choose to intervene, and we cannot escape the moral responsibility for their occurrence.

The system needs to take a hard-headed approach to this issue, an approach that balances the chances of making things worse with the chances of making things better, and one that involves the patient to the point where he or she can make a truly informed decision. This is extraordinarily difficult for the patient to do under the pressure and anxiety that evoked by the sense of unwholeness that follows labeling with a dread disease.

There is a second reason why the problem looms large for us, and that is because of confusion in the health professions about what is the real purpose of medical intervention.

Most of the interventions we are talking about, particularly with serious disease, have as their ostensible goal cure or life extension. It might seem, at first blush that these are reasonable objectives. But over and over again, in application, they are seen to break down, to be inadequate. They are inevitably inappropriate when we confront the reality of our inescapable dissolution and death, with all the human needs that attend both. A moment's reflection reveals that they are equally ill-suited for many of the problems of the elderly and for dealing with most chronic diseases.

Many would suggest, and I among them, that a more appropriate statement of the purpose of medicine — and therefore to some extent of all of the health professions — is not the preservation of life, but the maintenance

and restoration of health, of functional capacity, of relational capacity even. And I would add that no therapeutic intervention should be undertaken that does not have such restoration as its object, and no action counseled that does not have a reasonable probability of achieving that end — of sustaining or improving the health status of the patient. But we don't do that. If you look at how we act you could draw only one conclusion: that we are locked in combat with death, with the ultimate purpose of medicine, therefore, being the extension of life, holding death at bay for as long as possible. Michael DeBakey expressed this attitude very clearly in a recent interview.[4] He said, "You fight all the time, and you never really can accept it. You know in reality that everybody is going to die, but you try to fight it, to push it away, hold it away with your hands."

Of the many problems with this approach, not least is the fact that center stage is occupied by the technology, by the health care providers, by the struggle itself, and only rarely by the patient. The dignity and worth of the individual human being become distinctly marginal. The patient becomes both battlefield and prize. Fuchs argues that nations involved in all-out war provide the only analog to this operation of the technological imperative in medical care. In both situations — nations at war with enemies and physicians at war with death — a single-minded purpose — to win — stands above all others and eclipses them completely. The patient has become a means to an end...winning. It is entirely like destroying Vietnamese villages to save them from communist domination.

To sum up, the technological imperative is a problem both because we are confused about our purposes and because we have failed to appreciate the inherently probabilistic nature of the outcomes of our interventions, and have concentrated only on the outcomes we intended. The results, as I have already noted, are that — despite good intentions — we are too often doing more harm than good. Further, such interventions are inherently expensive, contributing to the runaway cost problems that beset the system.

Potential solutions

Given the cost pressures alone, it seems inevitable that the system will find ways to regulate the use of the technology. But it is not at all certain that that regulation will be of the right sort, or that it will not simply add new problems as it seeks to solve old ones. One is put in mind of the many attempts to cap expenditures, of recent experience with regional health planning councils and their attempts to control, for example, the proliferation of CAT scanners. But whenever costs are the primary motivating factor for such regulation, the outcome will almost always be bad.

What the system needs instead is a patient care manager — someone who combines the roles of patient advocate, knowledgeable advisor, and channel of access to the system — someone to help patient and family choose wisely when they are unavoidably disabled by both the unbridgeable knowledge gulf between them and the health care professionals and the anxiety always evoked by illness, particularly illness that is actually or perceptually serious. What is needed is someone who knows the system, knows what the technology can and cannot do, and yet can stand back from it far enough to have a reasonable perspective.

Who can be found to do this?

[Masters-prepared social workers], in some quarters, are seeking to move into this role. It is entirely possible, even, that MBAs may come to function in this capacity, though the reasons for their involvement would, in my judgment, be all the wrong ones, and I would suspect that the results would be quite unsatisfactory. (Nevertheless, I am realistic enough to recognize that cost pressures alone may produce precisely this outcome.)

Physicians taken as a group will surely *not* be the ones to meet this need, though they clearly claim this activity as part of their turf. The reasons are many.

First is the context of uncertainty in which all physicians must operate. This uncertainty tends to be interiorized by the physician. We inevitably feel that if only we had read more widely, or remembered better, or studied harder, or simply had better skills, we would know what to do in this case, or would be able to do it better. We feel that both our own uncertainty and the patient's failure to do well are somehow our fault. They usually are not, but one can almost never be sure of that. This inescapably creates a great pressure to act. In effect, the technology, unused, reproaches the physician. It is precisely the physician's sense of duty, of professional responsibility, the physician's awareness of his or her own too palpable limitations, which fuel this urge to intervene.

A second reason is the dominance within the profession of medicine — and indeed the success therein — of the illness-cure paradigm — identifying and fixing what is broken. The associated mechanistic view of human illness inevitably reinforces the technological imperative. We may rightly criticize the paradigm; we may cite instances in which it is not applicable — such as in dealing with many of the problems of the elderly. But we would be seriously mistaken if we denied either its power or its success. Nevertheless, while it has worked wondrously well, it is not the only approach, nor is it the best one for all situations. But all too often physicians cannot conceive of any other approach: they have *the* way of truth. Illness-cure is the dominant paradigm out of which medicine now operates.

Physicians are thus socialized into a culture formed by this paradigm and dominated by the very technology we are talking about. Inevitably therefore, they tend to define problems in the terms of that technology — what it can and cannot do. "To a hammer all the world looks like a nail." This is not to ridicule my professional colleagues; rather it is to point out why we should no longer expect them to be able to fill this patient advocate, knowledgeable advisor role.

Finally, there are two more reasons why physicians are not likely to fill this role. These reasons are not inherent in the patient-physician transaction, as are the two I have just described, but they are very much involved in the way we practice medicine in this country today. They are, first, conflicts of interest, and second liability pressures. Doing more than is good for the patient is almost always personally remunerative for the physician, and at the same time it is also a better defense against malpractice litigation.

If not medicine, who then? This brings us, inevitably, to nursing. Of all the health professions, nursing seems clearly the one best suited to move into this role. It fits nursing's paradigm like a glove. It emphasizes enabling patients in their own decisions, reflecting and respecting the patients' own values. To paraphrase Virginia Henderson, it is doing for patients what they would do for themselves if they could.[5] The role of care manager would not of course be nursing's only role, and not every nurse would want, or could carry, the responsibility. Nevertheless, I see it to be an extension of contemporary professional nursing. Further, it would not take major changes in the nursing curriculum to prepare professional nurses for this role.

Unfortunately, professional nursing is in a state of flux, and has been consumed, for good reasons, with intraprofessional issues for at least the past 20 years — perhaps longer. While I am personally convinced that nursing could fill this need, I am not at all certain that the profession will be able to position itself appropriately within our system. Frankly, I don't know what its best strategy may be. Possibly, rather than trying to change the whole profession — which may not be feasible — it may be better for a single school of nursing, together with a large health care system such as a well-established, population-based HMO, to commit itself to experimenting with such a solution.

In any event, I am persuaded that the system needs this role. I can only hope that nursing will rise to the challenge.

REFERENCES

1. Fuchs, V.R. The growing demand for medical care. New Engl J Med 279:192, 1968.

2. Pellegrino, E. Toward a reconstruction of medical morality: the primacy of the act of profession and the act of illness. J Med Phil 4:32-56, 1979.

3. White, R.J. Bioethical Shock. America, Feb. 28, 1987, pp. 174-176.

4. DeBakey, M. Lifesaving Michael DeBakey, St. Louis Post Dispatch, March 18, 1987.

5. Furukawa C. and Howe J. Virginia Henderson. In: Nursing Theories, pp. 49-72. Prentice-Hall, Inc., Englewood Cliffs, New Jersey, 1980.

U N I T   T H R E E

Study questions

Chapter Eight

As you read these articles, distinguish anticipated impacts from actual impacts. Try to distinguish actual policy from the way health care
administrators implement it.

1. Do you support government involvement in
the financing of health care? If so, why? If not,
why not?

2. Do you support government involvement in
establishing health care policy? If so, why?
How should this be done? If not, why not?

3. In your opinion, have prospective payment
systems (PPSs) adversely affected public
health?

4. How have PPSs changed nursing practice?

5. Does your philosophy of nursing include responsibility for cost-effectiveness?

6. Should nursing support a PPS approach for
all insurers of health care?

Chapter Nine

7. Why do you believe the current nursing
shortage exists? Which authors in this chapter
present the most convincing data and arguments? Which authors present the least convincing data and arguments?

8. Which authors' solutions to the nursing
shortage do all or most of the others agree

with? Which solutions are unique to a particular author or group? How would you prioritize
the Commission on Nursing's recommendations?

9. Should nursing education be modeled after
medical education? Do we need fewer better-
trained nurses and more less-well-trained assistants? Can technology replace some of the
work of nurses? What will improve nurse-physician working relationships?

Chapter Ten

As you read these articles, answer the following questions:

10. Who should resolve the conflicts and turf
battles that are emerging as the nursing profession changes to conform with societal
changes? Who does resolve them? Does organized medicine have too much control over
the health care system?

11. Is the "knowledge gap" between changes
in nursing practice and nursing faculties' subsequent perception of them just a natural part
of life, or can nursing do something to bring
practice and education closer together? What
would you propose? How would you ensure
that schools of nursing produce nurses with the
skills needed in the work place?

12. What data should be collected, and from
whom, to determine the desirability of new
roles for nurses?

Chapter Eleven

As you read these articles, reflect on the following issues:

13. Under what circumstances would you recommend the introduction of a new medical technology?

14. Under what circumstances would you support the use of a new (or old) medical technology for an individual patient?

15. If charting can be done more effectively through computers, who should decide whether or not it will be done that way?

16. How have you been prepared to use and evaluate new medical technologies?

17. In your opinion, what nursing functions will soon be done through robotics? Will technology replace nurses?

18. How can nurses ensure meaningful and safe use of new technologies in the current health care system?

19. Under what circumstances might a nurse see technology as "the enemy"?

20. Under what circumstances might a nurse see technology as a friend?

U N I T   T H R E E

Additional assignments

1. Identify one new medical technology introduced in a hospital unit, nursing home setting, or home care service. Interview the nursing staff to determine their understanding of the new technology, including its development, evaluation, application, contraindications, and side effects. Also ask the staff about their roles in decision making regarding the use of the technology and its applications for individual patients. Do their answers indicate the institution has adequate policies for using new technologies? Is anyone evaluating the cost-effectiveness of the technology?

2. Is your state experiencing a nursing shortage? If the answer is yes, talk with several directors of nursing service from various settings and determine how the shortage has affected patient care. Compare the strategies used locally to mitigate the shortage with those recommended by the Secretary of Health and Human Services' Commission on Nursing (see Chapter Nine).

3. Interview the presidents of your state medical and nursing organizations regarding the American Medical Association's proposal for a new health care worker, the registered care technologist (see Chapter Nine). How do their positions compare with those of the national leadership? Are new categories of personnel being used in your area? If the answer is yes, compare those workers to nurse's aides and licensed practical nurses.

4. Interview staff nurses from a local hospital regarding the impact of prospective payment systems. Compare their responses to those of staff from magnet hospitals (see Chapter Eight). Explain the similarities and differences in the responses you receive.

5. Write a letter to the editor of *Academic Medicine* regarding Kassebaum's and Pounds' perceptions of the profession and of nursing education (see Chapter Nine).

UNIT FOUR

The sociopolitical environment and nursing practice

EVERY SOCIOPOLITICAL TREND and phenomenon directly influences the practice of nursing. Yet nurses stood poised in the sociopolitical wings for many years, observing others playing major roles in the formation of health policy and benefiting their own professions and organizations. Eventually, that "understudy" experience made clear to nurses the advantages of active participation in the political process; for some, it provided the skills and courage needed to go "onstage" alone.

These courageous pioneers inspired many other nurses to become politically active and to focus not only on the "why" of politics but also on the "how." In many instances, the results have been gratifying: Nurses are interacting with members of Congress and with policymakers at state and local levels, developing networks for influencing the policymaking process at the most opportune times.

Assuming leadership roles
As reported in Unit Three, although nursing did not assume the leadership for change in health care financing, it did adopt a stance of maintaining concern for patient welfare as a higher priority. This safeguarding of nursing tradition is vital to our view of ourselves as nurses — but there are times when nursing

needs to assume the leadership role, and even take political action, to bring about change. This is true not only in the health care community but also in the political community.

Political involvement of nurses is not new, but it is not as strong as many think it should be. This unit focuses on trends in society that will affect nursing practice and that may force more nurses to assume political leadership.

Issues to be addressed include the following:

1. Certain groups in today's society, such as the elderly, the homeless, the poor (especially in the area of prenatal care), and the increasing numbers of AIDS patients, are underserved in our health care system. Is nursing's role not only to provide care as needed but also to change the inequities in the system?

2. Major demographic changes are occurring in the United States. What are the implications of these shifts for nursing practice and education?

3. America has changed from an industrial society to an information society. In this new sociopolitical environment, should we categorize ourselves as "knowledge workers" or "technology workers"? What does today's society need from nursing?

4. Many people view politics as a corrupt

process. How can nursing become involved in the political process without compromising its standards? What are the professional and personal benefits associated with being politically active?

Nursing's past political involvement

As long ago as the late 19th century — when women did not even have the right to vote — some nurses used the political process to improve public health by initiating legislation to create state nurse practice acts. The first nurse practice act was passed in 1903; by 1914, 40 other states had passed similar legislation. During the same era, nurses such as Lavinia Dock and Lillian Wald were visible forces for social change, advocating hospital reform, child labor legislation, and minimum wage standards for working women. These leaders felt that nursing needed to include social issues in its political agenda, not just professional ones.

By the 1950s, nurses were firmly entrenched in political activity, with an office of the American Nurses' Association (ANA) established in Washington to provide increased political support and visibility for nursing. By the 1970s, state nursing groups were establishing liaisons with the ANA to form nonpartisan, voluntary political action units for nursing. The units' goals included: educating nurses on political issues, helping nurses organize to take political action, and raising funds for selected candidates for public office.

Today's sociopolitical issues in health care

According to the ANA (1980), nursing has leadership responsibilities in five major sociopolitical areas today:

1. Organization, delivery, and financing of health care

2. Continuing development of health care resources, including technology and human resources

3. Implementation of preventive and environmental measures to protect public health

4. Development of new knowledge and technology through research

5. Health care planning as a matter of national policy under the National Health Planning and Resources Development Act of 1974 (Public Law 93-164).

Many legislators view nursing as a profession that is genuinely concerned with the health of the American public, even when that stance places nursing in opposition to the vested interests of other major health care professions. For example, in contrast to the American Dental Association, nursing favored water fluoridation legislation. And in contrast to the American Medical Association, nursing favored Medicare legislation. Nursing has also supported federal funding for nursing education, nursing research, and health care financing that would allow direct reimbursement for nursing services.

Nurses are also highly aware, and must make legislators more aware, of the growing problem of inadequate access to health care for many of our nation's citizens. Without significant alteration in our current health care policy, the number of Americans with little or no health insurance or access to health care is likely to increase because of changing demographics and rising health care costs. Will nurses care enough about health care as a basic human right to formulate and advocate new, more equitable health care policies?

In the ANA's *Nursing: A Social Policy Statement,* published in 1980, the authors clearly established the interrelatedness of nursing, society, and politics:

> Nursing, like other professions, is an essential part of the society out of which it grew and with which it has been evolving. Nursing can be said to be owned by society, in the sense that nursing's professional interest must be

and must be perceived as serving the interests of the larger whole of which it is a part.

As noted in the ANA's *Social Policy Statement,* the profession of nursing has leadership responsibility for influencing public health policy in directions that serve society's interests. This can be difficult when health care is viewed as a for-profit industry in which vested interests wield strong influence. For example, some sectors of the industry want health insurance to provide reimbursement only for care provided by physicians, not by nurse practitioners, regardless of the quality of care nurse practitioners can provide.

Aiken (1982), a nurse actively involved in influencing federal health policy, describes public policy and nursing's efforts as follows:

Public policy in health is the continuous process whereby health professionals, institutions, and industry interact with legislators, the executive branch of government, and the judiciary to determine the role government will play in the health sector. The process and products of federal health policy are aimed at improving the health care of the public and shaping the environment of those who work in health care.

Public policy formulation includes the following: the way issues are raised on the public agenda; the process by which laws are passed committing resources to programs that affect people; the development of rules and regulations that interpret statutes; the actual process of program implementation; and the evaluation of the usefulness of the program that provides the basis for continuing program revisions. Policymakers are not faced with a given problem; rather, they have to identify and formulate each problem to be addressed. The interaction that results in the formulation of the problem is a critical stage in the public policy process. Once the problem is formulated and moved to the public agenda, the re-

sulting programs are incremental in nature rather than total reformulations of previous programs or policies....

Federal health policies affect health care providers in four ways. The first and most important is that the federal government pays for health care for the poor and the elderly. Second, federal health manpower programs support the training of health care providers in order to influence the supply, composition, or distribution of the work force. Third, many of the new ideas and innovations in clinical care come from federally supported research, and fourth, federal programs provide capital support for new and renovated health care facilities, including nursing and medical schools, hospitals, community health centers, and rural clinics.

The nursing profession has attempted to leverage these four types of federal strategies to bring about improvements in areas of prominent concern to nurses. Six issues that have been the focus of concern are as follows:

1. Removing financial barriers to health care. A major public policy goal of nurses has been to achieve universal health insurance coverage so that no American is denied access to health services because of the inability to pay for needed care.

2. Improving the quality of nursing care available. The primary strategy advocated by nurses to improve quality has been to broaden the education of nurses and change the mix to include a higher proportion of nurses with baccalaureate and higher degrees.

3. Ending the shortage of hospital nurses. Since World War II there has been a persistent shortage of hospital nurses that has in recent years become more acute despite a doubling of the number of nurses in practice. Given the failure of local institutions or state groups to resolve the shortage, nurses (and other providers) have looked to the federal government for

assistance in finding a national solution.

4. Improving nurses' economic rewards. Nurses' incomes have not kept pace with incomes of comparable professional groups. Low relative incomes are associated with high levels of dissatisfaction, problems with nurse retention, and declining enrollments in nursing schools.

5. Expanding nurses' independent roles within hospitals. The rapid growth of knowledge and technology and changing medical practice patterns have made the traditional social contact between nurses, physicians, and hospitals incompatible with nurses' changing responsibilities in hospitals.

6. Developing new professional roles outside the hospital. National concerns about the delivery of effective and affordable health care have resulted in the evolution of new roles for nurses in ambulatory care and research.

Aiken's six areas of public health policy parallel the major issues presented in this book and particularly in this unit, which stresses that nursing continues to speak for those who are underserved in the health care system both directly and through action to change public policy. Nurses can be proud of these important contributions, but we must recognize the need for more nurses to be involved in the political process at every level of government. In particular, the poor, the homeless, and AIDS patients need health care professionals who will serve as advocates for their cause.

Our evolving society

Naisbitt (1982), in calling attention to 10 new directions that were transforming our lives, provided an excellent picture of how society evolves — and accurately predicted some phenomena that have occurred since 1982. Naisbitt's 10 megatrends and their implications for health care follow.

Trend 1. From an industrial society to an information society. In this new era, the strategic resource is information; it is in this context that nurses must identify themselves as either knowledge workers or technology workers.

Trend 2. From forced technology to "high tech/high touch." Advanced technology must accommodate basic human needs and emotions; otherwise, society will reject the technology. For example, in health care, at the same time that high tech was being advocated in all labor and delivery rooms, home births became more popular. Then, low-tech birthing rooms were developed in hospitals.

Trend 3. From a national economy to a world economy. Our changing economic position in the world market is made even more complex by production sharing — manufacturing taking place in countries around the world regardless of where the products will eventually be sold. In health care, drugs and technologies developed in France or Japan are used in many different countries, and American physicians and nurses assist wherever health crises arise, such as after the Chernobyl incident in the Soviet Union.

Trend 4. From short-term to long-term. In the short-term business approach, predominant in the United States, them future is sacrificed for this years' bottom line. This contrast sharply with management practices in countries such as Japan, where a healthy future is the goal. In the long-term view, business survival depends on constant strategic reconceptualization to prepare for change. For example, if nursing defines itself only in terms of illness care, and disease-free environments are developed, nursing could become obsolete unless long-term planning has been done.

Trend 5. From centralization to decentralization. Centralized structures are disappearing and America is being rebuilt from the bottom up into a stronger, more balanced, more diverse society. Decentralization empowers people at the grass roots level and is the great facilitator of social change. In health care, hospitals are reducing top-level managerial staff and increasing the authority of the department heads, many of whom are head nurses.

Trend 6. From institutional help to self-help. America's traditional sense of self-reliance has come full circle after a period of dependence on the government, the medical establishment, the school system, and other institutions. In health care, people are moving away from dependence on the medical profession to a self-help approach stressing health promotion and disease prevention, diet, exercise, reduced stress, and healthy life-styles.

Trend 7. From representative democracy to participatory democracy. Instead of electing someone to represent them, Americans are demanding and getting a greater direct voice in the institutions and organizations that surround them. Furthermore, consumers are voting with their wallets, and the business sector, from car manufacturers to fast food restaurants, is listening. Even hospitals have become more responsive to patient complaints and patient satisfaction surveys.

Trend 8. From hierarchies to networking. In our formerly industrial society, American businesses and institutions tended to be organized in hierarchical structures, with power and communication flowing down from the top. Today, a nonhierarchical peer networking model is replacing the hierarchical system, which was associated with frustration, impersonality, inertia, and failure. In health care, some hospitals in the United States have implemented quality circles and are eliminating middle managers by designating head nurses as department heads.

Trend 9. From North to South. America is restructuring from North to South in terms of population, wealth, and economic development. According to Naisbitt, California, Florida, and Texas are the three megastates, and a Los Angeles/Houston "axis" for the flow of jobs, money, and influence will replace the economic and financial axis that tied business activities between New York and Chicago. In health care, it will be interesting to see if the major hospitals of the future will be in the megastates.

Trend 10. From either/or choices to multiple options. The social upheaval of the late 1960s paved the way for the less restrictive, multiple-option society of the 1980s. No longer do people rely on strictly "either/or" choices, such as male or female for certain types of jobs. In health care, nurses no longer have to stop working to raise families or go to school, and they can hold leadership positions regardless of their gender or marital status.

The influence of current health care concepts and conditions

As Naisbitt reminds us, times change. Today, we are witnessing profound changes, such as the prevalence of certain types of diseases, the demographic changes taking place in our society, and the problem of entire subpopulations whose health care needs are not being fully met. Just as Naisbitt's 10 trends are transforming our entire society, so these sociopolitical changes promise to transform our system of health care and particularly the practice of nursing.

Nurses must be ready to reconceptualize who we are, what we are, and where we are going — again and again. We must also develop a process for change that includes a strong grassroots base, reflects the needs of society, and has the support of practicing nurses.

Changing health care emphasis and costs

Fries (1985), speaking at a conference for nursing leaders, called attention to the natural evolution in health care and the expenditure of health care dollars. In the 20th century, we have gone from a period in the early 1900s when most medical expenses were used to treat acute infectious disease (such as scarlet fever, influenza, and tuberculosis) to more recent times when most medical expenses have been used to treat chronic, noninfectious illnesses (such as cancer, hypertension, diabetes, emphysema, and arthritis). That period is ending, says Fries, and we are entering an era when disorders related to aging and stressful life-styles will absorb most of our health care dollars.

According to Fries, the medical model — with its biomedical research base and its emphasis on curing disease — is totally inadequate for this new era of health care problems. Therefore, he believes, a window of opportunity may be opening for nurses.

Fries sees two new types of nursing careers, one based in institutions and the other based in the community. The first would involve helping patients learn self-care (particularly elderly patients, whose numbers will double by the turn of the century); the second would involve educating the public about good health care practices.

Nursing needs to respond to these opportunities quickly by ensuring that nurse practice acts incorporate these new roles, by establishing standards of practice for them, and by altering nursing education programs to include content and learning experiences appropriate to them. Furthermore, nursing must actively advocate the adoption of health care policy that provides for adequate financing for new and evolving nursing services.

Needed: Facts, figures, action

As nurses move onto the sociopolitical stage, they are recognizing that arguments cannot be put forth, opponents cannot be persuaded, and advantageous laws cannot be enacted without facts and figures demonstrating the value of nursing to the individuals and communities it serves. First encountered as nurses fought for recognition and reimbursement in service agencies, this realization is now being underlined as a basic tool in effective policy formation — which in turn will affect care in those same agencies (Phillips 1982).

Will nurses fight for more responsible roles in our changing health care system and for humanitarian health policy at the state and national levels? Will the present inequities in our delivery of health care raise the level of concern among nurses, shaping modern-day Florence Nightingales, Lavinia Docks, and Lillian Walds? We cannot afford to wait and see. We already see the need. And we need to begin the journey.

REFERENCES

Aiken, L.H. (Ed.). (1982). *Nursing in the 1980's: Crises, opportunities, challenges.* Philadelphia: Lippincott.

American Nurses' Association. (1980). *Nursing: A social policy statement.* Kansas City: American Nurses' Association.

Fries, J.F. (1985, July). *The future of disease and treatment: Changing health conditions, changing behaviors, and new medical technology.* Paper presented at "Nursing in the 21st Century," a conference sponsored by the American Association of Colleges of Nursing and the American Organization of Nurse Executives, Aspen, CO.

Lyon, J.C. (1988). AIDS: What are the costs? Who will pay? *Nursing Economics, 6*(5), 241-244.

Naisbitt, J. (1982). *Megatrends: Ten new directions transforming our lives.* New York: Warner.

Phillips, T.P. (1982). Foreword. In American Acacemy of Nursing, *From accommodation to self-determination: Nursing's role in the development of health care policy.* Kansas City: American Academy of Nursing.

Santi, L.L. (1988). The demographic context of recent change in the structure of American households. *Demography, 25*(4), 509-519.

Scearse, P.D. (1988). Public policy: AIDS: Policies and perplexities. *Journal of Professional Nursing, 4*(2), 79-80.

U.S. could become a nation of minorities. (1987, March-April). *The Futurist,* p. 57.

CHAPTER TWELVE

Health care access, costs, and policies

AT THE PRESENT TIME, some segments of the U.S. population have little or no access to health care: the poor, the elderly, ethnic minorities, and the increasing number of Americans who have no health insurance. Many legislators would like to take action to correct this situation, but they are stymied by the need to *reduce* the federal budget, with its staggering burden of health care costs, rather than *enlarge* it by allocating more money for the nation's health care. Furthermore, they are aware that health care costs are currently escalating faster than the inflation rate.

In some states, legislators are considering plans that would ensure equal access to health care for all citizens of the state. In Oregon, for example, the state legislature in 1987 chose to restrict the use of state funds for soft-organ transplants and allocate funds for improved prenatal care; faced with limited resources, the legislature chose to use them for prevention, an act of courage that reflected a set of values regarding state funds and health care.

In 1989, the Oregon legislature is taking another important step by formulating a plan to provide health services to all Oregonians — a plan with important implications for Oregon's nurses. The plan, which emphasizes health promotion, disease prevention, and low utilization of high-technology equipment, is expected to be implemented through contracts with health care professionals, including nurses. Thus, nurses and other health care professionals, such as physicians, will be able to bid for the contracts.

In anticipating the need to equalize health care for all citizens, the Oregon model epito-

mizes some of the major issues involved —access, cost, and public policy. Besides addressing these important issues, this chapter highlights the potential role of nursing under such a plan.

In the article "How Nurses Would Change U.S. Health Care," Huey discusses how nurses would improve access to health services, basing her projections on information from nurses who care for those with limited or no access to health care and from nurses who are trying to fix the system. Their stories are both depressing and anger-provoking, but these nurses also offer a variety of proposals for increasing health care access and financing.

Addressing the health care needs of the elderly is the subject of the next two articles. In "Who Will Care for the Old?" Kovar and Harris discuss the plight of the disabled elderly, who are almost invariably institutionalized in nursing homes despite the ever-rising cost of such care under our present system. Their article illustrates the type of data and data analysis that are essential in developing public policy. In "Health Care and the Aging Population," Dimond provides statistics regarding the health care needs of the elderly and the resources currently available; her article is filled with thought-provoking questions such as, "Given that society has limited resources and multiple goals, what kind of life are we willing to provide for the elderly when meeting their needs requires community funds?"

How do we care for the homeless? What are their major health care needs and problems? Who should pay for their care? In the article "Health Care for the Homeless," Lindsey describes the growing population of homeless people nationwide, then discusses these questions in the context of the Los Angeles program for providing health care for the homeless.

Chow, in "Nursing's Response to the Challenge of AIDS," reviews the AIDS crisis, pointing out the relationship between societal needs, health care, and the political process. She also describes the AIDS program in San Francisco, including the ways nurses in that city used the political process to elect a mayor who supported nurses' vision of health care.

Nothing about the delivery of health care stands in isolation, as these articles reveal. Given the close involvement of nursing in today's sociopolitical and ethical-legal issues, nurses clearly must view themselves and their practice as indissolubly connected to the needs of all our citizens.

How nurses would change U.S. health care

FLORENCE L. HUEY, RN, MA

UNITED STATES CITIZENS have the poorest access to the most expensive health care system in the world. Is our system the best? You'll probably think so if you're having a heart transplant. But if you are a pregnant teen, an unskilled worker trying to have your child immunized for school, or an elder who can't afford dentures, your judgment of the system might be less glowing.

If they could, how would nurses create a better health care system — and how would they pay for it? *AJN* asked nurses who care for those whom the system has failed, as well as nurses who are working on mending the safety net.

Part I: The problem list
For millions of Americans, getting in and through the health care system is a bewildering nightmare with no dawn. Charlotte Katzin, a home care nurse, describes a 50-year-old home health aide with diabetes who is married to a man with a heart condition. Their medicines alone cost up to $100 per month. Though the woman usually works 40 hours a week, she is not considered a full-time employee because she works only when the agency calls her. Thus she has no health insurance.

How often must this woman wince at the irony of providing health care in a system that has left her locked out?

You bet your life. Those who are insured have other nightmares. Consider, for example, an elderly woman who had chronic obstructive pulmonary disease and needed oxygen at home. Her private insurer would pay — but only for three months.

If she needed oxygen after that, she was told to seek Medicaid. "If I apply for Medicaid," she responded, "they will take a lien on my house — which is all I have to leave to my children. I would rather die." Two months later, she did die.

"How many politicians would give up *their* homes for health care?" asks Ora Strickland, professor of nursing at the University of Maryland. "Yet that's what we ask thousands of Americans to do every day to qualify for long-term care."

It seems the ultimate irony that we lack a coherent long-term care program in an era when cures help people survive to acquire chronic problems. Another major irony is that we offer Medicare to the elderly and disabled — those who most need chronic care — yet Medicare emphasizes acute care.

Where does the money go? Throwing money at the system obviously isn't the answer. We pay the most per capita of any industrial nation — $1,800 per person, 11 percent of our GNP goes to health care. Yet, 37 million uninsured Americans depend on health care handouts. Canada offers universal access for $1,300 per capita, 8 percent of its GNP. (See *Health care investments*, p. 323.)

What do we buy with our $500 billion a year? Hospitals and physicians together devour $3 out of every $5 we spend on health care.

While prospective payment may be getting hospital expenditures under control, notes former HCFA head Carolyne Davis, physician costs continue to grow. Medicare Part B, for example — the part that pays MDs — is rising by 17 percent a year.

Thus far, however, getting the acute care

Where our public money goes (calendar year 1987)	
National health expenditures $(in billions)	**496.6**
Hospital care	192.6
Physicians	101.4
Dentists	32.4
Other professionals	16.2
Drugs/supplies	32.8
Eyeglasses/appliances	8.8
Nursing homes	41.6
Other personal care	13.1
Administration and net cost, pvt. insurance	25.9
Government public health	14.4
Research, facility construction	17.3

dollars in hospitals under control really has only shifted the cost to ambulatory care. According to the *1988 Health Trends Chartbook* of the Health Insurance Association of America, as the number of days spent in community hospitals fell from 68 million in 1980 to 57 million in 1986, the number of outpatient visits rose from 55 million to 67 million.

To try to stem this service shifting, Congress directed the Secretary of Health and Human Services to come up with a prospective payment plan for ambulatory surgery by April 1989, and for hospital-based and free-standing clinic care by 1990.

While the squeeze is tightened on institutions, what about physicians? All except inpatient radiologists, anesthesiologists, and pathologists are on a diversionary course *away* from prospective payment. The PhysPAC (Physician Payment Assessment Commission) is mostly busy considering a relative value scale (RVS) that proposes to distribute income

more equitably among physicians. It's still a fee-for-service system by another name, however.

Gerrymandered competition. Related to what the system pays physicians is what it *won't* pay nurses and other providers. "We have 30 years of cost-effectiveness data on nurses as primary care providers," notes Claire Fagin, dean of the University of Pennsylvania School of Nursing. Yet nurses are shut out as competitors.

Ada Jacox, director of the Center for Nursing and Health Services Research at the University of Maryland, and Vivian DeBack, who heads the National Commission on Nursing Implementation Project, both point to the extra costs of a system that combines regulation and competition.

"Either one or the other might be more efficient," notes Jacox. Instead, "insurers and state licensing boards regulate who can compete, so nurses are not free to deliver all they can."

Cure wise, prevention foolish. We traipse merrily along, penny wise and pound foolish, cutting the front-end costs of problem prevention and gallantly embracing the rear-end costs of high tech cures.

Hurdis Griffith, now a health policy activist, recalls working as a community health nurse in the slums of Baltimore: "One infant was getting bitten at night by the rats that got into the crib. I could get that baby a CT scan for a headache quicker than I could do anything about the rats or the parents surviving on potato chips and beans."

Rae Grad, RN, executive director of the National Commission to Prevent Infant Mortality, points out that for every $1 invested in prenatal care, $3 to $10 are saved.

Custodial care over the lifetime of a low birth-weight (LBW) infant can cost $400,000, says the Commission. The nation spends about $2 billion on hospital care to keep LBW infants alive for their first year. For a quarter of that cost — about $500 million — we could provide prenatal care to all women who now go without.

When we overspend on high tech and get a cure, we feel we've gotten something for our money. But have we?

Linda Aiken, trustee professor at the University of Pennsylvania School of Nursing, points to William Kannel's classic study of the cost effectiveness of ICUs: "He discovered that about 25 percent of patients who receive intensive care in our hospitals don't benefit because they are not sick enough. Another 8 percent don't benefit because they are moribund, so the care will not change the outcome. That is one-third of all people who use intensive care."

Last but hardly least is how much we pay people to manage the system: Administration of health insurance in the U.S. costs about 22 cents on the dollar compared to about 2.5 cents in Canada.[1] The reason: Canada has essentially one payer — the government.

The U.S. government also pays for health services, but in fragments. For a monthly premium, Medicare Part B pays partial medical costs. No premium is paid for Part A, which partially covers acute hospital costs for the elderly and disabled. Less than half (44%) the hospital and medical charges are covered.[2]

Medicaid's maze. The federal government, matching what states put up out of their general revenues to fund care for the indigent, also pays for health care via Medicaid — a means-tested obstacle course through which those in need of care must pass to prove their eligibility of coverage.

The rules of the game and the benefits vary according to the largess and creativity of each state. For example, a couple is allowed to have no more than $167 per month income in Tennessee to qualify for Medicaid, while in California, the income limit is $634.[3]

New York has a Medicaid waiver program that will pay for a phone for an AIDS patient

receiving amphotericin at home. Other states offer no more than basic hospital benefits.

Besides the government, we have over 100 commercial insurers — which oversee and pay bills for Medicare, in addition to offering their own complex array of coverages.

Where's the Great Society? The uninsured are grabbing the headlines these days, but their plight is not new. The uninsured have an unbroken history of begging for health care in the U.S.

Until such cost containment strategies as prospective payment entered the picture, however, the leftovers were often generous. Well-paid physicians could afford an occasional bit of noblesse oblige, and hospitals could shift expenses for charity care to third party payers who reimbursed hospitals after-the-fact for their costs (plus a profit).

About the time the uninsured began to be squeezed out of acute care by prospective payment, the Reagan administration's New Federalism swelled their numbers: In one quick chop — the 1981 Omnibus Budget Reconciliation Act (OBRA) — one-half million people lost their eligibility for Medicaid. The Act also gave states more flexibility in cutting their health budgets.[4]

Some indigent families found themselves without health care coverage when Medicaid eligibility was tied to qualifications for other federal programs. When, for example, the allowable income for Aid to Families with Dependent Children (AFDC) was lowered, single mothers who no longer qualified became ineligible for Medicaid, as well.

Uncharitable acts. When an entire category of adults lost their Medicaid eligibility, according to a story told in *America's Health Safety Net,* at least one California private hospital distributed maps telling indigent patients how to take public transportation to the nearest county hospital. The "helpful" map even advised patients, "Don't forget to ask for a bus transfer, which is 10 cents."[5]

O Canada

Some look longingly at Canada's health care system as a model the U.S. should adopt. We don't hear stories from our northern neighbors of long waits for care delivered by too few providers as we do of the British system. So *AJN* asked the Canadian Nurses Association's Executive Director Ginette Rodger to describe how our northern neighbors run their system:

The system, set up in the 1950s to provide hospital care and expanded in the 1960s to include physician care, has five basic principles:
1. Universality: All Canadians have access to this service regardless of income or need.
2. Portability: When people go from one province to another, they have the same type of coverage.
3. Comprehensiveness: All services provided by the hospital—drugs, dressings, rooms, surgery—are covered. (Private rooms cost extra.) All physician visits—for anything from an ingrown toenail to open heart surgery—are paid by the government.
4. Accessibility: Health facilities, while not in everyone's backyard, are accessible to everyone.
5. Public administration: The system is run by the government, not by private enterprise.

Paying the bill
Through a contract with the provinces, the federal government refunds to the provinces about 50 percent of the cost of care. The provinces—through various methods, including taxation and premiums—pay the remainder.

Physician's fees are negotiated between each provincial government and the provincial medical association and thus may vary from one province to another. Long-term care and home care are not mandated, so services vary from province to province. In 1985, Canadian nurses asked the government to start insuring community health care providers other than physicians. While the government still doesn't insure community health services, national legislation now allows provinces to insure other health professionals. Unfortunately, the provinces haven't done so in a significant way yet.
Editor's note: A Canadian was good enough to check his pay stub and tells us what he pays for hospital and medical services: $7.44 every two weeks. That works out to $193 per year; with his employer contributing an equal amount, his total premium is $366 per year. The premium is not income related, and the provincial government pays the premium for those who can't pay it themselves.

As Linda Aiken notes, these uncharitable acts hit just as the recession of the late 1970s increased the number of people who lost their insurance along with their jobs.

When the 1981 budget reform consolidated 21 health care programs into four block grants to be administered by states, federal funding dropped 18 percent for such programs as maternal and child health, alcohol and drug abuse, and mental health services.[6] New federalism also brought cuts in nutrition: in food stamps and school lunches.[7]

What we save by limiting access to health care, we spend to treat the complications. In a 3-year demonstration project in California, for example, prenatal care doubled and prematurity rates fell by 40 percent when nurse-midwives provided access to prenatal care to a disadvantaged population. When the program ended (because of physician opposition to nurse-midwives), prenatal care again fell and the prematurity rate returned to the previous level.[8]

Part II: Now what?

In an era of cost containment, we need to reduce the federal deficit, but we cannot, as an affluent nation, notes ANA Executive Director Judith Ryan, RN, "tolerate the unresolved problems of the homeless and the large proportion of our population that has no access to

Health care investments

	TOTAL COST OF HEALTH CARE PER PERSON	WHAT THE GOVERNMENT PAYS PER PERSON	PERCENT PAID BY THE GOVERNMENT	PERCENT OF GNP SPENT ON HEALTH
Australia	$ 904	$ 666	73.7	7.6
Austria	850	575	67.6	7.9
Belgium	792	609	76.9	7.3
Canada	1,282	973	75.9	8.6
Denmark	755	633	83.9	6.2
Finland	832	643	77.3	7.3
France	1,072	763	71.2	9.4
Germany	983	768	78.1	8.1
Greece	252	247	98.2	4.2
Iceland	1,052	873	83.0	8.4
Ireland	536	466	87.0	8.0
Italy	678	569	83.9	7.4
Japan	783	570	72.8	6.6
Netherlands	938	739	78.8	8.3
New Zealand	559	447	80.0	5.6
Norway	917	875	95.4	6.6
Portugal	297	215	72.5	5.7
Spain	456	326	71.5	6.0
Sweden	1,172	1,067	91.0	9.3
Switzerland	1,144	784	68.5	7.9
United Kingdom	627	564	90.0	5.7
United States	1,776	720	41.1	10.8
Mean	$ 848	$ 646	78.1%	7.4%

In 1985, U.S. health care costs, at $1,776 per person, were the highest of the countries listed. Yet, the U.S. spent the smallest proportion of public monies on health—41%, compared with an average of 78% for the countries listed. And, despite our neonatal ICUs, the U.S. currently ranks 19th in infant mortality.

Source: Schieber, G.S. and Poullier, J. Trends in International Health Care Spending. Health Affairs, 6:105-112, Fall 1987.

health care. We need to figure out the most cost effective way to provide universal access to a basic level of services."

Well said, but how shall we proceed? Is there a new direction? Or shall we, as Hurdis Griffith puts it, keep "plugging the holes one by one?"

We put Medicare in place for the elderly and Medicaid for the indigent in 1965. Now, the Catastrophic Act will plug another hole for the elderly and disabled. If the Kennedy bill (for the uninsured) passes, we'll plug another

hole. Then, if we do a Medicaid buy-in (also for the uninsured), that would be another hole plugged. Then, we'll have to do something for the people who can't pay premiums for the Medicaid buy-in. It's a very inefficient way of providing universal access, to have to fight these battles bit by bit."

Beyond inefficiency, Lillian McCreight, director of public health nursing in South Carolina, sees dangers in a plan that "targets specific populations or health problems: As budgets get tight, each piece of coverage narrows and the gaps between coverages widen. We thus create new gaps, and just hope someone will fill them."

Women and children first

If we're going to tackle the problems one by one, Rae Grad wants universal access for maternity care to be first. As a model for what could be, the Commission to Prevent Infant Mortality describes Japan's progress from the rank of 17th in infant deaths, after World War II, to [the lowest infant death rate] today. The U.S. currently ranks 19th.

To follow Japan's lead, the commission wants every pregnant woman to be able to get health care without financial, geographic, or administrative barriers: "Where there are no services, public health departments or local hospitals should establish them. Where there are long forms to fill out, waiting lists, hard-to-reach clinics, poor transportation, lack of child care services, or other administrative barriers, agencies should knock them down," admonishes the commission.

Grad sees such a program as fairly straight-forward to put into place: First, require that private insurers provide maternity coverage. "In 1985, 5 million women had private health insurance that did not include maternity care."

For uninsured women, provide universal access to Medicaid. "Universal access for pre-natal care also means that any child born is eligible for well baby care, immunizations, and so forth. We could make a logical cutoff at 6 years because we could say that at least the child is in the school system. Or we might say 12, so 50 children will be cared for to adolescence. Or 18."

Also concerned with maternity care is Ruth Lubic, CNM, director of the Maternity Center Association in New York City and a pioneer in the development of free-standing birthing centers.

"The view of pregnancy and birth as ill-nesses has led us into an expensive kind of maternity care management," observes Lubic. "If you view pregnancy as pathology and birth as surgery, you obviously will need physicians to intervene." If the woman needs a cesarean section — and twice as many women who go to hospitals as those who go to birthing centers do — the costs can soar to $10,000.

The total charge for a normal delivery in a birthing center is under $2,500 — that includes all prenatal care, education, birth care, and follow-up.

In Lubic's ideal system, every pregnant woman would be triaged to the appropriate level of care through a neighborhood birthing center run by nurse-midwives. This would lower the number of women handled at a level of care they don't require, which should lower the cost of care, as well as the C-section rate, predicts Lubic.

"The provider of choice would match the mother's needs. At least 75 percent — and many estimate more than that — of pregnant women are going to have a normal pregnancy and birth that could be handled by nurse-mid-wives. All the statistics have demonstrated that birthing centers are at least as safe as and, in most instances, have better outcomes than the more conventional physician care."

In 1983, Lubic calculated the savings if even 25 percent of the 3.6 million pregnant American women used birthing centers. She concluded that $717 million to $3.3 billion could be saved.[9]

To test whether a birthing center can make pregnancy care more accessible — and accept-able — to disadvantaged families, the New York Maternity Center is adding a birthing center to a neighborhood primary care center in the South Bronx. Lubic expects to do much more than deliver babies. She thinks the center will eventually become a haven for neighbor-hood teens in trouble. A midwife assistant, a neighborhood woman, will always be present in the center on site, because "You don't always get thrown out of the house at 3 PM; sometimes it's 2 AM."

South Carolina already targets teen pregnancy problems, according to Lillian McCreight. More teens seek family planning — and fewer get to the point of pregnancy or abortion — since schools added the 3-R (reproductive risk reduction) curriculum to teach teens decision making.

For the teens who do become pregnant, resource mothers are extra support. These neighborhood women, trained in nutrition and "every mother" knowledge, encourage the teens to stay with prenatal care and then teach the young mothers baby care.

Over the long term
Linda Aiken, the Robert Wood Johnson (RWJ) Foundation nurse who conceived and nurtured the RWJ Teaching Nursing Home project, places long-term high on the health care agenda.

Aiken is quick to make the point that long term care is a problem not only of the elderly: "About 40 percent of people who now require long-term care are under age 65. Most of them are chronically mentally ill, developmentally disabled, or physically disabled.

"We know from research that between a fourth and a third of the homeless have a history of psychiatric impairment and have been in the psychiatric system at some point. The whole system of long-term care fails when these people end up homeless."

Reverse the incentives. Paying more comprehensively for hospital than for community care is a perverse incentive, especially with the mentally and physically disabled, says Aiken.

"Our insurance programs tend to pay for physician or hospital services. But what these people need most are supportive care and long-term drug management in their communities.

"If you took the same amount of money

that Medicaid is already spending on these people and developed a capitation program, for example, that amount of money could be given to providers who could have more flexibility about how to spend it, and the outcomes would be better.

"Wisconsin did just that. Instead of purchasing care from state hospitals and then giving whatever was left over to the counties to care for people in the communities, the state gave all those monies to the counties. Then, the counties purchased hospital care when they needed it. The less hospital care needed, the more money left to expand community services.

"Counties, therefore, had an incentive to keep people out of the hospital and develop their community services. Wisconsin's outcomes demonstrated that very severely ill people who were formerly treated almost entirely with long-term hospital care could be effectively treated in the community at about the same cost."

What about long-term care for the elderly?
One of the more rational approaches to financing, says Aiken, is to raise the social security tax so that everyone pays a modest amount to provide universal coverage for everyone who needs long-term care — a new "Part C" to Medicare. The primary advantage of a higher social security tax, believes Aiken, would be the formation of the "ultimate" risk pool. Like any other insurable risk, the cost of insurance is less the more you distribute the risk across the population.

The two-year limit. "An alternative, possibly an interim step, to a publicly financed long-term care program might be a public-private mix," suggests Aiken. "The public, via either Medicaid or in a new federal program, would assume responsibility for catastrophic expenses in long-term care. Individuals would pay the front-end costs — for example, the first two years of nursing home care or equivalent home care services — either out of their own pockets or by buying a private insurance policy to cover costs.

"After two years, the federal government, or Medicaid, would pick up the financing of their care without requiring them to 'spend down' to become eligible. Some states are now experimenting with this idea."

High front-end charges to patients would limit the government liability more than universal coverage does, says Aiken. "I believe it would make private insurance more affordable. Private insurers would not have to worry about the long tail of liability for someone, for example, who has Alzheimer's disease and might require 10 years of nursing home care. After the first two years, Alzheimer's would be a catastrophic event, and the public program would kick in.

"This would be a net increase over what is now being provided. Estimates by the Brookings Institution show that such a program would not cost the public budget as much as you might think.

"In our actuarial estimates on the (Joseph) Biden Commission — the Task Force on Long-Term Health Care Policies that reported to Congress last year — we calculated that if, for example, we had a three-year deductible, it would cost something like $3 billion a year in public dollars — that's not astronomical."

How to pay is one part of the long-term care agenda. What to pay for is another. Mathy Mezey, RN, who directs the RWJ Teaching Nursing Home program, points to San Francisco's On Lok program as one of the most imaginative models for long-term care. *Managed care.* On Lok (which is Mandarin Chinese for happy, peaceful abode) is a managed-care program that serves about 300 elderly who would otherwise be in nursing homes. Yet only 11 are in nursing homes now. Plus, On Lok elders average only 3.3 hospital days per year — which is down from 9.9 days in 1980.

At the hub of the program are three day-care centers open seven days a week. The subscription of $2,000 per month is paid one-third by Medicare and two-thirds by Medicaid or private payers. The subscription is still about $1,300 less per month than nursing home care would be in San Francisco, says On Lok's Kate O'Malley, RN.

The monthly subscription covers the day care — staffed with nurses, social workers, a part-time nutritionist, and health workers who assist with personal care — plus, as needed, physician services, home health transportation, hospital and nursing home care.

Best all around

Personally, wouldn't you like to be cared for under the health plan that Kristine Gebbie, RN, director of Oregon's health department, half-jokingly suggests? "At some magic point of debility or age, we would each get a public health nurse who would take care of us, hook us to the system and move us through." The complexity of the system wouldn't matter because we would each have a guide — our own case manager.

In Gebbie's vision, we would have free problem prevention for all, paid out of public health dollars and provided — who knows where? Schools, at the job, maybe in shopping centers. Imagine free stress reduction and nutrition classes, physical exams, prenatal and well child care, parenting classes, child guidance, and counseling.

Gebbie wouldn't expect insurers to pay for health promotion — that would be a public health responsibility. Only sickness care would be billable to insurers — and costs should be minimal for those who have taken advantage of free health promotion and problem prevention services.

Priority on child health. Judith Igoe, RN, director of school health programs at the University of Colorado, also has a proposal high on many nurses' lists.

Finding the funds

On average, industrial countries in the West fund 78 percent of health care costs from public coffers. In the U.S., however, the major burden for health care costs—60 percent—is borne by private insurers or patients themselves. Only 40 percent of health care costs are paid by federal, state, and local governments.

Whether we want to add universal access to health care for children or a coherent long-term care system for the elderly, or both, the bottom-line question is, how will we pay for it?

A federal case

If we go after more federal dollars, where might we find them? Consider the U.S. government's FY 87 income:

$392.557 billion from income tax
$83.926 billion from corporation tax
$303.318 billion from social security tax
$32.457 billion from excise tax (e.g., tobacco and alcohol)
$7.493 billion from estate and gift taxes
$15.085 billion from customs
$19.307 billion from permits, passports, and other miscellaneous receipts.

This total income of $854.143 billion fell about $150 billion short of the $1.004 trillion in 1987 expenditures.

Taking the $45,000 cap off the social security tax is part of several bills proposed as a way to fund long-term care. Now we pay 1¾ percent social security tax on earnings up to $45,000. Estimates of what taking that cap off would add range from a low of $4 billion to a high of $30 billion.

Increasing excise taxes on gasoline, tobacco, and alcohol is another potential federal revenue raiser. In fact, raising the "sin" taxes on cigarettes and alcohol is part of Sen. Edward Kennedy's (D-MA) Life Care Bill to help cover the cost of long-term care.

A very small increase can yield very big returns because of the volume of these items produced and sold. If the excise taxes on cigarettes, wine, beer, and distilled spirits had been raised even to keep up with inflation since 1950, the extra income from excise taxes would be more than $20 billion per year.

Value added tax, or VAT, is sort of a federal sales tax common in other countries. Robert Reischauer of the Brookings Institution suggests that we could totally fund Medicaid—offering national standards and shifting the $24 billion burden off the states—with even a 7% to 10% VAT. That would still give the U.S. a low VAT, especially compared, for example, to Ireland's 25% VAT.

Each percent of a broad-based VAT would bring in about $25 billion. To help poor people most hurt by a VAT, one proposal is to expand the earned income credit.

A designated tax, something like the social security tax, has been suggested as a way to fund universal health care. A designated tax would ensure that the dollars collected went to health care—which a general income tax rise would not do.

Taxing health care benefits, is an unpopular way to increase federal revenues from individual income tax. "No one wants to tax sick people," explained a researcher at the Health Insurance Association of America.

Removing the tax exemption employers now take for health care costs might raise $20 billion a year.

An uncompensated care pool filled with "contributions" from hospitals and insurers is a way many states pay for uncompensated hospital care. Some call this a hidden state tax that ought to be abolished.

Private sources

Americans pay for quite a lot of their health care expenses out of their own pockets. In 1986, for example, we paid 10.6 percent of hospital charges, 18.5 percent of physician charges, 51.5 percent of nursing home charges, 64.5 percent of our dental care, 66.8 percent of costs for eyeglasses and appliances, and 74.9 percent for medicines—all out of pocket.

Mandating employers to provide health insurance increases the private contribution for health care. On Capitol Hill, Kennedy's proposed Minimum Health Benefits For All Workers Act has been around since 1986.

In April, Michael Dukakis, governor of Massachusetts, signed a law that will do for the state what Kennedy proposes for the

continued

Finding the funds *continued*

country. The buildup to get to coverage for all employed people in Massachusetts starts with the establishment, by July 1, 1989, of a health insurance pool for small businesses. A program of tax credits for businesses providing health insurance for the first time also goes into effect in 1989. In 1992, the all-employee program starts.

Kennedy's bill proposes to cover 24 billion of the 37 billion uninsured and cost the taxpayers nothing. The likely reality, of course, is that we will pay through higher priced products. This is said to hurt the people it is intended to help—the working poor who already spend a high portion of their income on goods. Other criticisms are that small businesses will fail or be forced to reduce their work force. Proponents say this litany sounds a lot like the opposition to the minimum wage legislation.

The American Hospital Association, in its 1988 report on private coverage, *Promoting Health Insurance in the Workplace,* raises another problem: Even when health insurance is offered, many workers are unable to afford it. Three out of four uninsured workers earn under $10,000 a year, yet the average employee is required to pay up to 35 percent of the premiums for himself and may need to pay more than 40 percent of the premiums to cover his family. Two-thirds of uninsured workers have employers that offer health insurance, but one-third are unable or unwilling to purchase the coverage and the other third do not qualify for the plan.

Medicaid buy-in, a program that would allow the uninsured working poor to pay premiums, on a sliding scale, to enter the Medicaid program, has been advocated by George Bush. But even with a sliding scale, how many will be able to buy in?

In a 1984 Gallup poll, one out of five families said they couldn't always afford food. When the poor have to decide what top two or three items—food, shelter, clothing, or health insurance—will be purchased, who really believes it will be health insurance?

Long-term IRAs sound like a better approach to funding long-term care than they, in fact, turn out to be. First, this approach only proposes to solve the funding problem for a small portion of those in need. Second, whether or not the amount needed was there would depend a lot on such factors as the inflation rate of long-term care costs in relation to the return on investment.

Private long-term care policies cover less than 1 percent of the elderly, and a 1987 Brookings Institution study estimates that 55 percent of the elderly will never be able to afford private long-term care insurance policies.

To limit liability, Sen. George Mitchell (D-ME) proposed that the federal government pick up 70 percent of the nursing home tab after the first two years. The legislation could spur sales of long-term care insurance policies and thus (it is expected) reduce premiums.

Kennedy's Life Care Bill would make Medicare a long-term care policy by allowing Medicare recipients to purchase optional Medicare coverage for 65 percent of the nursing home bills after the first six months.

About one in four of the 37 million uninsured are children. Because they have no primary care provider, when these children develop health problems, they aren't treated until the problems become severe. And, says Igoe, "when children who have not had ongoing care are hospitalized, they stay twice as long. This not only means cost to the system, but think of the consequences: so many more sick days for children who are poor raises their risk of dropping out of school."

Igoe's idea? A comprehensive school health program with nurses as primary providers. At the core of her proposal is primary care for every child, both to prevent complications and to treat problems early. The second piece is education to promote health. Third is a physically and psychologically healthy environment.

"In a national health care plan, we need to include the fact that nurses do a better job than any other providers in the area of primary care." As one proof, Igoe points to an RWJ study of school health programs that showed school nurse practitioners able to handle 87 percent of the problems with 96 percent resolution, no duplication of services, and for one-quarter of the cost of conventional end-stage care.[10]

Home for health. It is also comforting to think what health care would be like if Elsie Griffith, head of the New York City Visiting Nurse Service, had her way. Griffith agrees with Igoe that we need to care for people where they are. To her, that means at home. In her national health plan, she would make home care the first choice instead of the last resort.

Griffith's home care plan would contain two pieces: one, services and products — all the things people need to stay home — and two, payment based on acuity instead of service.

We would have well refined tools to determine patients' needs and whether the family, alone or with support, could meet the needs. Nursing homes would be only for the excessively frail who could not be cared for at home.

Griffith sees a need for physicians in home care to do diagnostic workups, make prognoses, and chart disease courses. "But it is not the role of the physician to order services. He doesn't do that now. He gets a typed sheet of what the nurse wants and signs it," explains Griffith. A nurse in HCFA agrees: "There is nothing medical in home care. After hospitalization, the physician should discharge the patient to nursing care."

Griffith suggests that a practical funding cap might be whatever home care services the patient needs as long as the cost does not exceed nursing home costs.

That approach apparently has worked in South Carolina where, Lillian McCreight reports, Medicaid pays for whatever services people need to stay at home — as long as the cost does not exceed 75 percent of the cost of nursing home care. That saves money up front, McCreight notes.

National health insurance. That's DRG inventor John Thompson's answer. "It can't be any more expensive," predicts Thompson, "and it would be easier to control costs with one payer. Insurers could process claims like they do for Medicare now."

How would we fund this NHI? "By putting taxes on industry for the amount they now pay for fringes, and supplement that with a general tax like Medicare. Medicaid would no longer be a state program so we could take a portion of funds that states now put toward Medicaid."

Since businesses can deduct what they pay for fringes now, however, Thompson's plan would do more than shift money. It would cost industry a write off.

A tiered system is what we have now — we just hate to admit it. Uwe Reinhardt suggests that the best hope of the poor is for an overtly tiered system that offers universal access to a basic "tourist class" health package, publicly financed as Medicaid is now. Care would be paid for through competitively bid, prepaid capitation plans. "Business class" health would be financed as now, through employers, and would be paid for under a mixture of prepaid capitation plans, PPOs and traditional fees-for-service. "Designer class" would be privately paid for and delivered in luxury hospital suites or fashionable health resorts.[11]

Among those who think Reinhardt's concept is the most practical way to sew together the fragments into a more substantial safety net for health care are ANA President Lucille Joel, ANA Executive Director Judy Ryan, and NLN President Sr. Rosemary Donley.

Joel points out, "Yes, 'all men are created equal.' That is the basic standard. On top of equality, there are those who work to achieve more and we offer personal rewards to them. No matter how committed we are, it is unlikely that we will change this basic ethos.

"We need a basic level of health care for everyone. In our country, I feel it will be done by public and private programs coming together, by legislation that may look like patching the tire."

It would be ideal if we could restructure the existing financing system, says Ryan. A more likely plan, however, would be a general income-tax-supported system of universal access to essential health and social services, complemented by supplementary private health insurance that would pay for access into additional services.

For universal access, Ryan suggests that the government estimate the cost of care per person. Then, it could give each person a voucher to buy into the system of his choice.

Essential services, Ryan thinks, should be provided by a managed care system that offers access to services across existing settings. Patients would be able to move unencumbered among hospitals, nursing homes, homes health care agencies, rehabilitation centers and prevention sites, as needs change.

Ryan doesn't propose assigning a case manager at a magic age, as Gebbie does, but she does suggest central referral and case management services, as part of the essential package of prevention benefits, to connect people to the appropriate services.

Other prevention benefits would include prenatal care and parental guidance, infant health supervision in the first year, health exams for children up to 5 years, then a full school health program, immunizations, dental care, and screening for early detection and management of potentially high-cost illnesses.

Home care, in Ryan's plan, would include chore services, transportation, and respite care, as well as nursing care.

Ryan also envisions having physicians share gate-guarding duty. "In acute care, the medical plan of care — the diagnosis and treatment — ought to be determined by a physician in primary practice," comments Ryan. "For home care, why shouldn't nurses be the gatekeepers?"

Whether we are talking tiers or tots, the common thread in what nurses want is universal access to ensure that all Americans can get the essential health services they need. Since we are so far behind, should we begin with prenatal and infant care? Or, since we have moved from an era of acute care to chronic care, should access to long-term care for AIDS victims, the elderly, and the physically and psychologically disabled be first on our agenda?

Nurses are no more certain of the single, sure way than anyone else in a pluralistic society. But nurses are painfully certain that our nation's health priorities are wrong: We need to shift emphasis away from the expensive settings — institutions — and the most expensive providers — physicians. Some say we have the money we need to offer basic health care to every American — if we just move the money in the most cost-effective direction. And, to many, that means deciding how much we will pay for each American's health care and then forcing providers to stay within that budget — or go out of business.

REFERENCES

1. Grey Panthers of Austin. *It's Time for a National Health System,* Austin, TX, The Association, p. 1, 1988.

2. Mechanic, David. Challenges in long-term care policy. *Health Affairs* 6:26, Summer 1987.

3. Pierce, Robert M. *Long-Term Care for the Elderly: A Legislator's Guide,* Washington, DC, National Conference of State Legislatures, 1987, pp. 22-34.

4. Omenn, G.S. Lessons from a fourteen-state study of Medicaid. *Health Affairs* 6:118-122, Spring 1987.

5. Gage, L.S., and others. America's Health Safety Net: A Report on

the Situation of Public Hospitals in Our Nation's Metropolitan Areas, Washington, DC, National Association of Public Hospitals, Oct. 1, 1987, p. 20.

6. Dutton, Diana B. Social class, health, and illness. In *Applications of Social Science to Clinical Medicine and Health Policy*. Ed. by L.H. Aiken and D. Mechanic, New Brunswick, NJ, Rutgers University Press, 1986, p. 31-62.

7. Popp, R. Health care for the poor: where has all the money gone? *J. Nurs. Admin.* 18:8-12, Jan. 1988.

8. Pagin, Claire M. Nursing as an alternative to high-cost care. *Am. J. Nurs.* 82:57, Jan. 1982.

9. Lubic, R.W. Childbirthing centers: delivering more for les. *Am. J. Nurs.* 83:1053-1056, July 1983.

10. Meekes, R.J., and others. A comprehensive school health initiative. *Image* 18:86-91, March 1986.

11. Reinhardt, U.E. Rationing the health-care surplus. *Nurs. Economics* 4:101-108, May-June 1986.

Who will care for the old?

MARY GRACE KOVAR; TAMARA HARRIS

ONE OF THE THORNIEST issues facing the health-care industry is providing long-term care for the disabled elderly. Health-care expenditures for older people are rising, and one of the most rapidly increasing costs is for nursing-home care. Projections show that nursing-home costs are rising at an average annual rate of 12 percent. At the same time, one of the greatest fears of the elderly is the fear of going to a nursing home.

Businesses that can postpone or prevent an older person's institutionalization may find a profitable market in home-based care. Though families provide much of this care today, as more middle-aged women — the traditional caretakers — go to work, families may need to turn to other providers.

Because of the public outcry over nursing-home costs, many Americans believe that most long-term care of older people is provided by nursing homes. But the family still provides the majority of long-term care for older people. This means that more information on who gets and who needs home-based care is needed. Potential providers of home-based care need estimates of the size and characteristics of the market — those who already receive or who might need long-term care outside of nursing homes, as well as the families who now care or would care for them. These estimates will help potential providers to develop services for today's elderly and to prepare for the long-term care needs of the baby-boom generation when it starts to turn 65 early in the century.

This article provides national estimates of the size of this market. It also investigates some of the characteristics of people who currently need, or are at risk of needing, home-based care.

Information on the elderly who receive long-term care outside of nursing homes is available from the Supplement on Aging to the 1984 National Health Interview Survey. The Supplement on Aging is a national household survey of 16,000 people aged 55 and older. The analysis in this article is restricted to the 11,500 respondents to the Supplement on Aging who were aged 65 or older and living in households in 1984. They represent the nation's 26 million noninstitutionalized elderly.

The Supplement on Aging asked respondents whether they had difficulty in doing any of seven daily activities: walking, bathing, dressing, eating, going to the toilet, going outside, and getting in or out of a chair or bed. If respondents had difficulty with one or more of these activities, they were asked whether they received help from another person in doing the activity. Those who lived with someone other than a spouse were asked whether they lived with that person because of their own health. Everyone was also asked whether someone was available to care for them if they became ill for a few weeks.

We used the answers to these questions to divide the elderly population into risk categories. The first category consists of people who currently receive care. We subdivided this group into those who live with someone because of their own health but who do not receive help with any of the seven daily activities, those who receive help with a daily activity but who do not live with someone because of health, and those who need help with a daily activity and live with someone because

Living arrangements

The chart below indicates the number of people aged 65 and older living in households in 1984, grouped by health status. Numbers are in thousands.

	TOTAL	65-74	75-84	85+
Total	26,433	16,288	8,249	1,901
Receiving help	3,247	1,247	1,278	728
Help with daily activities	1,781	782	694	305
Lives with others for health	699	273	292	134
Both	768	199	292	284
Not receiving help	23,186	15,041	6,971	1,173
Someone available to provide care	19,862	13,259	5,684	919
No one available to provide care	3,324	1,782	1,288	254
Percent distribution				
Total	100.0%	100.0%	100.0%	100.0%
Receiving help	12.3	7.7	15.5	38.1
Help with daily activities	6.7	4.8	8.4	16.1
Lives with others for health	2.6	1.7	3.5	7.1
Both	2.9	1.2	3.5	15.0
Not receiving help	87.7	92.3	84.5	61.9
Someone available to provide care	75.1	81.4	68.9	48.5
No one available to provide care	12.6	10.9	15.6	13.4

Note: Numbers are based on a sample. Small numbers may not be reliable. Source: National Center for Health Statistics, National Health Interview Survey, Supplement on Aging, 1984.

of their health. People in any of these three subgroups are at high risk of going to a nursing home if the burden on caregivers becomes too great or if their level of disability increases.

Our second category is the healthy elderly — people who do not currently receive long-term care. We subdivided this group into people who have someone available to care for them if they ever need it, and those who do not. The people who do not have someone to help them may be at a higher risk of institutionalization than those who do. Because this group does not currently receive care, it might be possible for businesses to prevent these people from ever going to a nursing home by providing home-based services.

A needy market

Overall, 3.2 million people — or 12 percent of the 26 million noninstitutionalized people aged 65 and older — received some sort of long-term care in 1984. Among those receiving help, a minority lived with someone because of their health problems. Though most of the 3.2 million received help in doing one

Diminishing independence

Among people aged 70 and older who were not receiving help in 1984, those who had no one available to help if needed were more likely to be in nursing homes by 1986 than those who did have someone available to help out.

STATUS IN 1984	TOTAL	STATUS IN 1986		
		IN HOUSEHOLD	IN INSTITUTION	DECEASED
Total	100.0%	88.6%	2.2%	9.2%
Someone available to help	100.0	89.1	2.0	8.9
No one available to help	100.0	85.9	3.3	10.7
Living alone	100.0	87.3	3.7	9.0
Someone available to help	100.0	87.3	3.6	9.1
No one available to help	100.0	87.3	3.8	8.9
Living with others	100.0	89.5	1.3	9.3
Someone available to help	100.0	90.0	1.2	8.8
No one available to help	100.0	82.4	2.1	15.5

Note: People not located in 1986 are excluded. *Source:* National Center for Health Statistics, Longitudinal Study of Aging, 1986.

or more of the seven daily activities, few had changed their living arrangements because of these problems.

The majority of the older people in this country live independently and care for themselves. Eighty-eight percent of people aged 65 and older who live outside of institutions neither receive help with any of the seven daily activities nor live with another person because of a health problem.

Among these healthy elderly, 86 percent have someone who could care for them if they became ill. But an estimated 3.3 million of the healthy elderly do not. This group is at high risk of going to a nursing home if they become ill.

We reexamined the status of the respondents to the Supplement on Aging two years later, using data from the 1986 Longitudinal Study of Aging, the first of several projected follow-ups of the people who were interviewed in the 1984 Supplement on Aging.

This follow-up allowed us to determine whether those we had defined as being at great risk of institutionalization actually were more likely to be in nursing homes two years later.

The 1986 data show that the people aged 70 and older who received help in 1984 were more likely to have been institutionalized or to have died than those who did not: 10 percent were in nursing homes, and 27 percent had died. In contrast, among those who did not receive help in 1984, only 2 percent were in nursing homes, and only 9 percent had died.

The current market for home-based services includes the 3.2 million people aged 65 and older who currently receive some kind of help as well as their families. It also includes another 3.3 million who don't need help yet but who don't have anyone to care for them if and when they do need help.

The people living with someone because of their health or who receive help with a daily activity are older, more likely to be women,

The needy

Between 1984 and 1986, 10 percent of those aged 70 and older who received help became institutionalized. Some of these old people might have been able to remain at home if services were available to ease the burden on family caregivers.

STATUS IN 1984	TOTAL	STATUS IN 1986		
		IN HOUSEHOLD	IN INSTITUTION	DECEASED
Total	100.0%	63.2%	10.3%	26.5%
Living with others for health reasons	100.0	75.1	6.9	18.1
Needing help with a daily activity	100.0	62.4	10.4	27.2
Both	100.0	54.7	13.0	32.4
Living alone				
Needing help with a daily activity	100.0	59.1	15.9	24.9
Living with others	100.0	64.1	9.1	26.9
Living with others for health reasons	100.0	75.1	6.9	18.1
Needing help with a daily activity	100.0	64.1	7.5	28.4
Both	100.0	54.7	13.0	32.4

Note: People not located in 1986 are excluded. Source: National Center for Health Statistics, Longitudinal Study of Aging, 1986.

and more likely to be widowed than those who are not receiving such help. Though their families are helping out, the burden may become too great for some families.

Among the majority of older Americans who are not currently receiving help, those who have no one to care for them if they become sick are older and more likely to be women than those who have someone to care for them. They are also much more likely to be childless, to have no siblings, and no spouse. They are twice as likely to be living alone.

Our data show that the 3 million elderly who need help because of health problems are more likely to be in institutions two years later. The same fate could await the 3 million healthy elderly who have no one to help them if they ever need it. This market of 6 million Americans and their families could benefit from a network of home-based services, creating an opportunity for the nation's businesses.

Health care and the aging population

MARGARET DIMOND, RN, PhD, FAAN

BY THE YEAR 2000, the number of persons 65 and over in the U.S. is expected to double, to some 45 million; the number of those over 85 will triple. And by 2030, the over-65 will make up 21 percent of our population.

The rapid aging of our society is already placing great stress on our health care system; although the over-65 made up only 12 percent of the population in 1984, they accounted for 31 percent of the nation's total health care expenditures. Most older people have at least one chronic condition, and many have multiple conditions. [1]

Efforts to contain costs have been only partially successful; health care costs rose to 10.7 percent of GNP in 1985 from 6 percent in 1965, despite the institution of prospective payment systems. Moreover, despite tightened regulations and service cuts, the cost of government health benefits has continued to rise. According to the American Association of Retired Persons (AARP), the average annual health expenditure for those over 65 is $4,202, of which state and federal government pay about two-thirds. Yet in spite of Medicare, Medicaid and other health insurance programs, the average annual out-of-pocket health care expenditure for the elderly is $1,000 — more than their total average health expenditure before the enactment of Medicare. Since over 21 percent of the elderly are poor or near poor, meeting these expenses is difficult. [1]

Exacerbating this situation is a grave mismatch between help needed and available services. Our health care system emphasizes acute medical care and care given in institutions, both in terms of services and in terms of financial coverage. This emphasis benefits two groups of the elderly: those who need only occasional acute care and those who are so impaired that they need to be in a nursing home. The great majority do not fall into either group; most need long-term rather than acute care. Furthermore, much of this care could be home-based, for many of the elderly need help only with functional, day-to-day activities to avoid institutionalization. Both provision and financing of services are highly fragmented. In addition, the current system relies heavily on the family for regular assistance, but many of the elderly do not have family or friends who are able to help. Formal services often are inadequate for those who have no family or friends to sustain them. [2]

The problems involved in the care of the elderly offer great challenges and opportunities for nurses. Yet if we are to find solutions to these problems, as nurses we must consider the interlocking cultural, economic and political forces that have created them. Let us look at the effects of these forces on several aspects of health care for the elderly.

Allocation of resources

Increasing longevity and advances in health care technology are forcing health care providers and policymakers to confront two key questions: Given that society has limited resources and multiple goals, what kind of life are we willing to provide for the elderly when meeting their needs requires community funds? How can we be sure that the wishes of the competent elderly are respected, the interests of the incompetent are protected, and determination of competence is made responsibly?

As all public expenditures come under increasing scrutiny, disagreement has arisen over whether society should make use of all the available, although expensive, medical technology to prolong life for those at advanced ages. At the other end of the life cycle, such decisions are increasingly being made with consideration for quality of life. Should this standard also be applied to life-and-death decisions involving the elderly? The danger of such reasoning is that quality of life may come to be viewed as synonymous with worth of life. If this occurs, the elderly will almost always lose out to the young, who are usually viewed in our culture as having greater worth to society. [3]

There are also disagreements over what conditions should be treated at public expense and to what extent. For example, senile dementia is a chronic, disabling condition that strikes one of five individuals over 80. The cost of treatment is high, averaging $26 billion annually.

Are the costs of senile dementia too catastrophic and unpredictable to be borne by the individual? If they are instead to be borne collectively, what can society afford? Do we know enough about the possible long-range societal repercussions of legislating various types of family involvement? Can we make long-range projections about the impact of such policies? Should policymakers capitalize on the current interest in Alzheimer's disease by proposing separate programs and benefits for senile dementia? [4]

Long-term care
Of all the deficiencies in the U.S. health care system, perhaps the most serious for the elderly is the lack of adequate provisions for long-term care. Among those over 85 years old, 33 percent are ADL (activities of daily living) disabled. [1] Yet, unlike Western Europe and Canada, the United States lacks a well-developed system of personal social services for the functionally impaired. According to a recent article, "All industrialized countries with the exception of the United States and South Africa now have in place reasonably generous pensions and health care programs through social security systems. These, together with a variety of housing options for older people, are usually considered the mainstays of long term care policy." [5]

Among the strategies currently being discussed in the literature are rationing, targeting, reallocating some acute care funds to long-term care, and increasing the emphasis on informal services, particularly those provided by family. Although our first concern should be quality of care, current discussions are frequently dominated by cost of care. As the Kanes remark, "the greatest challenge of all is to temper our passion for cost-effectiveness with a continuing concern about the purpose of the effort." [4]

Women and aging
The problems of aging are increasingly women's problems. More likely than older men to have inadequate retirement income, to be widowed, divorced, and alone, and to be caregivers to older relatives, women make up 71 percent of the poor elderly. [6] The sexual division of labor and the dual labor market contribute substantially to the retirement experience of women in this country. As Estes points out, "the root of the income problem for women stems from the labor market, wherein differential pay, low-wage occupations, and episodic work participation have a combined and often devastating effect in later years." [7] Women not only enter old age poorer than men, but continue to grow poorer as a consequence of widowhood, inequities in pensions and social security, and higher health care expenditures. The poverty rate of black and His-

panic older women is more than double that of white older women and is even greater for those living alone. [6]

Older women have less access to health insurance than men and also have a higher incidence of chronic health problems. They frequently have few available resources for home-based care and are often unable to afford home health services. Thus, women are more likely than men to be institutionalized for social rather than for medical reasons, and they may be inappropriately placed in nursing homes when alternative community supports might have permitted more independent lifestyles. Indeed, about 70 percent of nursing home residents are women. [8]

The social role of caregiver is one of the factors contributing to women's impoverishment in old age. The graying of America has important implications for middle-aged and older women who have become the caregivers of older parents and spouses. Because the gender segregation of caregiving work (80% of caregivers are women) continues through the life cycle, the disadvantaged economic position of older women is compounded, and gender inequities are perpetuated by the lack of policies to support family caregiving. [9] Because their caregiving work is unpaid, but instead is seen as their proper social role, it is not recognized by society as a contribution entitling caregivers to support in their own old age. If women's social and economic status is to improve substantially, the welfare of family caregivers has to be a central goal of public policy, not just a means to low-cost care. [10]

Conclusion

As health care costs continue to rise, society must confront this basic question: Should health care be a market good to be purchased by those who can afford it, or should it be provided as a right or collective good, regardless of ability to pay?

We must not let ever-increasing costs and the need for fiscal austerity prevent us from taking the necessary steps to overturn existing policies. Indeed, the inequitable and unmanageable cost of health care for the elderly is the very reason we should take action. We can participate in efforts to create a health plan for everyone in this country. We can take the lead in assuring that the U.S. does not remain behind other industrialized nations in caring for its elderly. If we do not, if market forces continue to drive our health care policy, the vulnerable elderly in our society will suffer enormously.

REFERENCES

1. American Association of Retired Persons. *A Profile of Older Americans.* Washington, DC, The Association, 1987.

2. Reif, L. Epilogue: the future. In *Eighty-five Plus: The Oldest Old,* by S. Bould, B. Sanborn, and L. Reif. Belmont, CA, Wadsworth, 1989, pp. 173-197.

3. Moody, H.R. Ethics. In *The Encyclopedia of Aging,* ed. by G. L. Maddox and others. New York, Springer Publishing Co., 1987, p. 226.

4. Kane, R.A., and Kane, R.L. *Long Term Care: Principles, Programs, and Policies.* New York, Springer Publishing Co., 1987, p. 374.

5. *Ageing International* 15(1):31, Summer 1988.

6. Hooyman, N., and Kiyak, H. *Social Gerontology.* Newton, MA, Allyn and Bacon, Inc., 1988, p. 500.

7. Estes, C. Health care policy. In *The Encyclopedia of Aging,* ed. by G.L. Maddox and others. New York, Springer Publishing Co., 1987, p. 211.

8. Kahana, E., and Kiyak H. The older woman: impact of widowhood and living arrangement on service needs. *J. Gerontol. Soc. Work* 3:17-19, 1980.

9. Brody, E. Parent care as a normative family stress. *Gerontologist* 25:19-29, Feb. 1985.

10. Hooyman, N. *Older Women: The State of Knowledge.* Paper presented at the Conference for Older Women, Salt Lake City, Utah, April 25-26, 1988.

Health care for the homeless

ADA M. LINDSEY, RN, PhD

AS THE NUMBER of homeless in our towns and cities continues to grow, the need for a coordinated effort to address the problem becomes increasingly urgent. To comprehend the complexities involved, it is necessary to consider why homelessness has emerged as a sociopolitical, economic, public health phenomenon; the magnitude of the problem; and the characteristics of this current homeless population.

There are numerous reasons for the increase in the homeless population. One of the most important is the economic climate. In most urban areas, the cost of housing has risen rapidly; federal subsidies for low-income housing have been slashed; and gentrification has replaced thousands of units of low-cost housing with more expensive units. The economic recessions of the late '70s and early '80s contributed to continued low or minimum wages, plant closures, and unemployment. The increase in homelessness may also reflect further disintegration of our family structure. Many of the homeless are indeed social isolates and are alienated from society. The homeless are different from those who are poor: the homeless are alone; they lack social connections/relationships with friends and family.[1,2] It has been estimated that 30 to 40 percent of the homeless are mentally ill; thus deinstitutionalization and a change in the laws governing commitment have contributed to the homeless population.[1,3,4] Alcohol and drug abuse also adds to the number of homeless. There are many fewer arrests for vagrancy and drunkenness because of the decriminalization of public drunkenness in the past 20 years.[2]

Estimates of the number of homeless people vary widely. In 1984, the U.S. Department of Housing and Urban Development gave a range of 250,000 to 350,000 homeless; in 1988, advocates for the homeless gave an estimate of 2 million to 3 million.[5,6] In Los Angeles alone, estimates range from 35,000 to 50,000.[5]

It is difficult to count the homeless; those who do count them use varying definitions of homeless. For example, are those who are temporarily housed in a shelter or in single room occupancy, voucher hotels for a few nights counted with those who are on the streets, in the parks, in tents, under scrap material covers, and under viaducts? Are those who spend the night in transportation terminals or in all-night movie theaters and those who live in cars (abandoned or their own) included? Others may be very temporarily, tenuously, housed with friends or relatives; these are the hidden, marginal, or borderline homeless. There is a turnover of homeless; some move into a residence while others become temporarily without housing.

Homelessness is also a major economic problem; for example, New York City houses about 10,000 individuals and 5,000 families each night.[1] The New York City budget for the homeless increased from $6.8 million 10 years ago to $312 million in 1988. To house a family of four in a welfare hotel, New York City spends $1,900 a month, with half the support coming from the federal government.[1]

The label homeless suggests a simple definition and an obvious solution: provision of housing. But the problem is not simple; the homeless are not a homogeneous group. Homelessness is a manifestation of extreme poverty, lack of some type of a permanent residence, and disaffiliation from friends and family. Fewer than 10 percent, however, are estimated to be long-term, antisocial street people. Today's homeless are different from those of previous decades, when this population was made up primarily of older male alcoholics. Males are still the great majority, but their average age has decreased to 34 years.[5] The fastest growing subgroup consists of women with dependent children.[3]

Social, ethical, and political issues must be considered in efforts to provide care to the homeless. For example, does personal freedom of the homeless individual preclude the involuntary commitment, the institutionalization of the homeless who are mentally ill? Does personal freedom of the homeless individual supersede public health and safety? Does personal freedom of the homeless individual take precedence over the personal freedom of individuals who own homes or businesses in communities where the homeless are congregating? Does every individual have a right to housing? What obligations does or should society have for the children of homeless families? Who should provide health care to the homeless, where should it be provided, and how should it be financed? These few questions suggest the complexity of the growing social phenomenon of homelessness.

As a consequence of the conditions in which homeless people live, their health problems are often exacerbated and sometimes become chronic. A study of homeless patients seen in a New York City free clinic identified diabetes, hypertension, and drug and alcohol abuse as their major chronic health problems.[7] The homeless population is at risk for communicable diseases such as TB, scabies, lice and AIDS; they are at risk for peripheral vascular problems, for hypothermia in the winter, for malnutrition, for dental problems, for drug abuse and alcoholism, for traumatic injuries, and for assault. Homeless children are at risk

for abuse and neglect. They also are at risk for missing their immunizations and thus becoming vulnerable to disease.

Health problems are more difficult to care for in the homeless. Homeless individuals are on a continuum of inadequacies, and many have multiple disorders.

Caring for L.A.'s homeless

In 1983, the Robert Wood Johnson Foundation (RWJ) and the Pew Memorial Trust announced a new initiative, the Health Care for the Homeless Program, which would fund four-year demonstration projects to provide health care to the homeless. Projects in 19 cities have shown that the homeless can be reached and that health care can be provided to them.[3] Los Angeles was one of the cities that successfully applied for funding under the Health Care for the Homeless Program. The Los Angeles grant proposal had three components: the University of California, Los Angeles (UCLA), School of Nursing Health Center, serving the Skid Row area in downtown Los Angeles; the Venice Family Clinic, providing health care to the homeless in West Los Angeles; and a third component, giving first aid and screening training for shelter workers, and selective case management and advocacy for benefits for the homeless.

The following description of the homeless population served and the care provided by the UCLA School of Nursing Health Center is an example of one model of delivery of primary health care to the homeless. UCLA's nurse practitioner faculty began providing primary care at the health center part-time in 1983, prior to the RWJ/Pew homeless program initiative. This activity provided an important community service, an opportunity for faculty to maintain their clinical skills and expertise, research opportunities, and clinical placement for students. Foundation funding in 1985 supported employment of a full-time nurse practi-

TABLE 1. Number of encounters by type of service, March 1985-December 1987

SERVICE	FREQUENCY	PERCENT
Primary care	15,744	72.5
Social service	1,013	4.7
Transportation only	4,946	22.8
Total	21,703	100.0

tioner, part-time physician coverage, a half-time social worker, and a full-time outreach worker.

The health center is located on the second floor of the Union Rescue Mission, which is in the Skid Row area of downtown Los Angeles. The building is almost 100 years old. The clinic has one large open room, a small pharmacy area, three small examining rooms, and one treatment room.

Over a 34-month period, 7,369 clients made 21,703 visits to the clinic (averaging 2.9 visits each), the great majority of which were for primary health care. In 1987, for example, the monthly average was 638 visits, of which an average of 387 visits were for primary care (see Table 1). Of these 7,369 clients, 85.3 percent had no benefits (i.e., no general relief, no Medicaid, no Aid for Families with Dependent Children, no veteran benefits, and certainly no private health insurance).

The age of the homeless clients ranged from less than a year to 87 years, with an average of 35.5 years. Most (80%) were between 19 and 50 years of age, with nearly 15 percent over 50 and slightly more than 5 percent 18 or under. More than half the clinic clients were white, with blacks making up almost 42 percent; 30 percent of these two groups were of Hispanic ethnicity (see Table 2). About 90 percent of the clients were men. Women have been hesitant to come to the clinic because the health center is in a shelter for homeless men.

Since 1987, however, the number of female clients has increased.

Because homeless clients move from the street to shelters or to other types of residence, the center recorded the client's place of residence at each visit. As Table 3 shows, the clients who made more than 11,000 of those visits (53.8%) were living on the street at the time of the visit; the clients who made more than a third of the visits (37.5%) were in a shelter.

The most frequent diagnosis (14.8%) was acute nasopharyngitis (see Table 4). The need for tuberculosis screening (to rule out the diagnosis of TB), including administration of PPD and, when indicated, referral for chest X-rays, was second. Open wounds and lacerations were the third most frequent diagnosis (10.4%). These included wounds from traumatic injury and from peripheral vascular problems. Respiratory conditions accounted for 20.8 percent of the diagnoses.

Acute nasopharyngitis was the most common condition in those aged 19 to 50 years, while open wounds and lacerations were the most frequently treated condition in adults over 50, and indications of a need for TB screening were the most frequently seen condition for those 18 or younger. Scabies was more prevalent among children, and hypertension was most frequent in those over 50. The two most common procedures were related to

TABLE 2. **Demographic characteristics**

GENDER	FREQUENCY	PERCENT
Male	6,659	90.7
Female	681	9.3
Unknown	29	
RACE		
White	3,773	51.2
African-American	3,084	41.9
American Indian	96	1.3
Pacific Islander	15	0.2
Southeast Asian	401	5.4

wound care and dressing changes. The three education or counseling topics that were most frequently reported were the plan of care pertinent to the current health problem, information about the diagnosis, and preventive health care practices.

After almost a quarter (23.4%) of the primary care visits, clients were requested to make a follow-up visit to the clinic. Referrals were made to the county hospital after 14 percent of the primary care visits. To make it easier for clients to get to the hospital and other health care or social services, the clinic purchased two vans from the City of Los Angeles for $1 each. Transportation to other services was provided after 22.8 percent of the client encounters.

What these data do not convey are the unique problems health care providers encounter when caring for homeless people. For example, although lice-infested clients can be sent to the mission shelter's showers for delousing treatment and then given a clean set of clothes, it is next to impossible to prevent reinfestation if the individual returns to his bedroll on the street. Homeless people who require

medication every four to six hours may not have a watch or clock, or even a safe place to keep their medication. Those referred to other services may be too debilitated, too ill, or too disordered to find the way or to negotiate whatever is required of them. Treatment requiring bed rest and/or elevation of the feet and legs may not be a plausible option for some homeless individuals. Another dilemma is how to follow up when an X-ray report on a homeless client comes back positive for pneumonia or tuberculosis. Given such challenges, the task of caring for homeless people has made special demands on the resourcefulness of the clinic's nursing staff.

Foundation funding of the Health Care for the Homeless demonstration projects ended in December 1988. Funding under the Steward B. McKinney Homeless Assistant Act, signed into law in 1987, has helped the clinic continue to provide services. In addition, over the course of the clinic's operation, both UCLA and the Union Rescue Mission have provided many hours of service, personnel and supplies; the County of Los Angeles has provided a full-time licensed vocational nurse and some medications and supplies; the City of Los Angeles

TABLE 4. Most frequent diagnoses (1985-1987)

DIAGNOSIS	FREQUENCY	PERCENT
Acute nasopharyngitis	2,694	14.8
TB screening*	2,066	11.3
Open wounds/lacerations	1,887	10.4
Skin	755	4.1
Tinea	718	3.9
Acute bronchitis	610	3.4
Hypertension	499	2.7
Acute pharyngitis	466	2.6
Scabies	452	2.5
Contact dermatitis and eczema	436	2.4

*Includes PPD testing and chest X-ray referral

TABLE 3. Residence status at each visit

RESIDENCE	FREQUENCY	PERCENT
Street	11,187	53.8
Shelter	7,796	37.5
Room	1,264	6.1
Apartment	474	2.3
Other	62	0.3
Missing data	920	—
Total	21,703	100.0

has provided two vans. A local hospital performs the requested lab tests and chest X-rays. The clinic has also received money from an organization called Comic Relief, which in conjunction with Home Box Office has raised funds for health care for the homeless through nationally televised comedy shows.

When the Division of Nursing issued a special projects initiative, UCLA pediatric nursing faculty submitted a grant application to add a focus on primary care for homeless children. Funds received through this program have allowed the clinic to provide care to more homeless children at a second downtown site called Para Los Ninos. The grant has provided a full-time clinic administrator, another part-time nurse practitioner, and an administrative assistant to help with the data management necessary to show the cost-effectiveness of nurse-provided care in a noninstitutional setting. The clinic has also received a few private donations.

In the fall of 1987, the health center was licensed as a community clinic, making it possible to bill for Medicaid; however, because most of the homeless people the clinic serves are not eligible, we collected only about $1,170 for fiscal year 1987-88.

This brings us back to the issue of who should provide health care for the homeless, where it should be provided, and how it is to be financed. And finally, how does health care rank in the context of other priorities for the homeless, such as food, shelter, clothing, social services, rehabilitation, long-term transition programs, job training, psychiatric counseling, education for the growing number of homeless children, and permanent housing? Homelessness is a complicated phenomenon; how to provide health care to this population is only one of the problems our society must address.

REFERENCES

1. Lockhead, C. All alone with no home. *Insight on the News,* May 16, 1988, p. 12-15.

2. Whitman, D. Hope for the homeless. *US News World Rep.* 104:24-28ff, Feb. 29, 1988.

3. Wright, J.D., and Weber, E. *Homelessness and Health.* New York, McGraw-Hill Book Co., 1988.

4. U.S. National Institute of Mental Health, Program for the Homeless and Mentally Ill. *The Role of Nurses in Meeting the Health/Mental Health Needs of the Homeless*, proceedings of a workshop held at American Public Health Association, Washington, DC, Mar. 6-7, 1988. Rockville, MD, The Institute, 1986.

5. U.S. Department of Housing and Urban Development, Office of Policy Development and Research. *A Report to the Secretary on the Homeless and Emergency Shelters.* Washington, DC, The Department, 1984.

6. Lockhead, C. Nowhere to go, always in sight. *Insight on the News*, May 16, 1988, pp. 8-11.

7. Brickner, P.W., and others, eds. *Health Care of Homeless People.* New York, Springer Publishing Co., 1985.

Nursing's response to the challenge of AIDS

MARILYN CHOW, RN, DNS, FAAN

In San Francisco, a Latino woman whose husband was an IV drug user becomes sick. She is diagnosed as having AIDS. She is terminally ill. Her husband leaves her. Her two small children are both infected with the virus and show some symptoms of clinical illness. She moves in with her mother. What bothers her most is not that she is going to die, but that no one wants her children.

A nurse whose brother is a physician discovers that another brother has AIDS. The physician is concerned because his stricken brother kissed the physician's newborn baby on the cheek. The physician knows his fear is irrational — "but this is my child," he says.

IN SAN FRANCISCO — and across America — we are watching this dread disease ravage the bodies of its victims and instill fear and prejudice in otherwise decent people. This fear is irrational and pervasive. Even nurses and other health professionals have refused to provide care to persons with AIDS. Fear of contagion is compounded by homophobia — an unreasonable bias and suspicion toward homosexuality. For many Americans, homosexuality is a moral and religious issue, and those moral or religious views too often affect the medical treatment people with AIDS receive.

The HIV epidemic is confronting America's health care system with a crisis of unprecedented proportions. Some 70,000 cases have been reported since 1981. It is estimated that 1 million to 1.5 million more people are now infected with the virus, and the number of cases is expected to reach 450,000 by 1993.

AIDS also threatens to overwhelm our health care system financially. It aggravates a burgeoning nursing shortage that already plagues communities across the nation. It forces all of us, as nurses, to face the fear and prejudice that exist within others — and even the bias that sometimes festers inside ourselves.

A few years ago, when Surgeon General Koop came to visit AIDS projects in San Francisco, he discovered that nurses are on the front lines in the war against this epidemic — ministering daily to the physical and emotional needs of those who are stricken; sometimes battling with physicians and administrators for the interests of people with AIDS; and developing successful programs such as the AIDS treatment unit established at San Francisco General Hospital in 1983 by nurse Cliff Morrison, formerly the unit's clinical coordinator (see box). Nurses played an instrumental role in developing the HIV programs in San Francisco. They are in large measure the reason why those programs, which now serve as models for the nation, exist today.

Three years ago San Francisco's nurses decided to elect a mayor who would support their vision of health care and social services delivery. Their candidate was Art Agnos, a state legislator and former social worker. Nurses served as precinct leaders, hosted hundreds of neighborhood coffees, labored as campaign coordinators, walked precincts, manned phone banks, worked at headquarters, raised money, and helped get out the vote. On election day, Art Agnos — a distant long shot early in the race — was elected mayor with 70 percent of the vote, the biggest majority for a mayoral election in this century. That victory

San Francisco General's special care unit

When plans for a Special Care Unit (SCU) for people with AIDS were being drawn up at San Francisco General Hospital in 1983, there were fears that the unit was to act as a kind of "leper colony," isolating those infected with HIV from other patients, doctors, and hospital staff. There were also concerns that the gay community would boycott the unit and that persons with AIDS would not want to be placed in the unit because of the stigma attached to it. But the difficulties of caring for AIDS patients scattered about the hospital eventually outweighed these fears.*

Staff for the unit were chosen through an intensive interview process. They were then given a formal orientation program with information on the disease itself, risk factors for contagion, infection control guidelines, and psychosocial issues.

To be admitted to the unit, patients had to have a diagnosis of AIDS or be in a high-risk group and have an AIDS-related condition. These guidelines were circulated to all medical staff and departments in the hospital.

The staff had been urged to establish and maintain good relationships with the rest of the hospital, a factor that was especially important in gaining acceptance for the unit. Although all support services had received the unit's infection control guidelines, some personnel over-reacted and came to the unit in masks, gowns, gloves and shoe coverings. The housekeeping staff, however, under-reacted, omitting the required practices. Eventually, a full-time porter was assigned to the unit and included in the staff to ensure that the guidelines were followed.

Problems followed with the hospital pharmacy, surgery, recovery room, laundry, X-ray, and other departments. Most of the issues involved handling patients or specimens. Resolutions often involved teaching staff to consistently follow the infection control guidelines. The infection control coordinator acted as a consultant to the unit staff and taught other departments. An AIDS educational coordinator was added to the hospital staff to teach support services and other department personnel about AIDS and its risks to health care workers.

The SCU staff had to survive a difficult period in which their sexuality was questioned and they were subjected to attitudes and comments springing from fear and hostility. Support groups helped them weather the initial tension. In spite of such problems, there is a high level of job satisfaction and camaraderie on the unit. The idea that once raised so many concerns has created a place where AIDS patients can receive expert, compassionate care from dedicated nurses who find their work satisfying and compelling.

*Viele, C. S., Dodd, M. J., and Morrison, C. "Caring for Acquired Immune Deficiency Syndrome Patients," Oncol. Nurs. Forum 11(3):56-60. May/June 1984.

was due, in no small part, to the role nurses played in his campaign.

As a result of these efforts, San Francisco now has a deputy mayor for health and human services — Myra Snyder, former executive director of the California Nurses Association — and nurses are being appointed to important city policy-making commissions. Now, when nurses in San Francisco battle for projects such as the AIDS treatment unit at San Francisco General Hospital, the administrators and the bureaucrats know that their voices are also heard in the places where decisions are made.

A second major effort was begun in 1986, when the California Nurses Association developed an innovative train-the-trainer program to educate providers about HIV infection and allay unwarranted fears. So far, the program has trained 1,600 individuals. Each of them, in turn, has provided AIDS education to an average of 35 health care workers in their places of employment. As a result, over 35,000 health care workers have been reached.

We have often had to overcome tremendous

resistance when attempting to provide sound information on AIDS. But by creating a comfortable learning climate, by assessing and addressing the fears of learners, by making learners active participants in the training process, and by making the content material clinically relevant, we have succeeded in breaking down barriers and overcoming anxiety and misinformation.

We still hear about persons with AIDS enduring bias and insensitivity at the hands of health care providers. But now we also hear stories about nurses who care.

One patient's dying wish is to be married to his male lover. The nursing staff, without telling the administration until the last moment, plan the entire wedding. They help organize the minister, the flowers, and the champagne. Other patients get involved. The patient dies shortly after the ceremony.

The nursing staff on that unit were able to set aside their own value judgments as to whether gay men should be married. Their only concern was the quality of their patient's life.

Nursing is about caring, about compassion, about concern. It recognizes that understanding is an important form of therapy, that sympathy is a vital part of care.

Nurses acknowledge the totality of the challenges their patients face and the anguish they feel. The physician gives the patient the diagnosis. But it is the nurse who picks the patient up after the diagnosis. It is the nurse who listens to the patient's fears and doubts. It is the nurse who talks with the family about the obstacles that must be overcome and the adjustments that need to be made.

With HIV infection, we nurses face a new and troubling dilemma. It challenges us to live up to our creed and to exercise strength and leadership wherever fear and ignorance abound. By caring for persons with AIDS, we can exemplify everything that we have always believed about nursing care, about quality of care, about cost-effectiveness, about prevention. With this disease, we can demonstrate that a nursing model of care is what makes the difference.

Nursing must establish a clear, simply stated health care agenda — a national nursing agenda — for the care of persons with HIV infection. This means that we, as a profession, must set objectives for ourselves: that by the year 1990, every RN shall be educated about HIV infection and its implications for nursing care; that by the year 1991, we shall have under way several key research projects examining the clinical aspects of nursing care and nursing delivery models of care.

It also means that we, as a profession, must reach agreement on the controversial issues and policies surrounding AIDS: voluntary versus mandatory testing, disclosure of test results, allocation of health care resources, dealing with discrimination, and using education to change people's behavior — including the behavior of many nurses and other health professionals.

Many of the problems we face today in addressing HIV infection spring from a political rather than a health response to the crisis. Therefore it is appropriate that nurses turn to politics for a solution.

Nurses involved in politics? Some may object. But what is the alternative? To leave decisions on the care and treatment of people with HIV in the hands of the politicians, some of whom see AIDS as just one more issue to exploit for partisan or political gain? Or get involved ourselves in molding the policies — and solutions — that we as nurses know are needed?

Daniel Inouye, senator from Hawaii, has described nursing as a sleeping giant. It is time for that to change. The challenge of AIDS demands it.

CHAPTER THIRTEEN

Influence of changing social patterns

CONCERNS ABOUT RISING health care costs have tended to obscure purely social issues as contributors to the problems of health care delivery in our nation today. Yet those issues, particularly changing social patterns, have far-reaching potential to hamper efforts at improving the nation's health care. The articles selected for this chapter address some of these critical social issues.

Eck et al., in "Consumerism, Nursing, and the Reality of the Resources," discuss the consumerism phenomenon by asking the reader to put consumers in the driver's seat and look at nursing care from their perspective. Referring to a study by Weisman and Nathanson that showed how managers of health care organizations can improve patient outcomes by providing working conditions conducive to staff satisfaction, the authors propose five strategies to bridge the gap among consumers' expectations, professional standards, and the reality of limited resources.

Aydelotte, in her article "Nursing's Preferred Future," offers a broad view of the future of society, health care, and nursing. Since the 1960s, this author has studied the relationship between nurse staffing and quality care, repeatedly challenging nursing with her concerns and criticisms concerning federal health care policy and the position nursing occupies within it. In this article, Aydelotte shares her vision of the future of nursing practice and proposes ways to accomplish that vision.

The article by Allen and Turner, "Where to Find the New Immigrants," details recent changes in U.S. demographics, based on immigration patterns, and discusses the health care implications of those population shifts.

In the final article, "The Challenge of an Aging Society," Longman writes of the challenge our society faces in balancing the ever-increasing cost of caring for the elderly against the shrinking population of younger workers who must bear much of that cost. This article is included here as an example of the complex ways segments of society interact, complicating the formulation of public policy.

Consumerism, nursing, and the reality of the resources

SHARON A. ECK, RN, MA; RACHEL R. MEEHAN, RN, MSN, CS, CCRN;
DIANE M. ZIGMUND, RN, MSN; LYNNE M. PIERRO, RN, CNA

CONSUMERS OF HEALTH CARE today are more sophisticated than ever before and are demanding the power to influence their own health care future. Acute care hospitals, which serve as the primary site of inpatient health care, may be viewed as the producers of a very important commodity, patient care. To compete successfully for the consumer's dollars, a hospital must be able to offer a product that is perceived by the consumer as being of high quality and fairly priced. This article will explore the reality and the ideal involvement of the public with the product of patient care and nursing's role in the delivery of that product. Strategies to bridge the gap between consumers' expectations, nursing's standards of practice, and available resources are presented.

Consumerism and patient rights

A consumer may be defined as one who uses a product. In the United States, consumerism, or the promotion of consumers' interests, has enjoyed considerable support, especially from the 1960s to the present. In the health care setting, all members of the population are consumers to some degree. As consumers, people have certain rights. President Kennedy in 1962 proclaimed four consumer rights to Congress.

These rights include:
1. the right to safety
2. the right to be informed
3. the right to choose
4. the right to be heard.[1]

In 1973, the American Hospital Association adopted a national policy statement on patients' rights.[2] These rights include, but are not limited to, considerate and respectable treatment, current information about one's diagnosis, informed consent, refusal of treatment to the extent permitted by law, and confidential handling of one's records and care. The National League for Nursing also recognizes the rights of patients and encourages the nursing professional to assume a greater sense of responsibility in informing patients of their rights and protecting their rights.[3] Aydelotte summarizes the patient rights literature and states the "four rights commonly accepted in our society: a. the right to the 'whole truth,' b. the right to privacy and personal dignity, c. the right to self determination, to make decisions that concern one's self, d. the right to complete records."[4]

Through the 1970s, the trend of consumerism continued to gain support. Information for the consumer on health care became readily available in local libraries, and the position of patient representative or advocate was established in hospitals and clinics. Representation on hospital boards by lay consumers, which had been in place since the 1940s, became more prevalent and powerful. In the 1980s, the rising costs of health care spurred consumer interest and participation in health care planning and implementation to new and greater heights.

Nursing's role in health care

Society establishes the role of nursing in health care.[5] People use or do not use the services of the profession. People support or do not support professional education. As stated in the American Nurses Association's (ANA) *Nursing: A Social Policy Statement,* a social

contract exists between nursing and society.[6] Nursing has the primary responsibility of meeting society's needs by alleviating suffering, promoting and restoring health, and preventing illness. Thus nursing is defined as the diagnosis and treatment of human response to actual or potential problems. The ANA has made the social policy more specific by:
- establishing a code of ethics
- fostering nursing research to guide nursing actions
- establishing standards of practice
- establishing educational requirements
- establishing a certification process.

By ensuring quality of nursing care, nursing strives to meet the needs of society. Society, however, may not always have adequate knowledge to realize the importance of certain standards of practice, especially in highly specialized, intense, or technological areas.

The consumer's role

The predominant role in which the consumer of health care has played a part is in the evaluation of services received. Volumes have been written about patient satisfaction, especially in relation to general health services or medical care. The validity of the concept of patient satisfaction becomes a central issue because of the unclear formulation as to whether it is from the professional or consumer viewpoint. The consumer movement to increase the rights and powers of the purchasers in relation to the sellers, however, is demanding a greater role than evaluation. Aydelotte, in her article on patients' rights, states, "Society, which pays for services and sanctions them, will continue to demand a larger role in the planning process, so that it will know to what it is committing itself."[7] In planning for health care services, does nursing know what society needs and wants in their nursing care? Virtually no literature addresses this issue directly. Clearly, consumers have played a rather limited role in voicing their expectations of health care.

Satisfaction with medical care

The majority of the research and literature on patient satisfaction has been in relation to general health care services or medical care. Ware, Davies-Avery, and Steward, in the mid-1970s, reviewed over 100 studies on patient satisfaction and cited two general purposes of the research: (1) to evaluate the provider service (most frequent), and (2) to predict consumer health and illness behavior (such as compliance with treatment or use of services).[8] General conclusions or comparisons are difficult to make because of the lack of reliability and validity measurements employed on the various satisfaction scales. The authors propose a taxonomy of patient satisfaction that identifies and defines the characteristics of patient satisfaction based on a content analysis of the literature and their own research. The eight dimensions of the taxonomy are:
1. art of care
2. technical quality of care
3. accessibility/convenience
4. finances
5. physical environment
6. availability
7. continuity of care
8. efficacy/outcomes of care.

Demographic and socioeconomic variables were also identified in the Ware patient satisfaction research.[9] Again, generalizations are difficult to make because of the variability in findings across studies. Some trends, however, emerged in relation to age, education, family size, income, occupation, and sex. For example, women tended to be more satisfied with general health care than men. No clear trends were identified with regard to marital status, race, or social class.

In a later article, Ware, Snyder, and Wright

present an excellent discussion regarding major issues in the study of patient satisfaction.[10] The authors provide future researchers with six recommendations in defining and measuring satisfaction. Articles of this nature facilitate the standardization of the research to generate findings that have greater generalizability and comparability and thus are more likely to influence health care practices.

During the 1980s, patient satisfaction studies have become more sophisticated and specialized. Greater attention has been given to the reliability and validity issues. Specialties have recognized the need to more precisely measure the satisfaction with their services. These studies have focused primarily on the physician-consumer relationship. Examples of these specialty areas include satisfaction with ambulatory care and obstetric care, parents' satisfaction with children's medical care, or satisfaction with the hospital emergency department.[11-15] Greater attention has also been given to the development of theory regarding patient satisfaction.[16]

Satisfaction with nursing care

In nursing, little attention has been given to consumer satisfaction and even less to consumer expectations. In a recent national study, Henry and colleagues delineate the nursing administration research priorities and found that a common thread throughout the top 20 categories was patient satisfaction. There was no mention, however, of looking at the consumer expectations of nursing care.[17] The President of the American Association of Critical Care Nurses, Sandi Dunbar, in her 1987 president's address, proposed seven expectations of nursing care by critical care patients and their families.[18] The methodology in determining these expectations was not stated, but they appear to have emerged through the perspective of the critical care nurse. According to Dunbar, consumers expect qualified and competent personnel, adequate nursing re-

sources, promotion of health, cohesive packages, congruence among authority, accountability and responsibility of nurses, high-quality health care and tech nology, and caring. The dual nature of quality nursing care is supported, that is, quality measurements based on clinical evaluation (standards of practice) and the patients' perceptions of satisfaction with their nursing care.

Some developments have been made in the exploration of patient satisfaction with nursing care. In the late 1950s, Abdellah and Levine presented the classic study that initiated tool development and testing in nursing.[19] Much rich, qualitative data were obtained, and in a later article they proposed five facets of satisfaction with nursing care. These include adequacy of the facilities, effectiveness of organizational structures, professional qualifications, competency in provision of care, and consumer outcomes.[20]

The tool developed by Risser in 1975 has been the major nursing measurement for satisfaction.[21] Satisfaction is defined as an attitude that reflects the degree of congruence between patients' expectations and their perceptions of nursing care received (ideal versus real). She identifies three aspects of patient satisfaction with nurses and nursing care. The first aspect, the technical-professional factor, refers to the technical activities or skills required to complete nursing care tasks. The second aspect, the educational relationship, is defined by the nurse's ability to provide information, answer questions, explain care, or demonstrate techniques. The third aspect refers to the trusting relationship between the nurse and patient and includes the caring aspects of nursing. The items on the Risser tool reflect a heavy emphasis on the dependent (physician-driven) functions, rather than on the independent or interdependent functions of the nurse. The Risser tool has subsequently been further tested.[22-24] To date, the emphasis in studying satisfaction with nursing care has been placed on tool development.

Professional and consumer satisfaction and consumer outcomes

Both consumer and professional satisfaction are typically viewed as outcomes of health care organizational effectiveness. In a unique study by Weisman and Nathanson, the relationship between job satisfaction of nursing staff and two client outcomes was examined.[25] This organizational analysis explored the relationship of nurses' job satisfaction across 77 family planning clinics and both the satisfaction of teenagers with the services and the rate of compliance with contraceptive prescriptions. The authors found that the job satisfaction of the nursing staff was the strongest determinant of the satisfaction of the clients, and the clients' satisfaction level predicted the rate of their subsequent compliance. The authors present significant implications for managers, stating, "The study suggests that managers of health organizations can improve certain client outcomes by providing working conditions conducive to professional staff satisfaction."[26] This startling study not only suggests the influence on health and illness behaviors that nursing possesses but also creates anxiety about what effects current nursing shortages and nurse job dissatisfaction are having on patients today.

Reality of resources

What are the available resources to meet consumer's needs? A review of nurse supply trends over the past two decades puts the present crisis in context. Work done by Aiken and Mullinix, recently published in the *New England Journal of Medicine,* identifies a correlation between depressed nursing salaries and vacant nursing positions.[27] Shortages in the early 1960s and mid-1970s were accompanied by a decline in nursing salaries. As pay levels for nurses rose in the mid-1960s and the late

1970s, the number of nurses entering the profession increased significantly.

As prospective payment became a reality in 1983 and 1984, nurses' salaries again fell behind. However, no problems with nurse vacancies were reported in the professional literature. With the advent of diagnosis related groups, nursing layoffs were a reported concern at the time. Concerns about shortages began to appear in print by spring 1986. By winter 1987, articles on the nursing shortage were appearing in major newspapers such as *The New York Times,* as well as in the professional literature.[28]

The number of registered nurses now exceeds 2.1 million. The number employed is at an all-time high of 1.5 million, which represents almost 80 percent of the total available pool.[29] Aiken and Mullinix suggest nursing is nearly at the maximum in terms of the utilization of available nurses.[30]

Such numbers have caused some speculation that a shortage does not in fact exist. A survey by the American Hospital Association, however, reported in the *American Journal of Nursing* in April 1987, reported 13.6 percent of the total number of registered nurse positions were vacant.[31] This is twice the number of the previous year. Critical care and medical-surgical staff nurse positions are the most difficult to fill, often requiring 60 to 90 days recruitment time.

This shortage has developed at an alarming rate, considering the high percentage of registered nurses currently employed in hospital settings. This increased demand for nurses can be traced to sicker patients requiring more care in shorter time frames. It is worth noting that the ratio of nurses to hospital patients has risen from 50 nurses for every 100 patients in 1975 to 875 nurses for every 100 patients in 1985.[32]

These changes reflect advances in health care and new technology, which then create demands for nurses with specialized skills, education, and experience. As Curtin states, "While financial and economic experts still presume that all hospital operations are physician-driven, some are becoming aware that... some of those operations are nurse-driven."[33] This has added significantly to the growing demand for nurses. Recognizing this need, hospitals have been replacing typically non-nurse positions with nursing personnel.[34]

In some areas, because of inadequate nurse staffing, hospitals have been forced to close critical care beds and to turn away ambulance admissions. Many are relying on nurse registries and agencies to provide minimal staff on all shifts. The impact on patients, physicians, and hospitals is striking. Waiting lists have grown for both routine and elective admissions, and the waiting time can be months. Many hospital departments are feeling the effect of this worsening shortage as they try to cope with problems resulting from fewer nurses.

How does this shortage affect the consumer? Clearly, there are fewer nurses available to meet consumer needs. This is occurring at a time when the college-age population is declining and the number of people entering nursing programs is diminishing. This has resulted in the closing of collegiate nursing programs, such as Boston University. Enrollments in baccalaureate nursing programs have decreased steadily since 1984. At the University of California at Los Angeles (UCLA), the number of women entering nursing programs is at an all-time low of 5.1 percent. By contrast, 23 percent are pursuing business careers, 11 percent are interested in teaching, 3.4 percent are pursuing medicine, 4 percent are seeking careers in law, and 2.8 percent are studying engineering. A survey of life goals of UCLA freshmen showed that "being well-off financially" was chosen by 70 percent of the freshman class, compared to 40 percent in 1970, while "helping others" rated 57 percent

and "developing a meaningful philosophy of life" hit a new low of 40 percent.[35]

What are some of the reasons nursing is not attracting students into the field? Federal support for nursing education has declined sharply over the past eight years. The availability of grants and scholarships has decreased, and eligibility requirements for loans are being tightened.[36] Other attractive career options are available to women that provide higher pay and more autonomy and control. Salaries are often cited as a major reason for not entering nursing. The average starting salary for a staff nurse is $20,340. The average maximum, however, for an experienced nurse is a low $27,744.[37] Recent severe shortages, however, have spurred salary increases, especially in the eastern and southern states. Other professionals have similar beginning salaries, but the salaries for the experienced persons are considerably higher. As a result, projected requirements for nurses with baccalaureate degrees are twice the projected supply for 1990 and 2000.[38]

Reports such as "The Nursing Shortage: Facts, Figures and Feelings," by the American Hospital Association,[39] offer recommendations that include a reevaluation of the reward system and incentives for nurses that recognize different degrees of education. Greater autonomy for nurses is needed in both patient care decision making and personal time management. Also cited are increased federal support for nursing education and greater public recognition of nursing's contributions.

Recently, some steps in this direction have been made by the introduction of legislation by Senator Kennedy (The Nursing Shortage Reduction Act of 1987) to develop an advisory committee to search out long-term solutions to recruitment and retention problems. At the state level, in Connecticut, Governor O'Neil has commissioned a Blue Ribbon Task Force to make statewide recommendations on the nursing shortage. Doris Armstrong, R.N.,

M.Ed., F.A.A.N., has been appointed cochair of this task force with Gardner Wright, the Commissioner of Hospitals and Health Care.

Bridging the gap

To bridge the gap between consumers' expectations, professional standards, and the reality of the resources, the following five strategies are suggested.

Nurse alliance with consumers. Recognizing the needs and wants of the consumer of nursing care will be vital to the survival and growth of nursing. Identification of the priorities and values that consumers place on their nursing care and integration of this consumer perspective with professional standards of care will strategically position nursing in the health care marketplace. Amidst the reality of a severe nursing shortage, knowledge about consumer expectation and satisfaction with care can facilitate priority setting and workload reallocation among nursing staff. Thus a marketing approach is proposed to explore the consumer perspective and create a greater alliance between nurse providers and nursing care consumers.

Kotler defines marketing as the exchange processes that occur in attempting to satisfy consumers' wants and needs.[40] Marketing is the link between, for example, nursing care consumers' needs and wants and the response by nurses in terms of goods and services that are provided. The goods and services that are capable of satisfying the needs or desires of the consumer are generally referred to as the product. The movement toward product line management, which is making management decisions based on the analysis of products, is the operational method for applying marketing principles in nursing.

A great deal of specific consumer data is needed on which to base management decisions. Market research collects, organizes, examines, and interprets data from the level of a large geographic area to a single clinical population or nursing unit. Nursing market research may be a formal inquiry into such questions as, What are consumers' expectations of their nursing care? What nursing activities are of greatest value or importance to consumers? What methods of certain nursing activities are most satisfying? What nursing activities are of least importance?

Some of these questions may be addressed in traditional and general patient satisfaction surveys used by hospitals. Nurse executives may find useful trends and issues, some of which may be useful for nurse managers at the unit level. For example, the tool used at Hartford Hospital provides useful information related to demographic variables such as age, sex, length of stay, number of hospitalizations, and education.[41] The specific open comments related to satisfaction and dissatisfaction with nursing care are extremely useful in identifying important nursing activities. The specific questions related to the nursing staff include explaining procedures, being kind and supportive, answering call buttons, and answering questions. These questions cover domains related to teaching, caring, and trusting nurse-patient relationships. These questionnaires are useful within the Department of Nursing at Hartford Hospital to identify annual trends and unit variations. The data, however, are not nearly specific or comprehensive enough to prepare a marketing plan.

Strasen, in discussing marketing skills for nurse administrators, suggests the following seven steps toward implementing a marketing plan in a nursing department:

1. develop a marketing team
2. select or develop a survey tool to obtain data
3. analyze data with regard to the internal and external environment
4. identify marketing goals and objectives
5. develop a marketing strategic plan to meet goals and objectives

6. develop a plan of action, accountabilities, time lines, resources required, promotion, pricing, place and product

7. evaluate and revise goals and objectives as appropriate.[42]

Unit-level nurse managers, clinical specialists, and staff nurses are key in integrating the marketing plan with professional standards of care. They can further explore questions such as the following:

• What professional standards of care are parallel to or in conflict with consumers' expectations?

• What activities that are of lesser importance to the consumer can be eliminated or delegated to support staff?

• What trends or aspects of the consumer perspective can facilitate setting priorities for nurse activity?

• What consumer expectations can or cannot be met within the current reality of human and financial resources?

At the executive level of nursing administration, a direct line of formal communication with a group of consumers, such as a patient advisory board, can be developed. The group can provide consultation on the planning level of nursing, such as in marketing, program, clinic, or service development.

A marketing approach can foster a greater nurse-consumer relationship. The marketing principles cannot be helpful in isolation and must be integrated in concert with professional standards and the reality of the resources. The challenge also prevails to identify and address the consumers' expectations of nursing care, rather than to merely be concerned with their satisfaction of care received.

Examining and restructuring nursing practice. In today's environment of high patient acuity and decreased staffing, it is imperative that nursing resources be utilized wisely and efficiently. Both the nurse manager and the individual nurse need to examine their daily practice and standards of practice to determine whether inefficient or redundant practices are present. In reviewing their daily tasks, nurses should ask themselves several questions, including the following:

• What is the outcome of a particular intervention or task?

• Is there a measurable impact on patient care or does the action merely represent a useless routine?

• What is the appropriateness of the nurse's doing a particular activity (does it belong to another individual or department)?

• Could the intervention possibly be done in a more efficient manner, utilizing less nursing time and, therefore, less cost?

• Could the intervention be delegated to a nonprofessional, thus freeing the nurse to perform more meaningful patient care actions?

• What technology could support the practice of the nurse?

Technicians or aides can assist nurses in doing routine care in many ways. In an intensive care unit or on certain units, there are often debilitated, immobile patients who require assistance with bathing, feeding, and repositioning. Support and nursing aide personnel can assist with these tasks, as well as with weighing patients, taking vital signs, ambulating patients, and emptying drainage containers. While technicians are performing the above-mentioned tasks, nurses are free to plan the care for their patients, direct and supervise the technicians in implementing the care plans, and evaluate the outcomes. Nonnursing personnel can also provide assistance with specialized equipment by ensuring its availability, setting it up and calibrating it, and checking the working condition of all materials. The role of the nonprofessional is to support the practice of the nurse, and it does not disturb the nurse-patient relationship.

Incorporating computer systems. A third strategy in "bridging the gap" in today's nursing practice is the incorporation of computer systems. Because of their capacity to perform certain tasks faster, cheaper, and more efficiently than humans, computers have been incorporated into businesses of all sizes and types. In nursing, the computer has many applications both for the nurse manager and for the staff nurse directly involved with patient care.

For the nurse manager, the computer can be used to facilitate the time-consuming process of preparing schedules. Maintaining a nursing database (employment record, educational level, clinical-ladder level, holiday and vacation time, etc.) and a patient census and acuity level allows personnel needs to be assessed and resources appropriately allocated. In addition, record keeping is made easier; clerical time is reduced; and report writing (budget and staff utilization) is improved and made easier.[43]

For the staff nurse, the computer can reduce time spent on clerical duties and thus free more time for direct patient care. Some of the ways this is accomplished is by facilitating communication and reducing duplicate logging and errors. The computer can be used to create, maintain, and update care plans and to assign automatic patient acuity ratings. Nurses' notes are made uniform and legible. Finally, the computer can be used to integrate patient data from a variety of sources (historical, ongoing physical assessments, and laboratory data) as they are accumulated.[44]

Promoting the self-care concept. In 1859, Florence Nightingale defined nursing as having "charge of the personal health of somebody, and what nursing has to do, is to put the patient in the best condition for nature to act upon him."[45] Now, almost 130 years later the same basic goal exists — for nurses to put their patients in the best condition they can. However, this condition has been expanded to include the patient's psychological and social, as well as physical, well-being. In addition, the role of the nurse as the active party who

does everything for the patient has changed. Nursing now acknowledges the benefits of having patients do for themselves.

The Orem Self-Care Model for Nursing Practice states that individuals initiate and perform self-care activities on their own behalf to maintain life, health, and well-being.[46] The patient is viewed as an active participant in his or her own care. Using the self-care concept, the nurse assesses the patient's capabilities and limitations to carry out therapeutic self-care demands and designs an appropriate system to meet these demands. In a wholly compensatory nursing system, the patient does not have the resources to meet his or her self-care demands; therefore, the nurse performs all the actions. In the partly compensatory nursing system, the patient performs those actions within his or her capacity, and the nurse performs those actions that the patient is unable to perform. In the educative-supportive nursing system, the patient is able to perform the necessary actions but cannot do so without the nurse's assistance. The nurse gives the patient guidance as it relates to decision making, behavior control, and the gaining of knowledge and skills. In the end, the patient is made responsible for meeting his or her self-care needs. Promoting this model clearly integrates the patient or consumer's viewpoint.

Incorporating guest relations for support nursing staff. Guest relations programs are aimed at increasing consumers' satisfaction with their health care. Specifically, the programs are aimed at humanizing the patient's hospital stay and being sure that the patient's nonmedical needs are met as well.[47] These programs may be particularly helpful for support nursing staff such as unit secretaries, nursing assistants, aides, technicians, and others. Programs may be developed in-house or purchased from numerous public relations firms. The content of most programs varies from basic courtesy tips to telephone skills. The guest relations movement fosters communication between patients and staff. Components of guest relations can easily be incorporated into the orientation of new nursing staff to create the climate of receptivity to patients' needs and wants.

For nursing to retain a favorable market position, the voice of the consumer must be heard. Consumers hold certain expectations about their nursing care, and the opportunity now exists to explore those expectations to create a new consumer-provider relationship. Nursing is faced with the challenge to integrate the consumer viewpoint within the profession's standards of practice and the reality of the human and financial resources. This is the era where only the strong will survive and continue to be self-regulated. The consumerism movement, the nursing shortage, and cost-containment efforts are driving forces for change. Now is the time to reach for new heights in the quality of nursing care services.

REFERENCES

1. Novello, D.J. "The Consumer's Role in Health Care." In *Consumerism and Health Care*. New York: National League for Nursing, Pub. No. 52-1727, 1978, p. 2.

2. Walsh, M.E. "Nursing Responsibility for Patient's Rights." In *Consumerism and Health Care*. New York: National League for Nursing, Pub. No. 52-1727, 1978, p. 23.

3. *Nursing's Role in Patient Rights*. New York: National League for Nursing, Pub. No. 10019, 1977.

4. Aydelotte, M.K. "The Patient's Bill of Rights: Implications for the Health Care System." In *Consumerism and Health Care*. New York: National League for Nursing, Pub. No. 52-1727, 1978, p. 36.

5. Ibid., 38.

6. American Nurses Association. *Nursing: A Social Policy Statement*. Kansas City, Mo.: ANA, 1980, 9.

7. Aydelotte, "The Patient's Bill of Rights," 38.

8. Ware, J.E., Davies-Avery, A., and Steward, A.L. "The Measurement and Meaning of Patient Satisfaction: A Review of the Literature." *The Rand Paper Series*. Santa Monica, Calif.: Rand Corporation, 1977.

9. Ibid., 19.

10. Ware, J.E., Snyder, M.D., and Wright, W.R. "Some Issues in the Measurement of Patient Satisfaction with Health Care Services." *The Rand Paper Series*. Santa Monica, Calif.: Rand Corporation, 1977.

11. Hulka, B.S., and Zyzanski, S.J. "Validation of a Patient Satisfaction Scale." *Medical Care* 20 (1982):649-53.

12. Linn, M.W., Linn, B.S., and Stein, S.R. "Satisfaction with Ambulatory Care and Compliance in Older Patients." *Medical Care* 20 (1982):606-14.

13. Zweig, S., Kruse, J., and LeFevre, N. "Patient Satisfaction with Obstetrical Care." *Journal of Family Practice* 23, no. 2 (1986):131-36.

14. Lewis, C.C., et al. "Parent Satisfaction with Children's Medical Care." *Medical Care* 24 (1986):209-15.

15. McMillan, J.R., Younger, M.S., and DeWine, L.C. "Satisfaction with Hospital Emergency Department as a Function of Patient Triage." *Health Care Management Review* 11, no. 3 (1986):21-27.

16. Linder-Pelz, S. "Toward a Theory of Patient Satisfaction." *Social Science and Medicine* 16 (1982):577-82.

17. Henry, B., et al. "Delineation of Nursing Administration Research Priorities." *Nursing Research* 36 (September-October 1987):309-14.

18. Dunbar, S. "Quality: From Imperatives to Innovations." *Heart and Lung* 16, no. 3 (1987):23A-40A.

19. Abdellah, F.G., and Levine, E. "Developing a Measure of Patient and Personnel Satisfaction with Nursing Care." *Nursing Research* 5 (February 1957):100-8.

20. Abdellah, F.G., and Levine, E. *Better Patient Care Through Nursing Research*. New York: Macmillan, 1965.

21. Risser, N.L. "Development of an Instrument to Measure Patient Satisfaction with Nurses and Nursing Care in Primary Care Settings." *Nursing Research* 24 (January-February 1975):45-52.

22. Ventura, M.R., et al. "A Patient Satisfaction Measure as a Criterion to Evaluate Primary Nursing." *Nursing Research* 31 (1982):226-30.

23. Hinshaw, A.S., and Atwood, J.R. "A Patient Satisfaction Instrument: Precision by Replication." *Nursing Research* 31 (May-June 1982):170-75.

24. LaMonica, E.L., et al. "Development of a Patient Satisfaction Scale." *Research in Nursing and Health* 9 (1986):43-50.

25. Weisman, C.S., and Nathanson, C.A. "Professional Satisfaction and Client Outcomes." *Medical Care* 23 (1985):1179-92.

26. Ibid., 1191.

27. Aiken, L.H., and Mullinix, C.F. "The Nursing Shortage, Myth or Reality?" *New England Journal of Medicine* 317 (1987):641-45.

28. American Hospital Association. *The Nursing Shortage: Facts, Figures and Feelings*. Chicago: AHA, 1987.

29. Iglehart, J. "Problems Facing the Nursing Profession." *New England Journal of Medicine* 317 (1987):646-51.

30. Aiken and Mullinix, "The Nursing Shortage, Myth or Reality?"

31. Curran, C., Minnick A., and Moss J. "Who Needs Nurses?" *American Journal of Nursing* (April 1987):530-31.

32. Iglehart, "Problem Facing the Nursing Profession."

33. Curtin, L. "A Shortage of Nurses: Traditional Approaches Won't Work This Time." *Nursing Management* 18 (September 1987):7.

34. Aiken and Mullinix, "The Nursing Shortage, Myth or Reality?"

35. "National Study Shows Drop in Number of College Freshmen Pursuing Nursing Careers." *American Journal of Nursing* (April 1987):530-31.

36. "Downturn in Aid Puts New Pressure on Students." *American Journal of Nursing* (April 1987):532.

37. Iglehart, "Problems Facing the Nursing Profession."

38. American Hospital Association, *The Nursing Shortage*.

39. Ibid.

40. Kotler, P. *Marketing for Non-Profit Organizations.* Englewood Cliffs, N.J.: Prentice-Hall, 1975.

41. LaBella, J. *Patient Attitude Survey.* Hartford, Conn.: Hartford Hospital.

42. Strasen, L. *Key Business Skills for Nurse Managers.* New York: Lippincott, 1987.

43. Kachhal, S.K., DeBlaise-Dietz, R., and Morris, M. "An Overview of Nursing Management Information Systems: Components and Capabilities." *Software in Healthcare* 3 (August-September 1986):41-43.

44. Kinch, R.E. "Bedside Patient Care Work Stations." *Software in Healthcare* February-March 1986):47-55.

45. American Nurses Association, *Nursing: A Social Policy Statement.*

46. Orem, D.E. *Nursing: Concepts of Practice,* 3d ed. New York: McGraw-Hill, 1985.

47. Stanford, G. "Psychological Care as a Marketing Tool: Gaining Hospital-Wide Commitment Through Guest Relations Training." *Children's Health Care* (Spring 1987).

Nursing's preferred future

Myrtle K. Aydelotte, RN, PhD, FAAN

The American Academy of Nursing has taken on itself the task of forecasting the future of the nursing profession. And in the acceptance of that task it has chosen to consider the preferred future, not a future that may happen because of lack of foresight or failure of strategy. To make strategic decisions, we need a vision of what is desirable, what is highly valued, and above all, what is most worthwhile to society. This paper, describing my vision, reflects my value system, especially as it relates to nursing, health and the clientele we serve, my knowledge of what is going on in the world, and my imagination. The papers that follow are the responses of some of my colleagues to this vision.

In the last 25 years, that is, since 1960, many events, discoveries, and natural upheavals have changed the world, such as the increase in air travel, the launching of satellites, the women's movement, the sexual revolution, the thrust of nuclear energy, the Vietnam War, and the growth of telematics.

Several trends and issues in the world will shape what it will be 25 years from now. These trends and issues reside in our social institutions, the economy, the demography of the population of the United States, science and technology, and the health care industry. To identify the forces giving rise to these trends and issues is difficult, because their interplay is complex.

Social institutions. Our social institutions are undergoing radical modification in almost every sector. Unless some social intervention occurs, we are drifting toward a distinct two-culture society, the rich and the poor, reducing the large middle class that has been dominant in our society. However, inherent in our very social and political structure has been a value system that emphasizes opportunity for work and education, mobility from one class to another, and fairness. I predict that the current trend toward benefitting the favored will not persist and that the pendulum will swing back to a balance assuring the maintenance of the large middle class and addressing the question of how to interrupt the culturization and socialization of the poor.

Currently, there is national concern over the quality of education provided both children and adults. The movement to improve the quality of teachers has caught the attention of legislators and political bodies, resulting in efforts to reduce large classes in elementary and secondary schools and stress basic skills. At the college and university level, the trends of corporatization and entrepreneurship are evident. Faculty members are caught up in the entrepreneur movement, and many are establishing their own businesses as consultants, inventors, and designers. The collegial system, which has developed for centuries, is giving way to the formal structure of business and to hierarchical decision making.

The costs of education will continue to rise. Growth in the number of well-educated blacks and some other ethnic groups has slowed. However, these trends will change over time. In 2010, individuals will be better educated, more informed, and more highly skilled in the use of the information available to them.

Changes are also occurring today in the structure of the family, especially in the role of women. There are now 63 million families in the United States. Currently, 54 percent of all married women with children are in the labor force, and the number of single-parent families continues to grow. Further, the number of women in the work force has increased by 20 percent over the past 25 years. Since 1970, the divorce rate has risen by 80 percent, and the number of women heading households by 84 percent. Women are marrying later or not all. Women still face pay inequalities, sex segregation in jobs, salary discrimination, lack of advancement in positions, and a lower standard of living because of divorce. The trends in the employment of women, both in numbers and in the percent of newly created jobs now occupied by women, are such that by the end of the century women will make up most of the work force.[1]

Unless there are some social interventions and value changes, it appears that these trends will continue. Further, children will be raised in households different from those of today. Although the traditional family pattern will continue, a new definition of family is emerging. Unmarried older women are choosing to have children. Selected intimate groups not connected by marriage or by genetics are seen as families. The extended family of today consists of several sets of parents, step-parents, the consequential grandparents and great grandparents, and intimate friends. Because divorce does not incur the social stigma it carried a few years ago, an individual may marry more often and for shorter periods of time.

The changes in family structure and lifestyle have given rise to family resource coalitions and religious groups wishing to strengthen the family. Attention is being given to the need for daycare centers and agencies, preparation for being parents, sharing of family responsibilities, and public policies to support family leave for child care, especially in the early years.

By the year 2010 A.D., with the increase of women in the political arena, I predict that child care will be addressed and advancement of a number of other issues concerning women will be apparent. I must temper that statement, however, because progress has been slow. The general societal attitudes toward women, child bearing and rearing, marriage and the family are deeply rooted. Further, there is little evidence that the socialization of girls has changed markedly. The present culture continues to stress femininity, male dominance, and womanly dependence. The myth that women will be cared for persists, even among women.

Demographic changes. By the year 2010, the increase in the elderly population will be substantial. By 2020, the baby boomer population (those born shortly after World War II) will have reached the age of 65. Over the coming decades, the proportion of society over 65 years of age will nearly double. The number who are young and who provide services to these groups will be relatively small, for the number of high school graduates, which peaked in 1977, will not begin to climb until the 1990s.[2]

Although the number of individuals 75 years and older will not constitute the majority of elderly until the year 2040, 30 years later than the date we are examining, the number of frail elderly will be high. An increasing number will experience limitations in activity and chronic disability in the decade that follows. The implications for society and nursing, at the present time and in future decades, are many.

Most current programs of caring for the elderly, especially the functionally disabled, have not been satisfactory; 22 percent of those over 85 years of age today are in nursing homes, and the care in many homes is suspect.

Currently, 1.2 million elderly Americans

live in the community and are cared for by family members. The "young old" are caring for the "old old," with only 10 percent using formal community services; families are caught up in the provision of care to older family members when their energies are needed for the care of children. With the increase in elderly in 2010, the matter is extremely important. Nursing must respond to meet the needs of this population.

Our society is becoming not only older, but more diverse. There is a rapid growth in both the Spanish-speaking and the Asian populations. Although currently the majority of people agree that integration of all people in our society is essential to our national development, there is not a state of real integration.[3] The caste system identified by Gunnor Myrdal continues. Within the next 25 years, we will see a pluralistic society of greater diversity and increased integration. I predict that the commitment to integration of all peoples will hold.

Information technology and bio-technology. Over the past 20 years, tremendous growth has taken place in technology, both that involving information and that concerned with living organisms. The current trend in the development of telematics and biotechnology will continue. These changes will be accompanied by both continuing and new legal and ethical concerns.

Telematics is the term applied to new information technologies. These technologies include machines and communication systems, bringing together video, computers, and satellites; networks, management systems, and artificial intelligence. There will be advances in the information technologies used in data bases, which will be clinical, epidemiological and environmental and will concern individuals and communities. Artificial intelligence will lead to highly sophisticated clinical and administrative decision making. Other systems will lead to management of complex ma-

chines. A major use in the health field will be the surveillance of clients and patients for clinical information and safety.

In the field of biotechnology, we have already seen major developments. Recombinant DNA research has led to genetic engineering, human gene therapy, and various molecular products. It has been legal to patent genetically engineered microorganisms since 1980. During the next 25 years, we will continue to see new pharmaceuticals and new chemical compounds resulting from biotechnology, and dramatic developments in gene therapy.

The risks, legality, and ethics of technology will continue to be subjects for debate. Consensus has not yet been reached on the ethics of abortion, surrogate mothers, fetal surgery, imperiled infants, maintenance of life in selected cases, elderly suicide and euthanasia. Government regulation of technology, especially biotechnology, will continue. Ethical concerns about confidentiality, mind control, gene manipulation, and ownership of genetic material remain. More attention to ethics and legal issues will be required of health professionals. Time will be required to reach consensus on ethical questions that deal with the beginning and ending of life in our pluralistic society.

Economy. Discussion of the future centers on consideration of the world economy and specifically on health care economics. Since the 1970s, the United States has lost 23 percent of its share of the world's trade market. The trade deficit is at an all-time high, as is the federal deficit. U.S. productivity has slowed down and U.S. invention has declined. I cannot predict the world economy in 2010, but there will be fewer young to carry the cost of health care and they will be burdened by a deficit incurred by this generation. Health care spending's share of the GNP reached a new high in 1985. Spent on health care was $425 billion, equal to 10.7 percent of the GNP. It rose 8.9 percent above the 1984 level and out-stripped the inflation rate (3.9%) and growth of the GNP (5.6%). One-fourth of the cost was the result of intensity of care and the length of stay of those over 65 years of age.[4] The forces that are driving costs upward are of two kinds: first, those of the cost of providing the service plus inflation and second, demand or use factors, such as the requirements of the aging population and number of individuals with increased insurance coverage.

The current administration's objectives are to redirect public responsibility, reduce controls and regulations on the health care market, and encourage competition and private enterprise. The changing federal role in health care financing has led to changes in Medicaid and the introduction of prospective payment.[5,6] But not yet addressed are questions of policy relating to chronic illness and disabilities or the social policy of health care — health as a social good — or the long-range financial impact of the lack of foresight directed toward health promotion and prevention.

Currently, the uninsured are a sizable minority. Approximately 15 percent of the population, or 35 million people, lack health insurance.[7] The impact of social and financial inequality results in distinct patterns of morbidity and mortality among different populations.[8,9]

With the changes in federal initiatives, several states have introduced strategies to restructure the state hospital payment system, using a competitive approach. The shift of the burden from federal to state to private payors and limiting choice of provider may not, however, be the answer to health financing or to the provision of care. Attempting to control the market through competition may in fact be even more costly unless regulatory controls are placed on medical technology, pharmaceuticals, and litigation, for example. The basic issue is what amount of the gross national product we should give to health care and how it should be rationed.[10] This basic issue in

health care financing focuses on serious questions of social ethics and government responsibility for access to health care as well as what that health care will be.

The current trend is moving us toward a multiple-tiered system in which the poor and uninsured will receive support financed by federal, state, and local government. The health care for these populations will be placed on the market for competitive bidding. Other groups will receive care through group insurance plans and private pay.

In my opinion, this trend will continue into the next few decades. Particular attention needs to be given to defining the basic package that will be given to the lower tier.

Health care in 2010 A.D.

The current trends in health care are corporatization and privatization. The provision of health care in the United States is becoming a health-industry complex, in some respects not unlike the military-industry complex. There is movement of units of service, including hospitals, into multi-institutional systems, especially those that are investor owned, but even the non-profit systems are using the same type of institutional structure and approaches.[11,12]

Currently, there are 250 multihospital systems in the United States.[13] Some are establishing HMOs and PPOs to lock up referral patterns so that all services in the system are used. Others have developed surgi-centers, nursing homes, clinics, various types of outpatient services, and emergency centers. The programs that these systems offer are highly diversified, including health education, counseling, screening, and public lectures. Some have further diversified by sponsoring insurance plans, hotel services, transportation, supply services, and management. Integration of financing, management and services has taken place. Marketing and advertising, unheard of a few years ago, are accepted practices.

Given the trend and the financial activity of the investor-owned multisystems, I predict the following future for the health care system.

• The health industry by 2010 will be controlled by a few dozen national and international companies, not unlike the airlines of today or large, diversified producers of service goods. These health industries will be highly diversified and will operate in a variety of settings. They will offer many different services and products related to their services, such as health products or related products, insurance, hotels and management.

• The systems will reflect a blurring of delivery models. Combined to capture the market will be HMOs, PPOs, independent surgicenters, clinics, and other types of health services.

• Nonprofit health care systems may convert to profit systems or increase the number or kind of subunits that produce a profit.

• The nature of the hospital will change. It will consist of multiple intensive care units offering highly specialized scientific and technological services. The case mix of patients will represent very complex conditions requiring sophisticated medical interventions. The patients will remain in the hospital for short periods.

• To capture the market, there will be new programs for individuals who wish to maintain their health and to delay the onset of chronic disease.

• The public hospital as it is today will not exist.

• The majority of physicians will be employees of chains or in group practices associated with chains. Today, over 50 percent of physicians are employees.[14]

Slowing these trends somewhat are countercurrents that reflect concern about the momentum of corporatization and privatization and what they represent. There is a growing concern about quality of service, brought about not only by the emphasis on restructuring to capture the market and to introduce efficiency, but also the economy and reimbursement policies. The concern about quality is expressed by purchasers of the services, the third-party payors, including businesses that are negotiating contracts. Although quality of services may be the most frequently verbalized concern, there are others.

• *Access and rationing of health services.* The development of multiple levels of services for classes of people — the poor and uninsured, the "coach" class, and the first-class luxury services — raises many ethical questions about the distribution of health services as a social good. Who will decide who gets what?

• *The impact of competition and economic restraints on the practice of health professionals.* Economic constraints are restricting practice interventions of nurses and doctors. If this is compounded by standards imposed from the executive level, how will professionals accommodate? If productivity is defined as the number of patients treated and the number of nursing care hours per patient or minutes per visit, what changes will occur in practice and how will they affect the health care professional?

• *The demise of the public hospital and care of the poor and the uninsured.* Because of the reduction of Medicare and Medicaid reimbursement, a few innovative state and community programs are being introduced. Few studies of the patterns of individuals seeking health care have been made, but one study indicates that education, income and geographic location of the health service unit are factors influencing choice of source of care.[15] Who will assume the care of the poor and uninsured? And how will it be paid?

• *Conflict of interest.* The health professional's involvement in the health care industry as a stockholder or owner when the service is operated as a business is in question. Full consensus has not been reached on what constitutes reasonable compensation for services rendered and whether these services are rendered for the primary benefit of the provider or the client. The purchase of expensive equipment for group or personal medical business in order to capture a market has been cited as leading to unwise and costly practices such as unnecessary tests and studies. No solution has been proposed to control these costs or to monitor use of equipment and testing in group and individual practice settings.

• *The ability of an institution or subchain to meet the specific needs of a particular community and the assurance of the permanency of the arrangement.* Some people are concerned that the participation of the community in decisions involving the health care system serving them may become increasingly restricted. Because of the elimination of competition, no other health care service may be available.

The restructuring of the current health care system has been widely criticized. Fragmentation and impersonalization are often cited as byproducts of this restructuring. The expectation that the customer is knowledgeable about the product (service) to be rendered may be unrealistic. Further, the recipient may not be the direct purchaser or the contractor because the arrangements are made through a third party, the business that contracts for its employees, the government that approves fees and arrangements, and insurers. Is it reasonable to expect that recipients of services will have a greater voice in services rendered? Since provisions for health care services are often made through third parties, how will the individual recipient participate in selecting the provider of care?

A fairly large proportion of individuals will be more knowledgeable about health and about necessary services. The emphasis on palliative measures and treatment of pathology is giving way to an emphasis on health and fitness. The stress is on the individual's responsibility for his or her health and on the larger community's adoption of programs to produce healthier living or healthier environments.

I believe this concern about health is not a fad. More and more individuals are becoming aware that they are responsible for the condition of their bodies. This awareness is beginning to be reflected in governmental social policy, such as the change in the Armed Services policy regarding smoking and the recent program on drugs.

With these trends and countertrends, what will the health system look like? I believe it will be divided into four branches. There will be a branch concerned with health promotion, health education, self-help, and health evaluation. Another branch's business will be chronic disease management, serving a clientele that will be fairly stable except for episodic illness when an omission or digression of treatment occurs in the management of the chronic problem. A third branch will be concerned with trauma and with severe illnesses in which pathology must be treated with highly sophisticated medical interventions. The system's fourth branch will concentrate on care of the frail elderly, the physically limited elderly, and the dying.

The services provided by these branches will originate in several types of structures, located in a variety of institutions. The majority of the structures will be in the community and readily accessible to the clientele served. Ambulatory services, home care, hospices, and protected homelike environments for the elderly and physically limited will dominate. Schools, industries, and social clubs will provide settings. The expectation that families will assume greater responsibility for family members will persist, but that expectation will be moderated by various types of program assistance and family resource centers. The hospital will be present but will hold a less central position. It will continue to be seen as a dramatic and overwhelming environment because of the high technology and scientific research in which the staff will engage.

A challenge to the executive and professional staff of these branches will be twofold. I predict that the current multiinstitutional systems will become repugnant to those served. The emphasis upon ability to pay, the perceived impersonality, the schedules and waiting time, the time constraints and pressures placed on professional staff will all lead to restructuring of services in the various settings. Smaller sub-groups serving groups of clientele and providing more personal and continuous interaction between the health provider and the recipient of services will be formed. Autonomy of practice will be returned to the practitioners. In addition, the linkage system among the various branches will be very complex and require highly sophisticated communication. Each person will own his or her own data base and will control additional input to it. Problems of data confidentiality and access will require thoughtful planning and a special staff to manage the data linkages.

Future nursing roles and nursing practice

The organization of health care into four main branches will appear fragmented as a result of attempts to make it more effective and personal, but the scope and nature of nursing practice will reflect the populations served in those four branches. Nursing practice will continue to reflect intimacy, helpfulness, and compassion. The knowledge base required for practice will be extensive, regardless of the branch of health care in which nursing operates. Further, I predict that the title *nurse* will be used for only one class, the *professional;* support personnel will assist the nurse. If one class does not emerge, the professional in what we perceive today as the occupation of nursing

will possess a new title. Skills in administrative and clinical decision making, human relations, interpretation of data, scientific inquiry, and communication will be needed. Nursing diagnoses and interventions will be well developed, and research and development will continue on these topics as well as on programs of health education, promotion, and maintenance for various population groups. Research and development of nursing will be a major concern within each branch (health promotion, chronic illness, trauma and severe illness, and the elderly).

The future roles of nursing will emerge from the needs of the clientele and the structure of groups of nurses in the branches. The services may not be connected administratively. Some of the services may be offered by larger systems; some by smaller professional corporations, whose specific mission is limited; and some may be offered by individual nurses on contract. The provision of links among units of branches will be challenging. Ideally, clients would enter the total system of health care through the branch of health promotion and health maintenance.

Nursing practice in the future will include the use of a number of functions, such as surveillance, diagnostic reasoning, provision of personal needs, and the care of the environment. Surveillance will involve the use of technology, especially telematics and machines not yet designed, for tracking individuals, for collection of data, and for orientation of families and individuals. The use of artificial intelligence will assist in diagnostic reasoning. Provision of personal needs will be made easier by the automation of systems to dispense medications and give highly specialized therapy, and to prepare materials for sustenance. Robotic equipment will assist in the maintenance of the environment. Individual automatic systems will monitor personal business relationships, such as tracking, ordering supplies, and correspondence. Scientific and technological advances will result in the design of devices that will enable the physically and mentally limited to be more mobile. The major role of nurses will be the assurance of personal interaction, support for coping and refreshing, and education of individuals on how to use programs and technology, including machines and telematics. Individuals will need help in making use of the media provided them.

Within each of the branches, at least four classes of roles are needed: the provider of direct services to clients; the researcher and developer of new knowledge and techniques; the case or panel manager; and the executive. The provider of direct services evaluates the health status of clients and patients, makes nursing diagnoses and plans interventions, designs nursing orders, executes selected interventions, makes clinical nursing decisions, and uses and evaluates support personnel, who may come from several professions and occupations. The researcher and developer uses various approaches and other personnel to develop new knowledge, educational programs, technology, media, telematics, and the like. The case manager in the health promotion and maintenance branch, who provides entry into the whole system, serves a panel or group of patients or clients. This case manager assesses clients and plans interventions to keep them well or refers them to other professionals or units of service, if necessary. The case manager in the health promotion and maintenance branch is, in a sense, the primary care giver and manages the health care of individuals. The functions of the role are concerned with health status assessment, health promotion, and health maintenance. The role evolves out of the current nurse practitioner role with major emphasis on prevention rather than remedy.

Executives will be needed to administer groups of nurses in the units. Their role will be concerned with securing resources; allocating resources; policy development, evaluation, and revision; and distribution of services.

Case managers in each of the other branches manage groups or panels of patients referred to them from nurses and physicians in other branches. They assess clients and make nursing diagnoses, then refer them to direct-care givers. The case manager views the panel of patients as a collective and serves as both the major coordinator of the information and the liaison with nurses in units of other branches. Case managers and direct-care givers will be scholarly clinical practitioners and scientists. The collection of information for assessment, diagnosis, and planning will be obtained by highly sophisticated methods and devices, many of which have not yet been designed or even thought of. The transmission of data will likewise be much easier and much faster. Nurses will provide these services through four different arrangements:

• Professional corporations headed by nurses who contract with populations or other organizations as a group to provide nursing services, such as intensive care, school nursing, hospice or home health care, or business.

• Nurse specialty practice groups that individually contract with clients or groups to provide special services, such as counseling, health maintenance, and technological services.

• Practice on an individual basis arranged by contracts to provide for highly specialized nursing service on a one-to-one basis or to give consultation to other nurses, professionals, and institutions.

• Employment in both profit and nonprofit health care systems operated by boards of directors. These will be chiefly oriented toward acute care.

Strategic decisions

Nursing practice in 2010 will be intimate, compassionate, empathetic and truly professional. The knowledge base of practice will be well delineated and unique; its use will enable the practitioner to offer services for which there is no substitute. Nurses will be well educated, highly skilled, and capable of managing their own affairs. They will practice in many types of settings and under varying contractual arrangements. Ethics and legal issues will be a major concern. Above all, nursing practice will continue to be directed toward helping others to live lives of the highest possible quality or enabling them to die with dignity and peace.

To achieve this preferred future of nursing, several strategies must be put in place now and in the near future. I am confident we can do the necessary work, but only if we have the necessary clarity of purpose and strong determination. Some of my proposals may be seen as elitist. That is my intent.

First of all, we must strive for clarification and understanding of the nature of the profession. Definitions and scope-of-practice statements are insufficient. A profession reflects the acquisition of knowledge and skills that no other group possesses. Consequently, there is no substitute for the professional. The knowledge of nursing must be exclusive. With our current egalitarian attitude and our eagerness to give content to others, we are impeding our drive to make our knowledge base exclusive and retain fully the skills that are needed to serve the public. We compromise our image, confuse the public, and most unfortunately, by default, make it possible for people to receive care, called *nursing care,* which is inferior and for which we are not responsible or accountable. But in the public's eye we are giving it. I am calling for a restriction on the practice of educating individuals to be less than professional nurses. In order to serve the public better, we need to garner our knowledge, refine it, and identify that which is exclusively ours. For example, I do not believe that the use of nursing diagnosis, diagnostic reasoning and nurs-

ing interventions should go the route of nursing process and be used by others. The professional in any field uses support personnel, but those individuals have a different knowledge base and different skills. Above all, access to those who are served is controlled by the professional. Further, the professional is accountable for support personnel.

Second, individuals entering nursing must meet high standards of intelligence and motivation. Public service motivation is paramount. Professions maintain control through admission to professional schools and through employment opportunities. I believe that we will not achieve the goal of excellence in nursing care for the public if we continue to be preoccupied by numbers and ignore standards. Neither can we attract talented individuals if we mix them with poor risks. For too long, nursing has been preoccupied with numbers. We are the most counted, most tabulated, and best described occupation in the United States. I believe that we must concern ourselves with building a cadre of true professionals rather than expend our energies in other directions. Furthermore, we need to learn how to use support personnel. There is a great need for excellence both in clinical nursing and in administration.

Third, a remodeling of nursing education is long overdue. The future calls for a different and much more extensive education than that currently in place. More depth in the sciences, a greater understanding of economics, emphasis on ethics and legal issues, introduction to management and business, understanding of information technology and artificial intelligence, and greater clinical application are all indicated. The future, although exciting, will not be easy. The student entering a profession today and graduating at the age of 25 may practice for 40 years. Many changes in the health field will take place. The educational foundation of the practice should be sound.

Fourth, the professional of the future needs preparation in self-governance and self-management. How can we provide that outcome through our present educational programs and current work experiences? Does our approach to teaching, especially in the practicum, allow the development of self-regulation? Only mature students can be prepared for self-governance and self-management. Opportunities for more responsibility in learning and in continuity of clinical nursing experiences are required. Avenues for the development of clinical nursing judgment must be explored and made available to students.

Fifth, our relationship with the public and the power elite and power brokers must change. Political action must extend beyond the legislative arena; it is not the only arena in which power brokers operate. We must learn the subtleties of power-brokerage. It can be done. We should move nursing into every aspect of community affairs. I suggest that nursing leadership make a concerted and calculated effort to move into powerful circles. There is no reason why nurses cannot become college and university presidents and vice-presidents, leaders in community and business affairs, heads of corporations, and chairs of boards.

Sixth, because money controls and dominates, let us get on with the costing out of nursing services, gaining reimbursement for our services, learning the management of contracts and business, and attaching value to services and quality. Many will say that what I propose will be too expensive for society, that we will make ourselves too costly. I disagree. The avoidance of the loss of functioning of others, the reduction of the length and cost of illness, and the value of rehabilitation of the sick will more than meet any additional cost. Further, nurses have always earned income; it simply has filtered to others disguised as hospital room costs or payments to non-nurse

supervisors. Let us recognize that a reimbursement system that pays directly to nursing services obtained by contracts may assist in identifying our worth.

These strategies are simply put, but they are not simplistic. To be effective, they need to be carefully fleshed out. Guiding us is a vision of nursing — a preferred future. Let us capture that vision and make it real, for not to do so places us among the oppressed. And it is time for us to carve out our own image and transform ourselves to that image. The public we will serve in 2010 will be better for it.

REFERENCES

1. Hacker, A. Women at work. *NY Rev. Books* 33(12)26-32, 1986.

2. Felton, G. Harnessing today's trends to guide nursing's future. *Nurs. Health Care* 7:211-213, Apr. 1986.

3. Pifer, A. *The Higher Education of Blacks in the United States.* New York, Carnegie Corporation of New York, 1973.

4. Health-care spending's share of the GNP reaches new high. *The Washington Post* p. A6, July 30, 1986.

5. Davis, C.K. The federal role in changing health care financing; Part I. National programs and health financing problems. *Nurs. Econ.* 1:10-17, Jul.-Aug. 1983.

6. _____. The federal role in changing health care financing; Part II. Prospective payment and its impact on nursing. *Nurs. Econ.* 1:98-104, 146, Sept.-Oct. 1983.

7. Jones, K.R., and Kilpatrick, K.E. State strategies for financing indigent care. *Nurs. Econ.* 4:61-65, 88, Mar.-Apr. 1986.

8. Robert Wood Johnson Foundation. *Special Report.* (Updated report on access to health care for the American people, No. 1) Princeton, NJ, The Foundation, 1983.

9. Aday, L., and others. *Health Care in the U.S.: Equitable for Whom?* Beverly Hills, CA, Sage Publishing Co., 1980.

10. Reinhardt, U.E. Rationing the health-care surplus: an American tragedy. *Nurs. Econ.* 4:101-108, May-June 1986.

11. Bauknecht, V.L. IOM study of "for-profits" finds care costs not very different. *Am. Nurse* 18:3-5, Jul.-Aug. 1986.

12. Institute of Medicine, Committee on Implications of For-Profit Enterprise in Health Care. *For-Profit Enterprise in Health Care.* Washington, DC, National Academy Press, 1986.

13. Brown, M. Multihospital systems in the 80s—the new shape of the health care industry. *Hospitals* 56:71-74, Mar. 1, 1982.

14. Relman, A.S. The future of medical practice. *Health Aff.* (Millwood) 2:5-19, Summer 1983.

15. Kronenfeld, J.J. Organization of ambulatory care by consumers. *Sociol. Health Illness* 4:183-200, 1982.

Where to find the new immigrants

JAMES P. ALLEN; EUGENE J. TURNER

IMMIGRATION IS AN IMPORTANT contributor to U.S. population growth, especially at the local level. Since 1965, changes in our immigration laws have increased both the numbers and the kinds of immigrants coming to the United States. But the size and the characteristics of immigrant groups differ greatly among American states and cities.

Businesses need to be aware that immigrant populations are growing at the local level because immigrants are potential markets and an important pool of labor. While many people are familiar with the pattern of immigration during the 1970s, there have been important changes in the 1980s.

Legal immigrants come to the U.S. with immigration visas, or they change their status to immigrant (or permanent resident) after arriving here as temporary visitors. During the 1980s, legal immigration has averaged 570,000 people a year — 30 percent higher than the average for the 1970s and substantially more than in any year from 1924 to 1978. In addition, hundreds of thousands of aliens with nonimmigrant status live legally in the United States. These include students, temporary workers, visitors, traders, and investors, as well as their spouses and children. Many become immigrants while they are here. After their legal status changes, they are included in the next year's statistics on immigration.

Annual immigration totals are well above the limits set by Congress of 270,000 worldwide and 20,000 from individual countries. These numerical restrictions do not apply to spouses, parents, and unmarried minor children of immigrants who have become U.S. citizens. Also, refugees who change their status to permanent resident after living here at least one year are not subject to the limits. As a result, over half of all immigrants arriving here since 1982 have qualified in nonquota categories.

In 1980, there were probably between 2.5 and 3.5 million illegal aliens here. Ideally, this analysis should account for illegals, but the lack of precise estimates of their numbers makes it impossible to include them. The number of immigrants who leave the United States each year is also unknown. But during this century, emigration flows probably averaged about one-third of immigration totals.

Net immigration to this country during the 1980s accounts for one-quarter to one-third of the nation's population growth, according to the Census Bureau. These figures — based on vital statistics, annual reported immigration totals, and estimates of illegal entrants and of emigrants to other countries — are arguably too low because U.S.-born children of recent immigrants are not included as immigrants. Moreover, the fertility of foreign-born women is somewhat higher than that of native-born women. The rate is especially high for Mexican and Indochinese women, which suggests that the cumulative effects of immigration are even greater than the official numbers imply.

Leaving home

To examine the characteristics of migrants to the U.S., it is important to know where the migrants come from. We use data on country of birth, collected by the U.S. Immigration and Naturalization Service (INS), whenever possible.

Between 1983 and 1986, Mexican-born immigrants made up the largest share of legal immigrants to the United States — about 60,000 people a year. The Philippines contributed about 46,000 immigrants a year. And immigrants from mainland China, Taiwan, and Hong Kong together account for another 45,000 annually. The next largest groups are Koreans and Vietnamese, with an annual average of nearly 35,000 immigrants each, and Asian Indians and Dominicans, averaging about 25,000 each. During most years, over 10,000 immigrants come to the U.S. from each of the following countries: Jamaica, Cuba, Iran, Cambodia, the United Kingdom, Laos, the Arab countries as a group, Canada, and Colombia.

The pattern of immigration in the 1980s is different from what it was in the 1970s. Immigration from Asia (which includes the Middle East and Pacific Islands) has risen so dramatically that the Census Bureau's estimates of the number of U.S. residents of a race other than black or white increased 45 percent between 1980 and 1986. The growth in the share of Asian immigrants is due to the settlement of many more Chinese, Vietnamese, Cambodians, Laotians, and Iranians in the U.S. during the 1980s. A small but growing proportion of immigrants are coming from Central America and Africa, while the share of immigrants coming from Europe has declined from 53 percent in the 1950s to less than 12 percent today. The share of immigrants coming from India has increased slightly, while immigrants from South Korea and the Philippines make up about the same proportion as they did in the 1970s.

In general, short-term shifts in the sources of immigrants are dependent on refugee admissions in previous years. Beginning with the Vietnamese in 1975, three Indochinese countries sent over 800,000 refugees to the U.S. as of 1986. Most of these people later adjusted their status to permanent resident. Laotian immigration was greatest in 1982 and 1983, following peaks of refugee admissions. The largest groups of Cambodian refugees began arriving here in 1981, resulting in rising numbers of Cambodian immigrants through 1986. More refugees have come from Vietnam than any other country in the 1980s, but there has been a steady decline in the number of Vietnamese immigrants over the decade.

Cuban immigration was especially large from 1975 through 1978. There also was a sharp increase in the number of Cuban immigrants to the U.S. in 1985 and 1986 as the Cuban "Marielitos" who came here as refugees in 1980 became immigrants. Haitian immigrant totals in 1986 and 1987 are twice as high as they were in the 1970s.

When a new group of refugees settles in the U.S., it can become a magnet for later immigration of relatives. Because of this, some countries that now send few people to the U.S. could become significant sources of immigrants. Ethiopia and Afghanistan, the source of 34,000 refugees early in the decade, for example, now contribute an increasing share of immigrants. Poland, Rumania, and the Soviet Union are also important sources of refugees, but these ethnic populations are already established in the United States.

Where to live

Nearly 90 percent of immigrants to the U.S. from 1983 through 1986 settled in only 20 states, according to intended destination statistics collected by the INS. Because of that, we focus this analysis on those 20 states. Though many migrants eventually move away from their intended destination, these data are useful for identifying major immigrant clusters in the U.S.

Between 1983 and 1986, California received the largest share of immigrants to the U.S., followed by New York, Texas, Florida, New Jersey, and Illinois. California is the most popular destination for most immigrant groups, adding to that state's ethnic diversity as well as to its population growth. By constructing an index of relative immigrant concentration, it is possible to discover where immigrants from a particular country of origin cluster in greater numbers than expected. Such an index is called a location quotient. The quotient equals 1 if the share of an immigrant group in a state's population is equivalent to the share of that group among immigrants nationally.

In many states, the location quotients are not surprising. New Filipino immigrants, for instance, are 6.8 times more concentrated in Hawaii than in the country as a whole. These variations in immigrant settlements occur because of the different historical circumstances that led to the first immigrant communities. San Francisco, for example, became a supply focus and retreat for Chinese gold miners and laborers, while Jamaicans first settled in Hartford in 1943 after having been brought to Connecticut to harvest vegetables and apples.

Typically, these initial settlements grow through "chain migration" — the arrival of friends and relatives who need the help of earlier immigrants in adjusting to the U.S. Because immigrants tend to go where others from their country already live, the destinations of large immigrant groups in the 1980s are likely to be where those from the same country settled in the 1970s.

Among professionals who speak English well, chain migration is not as important — provided the immigrant is willing to pursue opportunities without the social support of family and an immigrant community. This is why Chinese, Indian, Korean, Iranian, European, and Canadian immigrants tend to be more dispersed among the states.

There have been some changes in immigrant destinations over time. Vietnamese have been more likely to settle in Massachusetts and Georgia since 1982 than they were in the 1970s. More significantly, there has been a movement of Vietnamese already in the U.S. to California.

Before World War I, European immigrants established distinctive settlement patterns. But the correlation between immigrant destinations in the 1980s and these historic settlements is often low. This may be because many recent Europeans immigrants are not connected through family ties to Americans of European descent.

Metropolitan destinations

Almost 90 percent of immigrants choose to live in a metropolitan area. Most immigrants choose specific metropolitan areas because they have family and friends there.

We examined the 38 metropolitan areas that attract over 2,000 immigrants a year. New York City attracts more immigrants than any other metropolitan areas — over 90,000 from 1984 through 1986.

The greatest share of these immigrants were born in the Dominican Republic: more than one-sixth of New York City's immigrants come from this small country. The Dominican Republic's Caribbean neighbor, Jamaica, follows with over 10 percent of immigrants. People born in China, Taiwan, or Hong Kong make up the next largest share, about 9 percent. And immigrants from Guyana and Haiti each make up over 6 percent.

Los Angeles–Long Beach is second in the numbers of immigrants it attracts. An average of 58,000 listed it as their destination each year between 1984 and 1986. Over one-sixth of Los Angeles–Long Beach's new immigrants were born in Mexico, followed by Filipinos (12 percent), and Koreans (9 percent). In 1986 and 1987, Mexicans, Salvadorans, and Koreans were more likely to report Los Angeles as a destination than they were in 1984 and 1985.

Chicago gained more than 20,000 legal immigrants a year between 1984 and 1986.

Text continued on page 375

Destination, U.S.A.

New York is the most popular destination for new immigrants, but 37 other metropolitan areas receive at least 2,000 immigrants a year. Listed below are selected immigrant groups moving to major metropolitan areas, ranked by average annual immigrants received from 1984 to 1986.

METROPOLITAN AREA	TOTAL*	MEXICO	PHILIP-PINES	CHINA**	SOUTH KOREA	VIET-NAM	INDIA
New York, NY	92,345	478	1,761	7,823	2,641	832	3,036
Los Angeles-Long Beach, CA	57,912	10,026	6,680	5,081	5,092	3,200	1,139
Chicago, IL	21,620	4,105	2,178	1,021	1,366	445	2,372
Miami-Hialeah, FL	19,609	133	166	114	49	50	95
San Francisco, CA	16,521	705	3,563	3,793	467	1,200	242
Washington, DC-MD-VA	15,636	84	763	972	1,659	1,066	995
Anaheim-Santa Ana, CA	12,916	1,684	798	924	1,064	3,049	370
San Jose, CA	11,665	1,009	1,838	1,495	548	2,305	624
Oakland, CA	9,832	727	2,149	1,393	425	645	493
San Diego, CA	9,571	2,599	2,314	281	201	934	83
Boston, MA	9,325	29	143	905	233	746	374
Houston, TX	9,210	2,552	373	504	300	1,030	626
Newark, NJ	9,013	15	390	412	265	115	691
Nassau-Suffolk, NY	7,621	41	228	424	372	99	566
Bergen-Passaic, NJ	7,421	57	332	249	488	34	613
Philadelphia, PA	7,117	47	443	458	1,082	437	738
Jersey City, NJ	7,093	17	485	110	135	82	656
Honolulu, HI	6,849	12	3,403	757	888	451	13
Dallas, TX	6,378	1,781	205	303	300	494	438
Seattle, WA	5,248	84	758	497	553	675	185
Detroit, MI	5,116	84	395	217	380	78	508
Riverside-San Bernardino, CA	4,282	1,371	414	200	225	330	124
El Paso, TX	3,724	3,265	37	16	91	11	15
Minneapolis-St. Paul, MN-WI	3,697	78	121	154	468	363	164
Atlanta, GA	3,409	55	101	195	311	362	172
Phoenix, AZ	3,312	1,115	161	209	145	212	96
Sacramento, CA	3,181	396	373	343	122	523	92
Middlesex-Somerset-Hunterdon, NJ	3,058	22	137	225	168	45	487
Denver, CO	3,004	464	104	107	370	428	91
Fort Lauderdale-Hollywood-Pompano Beach, FL	2,910	19	57	53	32	33	72
Portland, OR	2,832	109	167	200	274	592	75
Baltimore, MD	2,785	10	215	177	595	67	252
New Orleans, LA	2,702	45	81	83	68	716	88
Tampa-St. Petersburg-Clearwater, FL	2,553	107	110	60	90	212	63
Fresno, CA	2,542	826	194	83	39	84	171
Fort Worth-Arlington, TX	2,513	704	69	138	90	274	135
Stockton, CA	2,431	449	398	104	24	340	62
McAllen-Edinburg-Mission, TX	2,296	2,189	9	10	7	—	2

*Total is the average annual number of immigrants moving to the metropitan area from 1984 to 1986.
**Includes immigrants from the Peoples' Republic of China, Taiwan, and Hong Kong.

DOM. REP.	JAMAICA	CUBA	IRAN	CAMBODIA	LAOS	COLOMBIA	HAITI	EL SALVADOR	GUYANA
15,554	9,415	647	807	497	39	3,610	5,947	1,162	6,510
32	227	1,402	3,883	1,697	122	393	28	2,953	84
62	323	243	314	185	111	232	207	136	30
436	1,153	10,571	66	5	7	1,162	1,067	179	94
5	22	42	410	341	114	48	17	904	11
188	613	66	901	318	168	201	125	1,066	277
4	17	113	696	498	250	90	2	101	4
3	14	15	491	413	85	20	3	111	8
2	24	16	324	143	197	32	3	133	12
9	9	33	353	343	320	30	2	26	3
435	404	56	231	466	114	168	718	90	45
33	95	144	277	160	98	169	10	308	33
263	556	701	63	13	1	579	763	188	360
578	640	63	282	13	16	364	274	574	251
914	460	178	150	6	1	637	28	106	88
42	429	23	144	380	54	77	69	25	39
716	34	1,924	36	—	7	448	64	192	141
1	2	1	7	31	219	2	1	2	2
9	33	74	281	245	174	44	4	42	14
1	6	6	150	451	319	25	—	9	2
6	87	14	100	18	42	26	9	11	12
2	17	51	92	66	22	27	1	56	12
2	—	6	21	1	—	7	—	7	—
3	13	11	108	259	607	56	1	8	93
9	90	86	154	237	89	62	15	15	13
1	7	9	71	67	15	23	2	23	7
3	9	5	92	20	255	7	—	28	1
425	95	89	34	5	14	85	12	25	59
2	6	13	94	115	164	19	1	8	2
28	637	260	30	—	1	172	227	26	33
1	4	16	119	194	217	17	—	8	1
13	172	3	146	11	4	25	11	16	23
24	17	175	29	53	34	39	5	49	17
26	125	355	52	42	43	66	40	8	16
1	2	1	60	88	610	2	—	10	1
2	9	16	93	98	117	19	2	10	3
—	1	—	4	404	294	1	—	6	1
2	—	7	3	—	—	4	—	7	—

Source: U.S. Immigration and Natralization Service

Immigrant clusters

The chart below shows the average annual migration and major concentrations of immigrants in the 20 leading state destinations, 1983 through 1986.

LEADING STATE OF DESTINATION	AVERAGE ANNUAL IMMIGRANTS 1983-1986	COUNTRY OF BIRTH AND LOCATION QUOTIENTS
California	149,818	(No group with location quotient greater than 2.5)
New York	103,791	Guyana, 4.2; Dom. Republic, 3.7; Ecuador, 3.2; Haiti, 3.2; Jamaica, 2.9
Texas	43,723	Mexico, 4.1
Florida	36,356	Cuba, 10.0; Haiti, 2.7; Colombia, 2.7
New Jersey	29,808	Ecuador, 3.1; Colombia, 3.1; Cuba, 2.6
Illinois	26,405	Poland, 5.0
Massachusetts	13,953	Haiti, 2.7
Pennsylvania	10,565	(No group with location quotient greater than 2.5)
Virginia	10,420	(No group with location quotient greater than 2.5)
Maryland	10,101	(No group with location quotient greater than 2.5)
Washington	10,055	Cambodia, 4.1; Laos, 3.5; Thailand, 2.8; Canada, 2.6
Michigan	8,336	Canada, 2.9; Poland, 2.8
Hawaii	7,945	Philippines, 6.8
Connecticut	6,899	Poland, 4.3; Jamaica, 4.1
Ohio	6,712	(No group with location quotient greater than 2.5)
Arizona	5,999	Mexico, 4.0; Canada, 2.7
Georgia	5,633	W. Germany, 3.0; Cambodia, 2.7; Laos, 2.6
Minnesota	5,383	Laos, 7.6; Cambodia, 4.0; Thailand, 3.2
Colorado	5,068	Canada, 3.0
Louisiana	4,449	Vietnam, 3.8; Guatemala, 2.7

Note: The location quotient is the share of immigrants from a specific country in a state's total immigrant population compared with the share of immigrant from that country nationally. A location quotient of 1 means that the share of immigrants in the state is the same as the national share.
Source: U.S. Immigration and Naturalization Service

Nineteen percent of these newcomers were born in Mexico. Asian Indians account for 11 percent, and Filipinos another 10 percent.

Miami ranks fourth partly because over 20,000 Cubans became immigrants in 1986. Over half of all recent immigrants in Miami were born in Cuba, and no other nation accounts for more than 10 percent of all immigrants to Miami.

In San Francisco, to which over 16,000 people migrate annually, those born in China, Taiwan, or Hong Kong are 23 percent. In California, four additional metropolitan areas — Anaheim, San Jose, Oakland, and San Diego — each average more than 9,000 immigrants annually. Other metropolitan areas receiving more than 9,000 immigrants a year include Washington, D.C., and Houston.

In 1986 and 1987, Koreans listed Baltimore, Maryland and the Bergen-Passaic area in New Jersey more often than earlier in the decade. Immigrants from Mexico and the Philippines have been much more likely to settle in San Diego during those two years than in 1984 and 1985. Cambodians have ben choosing Boston and Atlanta more frequently as destinations, and there was a decline in the number of new Laotian immigrants to Honolulu, Seattle, and Portland in 1986 and 1987.

Some areas that gain fewer than 2,000 immigrants a year are also worth mentioning. Providence, Rhode Island, for example, has attracted many Cambodians. Dominicans make up a considerable share of immigrants to the Lawrence/Haverhill area in Massachusetts. Jamaicans immigrate to Hartford, Connecticut, in substantial numbers, as do Filipinos to Norfolk–Virginia Beach–Newport News, Virginia.

The infusion of immigrants to the U.S. is transforming many metropolitan areas and affecting politics, the labor force, and consumer behavior. The best way to track where those changes are greatest is to know where the new immigrants are going. The best predictor of where immigrants are going is where they have gone in the past, but new patterns are emerging.

The challenge of an aging society

PHILLIP LONGMAN

THE AGING OF THE U.S. population, in combination with current low rates of investment in education and new technology, poses a severe threat to American industry's ability to compete in world markets. The shrinking supply of skilled young workers and the growing number of retirees may ultimately condemn the United States to becoming a second-rate industrial power.

Thus far in U.S. history, rapid population growth has provided American industry not only with an ever-expanding work force, but also with an ever-larger domestic market. But in the coming years, this will change dramatically. The American work force is aging rapidly. Not only is today's younger generation comparatively small — owing to the low birth rates of the last two decades — but an alarming proportion of American youth lack the basic skills that employers require.

At the same time, the trends toward early retirement and increased life expectancy among the old threaten employers with exploding pension and health-care costs. The declining ratio of workers to retirees means that business profits will fall, along with the American standard of living, unless the United States undertakes massive investments in raising the productivity of the next generation of workers.

The aging population

For the near term, the aging of the American work force has many positive aspects, for both business and government. Currently, one out of three Americans is between the ages of 27 and 42 — members of the celebrated baby-boom generation. As the youngest boomers move into their middle years, employers will have a vast pool of experienced workers upon which to draw. The boomers should also tend to borrow less and to save more as they become more established, which could provide American business with more and cheaper capital. Finally, so long as nearly all baby boomers remain at work, their taxes and pension contributions will provide a bulging source of cash flow for both public and private old-age benefit plans.

Yet, all these trends will be thrown into reverse in the not-too-distant future. The oldest boomers are now just 19 years away from reaching the current average age of retirement. In the meantime, the percentage of the population over 65, and particularly the ranks of the very old, will continue to grow rapidly.

Between just 1970 and 1980, life expectancy at 65 increased by more than 9%, while life expectancy at birth increased by only 3% and birth rates plummeted. As a result, the fastest growing segment of the population today is the age group over 80. At the same time, both the absolute number and the proportion of the population under 25 are declining. Thus, long before the retirement of the baby boomers, American business and government will be forced to pay much more for health and pension benefits, even as the supply of young workers is becoming scarcer.

The burden on business

Many businesses are already feeling the burden of an aging population. Service-sector companies have been struck by a severe shortage of entry-level workers. As recently as eight years ago, young people aged 16 to 24 made up a quarter of the work force. Today, this age group accounts for little more than a fifth of American workers — a percentage that will decline to 16% by 1995.

A decade from now, assuming sustained economic growth, the shortage of entry-level workers will extend to more senior positions. And the competition for qualified workers will be even keener because so many of today's young Americans lack basic language and math skills. Only 30% of today's 17-year-olds are classified as "adept" readers — competent enough to go on to college or to cope with business environments.

Meanwhile, many — if not most — manufacturing companies are faced with the more ominous burden of supporting a burgeoning number of retirees. In 1984, the Chrysler Corporation paid $530 in health benefits for every car it sold. Approximately 40% of this amount went to people who weren't even working for Chrysler — retired people and dependents. When the company first agreed to pay such benefits in 1966, it seemed a comparatively cheap and also humane way to buy peace with labor; paying the price would largely be the problem of the next generation of labor and management.

But no one imagined that the price would be so high. At Chrysler and throughout America's manufacturing sector, the ratio of workers to retirees has since declined dramatically, owing to layoffs, early retirement, and the increasing life expectancy of the elderly. The growing number of retirees has already severely reduced America's ability to compete in foreign markets and can only be compounded as the population continues to age.

At Armco Inc., a diversified steel company in Morristown, New Jersey, the ratio of active employees to retirees shrank from 5-to-1 in 1975 to 1.8-to-1 in 1985. During the same interval, Armco's annual retiree health-care

costs soared from $5 million to $40 million. The recent troubles of the LTV Corporation, which had been paying health-care benefits to more than 38,000 retirees, further dramatize the challenge that awaits all businesses in the years ahead. It is a challenge that is not confined merely to "sunset" or declining industries.

Post-employment health care is an open-ended promise, so no one is sure how to estimate the aggregate burden such benefits will present in the future. But some estimates put the total unfunded liabilities of America's private health-care plans higher than $2 trillion. Unless benefits are cut, this cost will come at the direct expense of the next generation of labor and management.

Private pension plans, while generally well-funded, will also come under severe strain if the aging of the population is not matched by increases in productivity. A sign of the trouble ahead is the yawning deficit of the Pension Benefit Guaranty Corporation, a little-known government corporation that guarantees the private pensions of more than 30 million Americans. Between just 1979 and 1984, the increasing number of failed pension plans caused the present value of PBGC's outstanding liabilities to more than triple. Despite recent steep premium increases charged to pension providers, the agency foresees itself becoming insolvent by 2005.

Death and taxes

The aging of the population, if unmatched by a rise in productivity, also threatens American business with an alarming spiral in payroll taxes to fund Social Security and Medicare. All but the most optimistic official forecast by the Social Security Administration (SSA) show, however, that for these programs to pay even reduced benefits to the baby boomers payroll taxes on both workers and their employers will have to rise dramatically.

Moreover, even these projections are based on what most informed Americans would consider rosy assumptions about the future of the economy: The SSA's so-called most-pessimistic model calls for the economy to perform better in the future than it actually has during the recent past.

If the economy behaves according to this "worst-case" scenario, the SSA predicts that, under current tax rates, the Medicare trust fund and the disability trust fund will be exhausted in the late 1990s and the pension fund by 2030 — assuming the pension fund's assets aren't used to replenish the shortfall in the first two funds. Moreover, all SSA projections are based on the explicit assumption that today's younger Americans will receive significantly fewer benefits than do today's senior citizens.

Educating the next generation of workers

Further underscoring the challenge of an aging population is the ominous increase in poverty among children. Senator Daniel Patrick Moynihan says, "It is fair to assume that the United States has become the first society in history in which a person is more likely to be poor if young rather than old." We don't know much about alleviating poverty, but we do know that poor children tend to grow up to be poor adults. Since 1973, the poverty rate among Americans under 18 has increased by more than 50%. More than one out of five children are now living in poverty. Experts predict that a third of all American children will experience poverty sometime before reaching adulthood.

The implications for American competitiveness are clear. "In the midst of our prosperity, we are facing the development of a potentially permanent underclass," says William Kolberg, president of the National Alliance of Business. "Most of our population, of whatever race or ethnic background, are making the transition from school to work and becoming part of society....Each year, hundreds of thousands of young people do not make the transition. They reach working age without the basic knowledge they need to learn even the simple skills necessary for success in an entry-level job."

Poor children are not the only ones growing up unprepared to compete in the world economy of the next century. A recent federal report on the state of public education, *A Nation at Risk,* observes that the United States has committed acts of "unilateral, educational disarmament." Between 1980 and 1985, while total federal outlays increased 21% in constant dollars, education outlays dropped almost a third. A 12-nation study of seven subjects (mathematics, science, reading comprehension, literature, English, French, and civil education) found that the U.S. average comprehensive scores were always in the lower third. In mathematics, American students were lowest among *all* nations tested.

Nearly all economists agree that the industrialized nations are moving toward an information-driven, rather than an energy-driven, economy in the next century. The intellectual skills of the labor force will thus become increasingly important to maintaining America's comparative advantage in trade, as well as to funding old-age benefits and other vital services. Yet, few observers take an integrated view of all the challenges that must be met.

"Scientific and technological decay, political neglect of education and the schools, and the juvenilization of poverty are related," says Donald Kennedy, president of Stanford University. "All form a trend in America's political economy that could, if we do not arrest it, become a death spiral."

Youth and capital

These social and demographic challenges to the American standard of living in the next century argue strongly for massive investments in raising the nation's store of both human and physical capital. Yet, far from investing adequately in its children's future, the United States continues in a myriad of ways to borrow against their anticipated future earnings.

The mounting federal deficits provide the most straightforward example. Viewed from a perspective of generational equity, the doubling of the national debt between 1981 and 1986 might have been justified if the money had gone toward purposes that truly benefited the next generation — such as education, research, and development.

Instead, the debt has largely been incurred to underwrite current consumption and to pay interest on previous deficits. In recent years, nearly 30% of federal spending has gone to pay old-age benefits to the 11% of the population currently over 65, while the amount spent directly on children is estimated at 3%-5%. Interest on the national debt is the fastest growing portion of the budget. Gross interest on the public debt skyrocketed from $80.4 billion in 1980 to an estimated $178.9 billion in 1986, which accounted for nearly 18% of all federal spending.

Yet, these numbers do not even begin to capture the magnitude of the costs that the United States is pushing into the future. Through Social Security, Medicare, and numerous "off-budget" loan guarantee programs, the federal government is each year incurring future obligations for which it possesses no capital or reserves. Instead, the next generation of taxpayers is simply expected to absorb these costs as they come due. Using the same "accrual method" of accounting that the federal government requires of private firms, the General Accounting Office estimated that the true national debt, as of the end of September 1984, was $4.7 trillion — more than double the officially admitted amount. Estimates by

the National Taxpayers Union have placed the number as high as $13 trillion.

Moreover, the debts of the people, as well as the state, are depleting the supply and running up the costs of capital available for productive purposes. Individual debt outstanding increased from 51% of gross national product in 1980 to 58% in 1986. In recent years, mortgage and consumer borrowing regularly absorb around four-fifths of all funds raised in the U.S. credit markets. Some of this debt goes for productive purposes, such as student loans, but most again goes to underwrite current consumption. Meanwhile, the nation's savings rate has dropped to its lowest level since the early 1950s.

Another measure of how America is borrowing from the future is provided by the declining investment in basic infrastructure. For more than two decades, per capita expenditures for public works have been declining. Thus, between now and the end of the century, the country will need to spend $1–$3 trillion just to repair and replace existing infrastructure, including thousands of miles of dilapidated interstate highways, railroads, and bridges. These figures approximate a form of borrowing from future taxpayers that, while off the books, is as real as each year's federal deficits.

An agenda for corporate America

By this late date, it is clear that America cannot borrow and spend its way to prosperity. If American industry is to compete in the world economy of the next century, business leaders must speak out on the need for policies that truly encourage thrift and investment. And there is no better way to drive this point home than to speak of our obligations to members of the next generation, who will ultimately be responsible for supporting us in old age. In an aging society, the need for increased capital formation and productivity growth becomes paramount, because there are ever-fewer workers available to support an ever-burgeoning number of retirees.

Ending age discrimination against older workers and discouraging the trend toward early retirement are important parts of this challenge. Of all *retired* workers covered by corporate health-care plans, half are not yet even 65 years old. The United States simply cannot afford to go on wasting the talent and experience of men and women who still, potentially, have many active, productive years ahead of them.

American business must also concentrate its political influence on advocating for the needs of children, who will become the next generation of workers. Again, as the population ages, the percentage of Americans living with children is declining. As a result, the political constituency for expenditures in education is also waning. American business must provide a countervailing force against this trend, in its own and in the nation's long-term interest.

Just as American corporations have a responsibility to overcome a bias for immediate results in design, manufacturing, and marketing decisions, they must also see to it that the business climate in which they operate is consistent with the long-term interests of employees, shareholders, and the firm itself. There is no more cost-effective investment a business can make, for example, than pressing for real reform of the nation's public schools.

But beyond this, corporations must assess the totality of public policies to see how they may be serving to push costs into the future. In the long run, the business climate is not defined solely by the government's tax and regulatory policies, but also by retirement, educational, and fiscal policies that serve to rearrange wealth and opportunity between the generations.

CHAPTER FOURTEEN

Nursing's role in formulating health care policy

POLITICS EPITOMIZES THE American way of life as much as apple pie and motherhood do. We constantly debate issues and policies, fret about funding for public programs, evaluate past actions, form coalitions, and try to advance society through political action. In other words, we experience politics as part of American life. And today, many nurses are learning to use politics effectively.

The first article in this chapter, "Nursing and Politics: A Forgotten Legacy" by Rogge, presents an inspiring account of the political power of individual nurses during the Civil War. The nurses described in this article saw clearly the link between politics and nursing; not content with the status quo, they were willing to do whatever they could to improve care at a time when primitive sanitary conditions prevailed and nursing was not yet recognized as vital to health care.

Within the United States Senate and House of Representatives, numerous members understand and value nursing's contributions to health care. In the forefront of these friends of nursing is Senator Daniel Inouye, Democrat from Hawaii, profiled in the article "Senator Daniel K. Inouye: A Champion for Nursing in Congress" by Kent and Canton. Senator Inouye's sincere and deep feelings for the profession and his exciting vision of nursing's role in health care are described vividly in this article.

The article by White and Hamel, "National Center for Nursing Research: How it Came to Be," is a success story that continues to impress members of Congress and the staffs of federal agencies. The creation of the National Center for Nursing Research is a major feat and source of pride for the nursing profession, which closed ranks and supported the project from inception to completion. Furthermore, establishment of the center reflects the value Congress places on nursing research.

Cohen and Milburn provide a very readable description of the political process in their article, "What Every Nurse Should Know About Political Action." Their examples help make the process very real for readers who seek to understand its complexities. The authors urge nurses "to rise to the challenge and bring their ideas to the forefront of American political discussion."

White, in her article "Involvement: Influencing the Delivery of Health Care and the Future of Critical Care Nursing," also describes the process of influencing health legislation — in this case, from the viewpoint of critical care nursing. This article provides explicit directions for proceeding through the political maze, including precautions for ensuring that a specialty organization's membership can be active politically without challenging the organization's nonprofit tax status. The author emphasizes that achieving the mission of critical care nursing means becoming involved politically at the state and national levels.

Nursing and politics: A forgotten legacy

MARY MADELINE ROGGE, RN, PhD

THE USE OF POLITICAL power by nurses is generally regarded as a recent development within the profession. Frequently nurses' effort to use the political system to shape health policies to improve patient welfare or nurses' working conditions appear nebulous. The majority of nurses resist participating in political activities, contending their purpose is to care for patients, not become embroiled in politics. Yet, nurses' use of political power is not a new phenomenon; it is not even a product of this century. Political power, simply defined, is the ability to influence or persuade an individual holding a governmental office to exert the power of that office to effect a desired outcome.

The Civil War revolutionized nursing care in the United States. For the first time in American history, well-educated, respectable, middle-class women were encouraged to use their knowledge of nursing to care for ill, injured, or infirm military personnel outside their own circle of family and friends. The war generated an increase in the demand for systematic educational programs designed to inculcate in women a knowledge of the principles of nursing care. Women breeched the social barriers to practicing nursing in hospitals, never again to be barred from the wards by social conventions. They won the grudging respect of surgeons and were often idolized by their patients. Many of the women became regional heroines and a few became national legends.

A major factor in the success of the women as nurses and their radical transformation of American nursing was the use of political power by individual Civil War nurses to bring about changes in the care of hospitalized soldiers. The results of their efforts were often immediate. Their examples of political power in nursing practice are part of the nursing profession's forgotten heritage.

The social context

The politically powerful nurses of the Civil War were women who had previously been excluded from hospital nursing practice by the prevailing social strictures and whose presence in the hospitals continued to be challenged by military medical authorities. However, the success they achieved and the public support they garnered in their new role are largely attributable to the political acumen they displayed.

Ironically, no one expected them to wield so much political clout. As women, they were not regarded as intellectually endowed to comprehend the intricacies of the political system. Concern for political affairs, it was thought, would tarnish their womanly honor. They did not even have the right to vote.

During the war, more than 600,000 men died, two-thirds of them from disease rather than from wounds sustained in combat, and the troops experienced more than ten million episodes of illness, wounds, and injury. [1] Conditions for caring for infirm soldiers were appalling, due to the meager medical resources available at the outset of the war and the almost total absence of experienced nursing caregivers in the armies. Attempts to alleviate the nursing shortage by detailing cooks, bandsmen, and convalescents as nurses, failed. There was, however, one segment of the population that possessed the essential nursing expertise needed in the military hospitals — the women. The idea may have shocked Victorian sensibilities, but it was pragmatic.

From the beginning, the women had staunch advocates in high office. Confederate Secretary of War Leroy Pope Walker authorized the employment of women as nurses in military hospitals in the summer of 1861, although the Confederate Congress did not officially legislate their position until September 1862. The "Act to better provide for the sick and wounded of the army in hospitals" provided for hiring two matrons and two assistant matrons for each hospital, and two ward matrons for each ward.[2] In August 1861 the United States Congress, in an "Act for the better organization of the military establishment," provided for hiring nurses in the army's general hospitals. Prior to this legislation, United States Secretary of War Simon Cameron, on June 10, 1861, appointed Dorothea Dix as superintendent of women nurses.[3]

The women were able to claim and maintain nursing positions in the hospitals because of the support they received from the executive and legislative branches of government. The importance of governmental policies sanctioning the hiring of women nurses was not lost on Georgeanna Woolsey. "Government had decided that women should be employed," she noted, "and the army surgeons... [were] unable, therefore, to close the hospitals against them."[4]

Individual nurses apply political power to nursing care

The women were not content with just gaining entree into the armies' medical departments. Once they were a part of the system, they undertook the reform of the more unfavorable conditions of patient care. Although they lacked strength of numbers or rank, the women often successfully challenged the military medical bureaucracy.[5] Tenaciously, the nurses individually lobbied politically power-

ful men to attain changes in hospital conditions.

Clara Barton, a battlefield activist. Dramatically, Clara Barton exercised political power to evoke a major change in the care of wounded Federal soldiers following the Battle of the Wilderness, fought May 5-6, 1864. In the two days of fighting, more than 21,700 Union and Confederate soldiers were killed or wounded. From the battlefield, the Federal wounded were taken, amid torrential rains, to Fredericksburg, Virginia, where the inhabitants were predominantly Confederate sympathizers. Thereafter, the wounded were to be transferred to Belle Plain for evacuation aboard hospital transport ships to Washington-hospitals. Arriving in Fredericksburg, Barton found thousands of wounded Federal soldiers pouring into the city and the treatment the men received deplorable. The sufferings of the wounded were exacerbated by Union officers' failure to order the people of Fredericksburg to give the patients shelter because it "was a pretty hard thing for refined people like the people of Fredericksburg...to open their homes and 'admit these dirty, lousy, common soldiers.'"[6]

She wrote after the war, that while inspecting conditions in Fredericksburg:

> ...I saw crowded into one old sunken hotel, lying helpless upon its wet, bloody floors, five hundred fainting men hold up their cold, bloodless, dingy hands, as I passed, and beg me in Heaven's name for a cracker to keep them from starving (and I had none); or to give them a cup that they might have something to drink water from (and I had no cup and could get none)....I saw two hundred six-mule army wagons in a line, ranged down the street to headquarters, and reaching so far out on the Wilderness road that I never found the end of it; every wagon crowded with wounded men, stopped, standing in the rain and mud, wrenched back and forth by the restless, hun-

gry animals all night from four o'clock in the afternoon till eight next morning and how much longer I know not. The dark spot in the mud under many a wagon told only too plainly where some fellow's life had dripped out in those dreadful hours. [7]

Barton remembered an ally who could help her expedite the care of the wounded. She returned immediately to Washington and summoned Henry Wilson, Chairman of the Senate's Military Committee. To him she reported what she had witnessed and within two hours of her return to Washington, the senator confronted officials at the War Department with her report; these officials had themselves received no such news from Fredericksburg, and they doubted the reliability of his information. Recalled Barton:

It was then he proved that my confidence in his firmness was not misplaced, as facing his doubters he replied: 'One of two things will have to be done — either you will send some one to-night with the power to investigate and correct the abuses of our wounded men at Fredericksburg, or the Senate will send some one tomorrow.'
This threat recalled their scattered senses.
At two o'clock in the morning the Quartermaster General and staff galloped to the 6th Street wharf under orders: at ten they were in Fredericksburg. At noon the wounded men were fed from the food of the city and the houses were opened to the 'dirty, lousy soldiers' of the Union Army.

Barton knew Wilson from her days as a Patent Office clerk prior to the war, and she had developed a firm working relationship with him. For two years she had nursed Union soldiers at the front, and she had often furnished him with reliable information about hospital conditions and had sought his advice in regard to her own work. Their earlier contacts had laid the foundation for the senator's trust in the nurse when she notified him of the plight of the wounded in Fredericksburg.

Nor was the Fredericksburg incident the first time Barton had relied on political power to accomplish what she alone lacked the authority to enforce. The shy former schoolteacher had been working in Washington when the war broke out, and from her observations in the capital, she was disturbed by the neglect endured by the wounded. The men languished up to five days on the battlefield or in ambulances, without assistance, before reaching facilities where medical and nursing care might be obtained. By March 1862 she was making arrangements to take nursing care to the casualties at the front. To obtain the required governmental passes permitting her to travel within army lines, she sought a personal recommendation from Massachusetts Governor John A. Andrew. Andrew willingly issued the recommendation — he owed her a favor.

The previous fall, Barton had become aware of a secessionist organization in the Washington area engaged in a treasonable conspiracy. Under the guise of a relief association, the conspirators collected funds for the support of Confederate soldiers, manufactured Confederate uniforms, and purchased arms and munitions for the enemy. Barton attempted to warn other relief societies of the plot, but because she lacked definite proof of the conspiracy, her warnings were ignored. During the winter, at home in Massachusetts, she confided her suspicions to a long-time friend, Colonel Alexander De Witt, previously the congressman from her home district. De Witt introduced her to Governor Andrew, to whom she repeated the information. The governor followed up on her report, and on February 27, 1862, twenty-five of the principal conspirators were arrested in Alexandria, Virginia. On March 24, Andrew gave Barton his support for the travel passes. [9]

Despite Andrew's recommendation, Barton

was temporarily thwarted in her plans to undertake battlefield nursing when Dr. Alfred Hitchcock of Burnside's division denied her the permit because he believed the front was not a suitable place for a woman. Barton sought a higher authority. On June 11, 1862, she received the critical authorization to "go upon the sick transports in any direction — for the purpose of distributing comforts for the wounded — and nursing them" from Surgeon-General William A. Hammond. [10] For the next month Barton collected her own supplies. Then on August 11, 1862, she packed her stores and boarded a box car for the front to tend the wounded of the Battle of Cedar Mountain (Culpeper). Over the next seven weeks, she was to be found in the field offering nursing care in the field to casualties of the Battles of Second Manassas, Chantilly, Harper's Ferry, and South Mountain. By September 17, she had become so efficient that she arrived at the front before the opening salvo of the Battle of Antietam — the battle that became the bloodiest single day of the war. The nursing care that Barton was able to give to literally thousands of wounded men during those tragic weeks, and that laid the foundation for her subsequent life's work, was realized because she enlisted the aid of key governmental officials.

Hannah Ropes, a diligent crusader. Hannah Ropes, matron at the Union Hotel Hospital at Georgetown, effectively applied political pressure to rectify flagrant abuses of the patients at her hospital. Ropes, before the war, had been active in the abolitionist movement. She had lived in Kansas for six months in 1855-1856, and had first-hand knowledge of the violence attending the issue of extending slavery into the territory. One writer has speculated that a letter she wrote to Senator Charles Sumner in November 1856 influenced his "Crime Against Kansas" speech, delivered in the Senate on May 19 and 20, 1856. This address so inflamed South Carolina's Representative

Preston Brooks, nephew of South Carolina's Senator Andrew Butler, that on May 22, while Sumner sat writing at his Senate desk, Brooks accused him of libeling South Carolina and his uncle. Then he severely beat the senator over the head with a walking cane. Sumner became a martyr to the abolitionist movement, even as Brooks was hailed as a champion of the South. The incident deepened the rift between the North and the South. Upon Ropes' return to Massachusetts, she became acquainted with senators and congressmen, and campaigned actively in the Free-Soil movement. [11]

In the fall of 1862, Ropes discovered the hospital steward was stealing patients' clothing and misappropriating soap intended for the hospital laundry:

> Every day the inmates of the house bring charges against him to me: I have been to the head surgeon [A. M. Clark] but it makes not the slightest impression on him. I wrote to the Surgeon General [William A. Hammond,] but the letter came back to the 'Surgeon in Charge' [Clark], whereupon the last named functionary, living in the same house, sent a formal official notice to me that I must prove the grave charge against the steward!...I only reiterated my belief in his dishonesty, and declined to hunt for evidence which was plain in the kitchen, the larder, and every pinched face one meets on the stairs or in the wards. [12]

Neither Hammond nor Clark took disciplinary action against the steward. Two weeks later the steward assaulted one of the patients, and Ropes telegraphed the news to the soldier's father, who arrived at the hospital the next morning. By evening a general visited the hospital and made initial inquiries into the case. Again no action was taken to curb the steward's mistreatment of the patients. The following week, the steward cast a patient named Julius into a cellar prison.

Ropes resolved to report the matter to her

long-time friend, General Nathaniel Banks. The General was an outspoken opponent of slavery and had become Speaker of the House of Representatives in 1856. A native of Massachusetts, he was elected governor in 1858, and in 1862 he was in charge of the military defenses around Washington. Accompanied by another Union Hospital nurse, Julia C. Kendall, [Ropes] called at Banks' headquarters. Learning the General was out of town, the two nurses proceeded to the Surgeon General's office.[13] According to Ropes:

> Three chairs lined the side of the door and the rail of the stairs. I asked audience of the Surgeon General; the man at the door post said, 'It is three o'clock, and he is never hear [sic] after that time.' As he spoke, the Surgeon [General] walked in and, passing us without the Christian courtesy of a look or nod, or even the old time civility of raising the hand to his hat, he vanished behind the opening door of his inner office.
>
> ...The man at the staircase followed his master, then came back to ask if I could send in my message. 'No, it must be given in by myself.' He returned only to say we could see the Assistant Surgeon [General], but at his door in the rear of the entry we were met with the notice that we must wait, he was engaged.
>
> Two rebuffs seemed about enough for a woman of half century to accept...and answered too as sufficient spur to take us to the Secretary of War [Edwin M. Stanton] office.
>
> Here the tone of things was very much more genial: we...received the promise of seeing the Secretary as soon as he came to his room. Ten minutes passed...a large man with dark beard, bald head, and legal brow walked into the room, stationing hims elf in front of the desk. The gentleman who had so kindly greeted us when we came, told me who it was. I went to the end of the desk and...stated in the fewest words possible the facts about Julius. Secretary Stanton's eyes gleamed with the fire of a purpose.

> 'Call the Provost Marshall' was all he said, and went on writing. Before we had got hold of the importance of the order, that functionary appeared. Stanton lifted the pen from the paper and, looking at him, said, 'Go to the Union Hospital with this lady, take the boy out of the black hole, go into it yourself so as to be able to tell me about it, then arrest the steward and take him to a cell in the Old Capital Prison, to await further orders!'[14]

In her initial complaints against the steward, Ropes had tried to correct the abuses by following the chain of command, but her efforts were frustrated by the surgeons who failed to adequately investigate the report of the steward's theft, or his assault on a patient. Not only did Hammond not look into the initial complaint, he betrayed Ropes' confidential communication. Treated with contempt by the surgeons and officers who refused to intervene on behalf of Julius and the other patients, Ropes and Kendall could but appeal to another governmental authority.

Politically astute, Ropes would have known Stanton would be her best ally. Stanton, who had replaced Cameron as Secretary of War, was the second most powerful man in the Lincoln Administration. He was at political odds with Hammond, and the antipathy the two men shared was well known in Washington; he would not discount her report of misconduct at the hospital. Not only was the steward whisked off to prison, but Clark also occupied a cell in the Old Capitol Prison for almost a week. An investigation was conducted, and by November 8, Clark had been replaced as chief surgeon at the Union Hospital.[15] Within a year, Stanton was instrumental in having Hammond twice court martialed and finally dismissed from the service in disgrace for irregularities in letting medical department contracts. Clark subsequently became a leading New York neurologist.[16] Ropes derived no satisfaction from his dismissal; she died of typhoid fever at her hospital less than three months after her meeting with Stanton.

Cordelia Harvey, an outspoken nurse. The widow of Wisconsin Governor Lewis Harvey, Cordelia Harvey enlisted the support of President Abraham Lincoln to improve the care of patients in the Union armies west of the Mississippi. There was strong evidence that the hot, sultry climate of the southern states, where most of the war's maneuvers took place, extracted a heavy toll on the health of northern soldiers. The weather was especially problematic in the West, where steamy swamplands incubated malaria and other fevers. It was widely believed that "the enfeebled soldiers might be restored to strength," if they could be sent North to complete their convalescence. [17] However, there was no military hospital north of St. Louis where soldiers from the western front could be sent; and medical directors, afraid of mass desertions, were reluctant to issue disability furloughs to the men to allow them to recuperate at home.

Harvey, after nursing in several hospitals along the Mississippi, decided to petition Lincoln directly for the establishment of a northern facility. The President shared the medical authorities' dread of decimating the ranks through desertions, and he had earlier turned down similar proposals. He was annoyed with her pursuit of a cause he had already rejected and listened impatiently to her claim that the Union hospitals in the South were inadequate. She pointed out the army would in fact be strengthened if the patients were permitted to return North to recover their health and the loss of men through desertion would be less than through the prolonged disability, or death, of the men languishing in the hospitals further south. In three interviews with the President and one meeting with Stanton, she pleaded for consideration for the patients, arguing private citizens "cannot understand why their friends are left to die when with proper care they might live to do good service for their country," and that "a majority of them would live and be strong men again if they could be sent North." [18] Furthermore, she challenged the reports of Medical Inspectors, including those of Surgeon General Hammond, that Northern Military Hospitals were unnecessary. She told Stanton:

> Our western hospitals have never received any benefit from these inspections, and we have very little confidence that any good would result from them. Any person with discernment, with a medium allowance of common sense and humanity, who is loyal, and has been through our Southern river hospitals, knows and feels the necessity for what I ask, and yet you have never received a report to the effect. [19]

To Lincoln she was equally emphatic in refuting the evaluations of the medical inspectors:

> Now the medical authorities know as well as I do that you are opposed to establishing Northern Military Hospitals, and they report to please you....I came to you from no casual tour or inspection, passing rapidly through the general hospitals, in the principal cities on the river, with a cigar in my mouth and rattan in my hand, talking to the surgeon in charge of the price of cotton...and finally coming into the open air, with a longdrawn breath as though having just escaped suffocation, and complacently saying, 'You have a very fine hospital here; the boys seem to be doing very well, a little more attention to ventilation is perhaps desirable.'
> It is not thus; I have visited the hospitals, but from morning until late at night sometimes. I have visited the regimental and general hospitals on the Mississippi from Quincy [Illinois] to Vicksburg [Mississippi], and I come to you from the cots of men who have

died, who might have lived had you permitted. This is hard to say, but it is none the less true. [20]

The nurse's perseverance and plain speaking were rewarded. President Lincoln issued an order for the establishment of a general military hospital in Wisconsin. [21]

Southern nurses and political power

The surviving documentation of southern women using political power to achieve improvements in patient care is fragmentary. Nevertheless, evidence reveals that southern nurses were as skillful in drawing on their political connections to improve patient care and conditions affecting their nursing practice as their northern counterparts.

Juliet Hopkins, Superintendent of Hospitals. Juliet Hopkins began working in the hospital established in Richmond for Alabama soldiers as early as June 10, 1861, prior to the first major battle of the war. Her acquaintance with the governor of Alabama was undoubtedly the product of her marriage to Arthur F. Hopkins, formerly the Chief Justice of the Alabama Supreme Court and a United States Senator. Although his authority to make the appointment was dubious, Governor John G. Shorter named her the Superintendent of all the Alabama hospitals established in Virginia.[22] She maintained a steady correspondence with Shorter pertaining to the conditions and management of the hospitals. Other women, seeking nursing positions in Richmond, contacted Alabama's governors to further their aims. On June 4, 1862, Shorter telegraphed Hopkins that he had the offers of two ladies to go to the Confederate capital as nurses, and asked if she needed their services. Before leaving office, Shorter's predecessor, A. B. Moore, wrote Hopkins a letter of recommendation for one nursing applicant, and another woman named him as a character reference when she applied to Hopkins for a position. [23]

Sally Tompkins, "Captain Of Cavalry, Unassigned." Following the first Battle of Manassas (Bull Run), in July 1861, Sally Tompkins was one of countless civilians who opened private hospitals to care for Confederate military patients. Operating the hospital at her own expense, she established such a high standard of nursing care that the death rate in her hospital was less than 6 percent of admissions, the lowest of any Richmond hospital, despite some of the most seriously sick and wounded men being transferred to her hospital for the special care given.

Three months later, the Confederate Congress enacted legislation transferring the control of these private hospitals to the government. Soldiers could be treated only at a hospital under the authority of a commissioned officer holding a rank not lower than that of a captain. Tompkins appealed to Confederate President Jefferson Davis for an executive order to exempt her hospital from the new legislation: His solution to the dilemma was to have her commissioned as an officer so that her hospital would conform to the law and become a component of the military organization. Secretary of War Walker, on September 9, 1861, signed her commission as Captain of Cavalry, Unassigned. Affording care to 1,333 patients, Tompkins continued to administer her hospital and to provide nursing care until the last military patients were discharged June 18, 1865. [24]

Conclusion

Although their political shrewdness has long been overlooked by the nursing profession, the Civil War nurses' use of political power established a durable precedent for today's nurses. Far from not understanding the military-political bureaucracy or the intricacies of the political system, as was assumed of nineteenth-century women, the nurses applied the government's political intricacies to the advantage of the sick and wounded. They commanded the attention, respect, and cooperation of governors, congressmen, cabinet members, and presidents. Appealing to governmental authorities was successfully adopted as a strategy for improving patient welfare and removing impediments to practicing nursing. Their initial means of establishing contact with influential officials varied, but they shared in common the approach of personally contacting those political figures whose help they most needed to enlist. Armed with facts and a commitment to their patients, they discovered that their individual efforts to influence political officeholders could make a difference in the welfare of their patients.

Exercising political power has become not merely a legitimate option, but rather an essential strategy, for safeguarding patient welfare in contemporary nursing practice. A maze of local, state, and national bureaucracies dictate pervasive health care policies that have profound consequences for patient welfare and conditions of nursing practice. Notwithstanding the profession's recent attempts to marshall nurses' political resources through the organization of political action coalitions, the responsibility for exercising political power remains with individual nurses committed to improving patient care. It is imperative that individual nurses follow the examples of Civil War nurses and personally establish and maintain working relationships with both elected and appointed governmental officials. By sharing with influential officials their firsthand knowledge of the impact of governmental policies on the welfare of their patients, nurses can make major contributions to the shaping of future health care policies.

NOTES

1. Courtney Robert Hall, "Confederate Medicine: Caring for the Confederate Soldier," *Medical Life* 42(1935):477,452; George Washington Adams, *Doctors in Blue: The Medical History of the Union Army in the Civil War* (New York: Henry Schuman. 1952), p. 3; and Thomas L. Livermore, *Numbers and Losses in the Civil War in America 1861-1865* (Boston: Houghton Mifflin & Co., 1900), pp. 1, 8, 22.

2. Adjutant and Inspector General S. Cooper. General Orders No. 95. Richmond, Va.: November 25, 1862.

3. Julia C. Stimson and Ethel C. S. Thompson. "Women Nurses with the Union Forces During the Civil War. Part 1." *The Military Surgeon* 62 (January 1928):2. 6.

4. Georgeanna Woolsey Bacon and Eliza Woolsey Howland, *Letters of a Family During the War for the Union 1861-1865*, 2 vols. (Privately published, 1899), 1:142.

5. Mary Madeline Rogge, "Development of a Taxonomy of Nursing Interventions: An Analysis of Nursing Care in the American Civil War" (Ph.D dissertation. The University of Texas at Austin, 1985).

6. William E. Barton *The Life of Clara Barton: Founder of the American Red Cross*, 2 vols. (Boston: Houghton, Mifflin & Co., 1922), 1:277.

7. Ibid., pp. 277-278.

8. Ibid., pp. 278-279.

9. Ibid., pp. 156-160.

10. Ibid ., pp. 156-160.

11. John R. Brumgardt, ed., *Civil War Nurse: The Diary and Letters of Hannah Ropes* (Knoxville: The University of Tennessee Press, 1980), pp. 14-28.

12. Ibid., pp. 74-75.

13. Ibid., pp. 79-81.

14. Ibid., pp. 81-85.

15. Ibid., pp. 83-84, 86, 94.

16. Otto Eisenschiml, "Medicine in the War," *Civil War Times Illustrated* 1 (May 1962):6: and Margaret Leech, *Reveille in Washington 1860-1865* (Alexandria, Va.: Time-Life Books, 1962), p. 400.

17. Cordelia A. P. Harvey, "A Woman's Picture of President Lincoln," *The Wisconsin Magazine of History* 1 (March 1918):241.

18. Ibid., p. 248.

19. Ibid., p. 245.

20. Ibid., pp. 249-250.

21. Ibid., p. 252.

22. Lucille Griffith, "Mrs. Juliet Opie Hopkins and Alabama Military Hospitals," *The Alabama Review* 6 (April 1953):104.

23. Governor Gill Shorter, telegram to Mrs. Arthur R. Hopkins, June 4, 1862; Governor A. B. Moore, letter to Mrs. A. F. Hopkins, September 10, 1861; and Mildred Duckworth, letter to Mrs. Arthur Hopkins, November 11, 1861. Correspondence in the Hopkins Papers. Montgomery: Alabama State Department of Archives and History.

24. [Mrs. Fielding Lewis Taylor], "Captain Sallie Tompkins." *Confederate Veteran* 24 (November 1916):521-524; Sallie Tompkins. Robinson Hospital Ledger 1861-1865 in the Tompkins Papers. Richmond, Va.: Museum of the Confederacy; and Confederate States of America, War Department, Sallie Tompkins Commission. Richmond, Va.: Museum of the Confederacy.

Senator Daniel K. Inouye: A champion for nursing in Congress

VIRGINIA CLARK KENT, RN, MSN, CANP; DENISE S. CANTON, RN, DNSc

SENATOR DANIEL K. INOUYE (D-HI) has been a champion of nursing for the past decade and continues to be one of nursing's strongest advocates within the U.S. Congress. Senator Inouye was first elected to the U.S. Senate in 1962, following a two-year term as the first U.S. Congressman from the state of Hawaii. He was re-elected to the U.S. Senate in 1968, 1974 and 1980. Since 1978, Senator Inouye has been the third ranking Senate democrat, as secretary of the Democratic Conference. He currently is a member of the Senate Appropriations Committee and several other strategic committees.

Senator Inouye creates public policy which markedly alters the legal environment in which nurses function. His most recent efforts on behalf of nursing have been the passage of the Federal Employee Health Benefits Program (FEHBP), which was to authorize direct reimbursement for nursing services. This bill was vetoed by the president.

In this interview, the senator chronicles his efforts to obtain nursing reimbursement legislation and discusses the directions nurse practitioners should take in the future.

Senator, why have you been so interested in the nursing profession?

I was brought into the world by a nurse midwife, and most of my health care during my early childhood was provided by school nurses or public health nurses. I was brought up to believe that nurses are competent, independent and professional. Unfortunately, I have spent more than two years of my life in various hospitals receiving the services of nurses and physicians. During this time, I never found it necessary to complain about the quality of nursing care that I received. More important, however, is that I found nurses to be very professional in their conduct, educational preparation and general demeanor.

Like most legislators, I am concerned about the escalating cost of health care in our nation. We presently spend more on health care than any other nation in the world. In 1984 alone, our nation's health care expenditures reached $387.4 billion, or 10.6 percent of the gross national product. This expenditure was the highest in the country's history, and the overall rate of growth exceeded that of nearly every other segment of the economy. The nursing profession must be a pivotal force in our attempts to control the escalating costs of health care by ensuring that quality care is made available cost efficiently to those who need it. *Would you review the most important legislative initiatives concerning the delivery of nursing care within the federal government?*

There are essentially four programs that the federal government oversees as a purchaser or provider of health care: CHAMPUS, the Federal Employee Health Benefits Program, Medicare and Medicaid.

CHAMPUS

The Department of Defense Civilian Health and Medical Program of the Uniformed Services (CHAMPUS) has an annual budget of approximately $1.4 billion and serves 7.9 million dependents of active-duty personnel and eligible retirees. Today, all categories of nurse practitioners and clinical specialists are deemed fully autonomous providers and reimbursable under CHAMPUS.

Efforts to make the services of these providers reimbursable began in 1977 in the Senate Appropriations Committee. That year, we convinced the Senate to adopt legislation to provide for direct reimbursement for certified nurse midwives and for psychiatric nurses. The House conferees adamantly opposed the amendment, allegedly because of their grave concern regarding the role of psychiatric nurses. In 1978, we were again able to have certified nurse midwives, psychiatric nurses and, at that time, the more generic classification of nurse practitioner included in the Senate bill. This time, the House conferees expressed their willingness to accept the nurse midwife language, but again vehemently opposed the other two categories. Thus, during the fiscal-year-1979 budget deliberations, certified nurse midwives were granted autonomous functions under CHAMPUS (P.L.95-457).

The Department of Defense delayed administrative action on this issue for almost one year before finally issuing regulations to implement the bill; however, they made regulations retroactive to October 1978. During this process, I decided to ask the Department of Health, Education and Welfare (which became the departments of Health and Human Services and Education on May 4, 1980) why it was taking so long to review and comment on the proposed CHAMPUS regulations. The department's response was issued by one of their senior bureaucrats who told me, "We really can't believe that your committee means 'independent reimbursement,'...none of our other federal programs allow this." I assured her that that was exactly what we meant, and the regulations moved off her desk within the week!

During the subsequent two years (1980-82), we were able to develop for CHAMPUS a demonstration, independent nurse practitioner reimbursement project. After the project was successfully completed, the passage of P.L.

97-114 removed the experimental designation for CHAMPUS. It thus enabled all categories of nurse practitioners and clinical nurse specialists to independently assess or diagnose and treat patients under CHAMPUS and receive direct reimbursement for their services. P.L. 98-525 was the statute incorporating this language into the Fiscal Year Department of Defense Authorization Act.

Recent CHAMPUS regulations make it absolutely clear that nursing's professional autonomy exists on both inpatient and outpatient levels as long as the state nurse practice acts provide for such practice. That is the key. In order for us to continue our fight for direct reimbursement, you must, as a profession, ensure that your various state nurse practice acts legislate practitioners to be autonomous professionals.

Federal employee health benefits program

The second major federal health care initiative is the Federal Employee Health Benefits Program. This program serves approximately 10 million federal employees, annuitants and their dependents. At my request, the General Accounting Office (GAO) completed a study and concluded that about 91 percent of all federal employees are presently enrolled in health insurance plans offering the services of certified nurse midwives. Based on our CHAMPUS experiences, I testified in 1983 before the Senate Governmental Affairs Subcommittee, which has jurisdiction over this program, urging the chairman to include legislative language which would expressly ensure that all beneficiaries would have the right to select a nurse practitioner or clinical nurse specialist for any health care services covered under his or her individual plan. The chairman, Senator Ted Stevens (R-AK), a long-time friend of nursing, assured me that he was supportive of my recommendations. During this current session of Congress, another friend of nursing, Senator Albert Gore (D-TN), was appointed as ranking member of the Civil Service, Post Office and General Services Subcommittee. With both the chairman and his Democratic colleagues expressing their support, I am confident that we will soon be successful in including nurse midwives, nurse practitioners and clinical specialists in the "freedom of choice" provisions of the Federal Employee Health Benefits Program.

Medicare/Medicaid

These two programs account for nearly 90 percent of federal health expenditures. The federal government now has 20 years of experience in administering these programs, which may serve as the models for our forthcoming National Health Program. We are making steady progress to ensure that nurse practitioners and clinical nurse specialists will eventually be deemed truly autonomous professionals throughout the Social Security Act.

Nurse practitioners and/or certified nurse midwives and the generic term "nursing" are mentioned in three aspects of the Medicaid statute. In 1980, P.L. 96-499, revising the Medicaid Act, made the services of certified nurse midwives a mandatory and autonomous benefit under Medicaid. This benefit must be offered by the states, regardless of whether there is involvement by any other category of health care provider, i.e., physicians. Again, however, I would caution you that it is the individual state nurse practice acts which control how these services are to be provided under Medicaid.

We are now working to ensure that Medicare will also treat certified nurse midwives as autonomous providers under federal statute. During one recent Senate deliberation on the Omnibus Reconciliation Act of 1985, I asked the floor manager to accept an amendment on this issue. He expressed support but requested

that I wait for a more appropriate bill, and I agreed to do so.

These Medicare and Medicaid provisions which authorize reimbursement for independent nursing care are important because states often draw on the experience of the federal government when designing their own health care statutes. If the federal government has been successful in organizing and funding a new program, the states usually follow suit in drafting their own regulations. Therefore, it is critical to have federal statutes which authorize reimbursement of independent nursing functions to influence state laws to grant nurses greater autonomy. In short, I do not want any federal health care program defining nurse practitioners and clinical nurse specialists as being less than fully autonomous, and I am working to ensure this through legislative initiative.

Recently, when the Health Care Financing Administration (HCFA) attempted to require physician administration of all birthing centers, we used the provision providing for autonomy in the Medicaid law to again modify the "clinical services" section of the act to ensure that any health care practitioner could be the administrator of any facility providing clinical services. In 1984, P.L. 98-369 Medicaid Statute was amended to state that these clinics need not be administered by physicians. For the psychiatric nurse clinical specialists, this provision also applies to community mental health centers.

Under Medicare, nurse practitioners have been legislatively deemed autonomous providers within health maintenance organizations since 1982. Similarly, within the Rural Health Clinic Program and the Professional Review Organization legislation, nurse practitioners are also defined as autonomous professionals. Under these provisions, nurse practitioners can practice to the fullest extent allowed by their states' nurse practice acts. When physician involvement is required, it is only on a "circuit rider" (as needed) basis. Several of these initiatives were included at my request and reflect the growing appreciation for nurses by members of the Senate Finance Committee. I might add that it has definitely helped nursing that Senate Majority Leader, Senator Robert Dole (R-KS) has a nurse (Sheila Burke) as his chief health staff member.

There are still a number of additional elements of the Medicare and Medicaid statutes which we must amend in order to ensure nurses complete autonomy. In this session, we are hoping to increase the conditions under which nurse practitioners will be able to autonomously certify continuous "medical necessity" in the home health care program as well as in nursing homes. We will also be working on legislation to ensure reimbursement for geriatric, psychiatric and pediatric nurse practitioners/clinical nurse specialists under appropriate provisions of the Social Security Act, P.L. 89-97.

Through the appropriations process, I will be working with the HCFA to implement nurse practitioner demonstration programs similar to those of CHAMPUS. I have recently learned that under the provisions of the Rural Health Clinic Bill, a new nurse practitioner urban clinic demonstration program has been started. The Department of Health and Human Services is currently conducting a four-year, 40-clinic demonstration project, and a formal report is expected in Congress by January 1987.

Would you discuss the Office of Technology Assessment's findings on nurse practitioner effectiveness?

The Office of Technology Assessment (OTA) is the scientific policy arm of Congress and has truly impeccable research credentials. In July 1983, OTA completed a case study entitled "The Cost Effectiveness of Nurse Practitioners." After a very comprehensive review of the literature, it concluded that nurse practitioners were definitely cost effective and could not find any objective evidence of "lower quality of care." In July 1984, Senator Mark Hatfield (R-OR), chairman of the Senate Appropriations Committee, and I asked the OTA to provide us with an updated report on the status of public and private nurse practitioner reimbursement programs. This time, Senator Hatfield and I asked the OTA to look specifically at those federal programs, such as CHAMPUS, that now have a history of directly reimbursing nurses. When OTA's forthcoming report is completed, we will actively work to ensure that every federal health care program will seriously consider making nurse practitioners autonomous and essential providers.

I also hope that nurses across the nation will use this report to modify their own appropriate state statutes. Your profession is an honorable and distinguished one, with an excellent record of serving our nation, especially those who are most in need. You must now seek to ensure that those of us who are elected to political office will give you the legal recognition that you so richly deserve.

What is the status of funding for nursing research?

For the past several years, the Senate Appropriations Committee has been hearing testimony that nurses were not receiving their fair share of federal funding from the National Institutes of Health (NIH), and that insufficient priority was being given to the psychosocial aspects of health care. For example, although directives from the committee were given to NIH asking it to increase its attention to nursing research, we were recently informed that only 0.6 percent of the public advisory committee members of the NIH were professional nurses and that of the more than $4 billion NIH annual budget, less than $1.5 million went to schools of nursing. With an aggressive effort by nursing using these statistics to educate Congress, we were successful during the closing hours of the 98th Congress, despite the administration's vocal opposition, in having legislation passed which would have established a new National Institute of Nursing (NIN). The president ultimately vetoed that bill, but Congress voted in November 1985 to override the veto, thus establishing the National Center for Nursing Research. The $5 million originally designated for the NIN was "earmarked" during conference deliberations on the Fiscal Year 1985 Appropriations Bill, so that the money will be released to fund the National Center for Nursing Research when the bill is finally signed into public law.

When I first began to focus upon nursing research, we faced a zero authorization request and a total annual research funding level of $1.4 million. Today, we have $14.4 million appropriated, including the $5 million that Senator Lowell Weiker (R-CT) and I have "earmarked" for the National Center for Nursing Research. My personal goal is to bring this up to $5 million for nursing research within the next decade.

What are some of your initiatives addressing the morale of military health care personnel?

At my request, the Senate Appropriations Committee held for the first time in over a decade, hearings in 1984 on the Department of Defense's health care programs and the status of nurses within the military. During those hearings, the department assured me that a nurse corps officer is in command of the naval hospital at Guantanamo Bay, Cuba, and another nurse corps officer is the regional medical commander for a portion of the United States under the Navy's new regional reorganization. I was very pleased with this progress.

However, at another point in the hearings, it became necessary for the committee to express its concern regarding a new Department of Defense directive requiring that nurse practitio-

ners, nurse midwives and nurse anesthetists in the military be supervised by physicians. We stated that this was not considered a progressive or appropriate use of nursing expertise and directed that the Nonphysician Morale Task Force, which the committee had established the previous year, examine the issue in depth. Military nurses, were, and are, active participants in this process, and I am optimistic that the department and the Congress will institute a number of recommendations that will be made by the task force.

Many don't realize that the real strength of our armed forces is its personnel, not its hardware. At my request, the Congress appropriated $12 million in fiscal year 1985 for the Department of Family Advocacy Program. The purpose of this initiative is to test various models of clinical intervention, to document cost effectiveness and to demonstrate the administrative efficiency of joint-service programs.

The Family Advocacy Program, now called Services Assisting Family Environments (SAFE), was begun as a three-year joint-service demonstration project in fiscal year 1982 under the Department of Defense's Office of the Secretary for Health Affairs. For example, in Hawaii, there are several SAFE teams operating. Each team consists of one registered nurse, one social worker and one outreach paraprofessional. The teams provide the following: aggressive family intervention, home health visits and crisis assistance. Generally, the project provides for prenatal care programs called "wellness in the home." All pregnant military wives in their first trimester attend a conference for two and one-half hours on prenatal care. They are asked to complete an assessment questionnaire to identify those at high risk. Home visits are made to these high-risk women by paraprofessionals under the direction of a maternal-child health nurse and a clinical social worker. Families exhibiting tendencies toward violent behavior are referred to SAFE teams for more intensive intervention. *What directions should nursing and nurse practitioners take in the future to assure cost-effective, quality health care for our citizens?*

One of the reasons I am so supportive of nursing is that nursing care is truly cost effective. I believe that the practice of defensive medicine is one of the main reasons why nurses have been kept from performing at the level of which they are capable. Defensive medicine results in increased costs to the consumer, due to the increased use of unnecessary tests and procedures. We must address this matter directly and not allow the fear of possible litigation to prevent nurses from practicing to their fullest capacities.

Americans are spending less than 50 cents per person on prevention, but we are spending $1,400 per person on curative care. The surgeon general of the United States has stated that of the 10 leading causes of death, seven could be significantly reduced if people would change their lifestyles, such as not smoking, getting more exercise, reducing weight, etc. The psychological and educational aspects of health care are clearly two of nursing's greatest strengths. I encourage you to document your research findings on nursing interventions in order to aid in marketing nurses as cost-effective health care providers. Also, we know, for example, that less than .001 percent of all nurses have specialized education in geriatrics. This is clearly another area in which nursing could increase its focus in the coming years.

The Congress and business leaders want to ensure that they are providing quality health benefits that are truly cost effective. Nurses need to continue to promote and market their skills as cost-effective providers. To succeed at this, nurses must work together. I fully understand that there is a difference between a certified nurse midwife, a nurse practitioner and a clinical nurse specialist; however, for the vast majority of my colleagues in Congress, a nurse is a nurse.

Please, don't continue to expect Congress to appreciate the subtle nuances of what are essentially intra-nursing issues. Do, however, continue your efforts on both a personal and an organizational basis to educate us as to the importance of quality nursing care! Meet your elected officials. Get to know them on a first-name basis. Those of us who get elected to the Congress want to serve our constituents. We do care! It is up to you, however, to let us know how we can be of assistance.

Aloha.

National Center for Nursing Research: How it came to be

DIANA L. WHITE, RN, BS; PATRICIA K. HAMEL, RN, BSN

POLITICAL SAVVY is perhaps the single, most important characteristic of a successful nurse leader. For nurse leaders who lobby at the local, state, and national levels, this savvy can be described as knowing the intricacies of the legislative process, being well read and informed about health issues, and having access to influential individuals and organizations.

Nurses in the federal health policy community recently demonstrated their increasing power and sophistication by using inside access strategies to successfully establish a National Center for Nursing Research. Amended to the National Institutes of Health (NIH) reauthorization bill, this legislation recently survived presidential veto and was finally enacted on November 20, 1985.

How did nursing promote the issue of a national nursing research center? How did nurses influence decision makers? This article examines how the National Center for Nursing Research achieved formal agenda status and how nursing accomplished its goal in the legislative arena.

Agenda-building

For nursing to accomplish its goal of establishing a national research center, it first had to participate in agenda building — the process by which an issue achieves formal agenda status.

Primarily, two types of agendas exist: public and formal. The public agenda includes visible issues of interest to the public. The formal agenda comprises issues that legislators have accepted for deliberation in a House or Senate Committee. Bills introduced to Congress that have symbolic appeal to constituents, but do not reach committee-level consideration, are labeled pseudo-agenda items. Once an issue reaches the formal agenda, the House and Senate act on it, resulting in a favorable or unfavorable outcome for the initiating group.

Three agenda-building models identified by Cobb, Ross, and Ross (1976) will help clarify this tedious yet critical process. In all models, the issue develops through four stages: initiation, specification, expansion, and entrance.

Outside initiative model. In this model, issues develop in nongovernmental groups. Through the agenda-building process, the issue first reaches the public agenda and then the formal agenda. For example, using this model, individuals helped establish the National Institute of Aging. Nongovernment groups, concerned about the increasing problems associated with aging, decided to inform the public of their concerns. Public pressure mounted, forcing government decision makers to respond in 1974 by establishing the most recent addition to the NIH (Lockett, 1984).

Mobilization model. In this second model, issues are initiated inside government and achieve formal agenda status almost immediately. The issue is then expanded and promoted to the public. An example of the mobilization model is the imposition of a population planning program in an underdeveloped country. After determining a policy to control population, the government must convince the public of the policy's merits before the policy can be effectively implemented.

Inside initiative model. In the third model, issues arise within the government sphere and are discussed by government employees, representatives, or those with direct access to governmental groups. These issues are not expanded to the public agenda because supporters perceive the issue as too complex or controversial. Public expansion would prevent the issue from reaching the formal agenda or would remove it after arrival. Through this final model, the inside initiative process, the National Center for Nursing Research has achieved formal agenda status.

Nursing's inside access strategy

Nursing leaders skillfully planned their strategy for promoting the issue of a federally funded National Center for Nursing Research. Their best option resembled the inside initiative strategy. Groups who opt for this strategy tend to have similar backgrounds, mores, and goals. Such similarity attracts support and decreases potential controversy. First, a group of nurses with access to government leaders articulated their frustration about the lack of nursing research support. Second, the nurses suggested a proposal to resolve the problem and benefit nursing.

Initiation. During the 1970s, nursing supported the growth in number of qualified nurse researchers whose work generated a growing knowledge base, leading to the use of the term "nursing science." Nursing research occurs in various settings and is currently funded by private, charitable foundations; nursing organizations; local, state, and federal agencies; and health-care facilities. Because no centrally located and adequately funded research center exists, coordinating ongoing research activities and disseminating information have been difficult.

Specification. To alleviate these problems, nursing mobilized to establish the National Institute of Nursing (NIN) within the NIH. In 1979, Congress requested the Institute of Medicine (IOM) to investigate nursing's status and needs. In spring 1983, the IOM published its report, *Nursing and Nursing Education: Public Policies and Private Actions.* Recommendation 18 of this report endorsed the establishment of an organizational entity to place nursing research in the mainstream of scientific investigation. The recommendation concluded that the federal government should fund a national agency to foster research that informs nurses and other health-care practitioners and increases the potential for discovery and application of various means to improve patient outcomes. The study's results and recommendations were reiterated by many nurse researchers and leaders as they lobbied for a nursing research center in the NIH.

In 1983, Leonard Heller, an IOM Robert Wood Johnson health policy fellow at the time, read the IOM report (Culliton, 1983). Heller brought the study to the attention of Rep. Edward Madigan (R-IL). Madigan's interest in the nursing research issue and his formal proposal for an NIN marked the end of the specification stage for the NIN issue. By amending the NIN proposal to the NIH reauthorization bill, the NIN issue achieved formal agenda status quickly and quietly.

Expansion. Despite access to decision makers, the originating group must compete with other issues and persuade influential legislators to move the issue to the top of the priority list. The originating group must then expand its support in a limited way by selecting persons who either identify closely with the originating group or who support the initiators and have influence with decision makers (Cobb et al., 1976). These individuals provide the necessary stimulus to garner a quick and favorable response. This is usually done privately; selective pressure is preferable to public pressure because the originating group remains accountable to the issue.

The cadre of nurse researchers, the initiating group, needed support to raise the priority of the proposal from several sources: the nursing political community, congressional decision makers, and agency heads in the Department of Health & Human Services (DHHS).

During the deliberations that led to the IOM's 1983 report on nursing, the NIN was discussed but not included in the report. The release of the IOM report, with its recommendation for an unspecified federal locus for nursing research, was swiftly followed by discussion in the nursing research community about the need for an NIN. This proposal was endorsed by the American Association of Colleges of Nursing (AACN), National League for Nursing (NLN), and American Nurses' Association (ANA), known collectively as the Nursing Tri-Council. During 1983-84, nursing publications shared progress reports, discussions, and analyses of the NIN issue.

Expansion of the issue occurred in the House due to the efforts of Reps. Edward Madigan and Henry Waxman (D-CA), as negotiations focused on the NIN and other NIH issues. Initial Senate support came from Sen. Daniel Inouye (D-HI), a long-time supporter of nursing research.

The NIN proposal did not fare as well in the DHHS administration. Principal parties interested in the NIN were former Secretary Margaret Heckler, the Division of Nursing, and the NIH. Heckler upheld the administration's position that new institutes were expensive and unnecessary. However, Heckler and the DHHS agencies remained sympathetic to the issue and used various strategies to meet nurse researchers' demands while preventing successful passage of the NIN. One strategy was to nearly double the funding for nursing research in the 1984 budget. Another strategy was to study the current federal effort and policy on nursing research.

Studying the issue. DHHS opposition to the NIN proposal spurred debate and two studies,

one conducted for the Office of Health Planning and Evaluation; the other for the NIH director. Both studies supported the present arrangements for nursing research, adding some modifications to give nurses more visibility and power.

A 1984 study done for DHHS staff (Gornick & Lewin, 1984) concluded that nursing's interests would be served best by keeping the nursing research functions in their present organizational location, the Division of Nursing within the Health Resources and Services Administration. In January 1985, Heckler established a center for nursing research in the Division of Nursing. The center was not funded by the Office of Management and Budget. Another option proposed in the Gornick and Lewin report was to elevate the Division of Nursing to bureau status, within which the center for nursing research would be housed.

The NIH director established a task force on nursing research in May 1984. The charge to this internal study panel was to examine the NIH's present and potential roles in nursing research. The task force concluded that, although the nursing research environment could be enhanced through administrative action, current nursing activities were consistent with the NIH mission.

The debate over the proposed NIN occurred within the context that Congress has repeatedly tried, sometimes successfully, to gain control over the NIH. In response to questions about the functioning of the NIH, DHHS contracted with the IOM to study the organizational structure of the NIH. The study was undertaken in 1983. During 1984, the administration repeatedly suggested that the creation of any new institutes be delayed until the IOM report was completed. When the report was released in late 1984, criteria for the development of new institutes were included.

Entrance and congressional action. The entrance stage of the inside initiative model is characterized by the attainment of formal agenda status. In this case, the NIN has achieved formal agenda status at the same time that limited issue expansion began to occur. Rapid entrance and limited issue expansion are hallmarks of the inside initiative model. During 1983 and 1984, the stages of expansion and entrance were occurring simultaneously. The fact that the NIN gained formal entrance quickly aided the process of limited issue expansion.

The House approved the amendment to create the NIN in 1983 through the efforts of Rep. Madigan, ranking minority member of the House Energy and Commerce Committee's Subcommittee on Health and the Environment, and Rep. Waxman, the subcommittee chair.

Senate support was not forthcoming until Fall 1984. The ongoing opposition from the Reagan administration was voiced by Sens. Orrin Hatch (R-UT), chair of the Committee on Labor and Human Resources, and Edward Kennedy (D-MA), ranking minority member of the committee. Despite lack of support in the Senate for the NIN, nursing leaders and researchers testified before committee hearings and continued lobbying for senators' support. Momentum in the Senate was lost when Sen. Hatch included in his nursing education bill a provision to elevate the Division of Nursing to bureau status and to include within it a new center for nursing studies and research. However, when House and Senate conferees met to resolve differences in the NIH bill, Hatch agreed to support the NIN, and it was then included in the NIH reauthorization bill which passed both houses. The president vetoed the reauthorization bill in October 1984.

In the 1985 session, the House proposed H.R. 2409 (The Health Research Extension Act of 1985), a similar version of the 1984 bill. Anticipating another presidential veto, nursing mounted an intensive override drive. Reagan did indeed veto the legislation; however, on November 12, the House overrode the veto 380 to 32. On November 20, the Senate concurred, overriding the president's decision by a vote of 89 to 7. Thus the National Center for Nursing Research was officially established.

The passage of H.R. 2409 authorizes the release of $5 million which had been appropriated in 1984 and extended until September 1986 under the Supplemental Appropriations bill. The release of this money was conditional upon legislative authority to establish a National Institute or Center for Nursing Research within NIH (Griffith, 1986). Funding authorized and appropriated under the Nurse Education Act will be used to fund research grants ($9.4 million) and training ($2 million).

Successful strategy

According to Dumas and Felton (1984), the process by which the NIN reached the formal agenda, here called the inside initiative model, has serious limitations because the larger nursing community was not informed nor part of the decision-making process. These nurses advocated organizational changes that would result in more communication and an increased use of democratic decision making. Their suggested strategies resemble the outside initiative model, in which an issue has broad-based support and is widely debated.

However, Cobb et al. (1976) described relationships between issue characteristics and issue expansion. Those issues for which wide support is likely to be sought are ambiguously defined, socially significant, and less technical. The NIN issue does not fit these criteria: It is narrowly defined, significant to a selected group, and highly technical. Given the characteristics of the issue and the nature of U.S. health policy, the process the nursing community selected to establish the NIN was the most likely to result in success.

REFERENCES

Cobb, R., Ross, J.K., & Ross, M.H. (1976). Agenda building as a comparative political process. T*he American Political Science Review, 70,* 126-138.

Culliton, B.J. (1983). A nursing institute for NIH? *Science, 222,* 1310-1312.

Dumas, R.G., & Felton, G. (1984). Should there be a National Institute for Nursing? *Nursing Outlook, 32*(2), 16-22.

Gornick, J.C., & Lewin, L.S. (1984). *Assessment of the organizational locus of the Public Health Service nursing research activities.* Washington, DC: Lewin and Associates.

Griffith, H. (1986). National center for nursing within NIH (Capitol Commentary). *Nursing Economics, 4*(1), 47.

Institute of Medicine. (1983). *Nursing and nursing education: Public policies and private actions* (p. 217). Washington, DC: National Academy Press.

Lockett, B.A. (1984). Setting the federal agenda for health research: The case of the National Institue on Aging. *Journal of Health Politics, Policy, and Law, 9*(1), 63-80.

What every nurse should know about political action

WILBUR J. COHEN; LONNA T. MILBURN, RN, PhD

ANYONE WHO WANTS to engage in the political process must accept the notion of perseverance. Without perseverance in the political process, all is lost, because the essence of this process — at least under the system of government in the United States — is that one has to overcome numerous obstacles that are presented by the political system itself. For example, a bill must pass through various congressional committees, the House of Representatives, the Senate, and the President. Each state is perilous, not only due to the controversies within the bill itself, but also due to surrounding circumstances — sometimes completely unrelated to the legislation at hand. Equally important is the power of lobbyists, whose goal is to promote their own interests by influencing policies.

Do not underestimate the fact that the political process increasingly involves important, well-financed, well-organized lobbies, directed toward pursuing the specific objectives of the group they represent. On the American scene, these organizations are becoming more important and more effective than ever before, and as a consequence, nurses also have to move into the political arena and organize their efforts effectively. When nurses are doing that, they must realize that others are doing it too — and often with more money, more members, and more political influence than they can develop at any given moment in time.

The need for nurses' involvement in the political process never has been greater. Budget cuts mandated by the Balanced Budget and Emergency Deficit Control Act of 1985

(Gramm-Rudman-Hollings) threaten survival of numerous programs that nurses have strived to establish. This legislation creates an automatic deficit reduction procedure for fiscal year (FY) 1986 through FY 1991 to ensure that at the end of FY 1991 the deficit will reach zero. In the event the deficit is anticipated to exceed the prescribed levels for any fiscal year, an automatic procedure will be used to achieve across-the-board reductions in the federal budget. Can there be a better example of the need for nurses to be informed and involved in politics and the formulation of national policy?

Legislation begins with both an awareness of the need for some kind of action to mitigate a problem and an idea for a solution. Although initially vague and at times controversial, the idea is the irreducible, irreplaceable first essential in the political process. It generates emotional response in the body politic and starts a large-scale public debate that escalates when people in power take a position.

Along with the controversial idea comes the period of germination. In this respect, nurses in their professional associations play an important role because they give a forum to the idea; they speak about it; they write about it; and by so doing, they aid in its development.

Organizations play an important part in this process for they can work the idea into a more widely accepted policy. The impact of the idea on organizations and persons within organizations is a significant factor in the development of public policy. The public may become aware of the need for some particular social action, but it is up to the organizations and interested persons in various groups to help develop the idea into a specific proposal on which the public can express its approval or disapproval so that a consensus, so to speak, can be obtained. At some point, somebody must transform the idea into a specific, viable legislative proposal.

The legislative proposal

Such a legislative proposal is necessary so that the views of organizations and individuals can be obtained; a wide consensus of opinion can be developed; and the proposal debated. Unless two conditions are met, however, the issue or the proposal will be stymied in the political process. First, the generalized idea must be converted into a specific proposal that can be discussed in detail, attacked, criticized, supported, and analyzed. Second, a dedicated legislative leader who commands respect not only of other legislative leaders, but the public, is needed to attract attention to the proposal.

Who the legislative leader of a proposal will be is essential to its survival. The fact that a bill has a high ranking leader automatically escalates its importance as a piece of legislation. To illustrate: presently, there is no legislative proposal on Medicare recipients' costs for catastrophic illness, one of the major ideas discussed during the past two decades. The idea of catastrophic-care insurance as a supplement to Medicare has received attention currently from President Reagan, such legislative leaders as Representative Pete Stark (D-California) and Senator Dave Durenberger (R-Minnesota), and U.S. Health and Human Services' Secretary Otis Bowen. In response to the insurance industries' concern about the government's involvement in Medigap insurance, the President initiated the creation of a task force under the auspices of the U.S. Department of Health and Human Services to study catastrophic care. Thus, this discussion on catastrophic-care insurance has reverted to the idea stage, and since there is no one legislative

leader giving the proposal momentum, there is no knowing at this moment whether the transformation of the idea into a new specific legislation proposal is a year away or five years away.

The period of conflict and public debate of an issue is probably the most exciting and distressing time in the whole process. During this period, advocates and opponents may make ridiculous statements: those in the debate may unleash all possible arguments pro and con, hoping that one will strike home. Often, issues become emotional rather than factual. The one thing to realize is that once the proposal is out and the conflict gets going, it is impossible to control.

This is a crucially important period also because it is when the reform or the piece of legislation jells, and this has serious consequences for the administration of the program once it materializes. In this way, an institution may become formed even before it is created.

An example comes to mind in connection with the administrative implementation of Medicare. It was initially necessary to spend a great deal of time in 1965 and 1966 correcting the views that physicians had formed of what Medicare really was. The physicians actually believed their own propaganda during the controversial period of the debate, when the Medicare proposal was characterized in unreal and unrepresentative terms. They subsequently had difficulty shaking off the negative image and the hostile feeling and the reactions engendered by their own spokesmen, who told them at the time that the program was going to regiment them, that it was going to tell them how to practice medicine. It was hard for the physicians to accept the fact that this was not so, but eventually they did. Facts superseded fiction in the long run.

The next element in the process is the forming of alliances. While a single group may successfully block a bill's passage, practically no piece of important legislation has been adopted by Congress because one single group, all by itself, unaided by anyone else, has tried to get it passed. American society is now so complex, so diffuse, so decentralized, so pluralistic that it is no longer possible for an American Medical Association or the veterans' organizations or the building and loan associations or the housing people to get controversial legislation through alone.

These alliances, however, always have a price that has to be paid — not only in money, as with a bribe or a transfer of funds, but also in modification of a group's own principles or priorities to accommodate those of other organizations in the alliance.

For example, the American Nurses' Association recently made an alliance with the American Association of Retired Persons, the American Hospital Association, the American Medical Association, and the Federation of American Health Systems to fight further cuts in the Medicare program.

This does not mean that nurses form an alliance with these organizations on every issue because their interests are not always of highest priority to nurses and vice versa. But in order to achieve a successful alliance with other groups, it should be recognized that often the priority or emphasis of one group must be tempered with that of the other group.

During the period of legislative debate, it often turns out that the objections offered are ones that the sponsors never even thought of themselves. The legislators and political parties who want to oppose a measure are absolutely ingenious in thinking up these objections. Professor Cohen illustrates from his own experience:

When I first returned to Washington in 1961, one of the programs I was most enthusiastic about was federal aid for scholarships to able but needy students. Ted Sorensen and I talked with President Kennedy about it; I had only been on the job as assistant secretary of HEW

[Health, Education, and Welfare] for a few weeks, and I was very optimistic. I said to the President: 'Well, this is one I am certain we can get through. We'll have a tough time on Medicare; we'll have a tough time on federal aid to elementary education, but federal aid for scholarships, Mr. President, that will be easy. We'll get going on that real fast.' The President approved our plan.

We managed to get the bill introduced, and the department had the support of many educational associations as well as other groups. I was called to testify before one of the congressional committees, and as was to be expected, the President's supporters gave a great deal of push to the legislation, and then a representative from the other political party turned to ask me some questions. The first one was: 'Well, Mr. Cohen, why are you so interested in federal aid for scholarships?'

I waxed eloquent and said: 'The national interest demands that we see to it that every single boy and girl of talent in our society has the opportunity to maximize his contribution to his family, to the economy, to the society as a whole. We just can't afford to let one single boy or girl in this nation, regardless of race, creed, or color, go without an education.'

I kept on in this vein — which I thought was very persuasive — and nobody interrupted me. Finally, the legislator said, 'Give me an illustration of what you think is a great shortage occupation that is in the national interest into which we ought to put a lot more money in scholarships.'

I replied: 'One of them is physicians. There is a tremendous shortage of physicians in the United States, and we can't have a great medical system that will bring the miracles of medical science to the American people even with all the billions of dollars we are putting into research unless there are more doctors, dentists, and nurses.' And he said: 'By the way, Mr. Cohen, how much do physicians get a year: What is their income?'

I responded that the median income then was about $25,000 a year net and he said: 'And you think we ought to start a new federal welfare program' — that's what he called it: *a new federal welfare program* — 'to help physicians get educated in order that they can make $25,000 a year or more?' "I said, 'Yes, I think we should. It's in the national interest.'

I knew then that we had lost. It took nearly two more years before the bill was enacted.

This amusing though lengthy story has in it two important lessons. First, the average congressman does not approach his political responsibilities in the same way that a national organization looks at national problems. He or she probably is a lawyer who came up the hard way, who may have gone to law school at night, who fought furiously in some small town or some small area or in a teeming metropolitan area to get nominated. He may have lost an election a couple of times. He may have had a tough time getting re-elected. He may have raised funds from a special interest group opposed to certain proposals. He does not always approach the problem from an intellectual point of view or from the standpoint of the national interest. This is not to imply that a congressman does not think of the national interest, but his conception of the national interest is influenced and molded in terms of the interests of his party and his congressional district. The second lesson: In legislative debates, expect the unexpected.

Here's an example of an unforeseen circumstance that, in this case, pushed a bill through. Disability insurance would not have been enacted in 1956 as an addition to the Social Security system if Walter George, dean of the Senate, was not going to retire. He wanted something in the nature of a great social reform to show his compassion for the unfortunate. If Walter George had not sponsored disability insurance in 1956, which won by the slim vote of 47-45 in the Senate, it is probable

that the whole development of Medicare would have been postponed by at least another five or ten years. This was because, in the sequence of events, the passage of disability insurance was the necessary precursor to the whole Medicare program since the determination of "disability" involved a medical examination and continuing governmental relation with physicians and hospitals. The Senate might have passed it later in 1958 or 1960 — no one knows. But it was passed in 1956 — even if by only two votes — and that would not have been possible if Walter George had not been willing at that moment in time to do something unexpected for social reform.

Although much of what transpires on the congressional floor may indeed appear haphazard, a basic premise stands firm: The American political process assumes that if each participant — lobbyists, congressmen, the President, etc. — pursues his or her own political objectives, out of this conflict of interest will come the national interest.

Once a law comes into being, the ideological antagonisms that occurred during the heated legislative debate must be forgotten. The key to future reform is the successful administration of those institutions that have just been created.

In America, nothing succeeds like success. If something works, people are willing to add to it, to build on it; even if the basic idea was faulty, they are willing to perfect it and expand it. But if the idea does not work out in practice, the political process will not tolerate future reform that tries to build upon it.

If Medicare continues to work well under the stress of the current budgeting crises and if physicians and hospitals say it is workable and practical with changes here and there to make it work better, then the idea probably will continue to be expanded and developed. Thus, cooperation in the administration of a program once it is launched is obviously an important element in developing legislation in this country.

In any case, there is a natural antipathy among the practical politicians to social legislation. But the same practical politicians will forego their opposition if the principles work out in practice and are administratively feasible. It is important to keep in mind what is feasible, when institutions are molded, new legislation is proposed, and new programs developed. It is disastrous for future reform as well as the maintenance of economic and social goals to find that a great idea has been developed into legislation, has been enacted into law, has overcome all these obstacles, and that it cannot be put into effect.

With all this in mind and given the current political climate that advocates great reductions in social and welfare programs, now is the time for nurses to develop priorities about further social and economic goals. The ideas developed by nurses and placed in the hands of the proper political leaders today will become the legislative mandates of the future. The next big opportunity may come between 1992 and 1995, and it is up to nurses to rise to the challenge and bring their ideas to the forefront of American political discussion.

Involvement: Influencing the delivery of health care and the future of critical care nursing

SUZANNE K. WHITE, RN, MN, CCRN

THE REVOLUTIONARY CHANGES in health care in this country are occurring in response to the need to improve our health care delivery system and to control spiraling health care costs. These dramatic changes have caused the American Association of Critical-Care Nurses (AACN) to examine its involvement in the legislative decision-making process. This article is written to stimulate your interest in becoming involved in the legislative arena, and to give you some member and chapter guidelines for involvement, particularly at the local and state level. Your involvement can have a tremendous impact on health care delivery and critical care nursing's future. According to U.S. Senator Edward Kennedy, nursing's major contributions to health care in America are probably the profession's best-kept secret.[1] Nursing professionals have also been described as the "invisible healers" and the "sleeping giant." Descriptive terms such as these have been used because of nursing's lack of interest and involvement in [legislation].

Some nurses have expressed disinterest in politics, claiming that they "don't know too much about politics" and "can't do much to change the outcomes," or that in their opinion "legislative involvement is not appropriate for nursing." As a human service profession that addresses the needs of all people, however, nursing cannot separate itself from politics and public policy.[2] Those who assert that professional nurses should not be political are really saying that nurses should not try to influence their own practice and the care that patients receive.[3] Yet there is no doubt that legislative, regulatory, and judicial decisions influence our practice at the bedside and the health care that we are able to provide.

AACN was founded 18 years ago for the purpose of "promoting the health and welfare of patients who are critically ill." Initially, this purpose was accomplished by educational programming for nurses working in critical care. As AACN has grown, so have the activities to accomplish its goals. The Association has been confronted with legislative, regulatory, and judicial decisions that have affected the health and welfare of critically ill patients. For example, prospective payment legislation and the Gramm-Rudman Bill have had an influence on health care funding, which directly and indirectly influences the practice arena. Although AACN's mission remains primarily focused on education, AACN has realized the need for increased awareness and involvement in the legislative arena, particularly in areas and decisions concerning critical care.

In 1979, with the realization that members need to be more aware and involved, AACN established the Committee on Public Affairs. This committee's purpose is to identify opportunities for enhancing AACN's outreach activities in public affairs. The committee's initial objective was to communicate information to the Board of Directors and members. Its objectives have now expanded to include not only information-gathering and communication, but also analysis of issues.[4]

In addition, in 1982 the Board of Directors unanimously passed a resolution stating, "AACN shall, in keeping with its stated purposes as a non-profit professional association, engage in activities to influence political decisions which affect nursing and health care."[4]

This resolution resulted in the deliberate exploration of ways in which AACN could play a more active role in Washington, D.C. AACN considered establishing an office in Washington, but because of the lack of financial and human resources decided not to pursue this further. AACN also lacked the historical perspective and networks necessary for direct influence. AACN strongly believes that the voice of and for nursing must be unified —one voice. In 1982, therefore, the AACN Board voted to support the efforts of the American Nurses' Association (ANA). In early 1984, AACN formalized a liaison agreement with ANA. AACN provides ANA with a monthly stipend to help defray operating costs in Washington and, in return, ANA provides AACN with weekly reports on the issues facing nursing, particularly those important to critical care nursing. This liaison arrangement has proved to be highly effective in bringing important issues to AACN's attention for action and input into ANA's efforts.

During the same year that the resolution was passed by AACN, the Committee on Public Affairs in conjunction with the Clinical Practice Committee developed a process for addressing practice, political, and professional issues.[5] This process was adopted by the Board of Directors in 1983 and provides an organized, thoughtful approach to a variety of issues including legislative ones.

In 1983 also, the Committee on Public Affairs developed the State Nursing Resource List. This list contains the names and addresses of state level and/or chapter presidents of organizations that make up the National Federation for Specialty Nursing Organizations. The State Nursing Resource List was developed to provide a networking mechanism that could be used to influence legislation.

Other events were also occurring at the same time. AACN always has encouraged chapters and members to be active at the state level with other nursing organizations. However, in about 1983, the Committee on Public Affairs began to receive letters from members who were participating in state federations, coalitions, and networks with other leaders or presidents of state nursing organizations. These members were being asked to represent AACN on the state level, and yet truly represented only one chapter within the state because of AACN's organizational structure. The Committee on Public Affairs also received letters from the Chapter Coordination Committee informing it of the concerns of members who were participating in state activities. These members needed direction.

At that time AACN recommended that the member "respond as an individual who has a critical care background, not as a state AACN representative." Subsequently, guidelines for such activities were developed and will be discussed later in this article.

Escalating local issues

The need for member involvement in decisions at the state level continues to increase not just in coalitions and federations but also in other legislative matters. Some trends creating the need include the following.

Reagan's "New Federalism." President Ronald Reagan was elected on a platform that promised to curb federal influence and the growing federal deficit. This platform included withdrawing the federal government from many local activities. With the "New Federalism," states have increased control over the allocation of federal monies and have developed policies for health and social services. Thus more decisions regarding health care are made at the state level. Nurses need to be involved in those decisions.

New development in health policy. Nurses need to expand their understanding of state government and increase their potential power at this level to influence health policy development and resource allocations. AACN recognizes that critical care practice is not independent of the environment in which it is practiced and that external forces are increasingly influential in changing our practice. Some state level issues and health policy developments that need nursing's immediate attention include tort reform, required request (organ donation) legislation, third party reimbursement, and access to care. AACN also recognizes that state level legislative action can set precedents. Eventually these collective actions may influence the national picture.

Such was the case involving the Missouri nurse practitioners in 1980. Two nurse practitioners in Missouri worked in a family planning clinic using standing protocols provided by physicians 40 miles away. Some of the nurse practitioners' responsibilities included performing pelvic examinations, inserting intrauterine devices, and prescribing birth control pills. The state medical board received complaints that the nurse practitioners were practicing medicine. Although the nurse practitioners suspected that the complaints came from physicians who were losing patients to the clinic, the questions considered by the State Medical Board, and later by the courts, focused on whether the nurse practitioners were competent to perform pelvic examinations and make diagnoses.[6] In this case, a judge was literally in a position to determine the future of nursing. The issue included scope of nursing practice, limits of medical practice, and the state board of nursing's authority to interpret and enforce nurse practice acts. Many nursing organizations, including AACN, worked successfully to ensure that the nurse practitioners won this case.

If that battle had been lost and the precedent set, nurses would have been unable to interpret and act on the data that they gather in providing care to patients. Nurses would have been unable to respond to patient situations unless a physician was present to validate their assessment. Not only nurse practitioners but also critical care nurses would have been affected. It would have been possible that when a code occurred in the intensive care unit the nurse would have been unable to respond even in the presence of standing protocols unless a physician was present to validate that an arrest had occurred.

The American Medical Association House of Delegates at its annual meeting in December 1982 adopted a resolution urging state medical associations to oppose enactment of legislation to authorize the independent practice of medicine by individuals not licensed to practice.[7] The [delegates] vowed to fight incursions of midwives, nurse practitioners, physician's assistants, nurse anesthetists, and others via efforts to oppose prescribing privileges, independent practice, mandated third party reimbursement, and other expansion.

Jurisdiction over the profession. States continue to define and regulate the practice of nursing through nurse practice acts. A current issue that explains the need for involvement related to professional regulation at the state level is entry into practice. Entry level into nursing practice is a professional issue and not one that belongs in the courts. However, it is a state regulatory issue, which is sure to affect practice in all settings.

An example of why we need a defined and consistent level of academic preparation for entry into professional nursing practice was evident in 1985. A federal judge ruled on a sex discrimination suit filed by six nurse practitioners. Because of the great variation in the educational background and training of the nurses, the judge found that the higher paid physician's assistant provided a higher level of care.[8] The case is being appealed, but the results of this case will weigh heavily on decisions in the future. Not only is this a professional issue, but it has set a precedent.

What can members and chapters do to influence legislation at the state and local level?

TABLE 1. Sources of information about legislation

Professional newspapers and newsletters
Examples
AACN News
American Nurse
SNA Newsletter
Capitol Update
The Political Nurse

Professional journals
Examples
Focus on Critical Care
American Journal of Nursing
Nursing Outlook
Nursing Management
Nursing Success Today

Political journals

Organizations
Examples
AACN
League of Women Voters
ANA
Women's Political Caucus

News magazines

Local newspapers

Legislative bills

Other
Legislative Network for Nurses
Washington Actions on Health
Health Legislation and Regulation

Personal involvement

First, members should get personally involved by participating as voters. Nurses cannot influence anything unless they are registered and vote. Voting is the first political act. Congressional elections are often won by 2000 votes. Today, there are an estimated 47 million unregistered eligible voters in this country. Thirty million women are not registered to vote; millions more do not vote in each election. Four-teen million young people between the ages of 18 and 24 are not registered.[9]

For success in the legislative arena, a certain amount of homework is needed. This is true for letter writing, personal contacts, preparing testimony, and obtaining support. An individual nurse or representative of a nursing special interest group must be knowledgeable of the issue or piece of legislation. Sources of information...are listed in Table 1.

Other ways to obtain information include contacting an organization that is likely to be involved with the issue. The nurse should meet or speak with the organization's government relations staff and ask what written information is available on the issue. State nursing associations are also excellent resources. The nurse seeking information may ask where they are targeting their legislative action and what are the most recent strategies. Sometimes organizations have copies of written testimony. Organizations like the League of Women Voters and the Women's Political Caucus offer information on issues, local elected officials, and specific information about city and county government. The nurse should find out about a legislator's background: what issues has he or she supported? Does he or she support health care or nursing issues?

Write your legislators. Guidelines for writing legislators are included in Table 2.

Meet your legislators. Make an appointment with your legislator. Prepare for the meeting by identifying the issue that you wish to discuss. A fact sheet can be formulated with written information to leave with the legislator. Do not try to cover too much material. It is better to discuss one issue in depth. Today, more than ever, when discussing a piece of legislation, think about the cost. What are the cost implications? That information can definitely influence the decisions. Follow up your visit with a thank-you letter and maintain contact with the legislator at least every 6 months. Developing a relationship of trust is important

---

TABLE 2. Guidelines for writing your legislator

1. Address your legislator by name. The use of *Representative* and *Senator* shows respect.
2. Write the letter in your own words.
3. Use your own stationery and stamps, not hospital or agency stationery.
4. Identify the bill or issue by bill number or describe it by popular title.
5. Identify yourself in terms of your position and basis for interest.
6. Be reasonably brief and as factual as possible. Never give misleading or exaggerated information.
7. Do not threaten the legislator with political retaliation if he or she votes against your wishes.
8. Express appreciation for consideration of your request in the conclusion of the letter.
9. Sign your full name with RN after it. Be sure your correct address is on the letter as well as the envelope.
10. The letter should be timely.

Address written correspondence as follows:

U.S. Senator	*U.S Representative*
Honorable John Smith	Honorable John Smith
United States Senate	House of Representatives
Washington, D.C. 20510	Washington, D.C. 20515
Dear Senator Smith:	Dear Representative Smith:

Use the same format when writing local and state officials.

---

and can help to establish credibility.

Another way to meet legislators is to go to the capitol. Many states have special-interest visitation programs that are fun, rewarding, and educational. Very few legislators have a health care background; therefore, their knowledge is limited regarding health care services and, like it or not, their decisions affect you and your patients at the bedside. Congressional representatives need your expertise. If nursing does not influence these actions, others with different interests will. If you are in nursing education, involve students in the legislative process. Take students to the capitol to meet legislators and to lobby an issue.... Students will realize that legislators need, want, and will use their information when voting.

Writing and presenting testimony is another way to demonstrate your expertise. Discuss the issue with your peers and consult others in your organization to see whether your testimony agrees with organizational priorities and current thinking. These skills require practice and experience. Do not hesitate to seek advice.

You can also become actively involved by registering voters at registration drives, participating in a campaign, or, better yet, running for an office.

Organizational involvement

With the New Federalism in mind and realizing that state level legislative actions can set precedents that other states follow, in 1985 the AACN Board of Directors directed the Committee on Public Affairs to explore the need for guidelines for involvement in legislative activities at the state level. In May 1986, the AACN Board of Directors approved the "Guidelines for AACN Member and Chapter Involvement in Legislative, Judicial, Regulatory and/or Organizational Health Care Issues." These guidelines encourage members and chapters to participate in legislative, judicial, regulatory, and organizational health care issues that promote the purpose and goals of the American Association of Critical-Care Nurses. The guidelines contain six sections that provide direction for chapter and member involvement in health care legislation and specify activities that are prohibited because of AACN's nonprofit tax status.

Section I lists prohibited activities that may be construed as supporting partisan political motives. These activities include:
• Support of any political candidate on behalf of AACN
• Political fund-raising
• Listing the Association's name on campaign literature.

Sections II through VI discuss the mechanisms for involvement in community, state, local, and national activities. Specific guidelines are included for involvement in state coalitions, committees, and federations. Members and chapters need to become familiar with the guidelines and AACN's position statements. A copy of the guidelines may be obtained from the National Office, AACN, One Civic Plaza, Newport Beach, CA 92660. The director of chapters and director of public affairs are available to members for information and guidance related to these guidelines.

Conclusion
Nurses are America's largest group of health professionals (1.9 million) and have enormous and untapped potential to play a proportionate role in helping to shape health policy. We are the sleeping giant whose health knowledge and influence is sure to become a valuable resource to legislative decision makers.

The "Guidelines for AACN Member and Chapter Involvement in Legislative, Judicial, Regulatory and/or Organizational Health Care Issues" provide a framework; however, you must be willing to do and act. Power is never bestowed; it must be assumed. No one will give it to you. You have the power and you must be willing to use it to help shape health policy. If not, the end result of powerless, po-

litically naive, frustrated nurses is inadequate nursing care.[3] Our patients' health and welfare suffer in the end.

As more issues are decided at the state level, chapters should gain consensus on issues and work together to influence public policy. On a personal level, a member may become involved, as an individual, a nurse, and an AACN member. Becky Kuhn, a past president of AACN, describes AACN's position:

During this time of increasing external influence in health care, ways and means to optimally influence the legislative arena will continue to be a focus for AACN, a focus consistent with and necessary to achieve AACN's mission of promoting the health of those experiencing critical illness.[4]

If we work together, we can achieve AACN's mission by influencing the delivery of health care and the future of critical care nursing.

REFERENCES

1. Kennedy EM. Foreword. In: Mason DJ, Talbott SW, eds. Political action handbook for nurses. Menlo Park, CA: Addison-Wesley Publishing Co., 1985:xxi.

2. Cole ER. Introduction. In: Mason DJ, Talbott SW, eds. Political action handbook for nurses. Menlo Park, CA: Addison-Wesley Publishing Co., 1985:xxix.

3. Mason DJ. The politics of patient care. In: Mason DJ, Talbott SW, eds. Political action handbook for nurses. Menlo Park, CA: Addison-Wesley Publishing Co., 1985:38.

4. Kuhn R. AACN's legislative involvement: past, present, and future. Focus Crit Care 1985;12(5):55-8.

5. Blichfeldt MP, Fredin N. Addressing controversial issues. Focus Crit Care 1984;11(3):68-9.

6. Hunter ML. These nurses weren't practicing medicine after all. RN 1984;47(1):69.

7. Calderson E. The organization in action: Washington (DC) nurses work for practice privileges. In: Mason DJ, Talbott SW, eds. Political action handbook for nurses. Menlo Park, CA: Addison-Wesley Publishing Co., 1985:473.

8. Long M. Titling and licensure. Ga. Nurs 1985;2:2.

9. Ford-Roegner P. Voter participation and campaigning. In: Mason DJ, Talbott SW, eds. Political action handbook for nurses. Menlo Park, CA: Addison-Wesley Publishing Co., 1985:398.

UNIT FOUR

Study questions

Chapter Twelve

1. After reading these articles, how do you feel about the American health care system? Does it match the values you ascribe to our country?

2. How do the problems and solutions listed by Huey compare with your own experiences with the health care system?

3. Can you formulate some solutions to the problems of limited access and rising costs of health care in this country? What would be required to implement your solutions?

4. What health care legislation is being enacted in your state? Are nurses involved?

5. Do you support a public policy of health care as a right for all citizens, including the homeless and people with AIDS? If so, why? If not, why not?

Chapter Thirteen

6. Is the consumer always right? What strategies would you add to those of Eck, et al. to bridge the gap between consumers and providers? Does their conclusion that improving staff satisfaction can improve patient outcomes surprise you?

7. Consider Aydelotte's vision of nursing. Where do you agree and disagree with her? Has she neglected some major trend?

8. After reading the article by Allen and Turner, ask yourself these questions: What do you know about the health beliefs and practices of the major groups of immigrants? What changes in morbidity patterns are likely to occur with changing demographic patterns?

9. After reading the article by Longman, do you support early retirement? Does your school or health care institution advocate early retirement?

Chapter Fourteen

10. The Rogge article and the interview with Senator Inouye were included for their motivational impact. After reading these articles, how do you feel about the need for nurses to be involved in the political process? Do you identify with any of the nurses described by Rogge? What reasons could you list as justification for not being politically active?

11. How would you link creation of the National Center for Nursing Research with the current efforts to develop the discipline of nursing, as described in Unit Two?

12. After reading the Cohen and Milburn article, mentally role-play the process of testifying for your bill in front of a legislative committee. What bill did you choose to defend? What questions were you asked? What data did you use to respond?

13. After reading the article by White, select a current legislative proposal that you strongly support or oppose. What guidelines in the article would you use to write letters to your legislators?

U N I T   F O U R

Additional assignments

1. Analyze data regarding the demographic characteristics of your city in conjunction with morbidity and mortality data. Compare it to national data. Do significant differences exist? Do any of the morbidity data or statistics regarding health care concern you? What strategies could change the situation?

2. Role-play a legislative hearing on a legislative initiative regarding health care for the uninsured. Collect data, draft legislation, and hold a hearing.

3. Identify a current bill concerning health care. Who initiated it? What is the data base? What is the underlying policy? Who will benefit? Who will not? Who will pay? What alternate bills were discarded in favor of this bill?

4. At the state level, is health care an issue? Who are the advocates in the Senate? In the House? What community groups are involved?

5. Interview faculty regarding their involvement in the political process. How many have testified before a legislative committee? How many view involvement as part of their responsibility? How many have worked with legislators to develop legislation? How many write routinely to their state and national representatives?

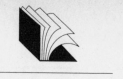

Legal and ethical issues

NURSES NEED TO BE as knowledgeable about legal and ethical issues as they are about techniques of client care. Why? Because virtually every nursing decision has a legal or ethical component, or both.

In addition, each year an estimated 1,900 nurses are named in malpractice lawsuits. Legal problems can even result from decisions made to resolve ethical issues! Furthermore, avoiding the risk of involvement in a malpractice lawsuit is becoming more difficult as nurses assume more and more responsibility for complex aspects of client care.

What can nurses do to give themselves maximum protection against legal liability? They can become knowledgeable about which nursing situations carry a high risk of liability (such as administering drugs and withdrawing life support) and take special care when working in those situations. Of course, probably the best form of self-protection against liability is possession of top-notch nursing skills: Such a nurse is simply less likely to make a mistake.

But nurses are not just affected by laws — they can and should help to create laws, particularly laws that help nurses take control of their practice. By participating in the legislative process at the local, state, and federal lev-

els, nurses will come to know and understand how laws are enacted, what bills are under consideration, and what they can do to protect clients' rights, particularly in this dawning era of rationed access to health care.

Law and ethics

The legal aspects of nursing were first emphasized in the late 19th century, when nursing leaders worked toward establishment of licensing and registration of nurses. Ethics has assumed major importance since the Nuremberg trials after World War II and with the advances in and complexity of medical technology. Among those tried at the Nuremberg military tribunals were Nazi physicians who, under the guise of medical experimentation, committed atrocities. The trials resulted in the Nuremberg Code, which guides ethical medical research. Today, law and ethics are having increasing impact on every area of nursing practice; more than ever, nurses need to understand the role of legal and ethical factors in clinical decision making.

Understanding and following the law as applied to nursing, although never easy, is at least a matter of interpreting facts — what the law says — within the clinical context. Not so with ethics, which involve the nurse's personal values and beliefs as well as her professional judgment in determining whether a decision is in a client's best interest. The chapters in this unit provide a thoughtful grounding in nursing law and ethics, explaining how they differ and how they can overlap. Also provided are vivid examples of nurses dealing with legal and ethical problems in practice.

What are the implications for nursing of rationed access to health care?

Biomedical and technological advances in health care have now surpassed our society's ability to provide them on an equal basis for all citizens who need them. As a result, our society is faced with the increasing likelihood of health care rationing — of allocation of health care to those who can pay for it and allocation of health care dollars to those most likely to benefit from treatment. As the chapters in this unit demonstrate, this emerging area of health care controversy has the potential to transform nursing by altering society's view of nurses as caring professionals. In addition, the legal and ethical implications of health care rationing have the potential to directly affect nursing practice.

Nursing law "basics"

Nurse practice acts are the foundation of nursing law, defining nursing and nursing's scope of practice in every state. Nursing law also applies in other nursing areas, such as nurse registration and the setting of educational standards in nursing schools. Today, as we read in the chapters in this unit, these "basics" of nursing law are the bulwarks of the profession's defense against encroachment — for example, movements for institutional licensure and for creation of new health care workers who would do some of the work of nurses.

The requirement for nursing licensure has tended to be questioned during periods of nursing shortages. One result has been occasional moves to initiate institutional licensure,

which would allow state governments to license health care agencies rather than individual nurses; the agencies could then use their own judgment in assigning workers to jobs (and job titles). So far, nursing has held off this movement, which the American Nurses' Association (ANA) has opposed in the interests of the client and of maintaining the quality of nursing care.

The state boards of nursing have a number of responsibilities, including involvement in disciplinary actions, such as license revocation and suspension, against individual nurses. Increasing malpractice litigation has forced institutions and nursing to recognize the legal risks of employing incompetent or physically or mentally impaired nurses. Disciplinary actions can also be taken against nurses for immoral, unethical, or unprofessional conduct and for use of fraud in procuring a license.

The challenge to nursing ethics

DeYoung (1985) quotes Wellman's definition of ethics as "a discipline in which one attempts to identify, organize, analyze, and justify human acts by applying certain principles to determine the right thing to do in a given situation." By this definition, ethics is a practical arm of philosophy and ethical decisions the action that translates ideals into the real world.

The early teaching of ethics in nursing schools emphasized loyalty and subservience — to the physician, the hospital, and the training school — rather than professional behavior and nurse-client relationships. The ANA's first constitution, in 1897, referred to the need for a code of professional ethics, but none was adopted until the first Code for Professional Nurses was published by the ANA in 1950.

According to Yeaworth (1985), the elimination of expected subservience of nurses, particularly to physicians, was prominent in this first code of nursing ethics. Revisions to the code, in 1956, 1960, 1968, 1976, and 1985, clarified concerns about nurses' competence and responsibilities, particularly in view of their increasing use of complex medical technology.

Another early factor in the formation of nursing ethics was the Florence Nightingale Pledge, a traditional part of many nursing graduation ceremonies:

> I solemnly pledge myself before God and in presence of this assembly;
> To pass my life in purity and to practice my profession faithfully;
> I will abstain from whatever is deleterious and mischievous and will not take or knowingly administer any harmful drug.
> I will do all in my power to maintain and elevate the standard of my profession and will hold in confidence all personal matters committed to my keeping and family affairs coming to my knowledge in the practice of my calling.
> With loyalty will I endeavor to aid the physician in his work, and devote myself to the welfare of those committed to my care.

Like all sworn oaths, the Nightingale pledge does not have any legal status. Instead, it is intended to serve as a nurse's sworn promise to always be moral and ethical and act in the best interests of the client. Another such writing is the "Patient's Bill of Rights," published by the American Hospital Association in 1973, at a time when the consumer movement was heightening public concern for the rights of hospitalized clients. The "Bill of Rights," reprinted below, is still used as a standard for minimum ethical consideration for clients, although it has been heavily criticized for its failure to recognize the rights to adequate medical care.

A PATIENT'S BILL OF RIGHTS

1. The patient has the right to considerate and respectful care.

2. The patient has the right to obtain from his physician complete current information concerning his diagnosis, treatment, and prognosis in terms the patient can be reasonably expected to understand. When it is not medically advisable to give such information to the patient, the information should be made available to an appropriate person in his behalf. He has the right to know, by name, the physician responsible for coordinating his care.

3. The patient has the right to receive from his physician information necessary to give informed consent prior to the start of any procedure and/or treatment. Except in emergencies, such information for informed consent should include but not necessarily be limited to the specific procedure and/or treatment, the medically significant risks involved, and the probable duration of incapacitation. Where medically significant alternatives for care or treatment exist, or when the patient requests information concerning medical alternatives, the patient has the right to such information. The patient also has the right to know the name of the person responsible for the procedures and/or treatment.

4. The patient has the right to refuse treatment to the extent permitted by law and to be informed of the medical consequences of his action.

5. The patient has the right to every consideration of his privacy concerning his own medical care program. Case discussion, consultation, examination, and treatment are confidential and should be conducted discreetly. Those not directly involved in his care must have the permission of the patient to be present.

6. The patient has the right to expect that all communications and records pertaining to his care should be treated as confidential.

7. The patient has the right to expect that within its capacity a hospital must make reasonable response to the request of a patient for

services. The hospital must provide evaluation, service, and/or referral as indicated by the urgency of the case. When medically permissible, a patient may be transferred to another facility only after he has received complete information and explanation concerning the needs for and alternatives to such a transfer. The institution to which the patient is to be transferred must first have accepted the patient for transfer.

8. The patient has the right to obtain information as to any relationship of his hospital to other health care and educational institutions insofar as his care is concerned. The patient has the right to obtain information as to the existence of any professional relationships among individuals, by name, who are treating him.

9. The patient has the right to be advised if the hospital proposes to engage in or perform human experimentation affecting his care or treatment. The patient has the right to refuse to participate in such research projects.

10. The patient has the right to expect reasonable continuity of care. He has the right to know in advance what appointment times and physicians are available and where. The patient has the right to expect that the hospital will provide a mechanism whereby he is informed by his physician or a delegate of the physician of the patient's continuing health care requirements following discharge.

11. The patient has the right to examine and receive an explanation of his bill regardless of source of payment.

12. The patient has the right to know what hospital rules and regulations apply to his conduct as a patient.

Current controversies in law and ethics

Technological changes in the health care system have profoundly affected nursing practice. The nursing journal *RN* conducted a survey in 1988 requesting information on ethical conflicts in nursing. The replies received from over 1,000 nurses identified the following ethics- and law-related conflicts:

1. The nursing shortage — its effect on reducing the quality of client care
2. Incompetence of peers — problems of reporting
3. Care of the dying client and prolongation of life or termination of life support
4. Informed consent and client advocacy
5. Risks in caring for AIDS clients
6. Abortion
7. Quality versus cost — implied implications for the rationing of health care.

These are only some of nursing's current ethical and legal concerns; others are reported in the chapters in this unit. As the authors of the articles in this unit make clear, successful coping with contemporary concerns requires, paradoxically, some of the most traditional characteristics of the professional nurse: knowledge, skill, and caring.

REFERENCES

1. DeYoung, L. (1985). *Dynamics of nursing.* (5th ed.). St. Louis: C.V. Mosby.

2. Yeaworth, R. (1985, summer). The ANA code: A comparative perspective. *Image: The Journal of Nursing Scholarship. 18*(3), 94-95.

CHAPTER FIFTEEN

Rationing nursing care

THE IDEA THAT nurses may have to participate in limiting health care to their clients is startling because nursing centers on providing the highest quality care to anyone who needs it. The ANA's *Code for Nurses* mandates that nurses base their clinical judgments on moral principles and the probable consequences of their actions. The first tenet of the code states that nurses must respect human dignity and each client's uniqueness, regardless of social, economic, or personal considerations or of the nature of the client's health problem. Obviously, a nurse confronting the need to restrict or refuse care will face an ethical and moral conflict, as well as a possible legal problem. The nurse who provides inadequate care may be sued for negligence or malpractice.

Health care is being rationed primarily through restricted federal and state funds for such health care programs as Alcohol and Drug Abuse and Mental Health Services, Aid to Families with Dependent Children, and Women, Infants, and Children Supplemental Nutrition Program. Elderly and poor clients particularly have been affected by the reductions. Furthermore, some states and counties limit or prioritize how state or local health care funds will be spent on indigent persons. Expensive medical procedures, such as organ transplants, may not be allowed or will have low priority, or youths may have care priority over elderly clients. Care also is rationed when health care agencies reduce the numbers of nursing and support personnel, which increases case load, and reduce equipment and supplies.

How will criteria for rationing of services be developed, and who will pay for the unemployed and the uninsured? How will nursing maintain a legal and ethical commitment to the client to provide quality care while reducing services? The answers to these questions are elusive. The articles in this chapter provide an overview of current thinking.

Popp, in "Health Care for the Poor: Where Has All the Money Gone?" addresses the adverse impact of federal budget cuts and health care rationing on health care delivery to the poor. "Rationing Health Care to the Elderly: A Challenge to Professional Ethics," by Fry, focuses on rationing care to elderly clients. Fry postulates that if rationing becomes policy, then nursing education, instead of focusing on critical care and life extension for elderly clients, will need to teach the student how to help the elderly live with suffering and pain and die with dignity. Ethics will also be taught differently, Fry forecasts, with clients' rights interpreted in terms of society's, rather than individuals', needs.

Richard Lamm, former governor of Colorado and currently director of the Center for Public Policy and Contemporary Issues at the University of Denver, is quoted in the Russell article "High Costs May Lead to Rationed Medicine." Lamm supports the concept that the older individual owes it to the younger generation not to overuse scarce health care resources, although he admits he is uncomfortable with the idea of a British-style system of rationing health care in part according to age.

In the same article, a Stanford University economist, Victor Fuchs, is quoted as saying, "Sooner or later, the only way to cut health care spending in a major way is to reduce the quantity of services delivered to patients."

The article's author states that we already have rationing through policies that discourage the poor from seeking medical attention.

What is the impact on the nurse who is providing direct client care in circumstances of personnel, equipment, and supply shortages? Collins tells us, in the article "When the Profit Motive Threatens Patient Care," that hospitals that try to reduce costs may jeopardize the quality of care and hurt themselves in the long run, when clients seek care elsewhere. She asks: Is the United States headed toward a system in which receipt of care is directly connected to the ability to pay?

Health care for the poor: Where has all the money gone?

SISTER ROSANNE POPP, RN, BSN

A PRIMARY CONCERN of the health care industry today is economics — particularly finding ways to decrease the cost of health care. Because nursing is an integral part of the health care industry, nurses must understand what changes in the economics of health care have occurred and how these changes affect the delivery of care, especially nursing care. This article will examine these economic concerns as they relate to federal budget cuts, health care rationing, and the impact these two events have had on health care for the poor.

The Reagan administration has been instrumental in bringing about changes in the distribution of health care in the United States. The "New Federalism" proposed by President Reagan has restructured the roles of state, local, and federal government in health care, [1] it has placed more responsibility on individuals and states. This shift in responsibility has focused on three major areas: Medicaid funding and regulation; conversion of health programs to state block grants; and cuts in nutrition funding. [2]

From 1983 to 1985, Congress reduced the Medicare/Medicaid budget by approximately $13 billion. The majority of the Medicaid changes were enacted as part of the 1981 Budget Reconciliation Act. This bill had several provisions that significantly altered health care delivery, especially to the indigent. It provided for new regulations that reduced federal monies to Medicaid by incrementally decreasing the amount of the federal contribution each year for 3 years.

This bill also reduced by one million the number of people eligible for Medicaid. This was achieved by tying Medicaid eligibility to qualifications for other federal programs. For example, the allowable income for obtaining Aid to Families with Dependent Children (AFDC) was reduced. When these indigent families, mostly single-parent women and children, no longer qualified for AFDC, they were also ineligible for Medicaid. [2]

More important than the direct reduction of funds brought about by this bill was the impact on the administration of these funds. The federal government gave states new powers to distribute funds and the flexibility to cut health care budgets. States could set limits on the amount of money and kinds of services for which they would pay; they could contract with less expensive health providers (and limit access to those resources in the process) and choose to cover community-based services as an alternative to nursing home care. [1]

The result of this legislation has negatively affected funding to the poor, but the most dramatic effect has been in the rate of decline of the program's growth. There had been an average of 15% growth in the Medicaid program since 1976; but in 1982, after the new formula for eligibility was established, the growth was only 9.8%.

The conversion of health programs to state block grants was also a provision of the 1981 budget reform bill. It provided that 21 health care programs be consolidated into four block grants to be administered by the states. The four grants were Preventive Health and Health Services, which funds a variety of public health and preventive health services for individuals and families; Maternal and Child Health, which funds a variety of services for mothers and children and services for crippled children; Alcohol and Drug Abuse and Mental Health Services, which funds programs that combat alcohol and drug abuse, provides services to the mentally ill through community mental health centers, and promotes mental health centers; and Primary Care, which funds delivery of primary care to underserved populations.[1]

The result of this consolidation has been 18% reduction of federal funding for these programs to individual states.[2] With the shift of responsibility to the states, there have been problems with the administration of the funds. Conflict over funding authority and expenditure has, at times, hampered effective use of the money that is available.[1]

The third area that has been adversely affected by the new federal health budget cuts is nutrition. These cuts were primarily in three areas: Women, Infants, and Children Supplemental Nutrition Program (WIC), food stamps, and children's nutrition. In 1982, Congress cut $1.7 billion from the food stamp program by restricting income levels of eligibility and disallowing food stamps for striking workers. WIC programs and child nutrition programs such as school lunches and breakfast programs were cut by $1.5 million. In 1982, there were one million fewer people receiving food stamps and another one million receiving fewer food stamps than previously.[2]

These budget cuts, the general mood of the Reagan administration, and other socioeconomic factors have brought us to the era of health care rationing. What is health care rationing and how does it affect the poor?

Health care rationing

Health care rationing can be defined as:

> ...limiting the consumption of medical care, so that a patient does not receive all the care that

he or his physician believes would be of some benefit to him. The denied benefit might be large, even life-saving, or it might be very small, but (qua benefit) is greater than zero.[3]

Rationing is determined by policy makers to be necessary when resources are scarce.

As a matter of principle, Americans have always been opposed to rationing of goods and services even when it was necessary, such as during World War II. Public opinion polls in the years 1982, 1983, and 1984 showed that Americans supported equal access to health care regardless of the ability to pay or the outcome of the illness. This unwillingness to limit access to health care has not been matched by the willingness of individuals or corporate groups to assume the extra costs of health care that equal access would entail. This reluctance and the support for federal budgetary reform have been interpreted as giving tacit approval to health care rationing.[4]

In actuality, health care rationing is not a new entity. The quality and quantity of care given have always been determined by the consumers' ability and willingness to pay for the services rendered. In effect, the marketplace, has, for centuries, been the arena for rationing not only health services but also other commodities and services that could be obtained by monetary means. It is only in recent years that the federal government has taken on the responsibility for providing equality in health care.

The marketplace and/or economic factors still play important roles in health care rationing. Economic rationing is determined by allocation of government funds and from third party payer decisions. Other economic factors that enter into the rationing of health care are the complexity of medical information that makes informed choices about the need for medical care difficult and the opportunity or capability for a person to make those informed choices. For example, most consumers must rely on the information given them by the physician, a provider of health care, to make choices about their need for health care, or decisions are made for them by the physician with minimal explanation or time for consideration.

Rationing can also take place by a number of other determinants. The individual characteristics of persons may be considered, such as social worth, residence, race, ethnic origin, and age. Health status has also been considered a factor as well as what have been termed "objective measures." These objective measures take into consideration technology's clinical efficacy, cost-effectiveness, and potential for enhancing life.[5] An example of objective selection might be choosing a transplant recipient who could be most productive after the procedure, or the odds that the time and technology used to perform an operation would produce a successful outcome.

Health care rationing produces what has been called a two-tiered or multilevel provision of health care which is controlled by the client's ability to pay. People who rely on public assistance for health care have reduced access to health services while those who rely on commercial or self-pay sources are privy to a larger number of services and resources. The two-tiered system has not taken definite shape yet but is developing rapidly with the formation of preferred provider organizations, health maintenance organizations, an increase in the corporation of health care systems, and a decrease in the amount of federal money available for health care.

Although President Reagan has assured the public that "safety net" measures would be undertaken to protect the programs that serve the truly needy, almost all of these programs have been adversely affected by the budget cuts. Medicaid, food stamps, welfare, maternal and child health, and community centers are among the programs which have suffered reduced funding. At the same time, many of the programs which serve nonpoor individuals such as the Veterans Administration were excluded from such drastic cuts. One study estimates that 60% of Americans below the poverty level received little or no benefits from those administration-defined safety net programs.[6]

Health care and the poor

Who are these poor whose health care services are being diminished by budget cuts and rationing of health care?

> The health care poor (are) those persons who are unable, through private resources, employer support, or public aid to provide payment for health care services, or those who are unable to gain access to health care because of limited resources, inadequate education, or discrimination.[7]

According to the census bureau, in 1982, 34.4 million people, or 15% of the population, lived in poverty. Of these, 11.1% were white, 34.5% were black, and 26.5% were of Spanish origin. About 40% lived outside the metropolitan areas and 45% lived in the south.[7] Other pertinent data are the fact that one of every five children lives in poverty and that this proportion increases to one of every two for black children. Over the past 5 years the disposable income of the poorest one-fifth of the American families (those headed by nonelderly black women) has dropped 9%. The poorest one-fifth of the population earn 4.7% of the total income in the country whereas the richest earn almost 43%.[8]

The poor/near poor population has increased by about 8 million in the same 5-year period. Most of these persons reflect the increased number of underemployed, and unemployed with their dependents. Of this population almost 60% are not covered by public or private insurance.[9]

When 15% of the population as a whole is without health care insurance, it becomes an issue that cannot be ignored. Studies have shown that insurance coverage is one of the major factors influencing the use of health care services.[9] It has also been shown that the increased use of such services is associated with increased health.[10] Health care insurance determines access to care and the type of care provided.

The two groups hardest hit by the Medicaid cutbacks and the resulting decrease in access to health care are children and the elderly. Children make up 40% of the poor population; of these, only one-third is served by Medicaid. Community health centers had been major sources of obstetric and pediatric care for the uninsured but as many as 250 of these centers were closed as a result of the 1982 funding cuts. This left 1 million people without a source of health services. Decreases in the funding for nutritional programs have also had adverse effects. Although it has been shown that participation in the WIC program by poor pregnant mothers can decrease the rate of low birth weight babies by 75%, the program has funds to serve only one-third of those who are eligible.[10] Several independent studies have shown that for each $1 spent on prenatal care and nutrition, $2 to $11 can be saved on care that would otherwise be needed later. For example, it has been shown that with a decline in prenatal visits there has been an increase of maternal anemia which has been associated with low birth weight and diminished intellectual and physical development in children.[10] There is also an increase in the incidence of chronic disease and poor health habits when prenatal care is inadequate.

The elderly have been limited to health care access mainly because of constraints imposed by Medicare. Higher deductibles and a decrease in the amount of reimbursement Medicare provides for health care needs result in increased expenses for which the individual is responsible. These increased expenses along with the proposal to limit Social Security cost of living allowances have the potential to increase the number of elderly who are below the poverty line by 72%.[10]

There is not only decreased access to health care for the poor but there is also evidence that the care received by these people is inferior to that being given to those people who have financial resources available.[7] Uninsured persons or those with public funding do not have access to primary or preventive health care. Because they may have fewer accessible paths into health care systems, they are less likely to receive timely and appropriate referrals, follow-up care, or the appropriate mix of services to best restore or maintain health. All these things lead to fragmented, episodic, and duplicated services.[7]

Health care institutions which provide services to the indigent population are experiencing increasing difficulties in funding these services. Recent changes in reimbursement policies, prospective payment, and cost shifting have all but eliminated the hospital's ability to provide voluntary, free care. In the past, care for the poor was mainly funded by private-pay and commercially insured patients through pricing structures that generated enough revenue to cover the provision of care to the poor.[7] Now, other ways of paying for indigent care must be found.

Rationing of health care is an alternative proposed to deal with the expense of free care that hospitals face. This can be done in two ways. The health care institution directly prohibits or discourages hospital use for people who are unable to pay, and the availability of services heavily used by the uninsured poor is reduced, especially if these services are unprofitable.[11]

An innovative plan for providing health care to Medicare/Medicaid recipients is outlined by Dunham et al.[12] These authors describe the proposal of Enthoven[13] to use vouchers which would allow Medicare/Medicaid recipients to select between alternative insurance packages. These vouchers, issued by the government, would have a certain dollar amount and the holder could choose where to use them to obtain health care. With more consumers having the freedom to choose health care providers, the competition among health care providers, especially insurance companies and health maintenance organizations, would increase. This increase would lead to reduced costs and encourage innovation.[12]

Two other proposed solutions for financing health care for the poor are to expand health insurance or to pay hospitals to deliver free care.[11] In the first instance the uninsured would be allowed to purchase, with government subsidy, insurance with minimum coverage. This insurance coverage could take various forms; it could be limited to catastrophic illnesses, be in the form of indemnity payments (*e.g.,* a certain amount to doctor and hospital per day), or be part of a public preferred provider organization which could share any cost-savings with the users of the programs.

In the second instance, hospitals would be reimbursed by the government according to the amount and kind of indigent care provided. Because 10% of hospitals give 40% of the nation's free health care, Feder *et al.* suggest that government reimbursement should go only to those institutions which provide substantial amounts of free care and are experiencing financial loss from these services. The money for the reimbursement could be provided through government grant programs or through upward adjustments to these hospitals' Medicare and Medicaid reimbursement rates.[11]

Sustaining delivery of health care to the poor and uninsured is a long-term problem. Changes in the number of uninsured vary ac-

cording to the status of the economy, but there will always be a substantial number of people whose health care needs are not met. Because equitable delivery of health care does not seem to be a priority for Americans, unequal access to services, quality, and quantity of care still remain.[7]

A comprehensive long-term solution to the problem of budgetary constraints, health care rationing, and their impact on the poor comes in the form of four recommendations presented by McIntire and Grueber. They propose that further work be directed by the following guidelines:

1. Establish a national health policy on the delivery and financing of health care for the poor.

2. Base public policy development on principles of equity and justice.

3. Establish an effective constituency or coalition that can serve as an advocate for the poor.

4. With health care professionals as leaders, develop and test models or programs that recognize the needs of both care recipients and providers and support recommended policy changes.[7]

Each of these proposed solutions highlights the fact that responsibility for health care of the poor is not only a complex task, but also one that must become the responsibility of the private as well as the public sector of business if the outcome is to be successful. Alternative plans for delivery of health services must be created to compensate for the traditional systems which have been severely curtailed with the budget cuts.

Federal budget cuts and the resulting health care rationing have had an adverse impact on the poor of our nation. Many of the avenues by which they obtained health care are no longer open to them. If adequate health care is to be achieved for all Americans, alternate ways of providing that care must be devised. In an era of economic and budgetary constraints this presents a powerful challenge to health care providers and consumers alike.

REFERENCES

1. Altman DE, Morgan DH. The role of state and local government in health. Am J Public Health 1985;2(4):7-31.

2. Haglund K. A new American body count? New Physician 1983;32(2):18-26, 25.

3. Baily MA. "Rationing" and American health policy. J Health Polit Policy Law 1984;9(3):489-499.

4. Friedman E. Two ties of health care: the unthinkable meets the inevitable. Hospital Medical Staff 1984;13(10):15-22.

5. Friedman E. Rationing and the identified life. Hospitals 1984;48(10):65-66, 68, 72, 74.

6. Dallek G. Who cares for health care? The first two years of Reagan administration health policy. Health PAC Bull 1983;14(1):7-17.

7. McIntire JR, Grueber CM. Health care for the poor: shaping public policy. Health Progress 1985;66(5):53-56, 68.

8. Aldis SS. Setting goals and priorities: 1984 presidential address. Am J Public Health 1985;75(11):1276-1280.

9. Wilensky G. Poor, sick, and uninsured. Health Affairs 1983;2(2):91-95.

10. Mundinger MO. Health services funding cuts and the declining health of the poor. N Engl J Med 1985;313(1):44-47.

11. Feder J, Hadley J, Mullner R. Falling through the cracks: poverty, insurance coverage, and hospital care for the poor—1980 and 1982. Milbank Mem Fund Q 1984;62(4):544-565.

12. Dunham A, Marone JA, White W. Restoring medical markets: implications for the poor. J Health Polit Policy Law 1982;7(2):488-499.

13. Enthoven A. Consumer choice health plan. N Engl J Med 1978;298:650-658-709-820.

Rationing health care to the elderly: A challenge to professional ethics

SARA T. FRY, RN, PhD

THE NUMBER OF PEOPLE over 65 years of age in the United States is rapidly increasing and is expected to continue to do so over the next 20 years. [1] Indeed, the elderly over 85 years of age make up the most rapidly growing age group in our society today. Because of the increasing number of elderly and their needs for costly and often limited health care services, it is not surprising that rationing health care to them is a current topic of discussion.

In a provocative book entitled *Setting Limits: Medical Goals in an Aging Society,* author Daniel Callahan develops a controversial rationale for limiting health resources to the elderly (those over the age of 65), "first at the level of public policy and then at the level of clinical practice and the bedside." [2] His book is one of several recently published that propose and defend a scheme for rationing health care. [3,4] Callahan's book is significant, however, in that it uses age, rather than need, as a principle for the allocation of health resources. The cost of health care for the elderly who are in the last year of their life, claims Callahan, amounts to about one percent (1%) of the gross national product each year. Because of these costs, Callahan argues persuasively, it is time for a shift in our attitudes toward aging, toward the goals of medicine and nursing, and eventually, toward rationing of our health care resources to the sick elderly.

Crucial to Callahan's argument is his theory of aging. The central axioms are that the young and the old need to understand that it is possible to live out a meaningful old age that is limited in time and that does not need medicine to make it more bearable, and that the primary orientation of the elderly should be to-

ward the care of the young and future generations and *not* the welfare of their own age group. Once the end and meaning of aging are refocused, claims Callahan, to the care and sustenance of the young, then it is possible to discuss the idea of a "natural life span" that is inevitably followed by "a tolerable death." Death should occur, states Callahan, at that stage in a life span when one's moral obligations have been discharged, the majority of life's possibilities have been accomplished, and it will not appear to be an offense to others. Callahan strongly urges that our views of aging in the United States change to allow individual acceptance of a tolerable death and the forgoing of costly health care to all elderly persons, but especially during the last year of life. The moral problem is how to "devise a plan to limit health care for the aged that is fair, humane, and sensitive to the special requirements and dignity of the aged." [2] It will require policy that provides the elderly with an honorable and bearable life in their remaining years, and that prevents the use of costly resources after a certain age.

In conjunction with this change in attitudes toward aging, he argues, medicine and nursing must refocus their efforts away from the cure of disease and the extension of life among the elderly. This is, perhaps, one of the more challenging aspects of Callahan's theory of aging and his rationing plan. What would a new view of aging and a readjustment of the goals of health care really mean for the education and practice of nursing?

First, it might mean that the content of many courses in nursing education would have to be changed or altered. Students would need to learn a new view of aging and the role of the elderly in our society. Instead of topics such as critical care in adult populations they would need to study topics such as suffering, caring, comfort, dignity, dying, and the like. More attention would need to be given to health care for children and the young adult and less attention to chronic diseases that primarily affect the elderly.

Second, the professional ethic would have to be practiced and taught differently than it is now. Instead of a focus on individual rights to health care, individual good, and the topics of advocacy, autonomy, and freedom of choice, the professional ethic would be taught with a focus on topics such as social welfare, societal good, the balancing and prioritizing of benefits, and aggregate good.

Third, instead of an appeal to the usual litany of ethical principles, rules, and theories for justification of individual moral judgments and actions, nurses would need to know about obligation theory, virtue theory, the principles of receptivity, relatedness, and responsiveness, and an ethic of caring for health care. Along with theories of justice for the distribution of health care resources, ethicists would need to articulate theories of compassion and suffering, and justifications for electing a tolerable death. Obviously, many changes might be required if a new view of aging and the rationing of health care to the sick elderly become a reality. Will nursing be willing? Will nursing be ready?

REFERENCES

1. U.S. Bureau of the Census. Projections of the population of the U.S., by age, sex, and race: 1983 to 2080. *Current Population Reports* (Series P-25, No. 952). Washington, DC, Government Printing Office, 1984, pp. 2-9.

2. Callahan, D. *Setting Limits: Medical Goals in an Aging Society.* New York, Simon and Schuster, 1987.

3. Churchill, L.R. *Rationing Health Care in America: Perceptions and Principles of Justice.* Notre Dame, IN, University of Notre Dame Press, 1987.

4. Daniels, N. *Just Health Care.* New York, Cambridge University Press, 1985.

High cost may lead to rationed medicine

SABIN RUSSELL

SEVEN-YEAR-OLD Coby Howard died of leukemia on December 2, six weeks after the state of Oregon refused to pay for a $72,000 bone marrow transplant that might have saved his life.

Oregon's welfare department also has denied funds to Donna Arneson, a 34-year-old single mother who needs a liver transplant. Coby died before public appeal could raise enough money for a private operation. Arneson has raised $200,000 and hopes to have the surgery performed in Texas.

Faced with a projected doubling every two years of its Medicaid costs for organ transplants, the Oregon legislature last July made a painful and controversial decision to ration medicine to the poor. The lawmakers cut organ transplants out of the welfare budget but added $5 million to finance prenatal care.

"These are very difficult decisions," said Herschel Crawford, assistant Medicaid director for Oregon's state welfare administration. "There are no winners. The department still feels the decision made was a correct one."

To Coby's aunt, Susan McGee, the boy's illness was a nightmare that lingers beyond his death. "In his last few weeks the family spent every minute trying to raise funds," she said. "We are bitter we had to market Coby Howard so the public would want to save his life."

With technology continuing to produce new and more costly medical breakthroughs, and public health budgets awash in red ink, the agony headlined in Oregon highlights the tough choices facing health policy makers across the nation.

"Sooner or later, the only way to cut health care spending in a major way is to reduce the quantity of services delivered to patients," said Victor Fuchs, a Stanford University economist.

Although most Americans are taken aback at the concept of health care rationing, the simple fact is that we already ration health care through policies that discourage the poor from seeking medical attention. Unaffordably high insurance rates, underfinanced state medical programs, and crowded clinics, in effect, ration care too. This hidden system of health care rationing allows us to duck the uncomfortable implications of a formal rationing program, which would allocate health care on the bases of:

• Age. In the United Kingdom, the National Health Service denies kidney dialysis to patients over the age of 55. Major surgeries are not available to patients over 70.

• Ability to pay. Transplants are out for welfare recipients in Oregon and Arizona. California denies Medi-Cal benefits to poor citizens who do not qualify for welfare.

• Lifestyle. Life insurance policies already limit coverage to people who have abused their bodies through smoking, improper diet, drugs or alcohol. Health insurers may be next.

• Diagnosis or treatment. Private insurers limit or deny coverage for many ailments. Kaiser Permanente, for example, will not pay for test-tube babies.

What are we buying?

Medical ethicists have begun to debate the morality of heaping the most expensive medical procedures on elderly patients who are gravely ill. Medicare pays out $21 billion, or

28 percent of its annual budget, for bills incurred by patients in their final year of life.

"With the amount of money we're spending for a small gain in life expectancy, I'm not sure we're buying very much," said Dr. Paul Ellwood, chairman of the Minneapolis research firm InterStudy. "We're reaching the point where spending money on something else might be more worthwhile."

John Golenski, a consulting ethicist to Kaiser Permanente and other Bay Area hospitals, believes that the heroic measures used to prolong the lives of dying elderly patients are the result of "bizarre and outrageous economic incentives," in the Medicare program. He likens the system to a factory that pays for piecework — the more procedures performed, the more a doctor is paid. "Since Medicare, we've seen a real corruption of the profession," said Golenski. "We've made it difficult for doctors to resist the habit of opting for the more expensive diagnostic procedure, even where there is very little benefit for the risk."

Many physicians are clearly uncomfortable with the prospect of prolonging lives of patients against their will. "Our society has valued continued life. We need to look at the quality of it," said Dr. Neal Cohen, chief of the intensive care unit at UC Medical Center in San Francisco. "Many elderly patients are very scared of being put on life-support systems that cannot be removed."

Richard Lamm, former governor of Colorado and currently director of the Center for Public Policy and Contemporary Issues at the University of Denver, believes age should be "a valid ethical consideration" in the delivery of medical care. "I feel it is morally repugnant if I use $100,000 or $200,000 of our kids' limited resources as I'm on my way out the door," he said.

Lamm admits he is uncomfortable with a British-style rationing system, where age strictly limits the amount of health care available. Most experts doubt such a system would ever be adopted in this country. "British physicians implement rationing in a humane way," said Princeton economist Uwe Reinhardt. "American doctors would say the government is murdering you."

Billfold biopsies

Whereas the Oregon transplant cases are graphic examples of health care rationing on the basis of income, the poor are often denied health care benefits on less dramatic terms. Five years ago, the California legislature removed 270,000 "Medically Indigent Adults" from the state's Medi-Cal program. These indigents were poor, but not poor enough to qualify for welfare.

Rationing of medical services for the uninsured begins in hospital emergency rooms, where one of the first procedures given is the "billfold biopsy," a test of ability to pay. In most cases, unless the illness is life-threatening, patients without insurance are sent to a public hospital.

Long waits at urban public hospitals — five hours on average nationally — discourage the poor from seeking medical attention. Hospital administrators call it "back-door rationing."

Five hours into her wait to see a doctor at the emergency room of Alameda County's Highland Hospital, Renee Anderson was upset. "I came in with just one ear hurting. Now, I've got two," she said. "It took me two hours just to get registered."

A study by the RAND Corp. found that six months after loss of their Medi-Cal benefits, medically indigent adults had a 40 percent greater chance of dying than the average citizen. "Hypertension is a big problem in this population," said Dr. Robert Brook, author of the report. "They stopped taking their medication. Blood pressures went out of control. They had heart attacks and they died."

Uninsured Americans with serious medical symptoms are half as likely to see a physician as those with insurance. They are also less likely to seek early prenatal care, immunize their children, or have their blood pressure checked.

"There is no question that the American health care system leaves a lot of misery at the bottom of the heap — physical and financial misery," said Princeton professor Reinhardt.

The burden of caring for MIAs has fallen on the county hospital system. Bad debt and charity care expenses among California's county hospitals have risen to $629 million from $158 million in 1982.

San Francisco General Hospital is in better financial shape than most county hospitals, but AIDS and the city's sudden budget crunch are straining the system. "Unless there is some additional support at both the state and federal level, we'll have a difficult time treating AIDS patients in San Francisco," said Phillip Sowa, S.F. General executive director.

Public health administrators believe that the growing financial crisis facing American medicine will force the issue of rationing from the back door to center stage. "It is a major policy issue that people either ignore or deny they have to face," said David Kears, Alameda County director of health services.

Lifestyle underwriting

Health insurers are battling to limit coverage of some costly new procedures. Kaiser Permanente changed its contract to explicitly exclude coverage of *in vitro* fertilization — test-tube babies — after a patient convinced a judge that the technique was no longer experimental and therefore ought to be covered under the existing Kaiser rules. "It's not an essential part of medical care," said Wayne Moon, manager of Kaiser's Northern California region.

Moon notes that Kaiser plans do not cover plastic surgery, unless it is being performed to repair tissue damage from burns. Kaiser will pay for heart transplants but does not do them

at its hospitals — it contracts for them at Stanford Medical Center. "We need to manage technology so we get the most out of the resources we have," said Moon.

Efforts by health insurers to permit AIDS blood-testing to screen applicants represent another from of health care rationing. But Ben Schatz, director of the AIDS civil rights project for National Gay Rights Advocates, sees such actions as an attempt by private insurers to back out of the century's biggest health crisis. "If insurance companies shirk their responsibilities to pay for AIDS expenses, these costs will be forced on to the public sector," he said. "This calls into question the very purpose of a private health insurance system."

Civil rights issues will also emerge if health insurers begin using lifestyle as a criterion for writing group medical coverage. "Very soon those who pay the biggest health care tab — corporate employers — will make cost-containment a personal issue for each employee," said Cleveland health care consultant Robert Carter. "The fact is that in health insurance costs, the majority are paying for the self-affliction of a minority."

Carter predicts that employers will begin using a "carrot and stick" approach, combining exercise and diet counseling with penalties for those who do not shape up. For example, employees who fail to meet weight reduction goals or who continue to smoke or abuse alcohol could be faced with paying deductibles as high as 50 percent.

"Abusers are dragging everyone else to the same cost mill," said Carter. "Companies must attack lifestyle abuse if they are to corral bulging health care costs during this century."

Many American health policy experts believe that the quality of medical procedures needs to be understood before we begin rationing the quantity of them. "We should eliminate classes of surgery that don't work before saying that nobody over the age of 90 gets a hip replacement," said InterStudy's Ellwood.

RAND Corp.'s Dr. Brook said doctors need to decide which surgeries are "medically appropriate" and which represent a form of medical luxury. "We should put a value added tax of 50 percent on luxury procedures and use the money to fund education," he said.

High on Dr. Brook's list of luxury procedures: carotid endarterectomies, an operation that clears blood clots from the principal artery in the neck. Independent medical panels have judged that two-thirds of such surgeries are of questionable medical value.

Dr. James Todd of the American Medical Association believes much unnecessary care can be eliminated by reducing doctors' exposure to malpractice lawsuits. "When patients are sick, the attitude is spare no expense, uncover every stone, because if you don't, I'm going to sue you," he said.

The counterrevolution

Rising doctor bills and rising insurance premiums may already be fomenting what Stanford economist Victor Fuchs describes as a "counterrevolution" in health care finance.

"If enough people lose their health insurance, it will have to be hurting the middle class," said Jonathan Showstack, associate professor at the USCF Institute for Health Policy Studies. "When that happens, we'll see a rethinking of where we're going in health care."

National health insurance, an issue placed on the back burner with the advent of Medicare in the 1960s, may resurface as a potent political issue as health insurance rates rise beyond the reach of the average American. "The next president, whether Democrat or Republican, will have to take that one on," predicts Ellwood.

The swelling number of Americans without health insurance has inspired a bill proposed by Senator Edward Kennedy that would require all businesses to provide health insur-

ance to their employees. Estimate of the cost of the program: $38.8 billion.

Small business groups are aghast at the proposal, which is backed by big U.S. corporations such as Chrysler and American Airlines. The National Federation of Independent Businesses, a small business lobbying group, estimates that 34 percent of its members cannot afford to provide health insurance. "Many employers would have to lay off employees to afford the insurance premiums," said Martin Hopper, California director of NFIB. "A mandated job benefit is no good to a worker without a job."

The Bay Area Health Task Force is completing a study to find ways of encouraging businesses to voluntarily provide health benefits. "There are at least 65,000 uninsured working people in San Francisco," said Susan Wilner, director of the study. "The costs for their care get passed on to people who do pay. Most people don't seem to understand that."

It may take tragedies like Coby Howard's death to drive home to Americans that our health care system has fallen into serious financial trouble. No matter how compelling a case can be made to limit medical expenditures, the reality of letting someone die to save money runs counter to our sense of fairness. "It's very difficult to deny technology, once it's out there and once the public can identify somebody who needs it," said John Gable of the Health Insurance Association of America.

Coby Howard's case emphasizes the ironies in our troubled health care system. High-technology medicine is outstripping our ability to afford it. We have a surplus of doctors and hospital beds, but large segments of the population are unable to get the most basic medical care. Americans are beginning to ration medical care like a precious resource, yet much of the care we provide is unnecessary. At a current cost of $499 billion, the system we have built to heal our bodies is sapping the economic strength of our nation.

When the profit motive threatens patient care

HELEN LIPPMAN COLLINS

"MONEY IS WHAT matters at my hospital, not people," a nurse from a large public institution bitterly complains. A colleague at a proprietary hospital agrees: "Dollars and cents matter more than the rights of nurses or patients."

Three out of five of the nurses who responded to our survey share the opinion that cost containment has hurt the quality of care provided at their hospitals — and that the situation is only getting worse.

Nurses are not alone in realizing the danger. A recently released, federally-funded study suggests a link between cost containment and higher death rates, particularly at hospitals that face stiff competition and stringent state regulations. Yet, in a recent survey of hospital executives — nearly half of whom are worried about fiscal failure — three-fourths agreed that there are times when care *should* depend on patients' ability to pay.

That view, and the increasing emphasis on the bottom line that it stems from, contradicts a basic tenet of nursing ethics — that care shall not be influenced by a patient's economic status. As a result, nurses face important ethical challenges: how to allocate limited resources and how to change the system over the long term.

High tech without high touch?

Nearly 75% of the nurses we surveyed agree that cost-containment measures have left them with "no time for a caring attitude." Typically, a med/surg nurse from a large community hospital laments the loss of "the little things" patients remember, like "psychological support, teaching, or frequent turning or repositioning."

In fact, such interventions aren't little at all, but an integral part of nursing standards and nurses' commitment to meet the physical and psychological needs of patients. Panelist Patricia Murphy finds it "tragic" that a "caring attitude" can be so compartmentalized, when "caring is part of everything nurses do." Still, since "the system places a much higher value on counting facts than on comforting," she's not surprised that caring is the first thing to go when times get tough.

"If the paperwork is done, does any supervisor ever ask who was with Joe when he died?" she demands. "How often do you find 'caring' mentioned on a nurse's evaluation?"

In spite of mounting pressure to keep costs down, hospitals that relegate caring to a back seat may be hurting themselves in the long run. Several surveys have shown that patients are more likely to choose a hospital on the basis of quality of care than on cost. Furthermore, much of what the public perceives as quality is one or another form of nursing. Yet, nurses we surveyed voice serious concerns about what's happening to nursing care.

An OR nurse, for instance, reports that her colleagues have grown accustomed to doing almost instantaneous assessments. The results? They "miss warning signs and symptoms, such as respiratory distress that signals pneumonia, or skin breakdown that, left untreated, becomes a full-blown decubitus ulcer." Yet, assessment-on-the-run violates the ANA's standards of practice, which call for "complete and ongoing data collection" as the basis for a nursing diagnosis and a plan of care. And the ultimate result when there's no time for thorough assessment is that, as a harried ICU nurse puts it, "the care we're giving isn't always safe."

Staff cuts are a major cause of the problem, according to nurses in every part of the country. Some hospitals try to make do with fewer RNs. Others eliminate ancillary staff, creating a situation that a weary med/surg nurse from the West Coast laments, "leaves no time to teach and do our regular chores, never mind give bed baths, empty the trash, do the job of a secretary, and still manage to get the work done on time or else be in trouble."

A nurse from the Southwest labels it "nurse abuse," but colleagues assert that patients are the real victims. One OBG nurse claims that institutional belt-tightening has led to "the poorest quality of care in a decade."

Working short without compromising care

Combine penny pinching and the nursing shortage and you get what panelist Mila Aroskar recognizes as "an untenable situation" that will not be resolved any time in the near future. In the meantime, she and our other panelists agree that there are steps nurses can take that will enable them to maintain a caring attitude, deliver adequate care, and deal with some of their own ethical distress.

Panelist Phyllis Taylor, for instance, asserts that nurses sometimes contribute to their high level of frustration and stress by *losing* opportunities to relate to patients. Aroskar concurs: "Studies show that even when nurses had the time, say, for two of them to make a bed or perform some other chore for a patient, they've more often talked to each other instead of to the patient."

Taylor's suggestion: Perfect the art of doing several things at once. For example: "I can look at skin integrity, talk about pressure sores, and explain why movement is necessary, all while I bathe a patient. Or remove an

IV and teach the patient to watch for signs of infection in the three minutes that I spend applying pressure to the site."

As both cost containment and the nursing shortage escalate, our panelists believe, nurses must redefine their image of themselves and their work: Taylor advises giving up some of the "need to be needed," and recruiting families, volunteers, or anyone else available to take over some of the non-skilled care of your patient.

Aroskar admonishes nurses to redefine the concepts of total care and primary nursing. "The acuity of today's patients, the emphasis on high tech, and the shortage of staff make it self-defeating and unrealistic for nurses to expect to give every bit of physical care and then to "feel inadequate if they can't give daily baths to patients who often don't even need them." Primary care, Aroskar points out, "doesn't mean nurses have to be everything to every patient."

Attorney Frank Reardon adds that modern technology demands a new attitude as well, particularly the recognition that there are many ways in which to care.

"Isn't running a machine caring for a patient?" he asks. "Or does it only count if you give a bath or sit and talk for a while?" Critical care nurses seem to accept his reasoning. Used to dealing with high tech equipment, they're the least likely of our respondents to complain about having no time to care....

When you don't have the right equipment

If time constraints don't compromise your ability to provide top-quality care, then problems with supplies and equipment might. Our respondents complain that they have to deal with "antique" equipment, monitors that malfunction, inferior products, and shortages of everything from bed linens to infusion pumps. A nurse at a community hospital insists the "administration cares more about beautifying

Quality vs. cost: 1987-1988

Three nurses out of five say that the quality of care at their hospitals has deteriorated in the past year because of cost-containment decisions. Far and away the biggest problems they see involve the quality of the care they're able to provide.

EFFECT OF COST CONTAINMENT	% REPORTING IT
Nurses have no time for a caring attitude	74%
Staff has been cut	65
Patients are discharged too early	63
Supplies/equipment are lacking	47
Outdated equipment is not replaced	29
Patients are admitted too late	27
Uninsured patients are turned away	13

*Percentages in all tables total more than 100% because of multiple responses.

its lobby than about providing up-to-date equipment."

In fact, nearly 30% of our respondents complain about the outdated equipment, and that figure climbs to 45% among employees of public hospitals. Nurses don't seem to be communicating such problems to hospital administrators, though: Only one hospital executive in 10 surveyed recently believes that the equipment at his institution is inadequate or out-of-date.

Shortages — of both supplies and equipment — are an even greater problem, reported nearly half the nurses we surveyed and as many as 62% of RNs at public hospitals.

At times, lack of supplies hinders basic nursing activities. A med/surg nurse reports "there aren't enough linens to let us change them often enough to prevent rashes."

Experienced RNs are adept at improvising: Neonatal nurses recall having to rip large diapers into miniature ones for preemies, for example. But coping with a lack of basic equipment requires a more organized approach.

Taylor urges nurses to use a "force-field analysis" for problem-solving. You begin by identifying, not the problem. but rather a "vision of what the nurses would like to see happen on their unit if they had the power."

Write that vision on one side of a chart, along with any forces at work that will help you move toward your vision and ideas that can strengthen those forces. On the other side, list the reality of the situation that you're trying to overcome and the forces that contribute to the reality. Also include ideas that will weaken those negative forces.

OB nurses, for instance, might begin a force-field analysis with the "vision" that all patients in labor will be adequately monitored for fetal distress — rather than starting with the problem of not having enough fetal monitors. Forces in favor of that vision might include accepted protocols — from NAACOG, perhaps — for determining when a patient *must* be placed on a monitor and when manual monitoring would be sufficient. Physicians might be listed as a resource as well, since their patients would benefit from improved

Where cost-containment measures are felt hardest

The problems that penny pinching causes for nurses clearly depend on area of practice. ED nurses, because they so often deal with situations in which every minute is crucial, are most apt to say they're working with too little time and too few hands—and to believe that cost cutting has led to a recent decline in the quality of care.

EFFECT OF COST CONTAINMENT	MED/ SURG	ICU/ CCU	GERI- ATRICS	OBG/ NEWBORN	ER	PEDS	PSYCH
Deterioration in care	66%	57%	65%	56%	76%	49%	70%
No time for a caring attitude	77	67	86	82	87	68	74
Staff has been cut	70	59	73	66	75	56	74
Patients are discharged too early	64	56	66	61	68	63	52
Supplies/equipment are lacking	48	50	59	51	45	49	48
Outdated equipment is not replaced	27	30	41	24	32	27	29
Patients are admitted too late	26	23	30	18	37	32	12
Uninsured patients are turned away	10	12	21	8	12	5	45

(% REPORTING IT WHO WORK IN)

monitoring. Something that would strengthen those forces would be the legal climate that leaves doctors and hospitals particularly vulnerable to lawsuits over obstetrical malpractice.

On the negative side, the nurses could list the lack of monitors, doctors who insist their patients be placed on monitors too early in labor, and hospital administration's claim that there's no money for additional equipment.

The analysis might well yield convincing arguments for purchasing additional monitors. On the other hand, it might lead to the conclusion that current equipment is being misused. The solution then would be to establish a system of priorities — agreed upon by nurses and doctors — to determine which patients get the

monitors and when such monitoring is needed.

Couldn't a physician with clout circumvent such a system and get whatever he wants for his patients? "Doctors aren't nearly as likely to get away with that sort of behavior anymore," asserts panelist Patricia Murphy. With hospitals under tremendous pressure from government, health insurers, and competing institutions, "physician power" is slowly becoming a thing of the past.

That's one reason why Phyllis Taylor encourages nurses that this is the right time to grab some of that power for themselves. "You can't do it alone, though" she cautions. Nurses will have to work together, using systems such as her force-field analysis to bring about change.

Where experience makes a difference

Although most of our respondents' views about cost containment aren't influenced by their level of experience, there are two areas in which experience makes a difference: The more experience nurses have, the more likely they are to believe that care has deteriorated in the last year, perhaps because they're comparing current conditions to pre-DRG days. On the other hand, nurses with the least experience are most apt to be troubled by shortages of supplies and equipment, suggesting that newer nurses may still be in the throes of reality shock or that older nurses are more adept at finding ways to make do.

EFFECT OF COST CONTAINMENT	% REPORTING BY YEARS OF EXPERIENCE			
	LESS THAN 2	3-5	6-10	11 OR MORE
Deterioration in care	52%	55%	59%	63%
Lack of supplies/equipment	57	52	47	43

Discharged too early, or admitted too late

Cost containment has had an impact not only on the quality of care, but on its quantity: Ever since DRGs, a patient's hospital stay never seems to be as long as it should be. A geriatric nurse from the Southwest claims she's "always being harped at to send patients home," whether or not they're ready to go. ED nurses, like the RN who "sends patients home, only to admit them the next day," are most likely to witness this revolving door syndrome.

What to do? "Holler," advises Phyllis Taylor: to your supervisor, to the physician, or to anyone who will listen, if your institution is about to discharge a patient you believe isn't ready to go. You'll not only be protecting your patient, but you could be saving your hospital from a lawsuit.

Still, Frank Reardon cautions nurses not to look to the courts for permanent solutions: "Malpractice trials don't provide clear direction. One jury today might say 'Yes, there is liability,' and award $500,000. Another jury tomorrow might take the opposite stance. They're not good policy makers."

Instead, policy needs to be based on the experience and opinions of caregivers, including nurses who speak out about early discharges as part of their ethical duty to be advocates for patients.

What about the opposite problem, when an HMO or other health insurer tries to save money by keeping people out of hospitals as long as possible? Just over 25% of our respondents claim that cost containment has delayed hospital admissions, a figure that reaches a high of 34% among nurses in proprietary hospitals and a low of 18% for those at public institutions.

Since you don't see these patients until *after* they've been admitted, is there anything you can do about it? An OR nurse reports how she and her colleagues keep the pressure on those responsible: "When a patient who should have been admitted earlier is brought to our hospital, we refuse to be involved. It's nursing supervisors, not staff RNs, who admit him and deal with the attending physician."

Mila Aroskar thinks that concerned nurses might find allies in the physicians employed by HMOs, who, she says, are often just as upset about inappropriately delayed admissions. Although they haven't found definitive answers either, "many doctors share the same

---

Where to get the best care

Every hospital in the country is under increasing pressure to cut costs, but each type of institution tightens its belt in different ways. Predictably, proprietary hospitals keep the closest eye on the bottom line, with nurses there most apt to say they see a deterioration of care in the past year. Nurses at public hospitals report the highest incidence of staff cuts. And RNs at non-profit institutions, especially university hospitals, most often report problems with premature discharge, perhaps because these hospitals face the greatest demand for beds.

EFFECT OF COST CONTAINMENT	% REPORTING BY TYPE OF HOSPITAL		
	PROPRIETARY	NON-PROFIT	PUBLIC
Deterioration in care	70%	57%	65%
No time for a caring attitude	87	73	69
Staff has been cut	67	63	74
Patients are discharged too early	57	65	51
Supplies/equipment are lacking	55	44	62
Outdated equipment is not replaced	36	25	45
Patients are admitted too late	34	27	18
Uninsured patients are turned away	31	13	4

---

pain, and like you, are looking for ways to take action."

Which patients get the beds?
Finally, with their eye fixed on the bottom line, some hospitals are turning away patients who have either no insurance at all or inadequate coverage. As Phyllis Taylor puts it: "If a patient comes in with private insurance, somehow a bed is found for him," she explains. "But if the patient has Medicare or Medicaid as his only insurance — or he has AIDS and third-party reimbursement won't cover the whole cost — then somehow the bed isn't there."

Is our country headed toward a system where care is directly connected to ability to pay? Apparently, judging from a just-released National Association of Public Hospitals report showing that since 1985 the caseload of AIDS patients has risen 101% at public hospitals but a mere 34% at private institutions. What's more, respondents to the survey of hospital executives express the almost unanimous belief that in the next few years, patients will have even less freedom to choose the kind of care that they receive.

Our survey points to a similar dichotomy: While only 13% of total respondents say patients are being turned away at their institutions, that number reaches 31% among nurses working at proprietary hospitals. Predictably, among those who work at public hospitals, the situation is almost non-existent.

Nurses can play an important role in assuring equitable distribution of care, says Frank Reardon, emphasizing that knowing the new COBRA law — "making it illegal for a hospital to dismiss a patient without stabilizing him first" — is one way to protect yourself and your patients.

Better yet, write to the Ways and Means

Committee of the U.S. House of Representatives in Washington for a copy of that portion of the law that deals with patient dumping and post it in your emergency department. A House subcommittee estimates that about 250,000 patients are being illegally "dumped" every year, Reardon points out, and arming yourself with the facts will make it easier to confront your administration.

You can make a difference

Together with knowing the law, Reardon urges nurses to keep documenting dangerous conditions — short-staffing, lack of proper equipment, inappropriate discharges, or whatever. He acknowledges that it's hard to do this when nobody seems to listen, but he points out that lack of response doesn't necessarily mean that nobody's listening. "Sometimes," Reardon says, "it may simply mean the real solutions have not yet been identified, even by management."

This state of flux is an opportunity for nurses, Reardon argues. "The way health care is delivered is going to change significantly over the next 10 years. And you have a real power base in those changes. Doctors work for HMOs now. They have less control over how they practice, while you're gaining more power in the health-care facility."

Patricia Murphy thinks nurses can build on that by digging out hard data and sharing solutions. She recalls how the recovery room in a large city hospital was being used as an ICU "with patients remaining on stretchers for several days." Nurses found local Board of Health regulations that prohibit the presence of people with sepsis in a recovery room. They not only presented those rules to the administration but also gave copies to the nurses facing front-line pressure in the recovery room.

Murphy's new law: "Do your homework. Somebody, somewhere has invented the wheel for just about everything. So if you're fighting inappropriate use of the ICU, write to nurses at Mass General where they addressed that problem and say: 'Listen, guys: Help! Send me your system.' Then present your data. Many times when you talk about what a Mass General or another top hospital does, the response is 'All right, do it that way.' It's true that many of these problems are not going to change today or tomorrow, but we've got to use these issues to get some kind of dialogue going and to get nurses on those hospital policy-making committees."

"That's working out your own power," adds Mila Aroskar. "If you wait for somebody to come by and hand you a basket of power, forget it, that won't happen." She urges nurses to build collective power through participation in national, state, and specialty organizations.

Phyllis Taylor agrees that breaking down the individual nurse's sense of isolation is crucial to finding solutions within a hospital and the basis for "working on a broad-based political-economic level. If the structure of health care and the allocation of funds are not fair, then we don't want people to adjust to that bad system."

Our panelists conclude that battles of cost over quality can be resolved ethically with a large dose of the basic nursing tenet that puts patients' interests first — and that only nurses can inject this solution into the health-care system.

CHAPTER SIXTEEN

The law and nursing practice

THE ACQUISITION OF a license to practice nursing is a satisfying and rewarding experience that the new nurse has worked and studied intensively to accomplish. Interestingly, it is also an experience in understanding the law and regulations governing nursing, which apply throughout the nurse's education and practice. To practice nursing most effectively requires that the nurse understand those laws and regulations, then practice as autonomously as possible within their limits.

The establishment of licensing laws for nurses (nurse practice acts) was an important step in the evolution of nursing and nursing autonomy. These acts specify the scope of nursing practice within each state and control the activities that a person licensed as a registered nurse (RN) may perform. Also closely regulated are the nursing educational programs, which must be approved by state boards of nursing and may be accredited by the National League for Nursing. In addition, nurses who participate in advanced education programs become eligible to participate in credentialing programs offered through professional organizations. (See Unit One.)

The articles in this chapter demonstrate that as complex as those regulatory frameworks are, they are only the beginning of the nurse's experience with laws and regulations governing or affecting nursing practice. The position statement of the California Nurses' Association, "Encroachment on Nursing Practice," reviews solutions to the autonomy problems confronting the nursing profession. It clearly delineates the reasons for the present-day increase in efforts to delimit registered nursing practice, particularly the proposal by the American Medical Association to develop the category of registered care technologist. (See Unit Three.)

Northrop, in "Nursing Actions in Litigation," discusses nurses' need to develop a strategy, which she labels "risk management," to avoid litigation in such circumstances as infections resulting from surgical procedures, client falls, administration of incorrect medications, and failure to implement medical orders properly. She emphasizes the need to know the standards of care for nursing practice and to know how the standards of care can be applied in each case.

Schulmeister, in "Litigation Involving Oncology Nurses," describes 12 incidents of oncology nurses who were involved in medication discrepancies, incorrect referral or follow-up, or injury to client's relatives, stressing the need for preventive and defensive nursing actions to prevent such lawsuits.

Yorker, in "Nurses Accused of Murder," describes cases in which nurses were charged with murdering clients and focuses on the fact that nurses make good targets for investigations: They are available 24 hours a day and are often the first people on the scene of an arrest when murder is suspected.

Cushing, in "Perils of Home Care," demonstrates the attention today's nurse must give to details of care in order to prevent legal problems. "When Nurses Must Question Doctors' Orders," by Tamelleo, emphasizes the need to follow accepted practices and protocols.

When nurses become substance abusers,

negligent practices (and lawsuits) can result, often involving the abusers' co-workers as well. Moore and Hogan, in "Substance Abuse in the Nurse: A Legal and Ethical Dilemma," discuss this issue and plead for humane treat- ment of substance-abusing nurses. These authors present the dilemma encountered in trying to assist abusers while simultaneously trying to protect clients and adhere to applicable laws.

Encroachment on nursing practice:
Position statement

TASK FORCE ON SCOPE OF NURSING

Introduction

ISSUES RELATING TO nursing practice encroachment have increased in intensity not only in the legislative and regulatory arenas but also in the practice settings. This increase in intensity prompted the California Nurses Association (CNA) to establish a Task Force on Encroachment of Nursing Practice in order to preserve quality of care and patient safety. This Task Force developed a resolution which was presented and debated at the CNA 1987 House of Delegates. The adopted resolution called for the establishment of a Task Force representative of all structural units of CNA in addition to nursing experts to develop a position paper that includes strategies to halt the practice of nursing without a registered nurse (RN) license.

Statement of problem

It is important to understand the statutory definition of nursing in the State of California in order to understand the issue of encroachment. Within the State of California, the Legislature clearly recognizes that nursing is a dynamic field, the practice of which is continually evolving to include more sophisticated patient care activities. The California Nursing Practice Act provides clear legal authority for functions and procedures which have common acceptance and usage. It recognizes the existence of overlapping functions between physicians and registered nurses and permits additional sharing of collaborative functions within organized health care systems. The California Nursing Practice Act defines the practice of nursing as those functions which help people cope with difficulties in daily living that are associated with their actual or potential health or illness problem or the treatment thereof including basic health care.

A more specific interpretation of the statutory definition is as follows:

> Nursing is the assessing, managing and caring of human responses to health and illness which requires a substantial amount of scientific knowledge and technical skills (core).
>
> Nursing practice includes, but is not limited to, assessment; diagnosis; planning; developing, implementing and evaluating programs, protocols and careplans; intervention and evaluation in the promotion and maintenance of health and wellness; the casefinding and management of illness, injury, or infirmity; the restoration of optimum functioning; or the achievement of a dignified death (patient).
>
> Nursing functions include provision of health assessment; direct care and treatment services; teaching; counseling; psychotherapy; applied psychotherapeutic techniques; psychosocial, psychological or mental health asessment; administration; supervision; delegation; and evaluation of practice (RN).
>
> Each nurse is directly accountable and responsible to the consumer for the quality of nursing care rendered. [1]

In the past decade there have been serious organized attempts to expand the role of allied health and other non-licensed health care providers into the scope of registered nursing practice, and to expand the role of the registered nurse so that it crosses intraprofessional as well as interprofessional boundaries. Such expansion is generally done under the guise of cost-savings, overlapping functions and perceived credentialing authority.

Encroachment, defined as the external infringement on registered nursing practice by others without the consent of the profession, has a historical basis. Additionally, encroachment seriously jeopardizes safe, effective, and appropriate patient care. Currently, encroachment is escalating and is supported by employers and other health care personnel.

The reasons for this escalation are:

1. A critical national demand for nursing services which created a shortage of registered nurses.

2. An oversupply of physicians and some health care providers.

3. Proposals by other health care professionals to solve the nursing shortage.

4. Shifts in reimbursement and changes in resource allocation.

5. Highly competitive strategies for profit-making by employer.

Types of encroachment. There are several types of encroachment which cross either intraprofessional or interprofessional boundaries. The most common form of encroachment is when another health care provider performs a task or function that is within the RN scope of practice and does so with perceived authority. For example: There have been frequent attempts by other categories of health care providers, e.g., home companions, respiratory care practitioners (RCP), designated school personnel and guards in correctional facilities, to either expand their authority or add on to their scope of activities such tasks as the administration of medications. Another common form of encroachment is when another provider challenges the authority of RNs to perform certain functions. For example, the question of whether or not a registered nurse not licensed under the Clinical Laboratory Law may lawfully perform certain standardized tests in

the hospital ward or a medical clinic. The Attorney General, in response to a request from a member of the Legislature, issued the following Opinion:

> When authorized by order of a physician or a standardized procedure a registered nurse not licensed under the Clinical Laboratory Law may lawfully perform a clinitest, acetest, a blood glucose dipstick test, a hematest or hemoccult, or a urine dipstick test in a hospital ward or a medical clinic. [2]

Another form of encroachment is when the employer or other health care provider decides to add functions and responsibilities to the current work of registered nurses without the consent of those nurses and/or the addition of appropriate resources. Examples include, (1) the elimination of respiratory care practitioner positions and the reallocation of respiratory care functions to registered nurses for cost containment purposes; (2) the elimination of Certified Registered Nurse Anesthetist (CRNA) positions that resulted in additional responsibilities of the Labor & Delivery (L&D) registered nurses for monitoring regional/epidural anesthesia generally performed by the anesthesiologist or the CRNA.

The last type of encroachment is forced interchangeability or substitutability of the RN. For example, the entire RN scope of practice has been usurped by Physician's Assistants (PA). The problem surfaced when certain counties in the state wanted to substitute Physician's Assistants for Nurse Practitioners (NP). In addition, employers and other health care providers in search of a solution for the critical nursing shortage are proposing down-substituting registered nurses by using personnel such as respiratory care practitioners, Licensed Vocational Nurses (LVN), Psychiatric Technicians (PT), Medical Assistants (MA) and nursing student workers.

Functions being reallocated. The most common functions being reallocated are the administration of medications and the performance of specific health and maintenance procedures.

For example, in the area of administration of medications, there has been a series of organized unlawful attempts to reallocate the administration of medication function to other categories of health care providers by either adding the route of administration or category of drugs to their responsibilities. The routes generally added are either topical, rectal, oral, intravenous, intramuscular, and subcutaneous. The most common categories of medications added to other health care personnel scope of activities are antibiotics, over-the-counter drugs, psychotropics, analgesics, sedatives and/or anti-convulsive drugs.

The most common health and maintenance procedures reallocated are nasogastric (NG) or ostomy feeding, tracheostomy suctioning, insertion of an NG tube, insertion/irrigation of catheters, sterile and/or unsterile dressing changes, handling of blood products, and changing of ostomy bags. Other examples of reallocation of procedures include the authorization, although uncommon, given to respiratory care practitioners to insert arterial lines, or the management of total parenteral nutrition (TPN) in the home care settings by non-registered nurses.

Patient assessment is another nursing function which has been reallocated to other health care personnel. For example, to promote access to comprehensive perinatal services, the Department of Health Services (DHS) promulgated regulations which amongst others stipulate that nutrition, psychosocial and health education assessment can also be performed by registered dieticians, clinical social workers and health educators, so long as they meet the definition of comprehensive perinatal practitioner.

Entities proposing reallocation. It is essential to understand that reallocation of functions is being proposed by private as well as public entities. For example, the California Medical Association introduced legislation to expand the scope of functions of Medical Assistants through regulations; the Board of Medical Quality Assurance (BMQA) supported the Respiratory Care Examining Committee (RCEC) Opinion on Parenteral Medications which includes the administration of dangerous drugs and controlled substances via parenteral routes, including intravenous; the Department of Health Services (DHS) attempted to adopt the concept of comprehensive perinatal practitioners that excluded registered nurses; the Sonoma County Department of Education sponsored the Geriatric Technician Health Manpower Pilot Project which created a new category of health care provider in long term care facilities (LTC) who is a Certified Nursing Assistant (CNA) with one year experience in long term care. The Geriatric Technician functions as a medication technician and is authorized to perform health and maintenance procedures (suctioning, catheter and wound care, etc.); and individual hospitals utilize nursing students to supplement the nursing staff by allowing them to perform licensed nursing functions outside the pre-licensure program.

In addition to these existing examples, there is a potential for another major encroachment associated with the American Medical Association's proposal for a new category of health care worker, titled Registered Care Technologist. The AMA proposal call s for the sponsorship and/or support of demonstration projects which will evaluate the efficacy, quality, and effectiveness of the RCT proposal. Private, for-profit hospitals purportedly plan to spearhead the implementation of the RCT proposal. *Reallocation rationale.* As the availability of the health care dollar tightens and priorities are shifting, administrators seek less costly alternatives to the mix of providers available to administer nursing care. Thus, the most frequent justification used for reallocation is economics. As registered nurses seek more equitable compensation and recognition of their value as well as increased status, employers strive for less costly alternatives. Examples include the return of certain functions, such as oxygen therapy, to nursing without providing additional RN staff; the requirement that registered nurses perform certain functions, such as the monitoring of epidural anesthesia, generally performed by other health care providers, yet reimbursement is not allocated to nursing.

Another frequent justification for reallocation is the common misconception that the registered nurse has the authority to delegate licensed nursing functions to unlicensed personnel. For example, the California State Department of Education issued erroneous statements to the County and District Superintendents and other interested parties that, under the Education Code, all personnel who provide specialized physical health care (NG/ostomy feeding, suctioning, catheterization, etc.) do so under the license of the school nurse and that the school nurse's license to practice covers the liability of the school district. The State Department of Education incorrectly required school nurses to delegate certain nursing functions to non-licensed designated school personnel and to provide general supervision.

This raises the issue of the meaning of delegation and supervision. In the case of delegation, the person in authority (RN) confers on another licensed health care provider the broad authority to perform specified functions in an autonomous manner and for which the person performing the function accepts responsibility. The person in authority (RN) also determines the level of competency and level of supervision required. In the case of supervision the person in authority (RN) directs and controls patient care by assigning a limited or specified procedure to one who is qualified to perform the procedure. As in delegation, the person in authority must also determine the level of competency and the level of supervision required for the performance of patient care, based upon the extent of scientific knowledge and type of technical skills required.

This very issue was brought to the attention of the Board of Registered Nursing (BRN) by CNA and very concerned school nurses. After examining the conflicts school nurses were experiencing regarding their authority under the Nursing Practice Act and their authority under the Education Code, the BRN ruled as follows:

> The extent of the nurse's authority in the Nursing Practice Act and the Education Code is to supervise and not to delegate or designate to non-licensed personnel specialized physical health care services. [3]

In the case of specialized physical health care services, the school nurse directs and controls the delivery of specialized services by assigning limited or specified functions to qualified school personnel, while the final responsibility remains with the school nurse who made the assignment. Additionally, the school nurse must determine the level of competency and supervision required.

It is important to point out that there is a distinction between the act of assigning and delegating, specifically as it relates to accountability and autonomy. The person assigned to perform a function has no authority to perform the function in an autonomous manner, thus, the RN who made the assignment remains fully accountable to the patient. On the other hand, the act of delegating confers on another person the broad authority to act autonomously. Such person, however, also accepts full responsibility thereby relieving the

RN of his or her primary responsibility for the welfare of the patient.

"Delegate" as used by medicine is similar to nursing use of "assigning." For instance, physicians are authorized to delegate medical functions to physician's assistants. However, such delegation does not relieve the supervising physician of primary continued responsibility for the welfare of the patient.[4] Furthermore, the supervising physician must make sure that the PA does not function autonomously.[5]

Recommendations

The practice of nursing without a license must be halted; it jeopardizes safe, effective and appropriate patient care. To accomplish this goal, a comprehensive plan must be developed focused on education; legislative, regulatory and judicial arenas; practice settings; and collective bargaining.

Education. Educate nurses, administrators, and faculty on the essential provisions of the Nursing Practice Act, other professionals' practice acts, each professional's role/function, and the implications of decisions made solely on the basis of economics.

Educate nurses, administrators, faculty and nursing students about the financial picture of health care organizations so that nursing dollars can be responsibly negotiated.

Information to include reimbursement methods, capital equipment and improvements, and allocation to nursing care.

Educate the public that the unique role and responsibilities of the nurse requires substantial scientific knowledge and technical skills. The public includes consumers, other health care providers, legislators, regulators, insurers, employers and media.

Educate nurses about the encroachment problem solving process.

Educate nurses to be proactive in influencing change within employment settings, legislative/regulatory arenas as well as the public and community.

Legislative, regulatory and judicial arenas. Continue to develop, monitor and influence legislation and regulations that affect nursing practice.

Identify areas which require legislative and regulatory changes that woudl clarify the practice of nursing.

Encourage the Office of Administrative Law (OAL) and other regulatory agencies to enforce existing statutes and regulations.

See Attorney General Opinions and judicial relief where appropriate.

Monitor pilot projects that affect nursing.

Practice settings. Enforce Title 22 Committee on Interdisciplinary Practice requirements in licensed facilities with staff nurse membership.

Utilize RN's skills, knowledge and experience effectively and efficiently by eliminating non-nursing tasks from RN responsibilities through the efficient use of traditional support personnel such as transportation escorts, housekeeping and clericals.

Place direct patient care personnel under control of nursing and utilize their skills appropriately.

Ensure that the RN controls the quality of nursing practice in the delivery of patient care in the practice settings by preserving the autonomy and the integrity of the nursing department within the organizational structure in the practice setting.

Increase nursing efficiency through the use of appropriate technology.

Institute and support Professional Performance Committees within the governance structure of the practice settings.

Encourage creative and contractual relationships between individuals or groups of nurses and health care agencies to assure control of nursing practice and reimbursement.

Review and analyze professional models of practice, for example, shared governance *Collective bargaining.* Negotiate provisions which implement recommendations regarding encroachment in the practice setting.

Administer and enforce existing nursing practice provisions included within collective bargaining agreements.

Education bargaining unit members on the nursing practice provisions included in the collective bargaining agreements.

Promote equitable compensation for registered nurses to assure recruitment and retention and to reward expertise.

NOTES

1. Adapted from the American Nurses' Association Proposed Draft of "Suggested State Legislation" Act I: Nursing Practice Act, dated May 18, 1988.

2. 70 Ops. Cal. Atty. Gen. 14.

3. See Board of Registered Nursing minutes, May 19-20, 1988, Sacramento, California.

4. California Code of Regulations Section 1399.542.

5. California Code of Regulations Section 1399.545(h).

Nursing actions in litigation

CYNTHIA E. NORTHROP, RN, MS, JD

In the following excerpt, the author provides an overview of legal cases involving nursing care, as reported in the 1985 issues of the Association of Trial Lawyers of America (ATLA) Law Reporter.

Summary of nursing actions

THE TYPES OF NURSING actions that led to allegations of nursing malpractice are listed in Table 1. As in all determinations of negligence or malpractice, all of the following elements must be established and proved: the duty to the patient, a breach of that duty, the proximate cause, and the injury.

The legal standard of nursing care is to provide reasonable and prudent care under the circumstances.[34,35] What is reasonable and prudent can be determined from a variety of sources. Some of the ATLA-reported case summaries identified the specific evidence used to establish duty, breach of duty, cause, and injury. The evidence included

• the *Physician's Desk Reference (PDR);*
• obstetrical nursing standards;
• written policies, rules, and protocols of the hospital;
• drug and equipment manufacturer's manuals;
• records of incidents involving machine failures;
• nursing and other health care literature;
• the patient's chart and medical record; and
• expert nurse witnesses.

Most of these cases involved the hospital (in one case a nursing home) as defendant, based on its liability as an employer for any employee's negligence. However, hospitals were also held accountable for their own duties and responsibilities to their patients, separate from employee actions (see Table 2). Tables 1 and 2 illustrate how an institution's obligations to patients differ from a nurse's individual responsibilities. Obviously, risk management strategies have to be developed for the entire institution, but this article deals only with risk management of nursing actions.

For discussion purposes, the nursing actions have been grouped into four main categories: treatment, communication, medication, and supervising/monitoring/observing. These categories relate to two primary standards of nursing practice.[36]

• Nursing actions assist the patient in maximizing health capabilities; and
• Collection of data about health status of the patient is systematic and continuous; these data are accessible, communicated, and recorded.

The standard of nursing care expected in practice can best be demonstrated through a closer examination of some of the nursing actions listed in Table 1.

Treatment. In one case a pediatric staff nurse administered an enema to a 7-month-old infant with a diagnosis of megacolon with vomiting.[1] The jury was informed that the *PDR* states that the type of enema used is contraindicated for a patient under 2 years of age with this diagnosis. Further, the *PDR* gives no dosage for a patient under 2 years of age. The nurse was held accountable for knowing what the *PDR* stated and for knowing contraindications to medica-

TABLE 1. Types of nursing actions involved in litigation

Treatment
- Gave enema to 7-month-old infant when contraindicated[1]
- Failed to test performance, take safety precautions, and properly connect machine, resulting in air being blown into bloodstream[7]
- Failed to cut jaw wires (respiratory distress)[8]
- Failed to respond to alarms, used malfunctioning equipment, and failed to supply oxygen when respirator could not promptly be reattached[10]
- Failed to implement orders for I.V. hookup and fetal heart monitoring[16]
- Failed to attach fetal monitor[19]
- Failed to manage infant's airway (brain damage)[23]
- Administered improper oxygen levels, failing to adhere to protocols[26]
- Fed infant with baby bottle warmed in microwave oven, resulting in burns[28]
- Failed to attend to patient during asthma attack[32]
- Allowed mother to walk for hours despite serious vaginal bleeding[33]

Communication
- Failed to notify or advise physician of
  a. changes in signs and symptoms and patient status[2]
  b. changes in a casted leg resulting from reduced circulation (circulatory compromise)[2]
  c. fetal tachycardia and meconium[4]
  d. pain and vaginal bleeding[5]
  e. increased pulse rate and lack of response to stimuli (intensive care unit)[6]
  f. dehydration, seriousness of condition[9]
  g. late decelerations that occurred during fetal monitoring[13]
  h. jaundice[25]
  i. excessive oxygen levels[26]
- Failed to chart vital signs for seven and three-quarter hours (labor room)[5]
- Failed to chart for three hours (labor room)[23]

Medication
- Gave wrong medication upon discharge (gave Alcaine, a topical eye anesthetic; should have given artificial tears)[3]
- Failed to discontinue oxytocin (Pitocin) as required by hospital policy when obstetrician was absent[4]
- Administered morphine without notifying physician[5]
- Failed to give diazepam (Valium) as ordered[6]
- Gave excessive dose of disulfiram (Antabuse)[11]
- Allowed inappropriate use of intravenous infusion equipment, which resulted in extensive infusing of fluids extravascularly into leg and foot[14]
- Gave thioridazine (Mellaril) at night, against physician order; mistakenly gave paraldehyde (intended for patient in next bed) with thioridazine (Mellaril)[17]
- Administered meperidine (Demerol) hydrochloride, clinically contraindicated[18]
- Administered potassium chloride improperly[24]
- Mishandled infusion pump[31]

Monitoring/Observing/Supervising
- Failed to recognize dehydration and electrolyte imbalance[1]
- Failed to observe changes in circulation due to leg cast[2]
- Failed to assess and record vital signs for seven and three-quarter hours[5]
- Discharged maternity patient upon order of physician who later denied giving order (should have notified supervisor)[13]
- Failed to periodically monitor, recognize misuse, and discontinue intravenous therapy[14]
- Improperly participated in obtaining father's signature on a consent form one and one-half hours after infant was born, before he had been apprised of the infant's condition[15]
- Failed to provide one-to-one monitoring in recovery room, which resulted in failing to recognize and respond to cardiac arrest[18]
- Failed to observe adverse reaction to meperidine (Demerol) hydrochloride[18]
- Negligently interpreted recovery room protocol[18]
- Failed to monitor fetal heart rate and contractions every 30 minutes as required by hospital policy[19]
- Was negligent in supervising a psychiatric patient who attempted suicide[20]
- Failed to notice hypoxia[21]
- Improperly assisted patient to bathroom (nursing home)[22]

TABLE 1. Types of nursing actions involved in litigation *continued*

- Failed to observe mother in labor for three hours[23]
- Failed to observe jaundice[25]
- Failed to recognize signs and symptoms of oxygen deprivation during surgery (nurse anesthetist)[27]

- Was negligent in assigning and supervisin a nursing student (student did not take bloo pressure for six hours)[29]
- Failed to observe head circumference, intracranial bleeding[30]
- Failed to monitor fetal heart rate[33]

---

tions and treatments under these circumstances.

In other treatment cases, the result of nursing negligence included death ,[7,8,12] burns,[28] anoxia,[16] hyperbilirubinemia ,[25] retrolental fibroplasia,[26] brain damage,[21,32] and stroke.[29] These results are obviously unacceptable in nursing practice.

Communication. Communicating changes in a patient's status to the physician and the nursing supervisor is an expected part of nursing practice, as is recording data in the patient's chart. In the cases examined here, charting and record questions arose in several ways.

In two cases no charting had been done for long periods of time under the circumstances.[5,23]

In one case a nurse obtained a new father's signature on a hospital consent form one and one-half hours *after* the infant was born and *before* he had been apprised of the infant's condition. Four obstetrical nursing experts testified that this action failed to meet the standard of nursing care.[15]

In another case, settled before trial, the original recovery room records had been destroyed.[21] This would have implied to a jury that the nurse had practiced below standard, that the facts of the case were being hidden, and that the nurse intended to lie and cover up what had actually happened. Altered records would carry the same implication.

Medication. The medication cases involved mistakes in dosage, in patient identification,

and in administration route. Some invol\ giving the wrong medication, failing to r the label, and failing to execute a medica order. The results of medication errors by nurses in these cases included death,[12] lo vision,[3] failed corneal transplant,[3] brain d age,[24] and cardiac arrest.[24]

The case that resulted in the highest aw to date against an individual nurse ($5 mil involved a medication error. An emergen room nurse received a proper medicatior from a physician for lidocaine, 75 mg, Failing to read the label, the nurse m picked up a 1-gram syringe of lidoca administered three-fourths of it — 1 the dose ordered. The patient suffere ate cardiac and respiratory distress a days later.[12]

The plaintiff's attorney investigat cidence of lidocaine errors reported Food and Drug Administration and i erature. Complaints to the manufactu doctors and nurses were also review argued that confusion about the colo and the label of the medication contr the nurse's error, thus implicating th facturer. Evidence was also presente hospital had recently given in-servic on medication administration to all r *cept* those in the emergency room, tl cating the hospital.

The jury found the nurse liable fo to administer the medication properl

---

2. Hospital liabilities other than nursing actions

- Failure to provide adequate staff to check plaintiff every 30 minutes as physician ordered[2]
- Failure to train emergency room nurses in the same manner as other hospital nurses concerning medication administration[12]
- Failure to establish a mechanism for ensuring that patients in labor have given informed consent to the method of delivery[15]
- Failure to establish a mechanism for prompt reporting of any life-threatening situation[15]
- Failure to provide adequate staff under the circumstances (nursing home)[22]
- Failure to supervise employees (impaired nurse)[28]
- Failure to enforce internal safety regulations requiring employees to test contents of heated bottles[28]
- Failure to provide immediate treatment of burns[28]
- Entrusting patient's care solely to a nursing student[29]

---

manufacturer, for failing to take corrective action after receiving complaints about confusion caused by its color coding; and the hospital, for the nurse's actions and for failing to train emergency room nurses properly.

Monitoring/observing/supervising. Nurses in several of these cases were held liable for failure to observe symptoms and signs, including jaundice,[25] increased head circumference,[30] and lack of response to stimuli[18]; failure to prevent a suicide attempt[20]; and failure to supervise nursing students.[29]

In one case, a nursing assistant informed a nurse who was taking report that a patient was having severe difficulty breathing. Rather than immediately investigating, the nurse finished the report; after a lapse of 10 minutes the patient was not breathing, and a Code Blue was called.[32]

In a case in which the hospital was not sued, the head nurse was found negligent for improperly interpreting written protocols as requiring continual cardiac monitoring only until the patient was stabilized: the nursing team leader, for administering 50 mg of meperidine (Demerol) hydrochloride 45 minutes prior to the cardiac arrest and for failing to detect clinically adverse reactions to the medication; the staff nurse, for failing to furnish one-to-one monitoring (as required by recovery room protocol), being diverted from patient care, and failing to detect and treat cardiac arrest (undetected for 5-10 minutes); and the cardiologist, for negligently clearing the patient for major surgery and failing to follow the patient's postoperative recovery properly.[18]

In these monitoring cases, the sources of standard of care most often referred to were protocols, rules, and policies and procedures of the hospital. Literature, education, and the usual and customary practice of nursing also help determine the standard of care. For example, in a case where an infant's jaundice was not promptly detected, the bilirubin level had climbed to 34 mg/dl. The literature on the care of infants indicates that jaundice is clinically observable at a bilirubin level of 10 mg/dl. The nurses had many opportunities to observe the patient and to act to prevent brain damage, and they were negligent to fail to do so.[25]

Risk management strategies

Based on these cases, the most important, overall risk management strategy is to know the standard of care for nursing practice, to know the source of that standard of care, and to know how the standard of care is to be applied to each situation. Nurses who can articulate the standard of care owed a patient under the circumstances in each clinical situation will not only be in a better position to defend themselves if things go wrong, but, more importantly, will also be able to improve the overall quality of patient care.

The four major categories of nursing actions discussed imply other, more specific strategies for risk management.

Treatment. To minimize the possibility of patient injury as a result of treatment, it is useful to

• adequately orient all personnel to a unit;

• test equipment regularly, provide routine maintenance for equipment, and keep records of equipment use;

• provide in-service education on treatment methods;

• organize a "buddy system" in which peers observe and evaluate each other's techniques and performance;

• provide close clinical supervision by peers and supervisors;

• conduct clinical audits of nursing practice;

• conduct periodic performance evaluations by supervisors, and self-evaluations;

• develop and support employee assistance programs; and

• urge prompt notification of any problems with a physician or other health care team member to the nursing administration.

Communication. The most obvious strategy in this area of nursing actions is prompt, complete, and accurate recording of data in patients' charts. Such a record makes it possible to recall the condition of the patient, the treatment given, the results of that treatment, and the follow-up. Failing to record data or altering a patient's chart implies a degree of negligence to a jury and certainly does not lessen risk.

To improve communication among nursing staff, nursing supervisors, and physicians about changes in patient status, a staff development program should be implemented that will sharpen the assessment skills of staff nurses, improve their ability to judge when a situation needs a physician's attention, and clarify the level of knowledge required by the

standard of care for nursing practice. (While nurses are not expected to have the same level of knowledge as physicians,[37] the nursing curricula provide evidence of the expected level of skill and knowledge.[38] Although three basic nursing education programs exist, each registered nurse is licensed by a state through a nationally standardized examination. This means that all nurses, regardless of basic educational program, are held to the same reasonable standard of knowledge. However, nurses with advanced or specialized education are held to the standard of that additional knowledge.)

Medication. Many of the risk management strategies already mentioned are also needed in the medication area: vigilance, accuracy, careful attention, and meticulous knowledge of medications and their administration.

In addition, nurses should conduct clinical research that examines modes of delivering medication to patients in order to answer questions such as the following:

• Do error rates differ when one nurse per unit is responsible for administering medications as opposed to several nurses administering medication to their assigned patients in one unit?

• Are there safer ways of giving medications?

Another strategy for minimizing risk of injury by medication error is to objectively evaluate labeling, packaging, coding, and other aspects of medicine identification. All members of the nursing staff should be encouraged to notify the nursing supervisor, the hospital, and the manufacturer, in writing, of any problems, questions, or concerns about the delivery of medications.

Monitoring/observing/supervising. Again, the best risk management strategies include vigilance, accuracy, careful attention, and meticulous knowledge. Specifically, the nursing staff should have a thorough knowledge and understanding of the hospital's protocols, rules, and policies and procedures. This could be encouraged by periodic review and/or testing. Nurses should be expected to follow the current literature in their primary area of practice. Workshops to enhance assessment skills and clinical judgment should be made available to all the nursing staff on a regular basis.

Conclusion

A hospital is liable for its employee's actions under the legal principle of *respondeat superior,* vicarious liability. However, every nurse is also responsible for his or her own actions under the legal principle of personal liability.

This brief survey of cases indicates that there is a movement toward individual nurse accountability in malpractice cases. (In light of this, nurses may want to review their need for professional liability insurance coverage.) Significantly, nursing standards promulgated by the nursing profession itself (the American Nurses' Association first issued professional standards in the early 1970s; these are currently undergoing major revisions) are being used by the courts to clarify, define, and prove the professional responsibility of nurses. The testimony of nurses as expert witnesses is being used more often as evidence in malpractice cases. These changes may well strengthen nursing as a profession and increase the quality of nursing care.

REFERENCES

1. Doerr v Hurley Med Center, NY, Genesee Cty Cir Ct, No. 82-67439-NM, Jul 5, 1984, 28 *ATLA L Rptr* 42, Feb 1985.

2. Jarvis v St Charles Med Center, Ore, Deschutes Cty Cir Ct, No. 33751, Aug 8, 1984. 28 *ATLA L Rptr* 86, Mar 1985.

3. Temple v St Luke's Hosp Inc, Ariz, Maricopa Cty Super. Ct, No. 449311, Aug 24, 1984. 28 *ATLA L Rptr* 87, Mar 1985.

4. Capaccio v Neuman, NY, NY Super. Ct, No. 21831/81, Oct 26, 1984. 28 *ATLA L Rptr* 89, Mar 1985.

5. Taylor v Richmond Meml Hosp, Va, Richmond Cir Ct No. LG—915, Dec 7, 1984. 28 *ATLA L Rptr* 136, Apr 1985.

6. Kuchak v Lancaster Genl Hosp, Ra, Lancaster City Ct of Common Pleas, No. 122, 1980, Dec 12, 1984. 28 *ATLA L Rptr* 136, Apr 1985.

7. Saylor v Good Samaritan Hosp, Fla, Palm Beach Cty Cir Ct, No. 83—6669 CA(L) 01 B, Nov 31, 1984. 28 *ATLA L Rptr* 137, Apr 1985.

8. Larrumbide v Doctor's Hosp, Tex, Dallas Cty 191st Jud Dist Ct, No. 81—5216—J, Nov 28, 1984. 28 *ATLA L Rptr* 184, May 1985.

9. Hicks v Santa Monica Hosp Med Center, Cal, Los Angeles Super. CT, No. WEC62328, Jan 29, 1985. 28 *ATLA L Rptr* 275, Aug 1985.

10. Lindsay v Meuller, Wash, Pierce Cty Super. Ct, No. 83—2—00271—6, Jan 9, 1985. 28 *ATLA L Rptr* 276 Aug 1985.

11. Sawyer v Tauber, NC, Buncombe Cty Super. Ct, No. 81CVS2567, Dec 18, 1984. 28 *ATLA L Rptr* 27, Aug 1985.

12. Woods v City of North Kansas City, Mo, Clay Cty Cir Ct, No. CV 182—267 cc, May 5, 1985. 28 *ATLA L Rptr 312, Sep 1985.*

13. Driml v Mission Community Hosp, Cal, Orange Cty Super. Ct, No. 39 40 00, Mar 8. 1985. 28 *ATLA L Rptr 326, Sep 1985.*

14. Ray v Tarrant Cty Hosp Dist, Tex, Tartant Cty 352d Dist Ct, No. 352—66487—81, Apr 1, 1985. 28 *ATLA L Rptr* 373, Oct 1985.

15. Campbell v Pitt Cty Mem Hosp, NC, Pitt Cty Super. Ct, No. 83 CVS 336, Apr 11, 1985. 28 *ATLA L Rptr* 419, Nov 1985.

16. May v William Beaumont Hosp, Mich, Oakland Cty Cir Ct, No. 81—230—540—NO, Apr 23, 1985. 28 *ATLA L Rptr 419, Nov 1985.*

17. Serota v Central General Hosp, NY, Queens Cty Super. Ct, No. 17029/79, May 14, 1985. 28 *ATLA L Rptr 467, Dec 1985.*

18. Torbert v Befeler, NJ, Union Cty Super. Ct, No. L—17463—81, Apr 24, 1985. 28 *ATLA L Rptr* 469, Dec 1985.

19. Herrup v South Miami Hosp Foundation, Fla, Date Cty Cir Ct, No. 83—37139, Oct 24, 1984. 28 *ATLA L Rptr* 89, Mar 1985.

20. Lasley v Jackson Park Hosp, Ill, Cook Cty Cir Ct, No. 78L10836, Nov 7, 1984. 28 *ATLA L Rptr* 89, Mar 1985.

21. Brown v St Vincent Infirmary, Ark, White Cty Cir Ct, No. 83—182, Nov 30, 1984. 28 *ATLA L Rptr* 136, Apr 1985.

22. Hernandez v Ara Living Centers, Cal, Los Angeles Super. Ct. No. C475 796, Aug 1984. 28 *ATLA L Rptr* 137, Apr 1985.

23. Schager v Davoli, NY, Bronx Cty Super. Ct, No. 16486/82, Nov 20, 1984. 28 *ATLA L Rptr* 137, Apr 1985.

24. Peltier v Franklin Foundation Hosp, La, St Mary Parish 16th Jud Dist Ct, No. 73—142—F, Jan 19, 1985. 28 *ATLA L Rptr* 182, May 1985.

25. Butts v Cummings, La, Caddo Parish 1st Jud Dist Ct, No. 234,350, Jan 30, 1985. 28 *ATLA L Rptr* 182, May 1985.

26. Willis v El Camino Hosp, Cal, Santa Clara Super. Ct, No. 468929, Nov 1984. 28 *ATLA L Rptr* 227, Jun 1985.

27. Montgomery v DePaul Health Center, Mo, St Louis Cir Ct, No. 832—04850, Dec 5, 1984. 28 *ATLA L Rptr* 276, Aug 1985.

28. Kozemczak v St Louis Children's Hosp, Mo, St Louis Cir Ct, No. 822—06798, Apr 29, 1985. 28 *ATLA L Rptr 418, Nov 1985.*

29. Venefra v Uhm, Wash, King Cty Super. Ct, No. 82—2—16570—1, Apr 11, 1985. 28 *ATLA L Rptr* 420, Nov 1985.

30. Harris v Skrocki, Mich, Macomb Cty Cir Ct, No. 84—2430—NM, May 30, 1985. 28 *ATLA L Rptr* 420, Nov 1985.

31. Jones v Samaritan Health Service, Ariz, Maricopa Cty Super. Ct, No. C 487995, Apr 5, 1985. 28 *ATLA L Rptr* 421, Nov 1985

32. Cauwenbergh v St Vincent Hosp, Wis, Wis Patients Compensation Panel, No. F4—1883, Feb 22, 1985. 28 *ATLA L Rptr* 228, Jun 1985.

33. Trevins v U.S., U.S. Dist Ct WD, Wash, No. C84—179T, Jun 7, 1985. 28 *ATLA L Rptr* 465, Dec 1985.

34. Prosser W: *Law of Torts*, 4th ed. St Paul: West, 1971, p 150.

35. Beardsley v Wyoming County Community Hosp, 453 NY 2d 793 (3d Dept 1982).

36. American Nurses' Association (ANA):*Standards of Nursing Practice*. Kansas City, Mo: ANA, 1973. (In addition, ANA has developed standards for many specialty areas.)

37. Fein v Permanente Med Group, 211 Cal Rptr 368 (1985).

38. Accreditation criteria used by the National League for Nursing to approve and accredit schools of nursing and state board of nursing rules and regulations under a state's nursing practice act are examples of the evidence that can be used to determine the content of basic nursing curricula.

Litigation involving oncology nurses

LISA SCHULMEISTER, RN, MS, CS

RECENTLY, MUCH ATTENTION has been focused on the legal implications of nursing. Basic tenets of the law reflect the professional role of the nurse in observing and evaluating a patient's condition, while providing reasonable and prudent care. Further, with increased recognition of professional autonomy the nurse is personally responsible for her own wrongful or negligent acts; as an employee or agent, she may render her employer liable as well.[1]

Suits based on claims of negligence or malpractice are brought in civil courts to recover damages for the injuries claimed. These claims give rise to such questions as whether or not the nurse is solely responsible for the alleged act, omission or other wrongs, and how the physicians and hospital are implicated, if at all.

Often, questions of liability are settled out of court. Therefore, the extent of litigious actions involving health care agencies and personnel is unknown.

In an attempt to identify incidents specifically involving oncology nurses, a review of cases was undertaken. Six cases citing nurses caring for individuals with cancer as defendants heard in trial courts in the southern U.S. were reviewed. In addition, the hospital records and legal proceedings of six additional incidents involving oncology nurses that were either settled out of court or dismissed were examined. Of the twelve cases, nine involved medication discrepancies. Of the three remaining cases, two involved a nurse providing incorrect referral or followup instructions and one involved a relative sustaining injury when a cot collapsed. Incidents involving restraints and falls are the most frequent accidents

prompting litigation involving health care agencies;[2] however, a fall occurred in only one case of the twelve reviewed.

Since care of the oncology client is complex, the variety and number of individuals caring for the patient may be extensive. Claims of negligence or malpractice usually involve all of the health care individuals in contact with the patient and are not limited to the direct care providers. Numerous other individuals and the institution itself may be involved.

Staff nurses, head nurses, and nurse supervisors were the nurses cited in the twelve incidents reviewed. Physicians, pharmacists, and hospital administrators were also cited in seven cases. In three of the cases, the hospital itself was sued. Because the involved hospitals were state supported agencies, two southern states were cited as defendants as well. Although a diversity of specific events prompted the litigations, several prevailing elements were identified.

Documentation of events

Although one case involved complete omission of documentation, the remainder of cases revealed that hospital records were either incomplete, inconsistent, or contradictory to the events witnessed by patients, family, or other hospital personnel. The patient's medical records were carefully scrutinized in all cases since they are legally regarded as an accurate report of the quantity and quality of medical and nursing care rendered.[3] In the cases that went to trial, hospital and office records were compared to the expert witness testimony concerning Joint Commission for Accreditation of Hospitals (JCAH) and institutional documentation requirements. Since institutional policies and procedures serve as internally imposed standards, they delineate the standards of care for that particular institution or agency and are above and beyond those imposed by external bodies, such as the State Board of Nursing.[4]

Although Nurse Practice Acts exist in every state and outline precisely what a nurse may do, they do not define or set forth a nurse's duties, except in general terms. Institutional policies and procedures are therefore regarded as the standard against which nursing practices are evaluated.

Particularly scrutinized were "late entry" nurses' notes and crossed-out notes. Notes written several hours after the incident that later prompted litigation were perceived (during a jury trial) to be an indication of some guilt. The jury felt that the late entry was an attempt to cover-up or minimize prior wrong doing, and deviated from the institutional standard of accurate, timely charting. Crossed-out notes were similarly perceived with suspicion. During one hospital inquiry, a nurse admitted to charting in advance of the procedure performed. When an adverse reaction occurred, her notes were crossed out and amended. Her actions were determined to be inconsistent with the established hospital policy of charting after completion of procedures. None of the incidents discussed involved "white out" on notes, although such notes have been deciphered in the past using X-rays.[5]

During the legal proceedings, nurses were given an opportunity to verbally clarify or supplement their notes. Since most cases were tried an average of fourteen months after the event in question, recall of specific events was limited.

Documentation of the events following a specific incident was also carefully scrutinized in all cases. For instance, in a case involving an analgesic administered to a patient with a similar sounding name and not to the intended patient, the attorney brought charges of harmful negligence against the nurse. The nursing documentation following this event was completed in both medical record and incident report format. When this documentation revealed no adverse physiologic changes, the case was dismissed.

Medication discrepancies

Medication errors are commonly occurring negligent acts.[1] Of the nine cases reviewed involving medication discrepancies, chemotherapy or narcotic analgesics were administered either to the wrong patient, via an incorrect route, in the wrong dose, or in an improper manner (extravasated).

In a case involving the administration of chemotherapy to the incorrect patient, charges of harmful negligence were supported after a jury trial. On a mixed hematology/oncology unit, a man with sideroblastic anemia received BCNU (carmustine) intended for his roommate. The man died two weeks later after a severe gastrointestinal hemorrhage. A lengthy trial ensued, and after much deliberations, the nurse administering the chemotherapy was found negligent. The hospital's insurance carrier made a large award to the patient's family. The nurse was also dismissed from employment.

"Reasonable and customary care"

Situations occur daily where the standard of care is not met, but fortunately, most of these situations do not result in injury or harm. When harm or injury is believed to have occurred, charges of failure to provide reasonable or customary care are commonplace. Provision of reasonable care has been defined as the activities that a reasonable person, guided by ordinary considerations that ordinarily regulate human affairs, would do.[6]

The majority of the cases reviewed cited

charges of failure to provide reasonable care following chemotherapy extravasations. Attorneys alleged that extravasations resulted in physical harm, ensuing pain and suffering, and reflected nursing negligence. In addition, allegations were made that interruptions in cancer therapy while extravasations were treated were life-threatening. All patients experiencing an extravasation following chemotherapy administration also requested remuneration for medical expenses incurred and recovery of lost wages. As a result of litigious actions, a definition of reasonable and customary care following extravasation has emerged. Because extravasation is a risk of vesicant administrations, it is reasonable to assume that it may occur, and sometimes does.[7] Despite variances in institutional policies, the generally accepted nursing action when extravasation is suspected or occurs is to:

1. stop the infusion;
2. notify the physician; and
3. document the event.

Documentation must include both incident report and medical record, although an incident report is not a part of the patient's chart.[8] When these three critical steps are not done, nurses may later find themselves defending their actions or lack thereof. If these steps *are* done, the nurse has provided what is generally considered to be reasonable and customary care. Also, if an institutional protocol for assessing and treating an extravasation exists, it is expected that the nurse be familiar with this policy and implement the treatment in accordance with the protocol.[9]

Referral or follow-up instructions

Unlike medication errors, charges of failure to provide referral or follow-up instructions often do not have an observable or measurable adverse effect. For instance, one case reviewed involved a patient with breast cancer who telephoned an office nurse about her back pain.

Calls were documented on only two occasions approximately one month apart, although the family testified that numerous telephone discussions between patient and nurse were witnessed. Nurse's notes described the nature of the problem as the patient described it but did not include instructions of any kind. The patient testified that she phoned the nurse weekly for almost three months and was even denied the opportunity to speak with the physician. She then changed physicians and was diagnosed with a vertebral bone metastasis. The physician employing the nurse denied any knowledge of the woman's complaints of back pain; the nurse, therefore, became the primary defendant. A jury subsequently decided that the nurse was negligent in providing appropriate referral or follow-up instructions.

In a similar case, a class IV Pap smear report was inadvertently filed without review in a busy clinic. When the patient requested a phone report, the oncology nurse stated that it was fine since all abnormal lab work was flagged and not filed. A month later, the oversight was discovered and charges were filed against the entire office staff. Although extensive legal action was threatened, the case was settled out of court after physicians' depositions supported the defense that delay did not affect overall patient outcome.

Responsibility and insurance

The "master-servant rule" (respondent superior) states that the master is responsible for the wrongful acts of his servants and applies to the relationship of principal and agent. Whenever a person is injured by an employee as a result of negligence in the course of the employee's work, the employer is responsible to the injured person. Since an employee is one who works for wages or salary in the service of an employer, the power to discharge is that of the employer.[10]

The effect of litigation on licensure rests with the individual's State Board of Nursing.

FIGURE 1. Preventive and defensive nursing action for avoiding litigation

---

Preventing medication discrepancies

A. Assure correct patient identification.
- Check arm band if worn.
- Ask for and verify name of patient, especially those patients without arm band identification.
- Ask for and verify birthdates of individuals with similar names, those with no arm bands, or those with language barriers.
- Identify and flag rooms and medical records of patients with similar names.

B. Assure correct medication.
- Review allergies verbally and as noted in the medical records.
- Verify physician's orders with drugs to be administered.
- Clarify orders with physician whenever unclear. Repeat the clarification or any additional verbal orders back to the physician for verification.
- Verify the dosage of drug ordered with the drug prepared by the pharmacy.
- Verify that dosage ordered is within the acceptable dose range considering the disease process being treated and size of patient.
- Verify the schedule and route of administration.
- Carefully select the site for I.M. or I.V. medications. For I.V. agents, observe the site during the infusion. Institute vesicant precautions if applicable. Instruct the patient to avoid arm movement if a peripheral vein is used.

Defending medication discrepancies
- Document the incident in the medical record and complete an incident report. Chart truthfully and objectively. Chart on time. Include documentation of any instructions given. Write clearly and legibly. Sign full name and credentials.
- Notify risk management or clinical supervisor depending on institutional procedure.
- Become familiar with institutional procedures concerning a medication discrepancy before an incident occurs.
- Summon such clinical assistance as necessary.
- Comply with accepted policies and procedures of employing institution.
- Even if employed in a setting that does not utilize a formal incident report, document the discrepancy clearly and completely in the patient's medical record. Also, make anecdotal notes for your own reference.

Preventing allegations of lack of referral or follow-up
- Verbally provide discharge instructions, even if short stay.
- Provide specific written take home or discharge instructions in addition to verbal instructions whenever possible.
- Instruct outpatients to call the office or hospital after procedures or treatments. Provide written phone numbers and procedures for contacting the appropriate health team member in the event of a problem or emergency.
- Elicit understanding of instructions from patients and families. Request that they repeat the information given.
- Whenever a patient is verbally referred to another health team member or agency, document the date of the referral.
- If referral instructions are given via telephone, briefly make a notation of the event in the patient's medical record.

The Board is empowered with both licensing and revocation of licensure and uses the state Nurse Practice Act as the standard against which nursing practice is measured.

Many nurses erroneously assume that they are protected by their hospital's professional liability policies, yet only about 10% of the hospitals in the United States insure their employees under a paramedical endorsement.[10]

An individual liability policy is needed, since a nurse may be sued individually as well as with her employer. Also, when the employer has to pay damages the insurance company may seek subrogation (restitution) from the nurse. Periodic review of liability insurance coverage by the nurse is also essential so that the amount of liability coverage is adequate for her professional role.

Conclusion

Despite increased awareness of the legal implications of nursing practice, oncology nurses are being sued or involved in legal proceedings. Several of the twelve incidents reviewed involved medication discrepancies, and investigation of these incidents was often hampered by deviation from institutional documentation requirements. Preventive and defensive nursing actions, including accurate and timely documentation of events and adherence to institutional protocol, are critical for avoiding potential litigation resulting from oncology nursing practice (Figure 1).

Although only a small number of litigious cases were reviewed and are not representative of all litigation involving oncology nurses, nor of oncology nursing practice in general, they are representative of common types of problems encountered. The cases should sensitize nurses to the legal issues within their practice by providing a beginning framework for examining the legal ramifications of suits involving oncology nurses.

REFERENCES

1. Creighton, H. *Law every nurse should know*. Philadelphia: W.B. Saunders Co., 1981.

2. Bell v. New York City Health and Hospitals, 456 N.Y.S. 2d 787.

3. Banyas v. Lower Bucks Hospital, 437 A. 2d 1236.

4. Rhodes, A.M.; Miller, R.D. *Nursing and the law*. Rockville, MD: Aspen Systems Corp., 1984.

5. Rocerto, L.R.; Maleski, C. *The legal dimensions of nursing practice*. New York: Spring Publishing Co., 1982.

6. Bullough, B. *The law and the expanding nursing role*. New York: Appleton-Century-Crofts, 1980.

7. Cullen, M.L. Issues in chemotherapy administration: current interventions for Doxorubicin extravasations. *Oncol Nurs Forum* 9(1):52-53, 1982.

8. Merryman, P. The incident report. *Nursing '85 48(12):57-58, 1985*.

9. Hemelt, M.D.; Mackert, M.E. *Dynamics of law in nursing and health care*. Reston, VA: Reston Publishing Co., 1982.

10. Fiesta, J. *The law and liability: a guide for nurses*. New York: John Wiley and Sons, 1983.

Nurses accused of murder

BEATRICE CROFT YORKER, RN, MS

WHEN CLUSTERS OF patient deaths are detected in quality assurance and risk management programs, epidemiological studies often trace the causes to infectious agents or chemicals.[1,2] In at least nine cases since 1975, however, such investigations have led to the indictments of nurses for the murder of patients in their care. Eight of the cases involved RNs and in one case in Texas, a licensed vocational nurse was charged.

In 1975, a case began when hospital administrators and medical staff in Michigan investigated a series of breathing failures and discovered pancuronium bromide (Pavulon) in several patients' bodies. The FBI and Centers for Disease Control (CDC) were contacted. As a result of an epidemiological study, the CDC traced the deaths to intravenous injections given in the ICU on the evening shift.[3] Two evening-shift nurses were convicted, but the appellate judge struck down the verdict because of procedural violations of the nurses' civil rights and violations of the rules of evidence.[4]

A 1980 case in Nevada began with rumors that nurses were running a betting pool on when patients would die. Murder charges were brought against one nurse who was accused of tampering with life support equipment to raise her odds of winning. However, no cluster of deaths was identified, and all charges ultimately were dropped because of insufficient evidence.[5]

Next, when infants on a cardiology unit in Toronto showed high postmortem digoxin levels following a series of 28 unexplained deaths over a nine-month period, the CDC correlated the cardiopulmonary arrests with the presence of a particular nurse on the night shift.[6] The judge, however, dismissed the charges against the nurse who was arrested, citing insufficient evidence.[7] Interestingly, the CDC study linked a different nurse to the suspicious deaths, but that nurse was never arrested.

Then came a California case concerning several patients who died with signs of lidocaine toxicity; postmortem reports revealed high concentrations of the drug. As many as 27 lidocaine-related deaths in two different hospitals were correlated with the presence of one ICU nurse. His home was searched, and vials of lidocaine were discovered. The nurse was found guilty on 12 counts of murder and sentenced to death. His case is on appeal and he maintains his innocence.[8]

In Texas, hospital administrators noted that a particular LVN was present during a high number of cardiopulmonary arrests.[9] Not wanting to risk publicity or lawsuits, the hospital set forth a policy excluding LVNs from the ICU. Unfortunately, the LVN took a job with a private pediatrician, and suspicious breathing failures started to occur among children in the physician's office.[10] A local hospital traced succinylcholine chloride (Anectine) as the likely agent, and the LVN was convicted of murder.[11]

In Florida, an RN was linked to a high number of insulin-related deaths in a nursing home.[12] The nurse pleaded guilty to four counts of second-degree murder and to one count of attempted murder. The judge sentenced her to 65 years' imprisonment.[13]

A Maryland nurse was acquitted because the judge said statistical evidence alone is insufficient to convict someone of murder. The nurse had been indicted in 1985 after a CDC study revealed her patients were 47.5 times more likely than other nurses' patients to suffer cardiac arrest.[14]

A Georgia case was noteworthy because of the hospital's response when suspicious cardiopulmonary arrests were detected on the evening shift. Within a month, a very tight protocol was in place to control use of potassium chloride (KCl). The drug had to be signed out, and potassium blood levels were measured on all patients who arrested. For the next three months there were no mysterious arrests. Then, a nurse was convicted of criminal assault when KCl was found in the IV tubing of a blood transfusion that the nurse had just started.[15]

This year, a New York case received national attention when a patient suffered a breathing failure immediately following an IV injection by a nurse. An investigation led to an indictment for one count of murder and three counts of assault. Although this nurse confessed, the admissibility of his confession has not yet been determined.[16]

Also this year, a nurse in North Carolina was convicted of second-degree murder after he was found to have deliberately omitted a prescribed dose of 1-norepinephrine (Levophed).[17]

The arm of the law

In order to arrest a suspect, probable cause (more evidence for than against) must exist. In the nine cases described, the correlation between a nurse's presence and a high number of suspicious deaths was deemed sufficient to establish probable cause and to bring indictments by grand juries.

Next comes the trial, which can take months and even years of preparation because of the extensive expert testimony required. The California case and the Maryland cases,

for example, each took two years of preparation.

Of the nine cases sine 1975, four led to convictions, and one nurse pleaded guilty. Charges were dropped against two and are still pending against one.

In six cases, the CDC was called in to conduct epidemiological studies. The length of time that hospital administrators formally investigated these "epidemics" varied from 1 to 15 months before the district attorney's office was called.[14,15]

Unless the nurse is caught in the act, proof of murder rests primarily on a statistical correlation. Typically, the events preceding identification of a suspect in the nine cases included some combination of the following:

• a significant rise in cardiopulmonary arrests or deaths in a particular patient population;

• an unusually high rate of successful cardiopulmonary resuscitation. (A patient in Georgia arrested eight times in one month. Ten patients in Maryland had multiple arrests even though most unwitnessed cardiopulmonary arrests do not respond to resuscitative measures.)

• cardiopulmonary arrests or deaths inconsistent with the patients' conditions;

• multiple cardiac or respiratory arrests in the same patient;

• cardiopulmonary arrests or deaths localized to a particular shift; and

• postmortem examinations revealing toxic levels of an injectable substance.

But why?

One of the most puzzling issues raised is that if indeed some of the nurses did hasten the death of patients, why? Only the three nurses in Maryland, Georgia, and New York confessed. None of the nurses had any history of psychosis. In only one case was an insanity defense used against the murder charges. (The Georgia nurse had been molested as a child and had had a history of entering dissociative states, a factor invalidating her confession. She was found guilty of assault. [18])

Euthanasia, or mercy-killing, emerged as a possible motive in the Georgia case. During the investigation, the nurse said she could not stand to see her patients suffer. In her confession, she said she thought the patients wanted her to help them die. She was described as a particularly compassionate nurse, and as a child she had seen her adoptive mother kept alive on life-support equipment. [19] The patients she was accused of murdering were either critically or terminally ill. Thus, an argument could be made that this nurse was motivated by compassion.

Another motive, hypothesized in the cases of nurses convicted in Michigan, California, and Texas, is psychologically complex. These nurses were described as being excited or exhilarated when participating in a code.[4,20,21] Indeed, it is satisfying to perform cardiopulmonary resuscitation well and see the patient recover. Thus, the prosecuting attorneys in the Michigan trial proposed that the nurses probably did not intend to have their patients die — they simply wanted to induce a cardiac or respiratory arrest. [22]

Another explanation offered is that some of these nurses wanted to justify the need for an intensive care unit. In Texas and Canada, investigators noted that suspicious cardiopulmonary arrests coincided with questions regarding the cost-effectiveness of pediatric ICUs.

Undue process

Another facet of these cases was the "witch hunt" atmosphere in the investigations. At least half the nurses in this study asserted due process violations. Sometimes the jury evaluated these violations during the trial, together with all other evidence, in an attempt to reach a verdict. In Michigan, the judge considered

the investigative violations sufficient to reverse the conviction. In the California case, evidence was deemed inadmissible because procedural safeguards regarding the search of the suspect's home were insufficient.[23]

In all the cases involving the media, hospital representatives may have felt compelled to provide the community with a plausible explanation for its increased death rate. Nurses can provide a ready target for investigations. They are in the hospital around the clock; they are usually the first people on the scene of an arrest; and they have access to the suspected agents. One attorney made the rather extreme comment that being accused of murder may be an emerging occupational hazard for nurses. [24]

The evidence used against these nurses almost always was circumstantial and statistical. In response, expert witnesses for the accused questioned the accuracy, for example, of postmortem toxicological examinations on bodies of patients who had died months before. Very little research has been reported on how drug concentrations change in tissues of patients after death.

Even the CDC reports include statements that limit their investigation strictly to epidemiological rather than criminal hypotheses. One investigator cautioned: "As an epidemiological study, our statistical analysis cannot answer whether intentional acts were committed against patients. No matter how strong the association between cardiac arrests and care by a specific person, a direct causal relationship cannot be proved by statistical association." [17]

These cases have had a profound impact on nursing. Communities served by the hospitals in question were understandably shaken. Families of patients whose deaths have been labeled suspicious find their grieving process interrupted for months and even years by the possibility of murder as the cause of their relatives' deaths. Trust in the care provided by these hospitals is eroded.

The whole state is usually subjected to detailed media coverage of each case. Brief and sometimes distorted vignettes of the trials receive national coverage. Follow-up, however, is often sketchy. Four times more stories were printed about the *charges* against the Nevada nurse than about her *acquittal*.

Beatrice and Philip Kalisch, discussing media coverage of the Nevada nurse's trial, pointed out that "Public reaction was no doubt further intensified by the natural sense of shock and outrage that occurs when a traditional source of good suddenly appears evil. Since nurses are entrusted with people's lives, the public has a need to believe not only that nurses are knowledgeable, but also that they are benevolent."[5] These reported scandals touch nearly everyone's perception of nurse-patient relations.

REFERENCES

1. Rothman, K.J. Sleuthing in hospitals (editorial). *N. Engl. J. Med.* 313:258-260, July 25, 1985.

2. Abramson, N.S., and others. Adverse occurrences in intensive care units. *JAMA* 244:1582-1584, Oct. 3, 1980.

3. Stross, J.K., and others. An epidemic of mysterious cardiopulmonary arrests. *N. Engl. J. Med.* 295:1107-1110, Nov. 11, 1976.

4. U.S. v. Narciso, 446 F. Supp. 252 (D.C. Mich. 1977). See also, Ann Arbor, VA nurses freed from charges. (News Section) *Am. J. Nurs.* 78:348, Mar. 1978.

5. Kalisen, P.A., and others. The angel of death: the anatomy of 1980's major news story about nursing. *Nurs. Forum* 19:212-241, Mar. 1980.

6. Buehler, J.W., and others. Unexplained deaths in a children's hospital: an epidemiologic assessment. *N. Engl. J. Med.* 313:211-216, July 25, 1985.

7. Timson, J. The anatomy of innocence. *McLean's,* May 1982, p. 17.

8. Skrove, T. Nurse could face death penalty in hospital murders. *Press Enterprise* (Riverside, CA), Nov. 24, 1981, p. A-1.

9. Istre, G.R., and others. A mysterious cluster of deaths and cardiopulmonary arrests in a pediatric intensive care unit. *N. Engl. J. Med.* 313:205-211, July 25, 1985.

10. Elkind, P. Death shift. *Texas Monthly,* August 1983, p. 106-196.

11. Nurse murders pediatric patient. *Regan Report on Nurs. Law* 27:1, Nov. 1986.

12. Sacks, J.J. *An Unexplained Cluster of Deaths in a Nursing Home.* (To be published)

13. Moss, B. Nurse pleads guilty. *Saint Petersburg Times,* Feb. 25, 1988, p. 1-B.

14. Sacks, J.J., and others. A nurse-associated epidemic of cardiac arrests in an intensive care unit. *JAMA* 259:689-695, Feb. 5, 1988.

15. Franks, Adele, and others. A cluster of unexplained cardiac arrests in a surgical intensive care unit. *Crit. Care Med.* 15:1075-1076, Nov. 1987.

16. Personal communication with the District Attorney's Office, Islip, NY, Feb. 26, 1988.

17. Downey, J. Shook convicted of first degree murder. *Winston-Salem Journal,* Feb. 26, 1988, p. 1.

18. Rachals v. State, 364 S.E. 2d 867 (GA 1988).

19. Beasley, D. Sanity expected to be key issue at murder trial of Albany nurse. *Albany Journal Constitution,* Sept. 14, 1986, p. 1-D.

20. Jones v. State, 716 S.W. 2d 142 (Tex. App. Austin, 1986), p. 158.

21. Gonzales, R: Diaz on 'emotional high' in emergencies, nurse says of Perris incidents. *Press Enterprise,* Dec. 22, 1983, p. B-3.

22. Jones, Ann. The Narciso-Perez Case—nurse hunting in Michigan. *The Nation* 225:584-588, Dec. 3, 1977.

23. Richardson, J. Diaz sues investigators, says his civil rights were violated. *Press Enterprise,* May 13, 1981, p. B-2.

24. Personal communication with defense attorney Fred Josephs, June 16, 1987.

Perils of home care

MAUREEN CUSHING, RN, JD

A CRITERION FOR measuring the cost-effectiveness of DRGs will be the incidence of readmission for the same condition or related complications. While health care executives accumulate data evaluating the wisdom of DRGs, home care nurses are left wondering whether their risk of liability has risen with the acuity of their patients.

When a patient leaves the hospital with medical problems only marginally resolved, the home care nurse's duty to thoroughly evaluate the patient, monitor any changes, and be able to recognize if and when the patient needs hospital readmission escalates. So do the liability risks of nurses caring for these "high-tech" patients on ventilators, chemotherapy, dialysis, or other regimens.

How can the home care nurse protect him/herself? At this time — which is early in the DRG movement — one has to rely on cases that are only marginally related to provide lessons for nurses practicing in patients' homes.

Is the patient OK?
In a recent case, a jury awarded a diabetic patient more than $1.5 million after he was discharged from the hospital clinically dehydrated and subsequently suffered a thrombotic stroke. [1]

The problems began when a pharmacist, refilling the man's prescription for acetohexamide (Dymelor) to control his blood sugar, accidentally gave him a bottle of the antihypertensive methyldopa (Aldomet). Within a day, the man's blood pressure dropped to 100/60; his pulse rose to 140; and his blood sugar was 307 mg/dl. His physician diagnosed that the man's diabetes was out of control and admitted him to the hospital.

At the hospital, in addition to a high blood sugar, the man had ketone bodies in his urine. At the trial, an expert witness who examined the admission lab results testified that the patient was dehydrated when he entered the hospital. Yet, he did not receive any hydrating fluids throughout his 10-day hospitalization. In fact, his dehydration was never documented on the record.

The day after the man's admission, his wife connected his illness with the prescription refill and brought the pills to the physician, who discovered the pharmacist's error. (The pharmacist also was sued.)

The man's blood pressure stayed below its usual level throughout the hospitalization, but no tests were done to determine a reason for the low blood pressure. On the evening of his discharge, the man suffered a thrombotic stroke with significant residual impairment.

The plaintiff's experts testified that, based on the patient's admission symptoms (elevated urine specific gravity, rapid pulse, abnormally low blood pressure, and fever), he was dehydrated and this had gone uncorrected. In addition, any diabetic out of control suffers from dehydration, which the high methyldopa dose would have worsened. These experts also testified that the prolonged dehydration reduced circulating blood volume, and that these circumstances combined to allow blood to clot in the small vessels of the brain, resulting in a stroke. If the stroke had happened a few days later, a nurse caring for him in the home may well have been included in the negligence claim.

What is the lesson for nurses practicing in patients' homes? When assessing this patient, the nurse would have needed to know the relevant history, including the drug error. Undoubtedly, an alert home care nurse examining the patient's lab studies would have seen, questioned, and documented what she did about the unresolved clinical findings.

In a case such as this, or where a marginally managed patient's condition deteriorates, the legal standard applicable to a nurse would be: was what the nurse did, or did not do, reasonable under the circumstances? A clear lesson is that the agency must have protocols that enable the home care nurse to get the patient back into the hospital if that becomes necessary.

Care plan. Since we don't have the scientific data needed to predict the problems most likely to occur in patients discharged but not fully recovered, a persuasive argument can be made that a reasonably prudent nurse will err on the side of safety in drafting a plan of care to prevent problems. Of course, the legal axiom that a hospital is not the insurer of patient safety can be argued so that the nurse is not the insurer against all harm that may befall a patient receiving home nursing services. In addition, the law recognizes that a home differs considerably from a hospital with all its resources to manage acute problems.

In the past, a time lag in communication between hospital care and home care was permitted. Arguably, in many instances today, written communication (alone), with its attendant delays, will be unreasonable.[2]

Who is watching?

Two physicians and a public health nurse were unsuccessful defendants in a malpractice suit in Tennessee. The facts presented at their trial offer valuable lessons in communication and patient monitoring.

In that case, a woman with diabetes and cataracts tested positive for tuberculosis.[3] The treating defendant/physician testified that he called the tuberculosis clinic at the public health department to obtain free antituberculosis medicine for the plaintiff. At that time, he spoke to the defendant/charge nurse, and they discussed the various drugs available for treatment. The nurse testified that the physician prescribed a standard combination of ethambutol and INH and that he asked her to take the drugs to the patient's home the next week.

The physician testified he told the nurse he had not treated anyone with tuberculosis for several years, and he said that he asked the nurse to place the patient on the public health department's protocol and treat her. He told the court that he believed he had turned the patient's tuberculosis management over to the public health department.

A few days later, the nurse wrote prescriptions for ethambutol and INH and took them to a part-time public health physician who signed them without seeing or talking with the primary physician. Nor did the physician ask the nurse whether the patient had any other medical problems; nor did he ask her to check the patient for contraindications.

In his defense, the public health physician successfully argued that no physician-patient relationship had been formed, thus his only possible negligence was for any breach in his duty to supervise the defendant/nurse's management of the patient. However, he could not be held vicariously liable for her negligence in failing to monitor the patient as he was not her employer.

The nurse testified that she went to the patient's home in early April and with the woman's sister present administered an eye test with a Snellen chart. She said she told the woman to watch for any loss of visual acuity and to notify the physician if she saw any yellowing of the whites of her eyes.

The woman and her sister, however, testified that the nurse did not tell the patient about blurred vision or that her eyes should be checked. In mid-July, the patient noticed she could not see aisle signs in the grocery store nor stop signs while driving, and she found that her vision was more blurred after a nap than before. She assumed that the rapid visual loss was because of her cataracts.

She did not notify anyone with the public health department and did not tell her primary physician of her eye problems until she saw him at her August checkup. The physician confirmed that the woman told him her vision was declining, but he did not refer her to her ophthalmologist.

Experts testified that if the woman's vision had been checked in August and if the ethambutol had been stopped, her vision loss probably could have been reversed. Instead, her vision decline was not evaluated until she saw her ophthalmologist two months later. He referred her to a neurologist, who immediately concluded that the ethambutol was causing her vision loss.

During the trial, the plaintiff's expert agreed that prescribing ethambutol was in accord with the standard of care, but especially because of her cataracts the woman's eyesight should have been monitored closely and any decline in vision thoroughly evaluated.

There was evidence that the standard of care required the defendant/primary physician to know which drugs the plaintiff was taking. The appeals court also said that when two or more physicians treat a patient, they are required to coordinate their findings and to communicate "in a manner that best serves their patient's well-being." The extent of the physician's involvement determines what effort he must take to satisfy his obligation to communicate.

Early discharge may increase the incidence of such unresolved medical problems, and nurses need to have solid assessment skills and professional decision-making ability to compensate for these potential problems.

REFERENCES

1. *Fultz v. Pearl*, 494 N.E.2d 212 (IL 1986).

2. *Mass. Gen. Laws Ann.* ch. 111 S51(d) requires that acute care hospitals provide written individualized discharge plans to Medicare patients or their representatives at least 24 hours before discharge.

3. *Bass v. Barksdale*, 671 S.W.2d 476 (TN 1984).

When nurses must question doctors' orders

A. DAVID TAMMELLEO, JD

MUST NURSES ALWAYS follow doctors' orders? The answer is a resounding no! In this interesting North Carolina case, a serious question arose as to whether a nurse should have questioned a doctor's order that she knew or should have known was wrong. As a result of the failure of the nurse to question the doctor's orders, the nurse's conduct was a key issue in this interesting case.

On June 29, 1981, Shirley York was 38 years old and was at term with her second pregnancy. Because her first pregnancy in 1970 required a classical Caesarean section, she was scheduled for a second Caesarean section at the hospital on July 1, 1981. She was informed by her obstetrician that in the event she should experience any sign of labor before the scheduled procedure, she should contact him and go immediately to the hospital. On June 25, 1981, Mrs. York contacted Dr. Guidetti, an Anesthesiologist and President of Piedmont Anesthesia Associates, P.A., in preparation for the surgery. She advised Dr. Guidetti that she was a repeat Caesarean patient and that she had been instructed not to labor. At 9:00 P.M. on June 29, 1981, Mrs. York began to experience labor pains and went to the hospital, arriving at approximately 10:15 P.M. She was taken to the labor room at 10:35 P.M. where she was attended to by Nurse Joan Vest. Nurse Vest took Mrs. York's history and was informed by Mrs. York that she was a repeat classical Caesarean section case. When Nurse Vest went off duty at 11:15 P.M., Nurse Shirley Danley began attending Mrs. York. Nurse Danley was likewise informed of Mrs. York's repeat classical Caesarean status.

At about midnight, Mrs. York's attending obstetrician was notified of her admission to the hospital. He ordered that she be given Seconal, a sedative, but did not come to the hospital. At approximately 1:30 A.M. on June 30th, Nurse Danley notified the doctor that Mrs. York's contractions had become stronger. The doctor arrived at the hospital sometime after 1:30 A.M. He ordered that Mrs. York be given fluids intravenously and that she be administered Stadol, a barbiturate for pain relief which has the effect of causing respiratory depression. By approximately 2:20 A.M., the fetal heartrate, which had been strong at the time of Mrs. York's admission to the hospital, could not be detected with a fetascope but could be heard with a monitor. Mrs. York was taken to the operating room at 2:35 A.M. At 3:04 A.M., Matthew Howard York was delivered by Caesarean section. He suffers from cerebral palsy and mental retardation.

The Yorks filed a complaint against the hospital, Dr. Guidetti, and other defendants, alleging that Mrs. York and her child sustained serious and permanent injuries as a result of negligent medical treatment rendered by the hospital, the anesthesiologist, and his professional association. The Superior Court, Surry County, entered Judgment for the hospital, Anesthesiologist, and Association on a jury verdict. The Court of Appeals of North Carolina held that the Trial Court's instructions on whether the child's injuries were proximately caused by the hospital's negligence were incomplete. Accordingly, the Court granted a new trial in part. The Court recognized that the thrust of the Yorks' complaint was that the rupture of Mrs. York's uterus occurred as a direct and proximate result of the hospital's failure, through its agents, to promptly and properly perform a repeat classical Caesarean section and to attend to Mrs. York's needs following the rupture of her uterus and to assemble a competent and adequate medical staff for these purposes.

The Court found merit in the Yorks' contention regarding the instructions given the jury as to whether the infant's injuries proximately resulted from the negligence of the defendant hospital and its agents and employees. Because the instructions given the jury were incomplete and potentially misleading, the Court was constrained to order a new trial on that issue. The Appellate Court noted that the Trial Court instructed the jury that if it found that the plaintiff had proven by a greater weight of the evidence that the hospital was negligent in that the hospital accepted Mrs. York for delivery of her baby by Caesarean section or that the hospital was negligent in failing to use reasonable care and diligence in treating this patient and failed to commence its duty within a reasonable time after notification, then there was a responsibility to find in favor of the Yorks.

The Trial Court's instruction specifically directed that the jury could find for the plaintiffs if the jury found that Nurse Danley breached her duty not to obey instructions of a physician which are "obviously negligent," which were deferring the immediate repeat classical caesarean section upon Mrs. York when she was in labor. This case illustrates the obligation that a nurse has to question a doctor's order when she knows or should have known that it was inappropriate. It was clear and unequivocal that Nurse Danley knew that the patient was not to go into labor and was a classical Caesarean section. (York v. N. Hosp. Dist. of Surry County—362 S.E. 2d 859—NC) (N.C. App. 1987)

Substance abuse and the nurse:
A legal and ethical dilemma

GARY MOORE, RN, PhD; RICHARD L. HOGAN, MD

RECENT PUBLICITY surrounding drug use in the U.S. has focused concern on the issue of substance abuse by nurses and other professionals. While there is little doubt about the nature of the confidential relationship established when a client presents with a substance abuse problem, dealing with a colleague exhibiting behaviors indicative of drug abuse raises a different dilemma. Disclosure of such a problem can result in consequences that range from prescribing a period of treatment and rehabilitation to having a nurse's license to practice revoked. The purpose of this column is to present a case for humane, ethical consideration of the substance abusing nurse while promoting compliance with the legal requirements stated in all state licensure laws to report such behaviors.

Fowler argues that the concept of nonmalificence and established ethical guidelines should be used by nurses in identifying and reporting colleagues with a substance abuse problem.[1] The American Nurses' Association *Code for Nurses* informs nurses that they must protect confidential information and protect the client and public from incompetent, unethical, or illegal practice by any individual.[2]

These standards are not difficult to uphold when a positive identification of drug abuse can be made from direct observation of the act of taking drugs. The public must be protected and the abusing nurse reported. Broad ethical guidelines relating to impaired nurses have been discussed. However, little attempt has been made to address how to handle individuals and individual situations. Fowler's article addresses situations where a nurse is a known drug abuser. In most situations, however, the only evidence that a problem may exist comes from observing a colleague's behaviors that are suspicious and point to the possibility of drug abuse. The nurse who suspects a colleague of drug abuse should look for changes in mood and appearance. Changes in mood generally reflect the effects of increased psychological stress, such as irritability, depression, angry or hostile behavior, self-excuses, or a blaming attitude. Changes in attendance and tardiness can also accompany drug abuse. Self-isolation is often observed at a later stage of development. Finally, and most importantly, the individual's professional performance decreases.

The individual working closely with a person in the practice arena will probably recognize these symptoms at an early stage. In order to establish reasonable grounds to show that a problem does exist, behaviors that indicate impairment must be documented. Once the behaviors are well documented, the observing colleague should share his/her observations with the individual in question while at the same time making it clear that the information must also be shared with the appropriate supervisory staff.

This initial confrontation with the nurse suspected of drug abuse can be critical for establishing either an advocacy or an adversarial relationship between the two involved parties. Fowler points out that, at this point, the nurse reporting behaviors enters into a professional relationship with the individual being reported, and suggests a stance that she labels "active advocacy."[1] Active advocacy involves the continued involvement of the reporting nurse by actively pursuing the cause of humane treatment for the offender. Such a stance serves two purposes: 1) the reporting nurse is in a position to follow through in the supportive professional relationship established with the substance abuser following the initial confrontation; and 2) the profession itself is served by identifying the impaired practitioner and protecting the public from faulty professional judgment and practice. Active advocacy permits the reporting nurse to assume a more positive role in the treatment process and allows the substance abuser to feel humanely supported throughout the treatment and recovery process.

In summary, nurses have a professional responsibility to protect the public from incompetent nursing practice. Nurses displaying symptoms indicative of drug abuse may jeopardize client safety. The nurse observing these behaviors should closely document the situation and work with the individual in a position of active advocacy to serve both as a therapeutic contact for the impaired nurse and as an agent for protecting the public and the practice of nursing.

REFERENCES

1. Fowler MD: Doctoring or nursing under the influence. Heart Lung 15:205, 1986

2. American Nurses' Association: Code for Nurses. Kansas City, American Nurses' Association, 1985

Ethical dilemmas

As NURSES, WE ARE daily confronted with ethical dilemmas — in both our work and our personal lives. Each ethical decision we make involves us in examining our personal and professional values, beliefs, and cultural backgrounds in addition to any ethics-based laws that apply to our care of clients. Thus, our ethical decision making, in contrast to our clinical decision making, derives in considerable measure from our personal and individual viewpoints on life.

When an ethical dilemma arises, the nurse caring for the client may either make the decision or assist and support the family in making it. In all instances, the nurse is required to know the law relating to ethical decision making, the options available, and the consequences of those options.

Sometimes, in order to face making a personal ethical decision, the nurse needs colleagues' support. The following vividly recounts the personal experience of a nurse when she assumed responsibility for the care of an elderly relative who had played a significant role in the nurse's life:

The telephone rang at dinner time: The nursing home was calling. My 93-year-old Aunt Emma had suffered a stroke, and I would be responsible for making decisions regarding her care.

Even though I was the responsible relative in this instance, I felt I should rely on my preparation as a health care professional in dealing effectively with the many questions that were sure to arise. My first decision was personal: to drive to the nursing home and speak with the staff in person rather than to use the telephone.

Once at the nursing home, I could see that my aunt was comatose, not responding to verbal stimulation. The staff shared data regarding her vital signs and told me that the speech therapist could find no swallowing reflex. I called the doctor, who left all the decisions to me in view of my aunt's cognitive impairment and fragile health status.

The first question was whether or not I wanted her transferred to a hospital. I chose not to hospitalize her; this meant my aunt would not receive food, fluid, or medication, because that would require new orders from a physician. With this decision made, I decided to hold all other decisions until the following day, when we could determine any change in her condition.

The next day, with one of my sons joining me for support, I participated in a conference with the staff, including my aunt's primary nurse, two clinical nurse specialists, a hospital administrator, a speech therapist, a social worker, and a chaplain.

The conference began with a review of my aunt's current medical situation. Were there any changes? What responses were noted? Then we talked about Aunt Emma's wishes. What would she want? How did we know that? What was the potential for her full recovery? How would she feel if her past condition were further compromised by this stroke? The staff shared their knowledge of similar past cases and reminded me that death is not more painful under those circumstances and may actually be less painful.

As we talked, I knew that within a few minutes I would have to decide whether or not to continue withholding food and fluids. And I knew what Aunt Emma would say. When the time came, I decided to continue withholding food and fluids. I cried, and the primary nurse cried.

I sat with Aunt Emma until she died, a day and a half later. At one point, the chaplain brought his guitar, and we held Emma's hand and sang hymns. At other times, we moved her into the day room where other residents could pat her hand. And then, around midnight, her respirations became very irregular, and in a peaceful, beautiful way, Emma died.

Have I ever regretted my decision? Never. I knew then and I know now that it was right for my aunt. Could I have made it alone? Maybe, but the support of the nursing home staff—in an important sense, my colleagues as well as caring professionals—was essential. They used their knowledge to help me make the decision that I thought Aunt Emma would want, and the group approach brought us all together in a supportive, unified way, free to *care* for Emma as she died. I know her death was more peaceful because of that group meeting.

The articles included in this chapter were selected to demonstrate the complexity of some of the major ethical issues that face the nurse — issues including caring for AIDS clients, withholding food and fluids, interpreting the dying process, telling the client lies, responding to nursing incompetence, and evaluating the ethical implications of organ donations from anencephalic infants.

The article by Brown, "AIDS and Ethics: Concerns and Considerations," discusses the need for a framework and guidelines to assist nurses in making ethical decisions regarding the care of AIDS clients. She reprints and discusses the *Code for Nurses* and explores three

controversies: individual and institutional value systems, confidentiality, and resource allocation.

Anderson, in "Death and Dying: Ethics at the End of Life," brings issues of death and dying to the fore in discussing a survey he conducted that revealed dissatisfaction among nurses with the way hospitals and society in general deal with death and dying. Besides indicating his belief that withholding information from clients and families is unethical, he details the problems confronting nurses caring for clients on ventilators and tube feedings who are irreversibly comatose, vegetative, or brain dead.

Schmelzer and Anema, in "Should Nurses Ever Lie to Patients?" review and analyze the dilemma nurses face in deciding whether or not they should lie to clients when they think the truth might be harmful. The authors cite the professional codes of the International Council of Nurses and the American Nurses' Association (ANA), as well as the Hippocratic Oath, to support their contention that nursing has traditionally tolerated lying in such situations.

Another ethical decision-making area is relationships among nurses. Cerrato, in "What to Do When You Suspect Incompetence," writes about "whistleblowers," those individuals who take the initiative in reporting colleagues' incompetent, unethical, or illegal practices. He reports the results of a survey he conducted, revealing a wide variety of nurses' reactions when confronted with incompetent co-workers. Cerrato also cites the ANA Code for Professional Nurses as a basis for making decisions about what should be reported, and when.

"New ANA Guidelines on Withdrawing or Withholding Food and Fluid from Patients," by Fry, and "California Nurses' Association Position Statement on Anencephalic Infants as Organ Donors" deal with professional guidelines for resolving ethical issues. In the former, Fry reports on the new ANA guidelines for withdrawing and withholding food and fluids from clients on life-support systems; in the latter, members of the Ethics Committee of the California Nurses' Association advocate expansion of the availability for transplantation of organs from anencephalic infants. This position statement is a good example of how state nurses associations are addressing ethical and legal issues, which often overlap.

AIDS and ethics: Concerns and considerations

MARY L. BROWN, RN, MS

SINCE ACQUIRED IMMUNE DEFICIENCY SYNDROME (AIDS) was identified and information was published by the Centers for Disease Control in 1981, about 35,000 people in the United States have developed the disease.[1] More than half were diagnosed in 1985, and by the end of September, 9563 patients had been diagnosed in 1986.[2,3] Centers for Disease Control officials predict that by 1991, the cumulative total will be 201,000 to 311,000. These same officials report that by the end of 1986, 18,000 people will have died from the disease.[1]

This epidemic and resulting public confusion create a difficult and challenging atmosphere for nurses. The decisions that need to be made regarding care of AIDS patients and the risks to health care providers and the general public force nurses to review their commitment to nursing and their individual values and beliefs. Since the demands of direct patient care and the demands of nursing management can create intraprofessional conflict, the specific concerns of staff nurses and nursing administrators need to be addressed. Ethical principles and the American Nurses' Association (ANA) *Code for Nurses*[4] provide a possible framework for decision making in considering the ethical issues surrounding the care of the patient with AIDS.

Ethical questions for staff nurses

Staff nurses in all settings may encounter patients with AIDS. The home health or hospice nurse may care for these patients in their own homes or in the homes of family or friends. The acute care nurse may provide care in a teaching institution, community hospital, or nursing home. The nurse clinician or nurse practitioner in ambulatory care may see AIDS patient in the physician's office, hospital ambulatory care facility, or community clinic. These nurses need to address the following concerns:

• What are the feelings of the individual nurse about alternative lifestyles, homosexuality and patients who abuse drugs?

• What are the consequences for nurses who refuse to care for AIDS patients?

• How can nurses examine their practices to provide confidentiality for patients with AIDS, those suspected of having the disease, or those with seropositive blood?

• How should the nurse respond to the AIDS patient requesting information about treatment or alternative therapies when recommended therapeutic interventions may be investigational or futile?

• What guidelines does the employing agency provide to assist in caring for AIDS patients?

Ethical questions for nurse administrators

Nursing administrators face other concerns. Competition for the health care dollar as well as pressure to contain costs will continue to cause stress at all levels of health care. The AIDS crisis has magnified the need to examine how shrinking resources can best be allocated. Long range planning in the face of this epidemic requires creativity, skill, and intuition. In addition, planning care for AIDS patients requires careful scrutiny of both institutional and individual values. The nurse administrator may ask:

• In this period of cost containment, how can optimum care be provided to patients who require significant resources?

• What value system does the organization have to help resolve conflicts involving the care and treatment of AIDS patients?

• What policies and procedures need to be in place to insure patient confidentiality?

• What direction is needed to provide staff nurses with guidelines and support for patient care?

• What community resources can be utilized to asist in long-term care to minimize the need for acute hospitalization?

• What guidelines need to be formulated for the staff person with seropositive blood, AIDS, or AIDS-Related Complex (ARC)?

AIDS-related ethical controversies

In reviewing the ethical concerns generated by the need to plan care for AIDS patients, three common themes are explored. These themes, though not a complete list, illustrate the controversies raised by both groups of nurses. The themes are: value systems (individual and institutional); confidentiality; and resource allocation (at all levels).[5]

The application of ethical principles can assist nurses in resolving some of these conflicts. The nurse may be further guided by the idea that ethical principles direct moral acts according to basic rational thoughts and are often used to address ethical problems in nursing.

Values: Definition, conflict and clarification

Values are the bases from which ethical decisions are made.[6] They are standards that influence behavior and are conceptions of what an individual feels is important. Nursing autonomy, professionalism and caring are examples of health care values.[7] Organizational values may often conflict with personal values. Complex health care institutions' need for efficiency, power, and authority may present barriers to the individual pursuing and perceiving nursing as a helping profession.

This incongruity between staff nurse and institution and between nurse and patient may surface when a nurse with a heavy patient assignment is asked to care for a very sick person with AIDS. The situation can be complicated by what the nurse terms as "poor staffing," but what the hospital management terms as "downsizing": the development of a sleeker, more efficient organization. Citing inadequate staffing, the nurse may refuse to care for the AIDS patient. The nurse's own knowledge about the nature of the disease, its transmission, and those who have it may create feelings of frustration and anxiety. The nurse could be caught trying to resolve conflicts in ability to provide care and conflicts in values surrounding the lifestyle of the patient. Furthermore, the nurse may be unable to conceptualize that responsibility is a value, and that it extends to patients, colleagues and the employing organization. If left unresolved, these conflicts can cause anxiety and frustration leading to increased turnover and less than acceptable levels of care.

In this situation, the nurse and nurse manager may turn to the ethical principles of nonmaleficence and beneficence. *Nonmaleficence* requires that others are not harmed (either intentionally or unintentionally) and that those who cannot protect themselves (due to age, illness or mental status) are protected from harm.[7] Unintentional harm occurs when nurses do not or are unable to practice with due care. As in the example of the busy and frustrated nurse, institutional barriers (the lack of staff) may be present, limiting the nurse's ability to practice carefully and thoughtfully.

Beneficence requires that harm is prevented; harmful conditions are removed; and good is done for the benefit of others.[7] Smith interprets beneficence as a duty by which patients are not harmed, and efforts are undertaken to benefit them as well.[7] In further attempting to resolve this situation, Item 1 of the ANA *Code for Nurses* may be considered. This statement defines the right to care: "Patients have a right to be cared for in a manner which respects their human dignity. Refusal to provide care, providing only minimal care, or making derogatory comments to or about the patient are clearly unethical. The rights of the patient and the duties of the nurse are clear (p. 28)."[4,8] Should a nurse refuse to care for a patient, provide minimal care, or treat a patient disrespectfully, the nurse manager should identify this behavior and the nurse be given assistance and the opportunity to change.

Should a nurse experience difficulty in caring for AIDS patients due to prejudices felt about homosexuality and drug abuse, the nurse is still required to provide competent and respectful care regardless of the prejudice. If the nurse expresses fears of contracting AIDS and states that there is a right to be safe from harm, it is the responsibility of the employer to provide accurate and current information, enabling the nurse to give care with minimal individual risk.

In these situations values clarification is needed; this process can be a rational one.[6] It involves developing options, deciding which option fits the needs expressed, and then making decisions based on the selected option. Making a change in values based on new information is difficult. As more is learned about AIDS, both staff nurses and administrators must think carefully about their perceptions and what risks they are willing to take as they demonstrate necessary changes in their behavior.

Managers need to be aware of the importance of values in the process of reconciling values conflicts.[7] The administrative goal can then be to develop a plan that looks for solutions and promotes positive individual and universal values.

Confidentiality: An inherent right to privacy

Many authors have addressed the issue of confidentiality and AIDS patients. While most nurses are aware of the long-standing professional obligation of patient confidentiality, the AIDS epidemic has forced this concept to the forefront of discussion. Item 2 of the ANA *Code for Nurses* expressly states that the nurse safeguards the patient's right to privacy by protecting confidential information.[4] Information may be revealed only if the patient gives permission, or if it is required by law.

Protection of patient confidentiality is a moral challenge.[9] Confidentiality is basic to interpersonal communication in general, and a respected aspect of nursing practice.[9] It enables patients to seek assistance without fear of public disclosure, preserves the patient's right to self-determination, and insures privacy. Distress can occur when confidentiality is broken to protect others. This may be in conflict with the law, and in the context of the AIDS epidemic, the issue is problematic, since physicians, hospitals and laboratories are required to report communicable diseases. Although the professional ethic is clear in matters of confidentiality, it may not be reasonable in the reality of nursing practice.[9]

Information for reporting. Confidentiality is critical for AIDS patients, as well as for those with ARC and seropositive blood. Controversy about confidentiality has arisen in two major areas: information gathered for reporting and information gathered for medical records. AIDS cases are reportable to the public health authorities in the United States, and failure to do so may result in a fine, incarceration, or loss of medical license.[10] Although states have enacted various statutes that govern reportability of patients with AIDS, ARC, and seropositive blood, problems remain. The first problem is that without comprehensive and compulsory screening, those reported would be self-selected and a small number of those infected. Second, since education has been determined as the only accepted method of controlling AIDS, the usefulness of reporting information would not outweigh the negative social and economic consequences for the infected person. [10] Revealing the identity of the AIDS patient to prior sexual contacts, to those with whom they have shared needles, or any others who may have had contact with their bodily fluids remains controversial and is not generally practiced. Further disclosure is not necessary since discrimination with regards to public services, insurance, etc. may occur. This may also be considered a fundamental violation of privacy.

Should a patient have positive HTLV-III blood test, information should only be reported to appropriate health authorities. A positive result in serologic testing for HTLV-III antibody "...should not be communicated by health professionals to any other party except the patient whose blood has been tested (p. 578)." [11] California is the only state that has enacted a law forbidding the disclosure of HTLV-III antibody tests without written permission of the person tested. This law conflicts with other legal rules permitting limited disclosure in cases of other diseases. Until this conflict is resolved, California physicians are seeking assistance from public health authorities if they believe contacts are in jeopardy. [10]

Medical records. Information gathered for medical records creates another dilemma. Patient records belong to the agency where data are collected, and the individual maintains the right of control over whatever information may be in the record. Many people have access to patient records, so institutional mechanisms to assure confidentiality need to be in place at every level. Smith believes that information needed for AIDS research (i.e., sexual preference, sexual practice, drug use) should be kept separately from the patient's record

and stored where access is limited. [8]

The nurse's ethical responsibilities to all patients are the same. To perform nursing care, nurses have a right to current and accurate information. Nurses also have a right to infection control policies which will allow them to care for persons with AIDS with minimal risk to themselves. [8] At the same time, however, nurses can function as leaders in this area, assisting AIDS patients in protecting and maintaining confidentiality. Too much may be at stake for the patient to allow this concept to be ignored.

Dwindling resources: Considerations and reality

Nurses have a moral responsibility to identify and resolve issues related to the allocation of scarce resources. How health care is distributed affects the public good, and benefiting (not harming) "...the public good in matters of health are moral obligations inherent in the social contract between nursing and society (p. 12)." [12]

Item 11 of the ANA *Code for Nurses* reinforces the concept of a social contract and the need for nursing involvement in resource allocation. This item discusses the collaboration needed between nursing, other health care professions and citizens to promote community and national efforts that will meet the health care needs of the public.

Access to even basic health care may not be economically feasible in the near future. [13] A major conflict can be predicted as society continues to demand access to health care and available resources become more limited. Many components of the health care system are under scrutiny by health care economists. Some ramifications of this scrutiny include: how the quantity and quality of resources allocated affects the health care industry; monetary losses related to illness, disability and death; and the advantages of scale economics (low costs and increased volume, costs of increased inpatient days). The AIDS epidemic, accessibility to care and cost containment are in conflict.

Ethics and access to resources. The principles of beneficence, nonmaleficence and utility may assist the nurse in coping with concepts surrounding the allocation of resources of AIDS patients. Beneficence and nonmaleficence were described earlier. The principle of *utility* may be defined by using the maxim, "One should produce the greatest good for the greatest number of people."[8] One must be cautious here, however, and it is likely that ethicists and health care providers will struggle over what goals are the most desirable, and what "good" will take precedence.

Since AIDS patients require tremendous human and monetary resources, and since the disease remains socially unacceptable, access to health care may be difficult for some patients. This accessibility, a strong value in our society, has been shown to vary in amount and kind among individuals, groups and communities.[9]

Because AIDS is currently fatal and incurable, decisions about long-term and life sustaining treatment (including cardiopulmonary resuscitation and intubation) may be influenced by the patient's decision making, socioeconomic status and response to previous therapy. Disagreements could arise among care givers who may feel differently about a 60-year-old woman with transfusion-related AIDS than they do about a young gay man with a history of IV drug abuse. Care givers should be encouraged to distinguish these value judgments from scientific facts as the goals of treatment are clarified with patients early in the course of the illness.[14]

Decisions about limiting treatment based on medical futility need to be distinguished from those decisions based on scarce resources, such as allocation of ICU beds. These decisions are probably best made through advance

planning by hospital administrators, physicians, nurses, and possibly local governments and regional health care networks.[14]

Financial considerations. Further considerations about resource allocation and the patient with AIDS center around financial implications of the disease. The American Hospital Association (AHA) estimates the average costs to be $140,000 for an AIDS patient. This includes an initial hospital stay of about 30 days, as well as other hospitalizations, ambulatory care, and home care. These cost estimates are based on increased staff time, increased use of expensive supplies, loss of revenue as hospital rooms are converted from semi- private to private, and the lack of ambulatory care options. IV drug abusers may need services related to drug use in addition to those related to AIDS care.[15] Prolonged hospitalizations are directly responsible for much of the cost incurred for AIDS patients. Few cities have community-based programs as available care options. In San Francisco-area hospitals, the availability of alternative care has decreased the average length of hospital stay to 12 days. This is in sharp contrast to New York City public hospitals that average a 50-day hospital stay.[15]

To illustrate costs even more, the AHA notes that the first 9000 AIDS patients cost about $1.25 billion, while cost for new AIDS patients this year will be about $2.25 billion. Revenue lost in the treatment of an AIDS patient is $5214 per admission, 3.4 times more than the uncollectible amount for an average patient with a different diagnosis.[15]

As the number of AIDS patients increases, few hospitals will escape the financial burden. Since hospitals are already feeling pressure about costs from government, third party payers and business, a disastrous outcome could occur if the insurance industry changes the benefit structure for AIDS patients.

When considering the ethical issues related to costs incurred by patients with AIDS, work is needed to identify what costs are appropriate and legitimate. Insurers using actuarial tables to set life insurance premiums are finding these tables to be distorted by AIDS, since the disease strikes a relatively young population (68% are between 20 and 39 years old).[15] Many insurers, interested in protecting themselves from claims involving policies issued to those already sick with AIDS or likely to contract the disease, have considered many people with AIDS antibodies as unacceptable risks.[15] Since seropositive blood indicates only exposure to the virus, this practice has led to the enactment of legislation in some states that forbids the use of blood test to deny insurance to people who have been exposed to AIDS. A major confrontation is likely to occur between insurance companies and those who say it is unfair to deny insurance to those at risk of contracting AIDS. The insurance industry claims that without pre-screening the financial impact will be crippling to their industry. As for concerns about privacy and AIDS testing, insurance industry leaders claim they have a good record for keeping confidential information.

Under the best circumstances, the AIDS patient will be working when diagnosed and will be covered by a company insurance policy for several months after quitting work. Many AIDS patients can work until the final stages of their illness. At the time, the patient may obtain state disability if that option is present in the state of residence, or the patient may be offered private rates to maintain coverage. This second option, however, is often too expensive. In many states, the patient must deplete all personal resources before applying for public assistance that will support health care costs for catastrophic illness.

Nurse's role. Nurses can make a strong statement about the process of distributing care. The nurse executive and staff nurse can work together to use ethical principles, the broad scope of nursing knowledge, and nursing care documentation to aid in determining accessi-

bility, how resources will be allocated, and how the safety of the patient and general public will be affected. If nurses do not actively participate in this process, other groups will develop resource distribution policies in which the AIDS patient may not be represented. This could have disastrous results, given what is known about the epidemiology of the disease and the predicted numbers of patients who will need care in the future.

A framework for decision making

Although Items 1, 2 and 11 have been previously discussed, the ANA *Code for Nurses* can be further utilized in helping to resolve dilemmas identified by nurses caring for AIDS patients.

The ANA *Code for Nurses* defines the primary goals and values of the profession. The preamble states that the code itself is, "...based on a belief about the nature of individuals, nursing, health, and society (p. i)."[4] It complements the definition of nursing in the ANA *Social Policy Statement*[16] and stresses that the "...goal of nursing actions is to support and enhance the client's responsibility and self-determination to the greatest extent possible (p. i)."[8] Given that the most fundamental moral principle is respect for other people, the Code and its interpretive statements provide behavioral direction for nurses performing nursing activities and responsibilities consistent with professional ethical obligations and high quality nursing care.

Each item in the Code may be pertinent to the AIDS patient at some point along the illness trajectory. While the Code does not assure professional practice for each nurse, it does provide general principles to guide and evaluate nursing actions. All of this can help reassure patients in general and AIDS patients in particular that ethical decisions are not made in a vacuum — that the professional nurse has the collective conscience and philosophy of nursing available as responsibilities are discharged.

The Code discusses respect, privacy, and patient safety. It provides support for the nurse assuming responsibility for nursing actions and judgments. It discusses the many roles of the nurse and encourages the individual nurse to contribute to the body of nursing knowledge. The Code voices the need for nursing standards in settings conducive to high quality care and it provides direction for nursing's effort to protect the public from misinformation while promoting health.

Conclusion

The obligation of health care providers in caring for patients who have a lethal disease is based on moral, ethical, and historical perspectives. Although nursing responsibilities to care for the patient are clear, many difficult times are ahead as the AIDS epidemic gains momentum.

Nurses in clinical and management roles will need to carefully evaluate ethical issues as they arise. Many of these issues will take long periods of time to resolve, since there are few precedents and few guidelines. Ethical theory can continue to provide the conceptual base and the ANA *Code for Nurses* can assist in providing a framework of general principles that can aid in directing actions.

Society will continue to look to the helping professions for support as more segments are affected by AIDS. Nurses can fulfill their professional obligations to patients and use the greater body of nursing knowledge to complement actions.

The nurse caring for AIDS patients requires two dominant characteristics: courage and impartiality.[17] Courage is needed to confront risks, particularly in facing an illness that poses a threat. Impartiality is needed to temper prejudice. The gay lifestyle and drug culture associated with most AIDS patients are not well understood or accepted by many people. The need is to provide astute clinical management without concern about the patient's lifestyle. The person with AIDS is an individual — an individual in need of a courageous and impartial nurse.

REFERENCES

1. Barnes, D. Grim projections for AIDS epidemic. *Science* 232(4):1589-1590, 1986.

2. Bennet, J. AIDS: epidemiology update. *AM J Nurs* 85(9):968-972, 1985.

3. Centers for Disease Control. *Mortality and morbidity weekly report (MMWR)* 35(39):615, 1986.

4. American Nurses' Association Committee on Ethics. 1983-1985. *Code for nurses with interpretive statements.* Kansas City, MO: American Nurses' Association, 1985.

5. McFadden, C. *Medical ethics.* Philadelphia: F.A. Davis Company, 1968.

6. Steel, S. AIDS: clarifying values to close in on ethical questions. *Nursing and Health Care* 7(5):247-248, 1986.

7. Binder, J. Value conflicts in health care organizations. *Nurs Econom* 1(2):114-119, 1983.

8. Smith, S. AIDS: ethical duties of nurses. (In) *Ethics: Principles and Issues.* San Francisco: California Nurses' Association, 1985, p. 28.

9. Fry, S. Confidentiality in health care: a decrepit concept? *Nurs Econom* 2(6):413-418, 1984.

10. Special Report: The acquired immunodeficiency syndrome: infection-control and public health law. *N Engl J Med* 314(14):931-936, 1986.

11. Health and Public Policy Committee, American College of Physicians and the Infectious Disease Society of America. Position Paper: Acquired Immunodeficiency Syndrome. *Ann Int Med* 104(4):575-581, 1986.

12. Silva, M. Ethics, scarce resources, and the nurse executive. *Nurs Econom* 2(1):11-18, 1984.

13. Curtin, L. Ethics and economics in the eighties. *Nurs Managem* 15(6):7-9, 1984.

14. Steinbrook, R.; Lo, B.; Tirpack, J.; Dilley, J.; Volberding, P. Ethical dilemmas in caring for patients with the acquired immunodeficiency syndrome. *Ann Int Med* 103(5):787-790, 1985.

15. American Hospital Association, Infection Control and Environmental Safety Committee. *AIDS.* Chicago, IL: American Hospital Association, 1986.

16. American Nurses' Association. *Nursing: a social policy statement.* Kansas City, MO: American Nurses' Association, 1982.

17. Jonsen, A. Ethics and AIDS. *Bull Am Coll Surg* 70(6):16-18, 1985.

Death and dying: Ethics at the end of life

DAVID ANDERSON

ISSUES OF DEATH AND DYING force more difficult choices on nurses than any other area of ethical decision making. The reasons are plain enough. The hardest cases present no comfortable alternatives.

Dedicated to relieving suffering, nurses experience distress when CPR and other traumatic interventions are used to revive patients whose subsequent condition allows neither satisfaction nor comfort.

Devoted to nurturing humanity, nurses can become frustrated when tending patients who are irreversibly comatose, vegetative, or brain dead on ventilators and tube feedings. A comment made by more than one survey respondent points to an even deeper psychological response to the situation they have been put in — loathing: "I have seen patients literally rot from the inside while on ventilators!"

Just as strongly, however, all nurses feel reverence for life. They can't forget there's no bringing a patient back once a decision is made to forgo or stop treatment.

Our survey revealed that most nurses are dissatisfied with the way their hospitals and this society deal with these issues. Our round table participants tell how thoughtful, engaged nurses can improve the lot of their terminally ill patients and their own as well.

Useless codes: torment and despair

Six survey respondents in 10 have participated in resuscitation efforts they considered senseless or hopeless during the past year. They gave many vivid examples:

"Premature infants weighing under two pounds are sometimes kept alive for several days when it's obvious they don't have a chance."

"A patient who had been in a coma for eight years began to have GI bleeding and was given pint after pint of blood."

"An 81-year-old man with cancer metastases to the brain came to the ED with a ruptured abdominal aortic aneurysm and they repaired it."

"A patient with end stage AIDS received multiple resuscitations."

No matter how futile some interventions seem, however, round table panelists caution nurses against projecting their values on patients. "In the eyes of the law," Frank Reardon stipulates, "it's what the person in the bed thinks, not what the nurse thinks. You could really say, 'Isn't this the nurse playing God by saying these things are senseless and hopeless?'"

Some survey respondents seem to be falling into this trap. Thus, one regrets that "In the neonatal ICU many infants are kept alive only to be severely retarded" — without stopping to reflect that some people want to parent their children whether they are handicapped or not.

Other nurses may be inappropriately dismayed to see, for example, "80-plus patients who lie in bed all day in nursing homes, no life to speak of, placed on ventilators, pacemakers, and dialysis." These nurses may be creating conflict for themselves by not understanding the range of accommodation people can make with advancing age.

Phyllis Taylor underlines the need to evaluate the person, as well as the diagnostic and prognostic information in judging whether a situation offers hope or not. She tells of once

---

Senseless codes: Specialty makes a difference...as does education

As might be expected, nurses who work in critical care and the emergency room are more likely to report having participated in what they consider senseless or hopeless codes during the last year than their colleagues who work in units where patients aren't so sick. Nurses in the ICU, CCU, and ER also report seeing more hopeless codes: The survey average is just under four such instances a year; yet 25% of ER nurses and 18% of ICU/CCU nurses report 10 or more.

SPECIALTY	% PARTICIPATING IN SENSELESS CODES
ICU/CCU	91%
ER	87
Geriatrics	77
Med/surg	66
Pediatrics	45
OBG/newborn	24
All respondents	**61**

LEVEL OF EDUCATION	% PARTICIPATING IN SENSELESS CODES
Associate	69%
Diploma	53
BSN	61

---

supporting aggressive coding despite knowing it could add no more than a few days to a cancer patient's life. "This woman desperately wanted to be able to hear Kol Nidre, which is the most haunting chant of Yom Kippur, the holiest day in Judaism. For her husband, too, this was terribly important."

Reasons for hopeless codes

Survey respondents report that superfluous, demoralizing life support measures are very common despite the fact that some 90% of their hospitals have policies concerning Do Not Resuscitate orders. Why?

Sometimes a DNR order doesn't accompany the patient from one area of the hospital to another, or go home with the patient. As a result, uninformed health-care workers in the other departments or EMTs are likely to attempt unwanted resuscitation.

To prevent this, hospitals are now developing systems whereby DNR orders physically travel with patients. When patients go home, Phyllis Taylor reports, "some physicians write the orders on prescription slips for patients to carry at all times. Other institutions coach families never, never to call for rescue.

"But none of these solutions is completely satisfactory. One problem is that new environments and the passage of time can bring new perspectives; how, then, can people be sure that the patient has not had a change of mind?"

Most misapplied codes, round table panelists agreed, come about because, in the words of Phyllis Taylor, "the vast majority of people are not being asked what they want for themselves in case of emergency — or else they're being asked in a way that sets them up to answer one way or another. For example, 'You would want us to help, wouldn't you, if your breathing stops or your heart stops...' Or, 'This is your mother; we have to do this for her.'"

How nurses view doctors' roles

Survey respondents report many reasons why doctors fail to discuss or implement DNR options despite official policy. Some are sympathetic, some understandable, and others reprehensible.

An OR nurse from the South notes that doctors' inaction is sometimes based on empathy: "Physicians keep 'dead' patients on life support until the family is ready to accept the situation."

Frequently, however, it is the doctor who can't accept the loss of a patient. "Doctors try to prolong life because otherwise they feel they are failures," says an OR nurse from the mid-Atlantic region, and that observation is echoed by other nurses throughout the country.

Unresolved personal attitudes about death and unrealistic expectations of oneself lead to impasses where, as an ICU nurse puts it, "Doctors are unable to approach the family for a DNR, thinking it will reflect badly on them."

"The fear of malpractice suits has caused doctors to go 'above and beyond' in caring for patients," writes another OR nurse from the South, expressing an insight shared by many. This self-protective rationale for overtreatment will become less attractive as the public learns more about the often violent or chilling nature of the interventions necessary to keep terminally ill patients going, Frank Reardon predicts. "Hospitals have already been sued for resuscitating patients against their will," he says.

A few nurses agree with some physicians who believe that the goal of medical progress

justifies using unknowing terminal patients for training or experimental purposes. "You know someone will die within a few days, and major teaching hospitals need pathology to work on," one nurse reasons. More, however, are justly horrified that, in the words of another, "many patients who have no relatives appear to be guinea pigs; if they have no money the attitude is, 'Let's try this!'" Subjecting patients to interventions that offer them no potential benefits clearly violates the Hippocratic oath.

Some nurses accuse doctors of denying patients death with dignity for reasons of self-interest. "Patients are being kept alive just to line the doctor's pockets," declares a New England pediatric nurse. "Some doctors perform unnecessary — and expensive — surgery after establishing that the patient is terminal," claims a med/surg nurse from the Far West.

Our panelists confirm that such unscrupulous practices exist. Referring to cases in which hospitals have sued to avoid a family's request to withdraw feeding tubes, Patricia Murphy summarizes an observation that's advanced by Frank Reardon: "The cases they bring to court are the ones where they're getting $150,000 a year from insurance, and if they give up that patient they might get a Medicare patient instead."

Whenever doctors withhold from patient and family the means to make informed decisions regarding their own best interests, it is unethical. When the reasons for withholding are unscrupulous, nurses are made doubly miserable. Not only are they ordered to inflict pointless indignities on their patients, but they must also witness a cynical subversion of the healing professions.

Individual nurses acting as patient advocates can sometimes help individual patients and families in such situations. More comprehensive and permanent improvements can be achieved by nurses working together with hospital ethics and quality assurance committees

---

When there's no DNR

Partial codes—chemical code only, code but no intubation, intubation but no compression—and "slow" codes are both ways of avoiding what otherwise might be seen as a hopeless code. The former lets everyone concerned feel like they're doing something. The latter puts the nurse on the ethical hot seat.

Fortunately fewer than three respondents in 10 have participated in slow codes in the past year. Partial codes are becoming more common, however, and in both cases, it's the nurses in critical care and the ER who are most likely to be in those situations.

SPECIALTY	% PARTICIPATING IN	
	PARTIAL CODES	SLOW CODES
ICU/CCU	87%	48%
ER	57	40
Geriatrics	50	41
Med/surg	39	30
Pediatrics	26	19
OBG/newborn	13	11
All respondents	**43**	**27**

---

to create and enforce rules against such practices.

Before concluding that a patient is receiving inappropriate treatment, however, make sure that you have all the relevant information. Sometimes poor communications can make things seem worse than they are. Phyllis Taylor illustrates that point: "A young man with AIDS was comatose, and the surgeon scheduled a brain biopsy. The nurses were furious. But when we told the doctor that we absolutely needed to know why he was going to do this, he had a good reason for this course of action. The biopsy would tell him if the patient had a lymphoma, which it would be pointless to treat given the extent of his illness, or toxoplasmosis, which might yield to quick treatment, improving the quality of the life he had left."

Partial codes and slow codes
Partial codes are designed to prohibit interven-

tions that patients deem to be intolerable — for example, ventilation or compression — but guarantee every other measure, including food, fluids, and meticulous hygiene, necessary for life support and comfort.

Physician, patient, and family alike are spared having to make an all-or-nothing, life-or-death decision. They're also relieved of a common fear identified by panelist Mila Aroskar: "In some institutions, patients with DNR orders legitimately worry that they'll be more or less abandoned."

Our survey demonstrates that partial codes are becoming common practice, with some 43% of respondents having participated in them. However, it does not indicate that partial codes are delivering the hoped-for benefits. Nurses in the South — with the highest percentage of nurses reporting involvement in partial codes — also report the highest incidence of inappropriate codes. Nurses in the West, who are least likely to report partial codes, also report the least number of useless codes. These figures suggest that nurses believe even the interventions performed in partial codes are unwarranted. It makes little sense, for instance, to continue pushing drugs when the heart is no longer pumping them into the body.

When doctors want to issue a DNR order but they're unable to persuade the family to agree, they sometimes pass along the word that the patient is a "slow code." Nurses are then expected to take their time responding if the patient arrests. Over the years, slow codes seem, unfortunately, to have become an entrenched bad habit in some hospitals.

One nurse in four says she participated in slow codes last year. Nevertheless our panel was unanimous in branding the process unethical. "I don't think there is any defensible rationale for a slow code," says Phyllis Taylor. "It's unfair to the nurse, wasteful of her time and skills, unfair to the patient, and financially wasteful." From the legal viewpoint, Reardon added, "It could be really hot. Anything that falls below standard medical practice is malpractice."

The nurse's role: Listen first, then act

The key to preventing superfluous codes is understanding that, in Frank Reardon's words, "It's not senseless or hopeless if the patient and family have dealt with it and said, 'I think this is good.'" As communicators, nurses have a vital role to play in implementing this principle for each patient.

First, they should try to see that every patient is assigned a code status. Patricia Murphy, for example, helped write a policy dictating just that for her facility. Healthy patients who come in for a minor procedure such as a tonsillectomy may be assumed to want resuscitation, but the onus is on physicians to ask patients with more serious conditions what their wishes are.

While nurses in some institutions fear disciplinary action if they initiate DNR discussions without a doctor's go-ahead, they can urge physicians to initiate such discussions and lobby for a team approach. The nurse can be effective, Murphy points out, whenever a patient alludes to the subject. "I write in black ink, on the chart, exactly what the patient has said: 'Mary said she does not want to be a vegetable.' And then I tell the doctor about it."

Phyllis Taylor offers guidance for instances when a doctor seems reluctant to raise the DNR issue. "I might approach him and say, 'So and so said this to me; it's clear he's thinking about these things; what is the status?' If the physician doesn't respond I might go to our nurse manager, then the ethics committee. I might work my way up the established hierarchy of the hospital, but I wouldn't let it drop. To do so would be to settle for what I feel is poor nursing practice."

When a doctor approves of the nurse discussing a DNR order with the patient, Taylor continues, it's important to frame the discussion in a non-threatening way. "Say: 'This is something to think about, not for now, but for the future. We'll do everything we can to make sure it's a long way in the future, but if it should happen, what do you want?'"

Second, nurses need to recognize the special contribution they can make to the often difficult no-code decision. As Patricia Murphy points out, "What we are about is assessing what patients and their families want and then helping them to implement those wishes. Some patients are especially eager to share with their nurses a lot of themselves, who they were and what they wanted to be, and what they want in relation to their disease." This relationship, together with superior interpersonal skills, make a nurse invaluable in patient care conferences, especially when there is a deadlock between doctor and family.

A prerequisite for success in such efforts is

Who makes treatment decisions?

Nurses believe strongly that a patient should decide ultimate questions for himself: 87% agree that terminal patients have the right to refuse all treatment. When it gets down to specific treatment measures, however, fewer are willing to grant the right to refuse tube feeding. Nurses who care for geriatric patients are most willing to recognize their patients' right of self-determination.

	% WHO BELIEVE PATIENTS HAVE A RIGHT TO REFUSE	
TREATMENT	ALL RESPONDENTS	GERIATRIC NURSES
Tube feeding	83%	94%
Mechanical ventilation	93	100
CPR	93	100

---

an ongoing relationship with your institution's ethical policy-making body, argues Frank Reardon. "What you want to do is work with generic issues, to try to get the institution to set up satisfactory guidelines for when it's appropriate to withdraw respirators from long-term care patients. Doing things on a patient-specific basis is the worst, the absolute worst, because emotions go right through the roof and everything blows up."

Today more than ever before, determined and skillful nurse advocacy can obtain better consideration for terminal patients, relief from the emotional burden of inappropriate codes, and curtailment of abuses. "Seven years ago," remarks Reardon, "most physicians would have seen sitting down with the patient and going through all of this as a waste of time. Now, I think they realize that it's part of medicine."

Patricia Murphy confirms, "It's been a long time since I ran into a doctor who refused to write a DNR order. Cost-effectiveness is making a big difference. Having these discussions prior to a tragedy or emergency saves money over the long run."

And Mila Aroskar remarks that, "More families are asking about DNRs before the health professionals bring it up." The public is also more willing to face the formerly unfaceable.

Soul searchers: Euthanasia, suicide

Nurses' most agonizing problems arise when patients refuse treatment or express the wish to terminate treatments that are keeping them alive. "I took care of a 94-year-old lady who was coherent and wanted to die but was kept on a respirator. Her hands were tied so she wouldn't pull out her trach." This writer is a med/surg nurse from New England, but such painful incidents occur everywhere.

Overwhelmingly, nurses believe that patients should have the right to refuse both CPR and mechanical ventilation. They express slightly more hesitation about the right to refuse tube feeding. Nursing's ambivalence seems to parallel that of the courts, which have sometimes held that removing mechanical ventilation *allows* a patient to die from his disease, but withholding nourishment more actively *causes* death from starvation. Significant opinions within the nursing community and the courts have recently rejected this stance, however.

Mila Aroskar and her colleagues, who were

Where nurses stand on active euthanasia

Eight out of 10 respondents agree that modern medicine needlessly prolongs the death of too many patients. Yet only two in five would approve a law that would allow terminally ill patients to request active euthanasia by lethal injection. Judging from the responses from the Far West, however, nurses who live in California—where such a law was recently proposed—might be more inclined to pass the measure.

	ALL RESPONDENTS	THOSE IN FAR WEST
Campaign actively for the law	4%	7%
Vote for, but not campaign	34	40
Campaign actively against	10	10
Vote against, but not campaign	41	37
Probably not vote	11	7

---

on the 1985-1987 American Nurses' Association ethics committee, adopted the position that, "since competent, reflective adults are generally in the best position to evaluate various harms and benefits to themselves...their refusal of food and fluid should generally be respected." In a landmark, right-to-die case, *Brophy vs. New England Sinai Hospital,* Frank Reardon successfully argued that a comatose patient's wife and family have the right to insist that feeding tubes be withdrawn on the grounds the patient would have wanted it.

The more active an intervention to effect death, however, the fewer nurses condone it. Euthanasia by lethal injection is certainly more active than terminating treatment, and only four nurses in 10 would favor its authorization in a bill such as the one that was recently petitioned in California.

Sooner or later, laws or no laws, many nurses face the question of euthanasia. A nurse from the Midwest, for example, gives a typically heartbreaking account: "An 80-year-old patient came to us last year bedridden, arms and legs contracted, weighing 80 pounds. When asked what we could do for her, she al-

ways answered, 'Put me to sleep.' She went back and forth between hospital and nursing home seven times before she finally died."

Round table panelists responded very personally to the question of active euthanasia.

"If you have somebody who literally is in unimaginable pain, where the very best pain control we have doesn't help, it's not clear to me that it's not the most humane thing to do," Mila Aroskar postulates. "But I still don't know that I would do it — probably not. On the other hand, it scares me to death that there seem to be a lot of people who have the impression that, if a person has had a long life, it's OK if they die. I think we have to have great concern about misuse of so-called mercy killing!"

"I've been asked to kill people," Phyllis Taylor says. "My position is that I have no problem providing whatever is needed to alleviate pain, even if it depresses respiration. But I can't administer a drug for the express purpose of killing. I've also heard the question raised about whether to help a patient set up IV lines or tell them what dosages will be lethal so they can take them on their own. Even though I think it would be ethical to do so if the patient was not coerced and understood what was happening, I could not do it. I might give such a patient the address of the Hemlock Society, however, since I believe in her right to make that decision."

"Sometimes," cautions Patricia Murphy, "patients who ask what drug dosage will kill them are really trying to communicate something else. Obviously, a person who's receiving a little bit of morphine every day knows that taking the whole bottle will do the job. It's the nurse's responsibility to recognize this and try to find out what's really going on in that patient's mind."

Two nurses, both from the Great Lakes states, neatly sum up the dilemma that modern medicine, with its ability to sustain bodily functions indefinitely, has presented to soci-ety. One writes, "Why prolong the inevitable? It only makes it harder on everyone." The other writes, as if in reply, "Life is precious, and miracles do happen."

It is in the area between these two attitudes that nurses must define their personal and collective convictions on the complex issues of death and dying. Once their minds are made up, they need to employ their skills as communicators to implement them into patient care situations, and to incorporate them in their institution's policy manuals and mechanisms such as ethics and quality assurance committees. Educating the public to express their wishes through such instruments as the Living Will and Durable Power of Attorney will impact forcefully in favor of appropriate and ethical decision making.

Should nurses ever lie to patients?

MARILEE SCHMELZER, RN, PhD; MARION G. ANEMA, RN, PhD

NURSES MAKE NUMEROUS value judgments in a day, sometimes after careful consideration, at other times with little thought. Schroeck (1980) noted that nurses give more attention to ethical issues such as abortion, organ transplants and human experiments, which they rarely confront, than to ethical problems involving patient rights and the abuse of professional power, which they confront daily.

One dilemma that nurses often face is whether or not to lie when the lie might benefit the patient. For example, Lemay (1985) tells of how he lied to his patient in order to support her in her grief. The author, a registered nurse, was caring for an elderly man who was dying; the man's wife had suffered a myocardial infarction and was in another part of the hospital. One day, seeing that Mr. Laning was about to die, Lemay called the wife's ward to have her come immediately, but he died before she arrived. Other members of the family were at the bedside. Remembering that Mrs. Laning was nearly blind, Lemay suggested letting her believe that her husband was still alive, and the family agreed. When Mrs. Laning entered the room in a wheelchair, Lemay brought her to her husband's bedside. She lifted her husband's still warm hand to her lips and said "Darling, I'm here with you." Lemay assured her that everything had been done to keep her husband comfortable and then said, "His respirations are going down. I think he waited for you to come." A few minutes later, Lemay said that Mr. Laning has stopped breathing.

Mrs. Laning began to cry softly and so did the other family members "after having been so brave during those long 10 minutes." As the woman left the room, she said to Lemay, "Thank you. I'm so glad George waited for me." The author described how he wept afterwards and added that he "couldn't regret the lie that had given Mrs. Laning a chance for fewer regrets in the lonely months of grief ahead."

Veracity and beneficence

An ethical dilemma is a conflict between two ethical principles, in this case veracity (truthfulness) and beneficence (doing good). The nurse was willing to lie, violating the principle of veracity, because he thought a lie would benefit Mrs. Laning more than would the truth.

Historically, there has been disagreement about whether or not such behavior should ever be condoned. Immanuel Kant believed that lying could never be justified because it was always harmful, if not to a particular person, then to mankind in general. Kant (1981) said that everyone has a strict duty to be truthful even if the truth might be harmful: if harm results from the truth, it is an accident, but if harm results from a lie, the liar is responsible.

Veatch (1981) agreed that telling the truth is essential for human interactions: "It is disturbing to see these fundamental elements of human interaction compromised, minimized, and even eliminated supposedly in order to keep from harming the patient" (pp. 57-58).

A contemporary ethicist, William Frankena (1973), makes beneficence one of the guiding principles of his ethical theory. Beneficence, he says, includes four components:

1. One ought not to inflict evil or harm.

2. One ought to prevent evil or harm.

3. One ought to remove evil.

4. One ought to do or promote good.

Frankena argues that #1 takes precedence over #2, which in turn takes precedence over #3, and #3 takes precedence over #4, other things being equal.

Rather than seeing a conflict between veracity and benevolence, however, Frankena (1973) sees veracity as being directly derived from the principle of beneficence. No rules are absolute, he says, including the rule that one must tell the truth. Yet according to Frankena some actions — for example, lying — are intrinsically wrong and can be made right only if they are necessary to avoid a greater evil.

Bok (1978) agrees that there are times when lying is justified; she describes a method of weighing the good and bad consequences of a lie to decide whether or not it can be justified. However, she also recognizes the difficulty of determining how much weight to give each consequence. Further, Bok views lies as being intrinsically wrong and suggests giving them a negative weight before comparing their benefits with those of the truth. In situations where a lie is one choice, she says, individuals must first seek truthful alternatives.

Bok (1978) notes the vast differences between how liars and those deceived perceived the benefits of a lie: liars believe their actions to be benevolent, but those deceived feel resentful, suspicious and distrustful when they learn of the deception. Initially, says Bok, the liar appears to have no self-interest in the lie. However,

> on closer examination...the benevolent motives claimed by liars are then seen to be mixed with many others much less altruistic — the fear of confrontation which would accompany a more outspoken acknowledgement of the liar's feelings and intentions...the urge to maintain power that comes with duping others (never greater than when those lied

to are defenseless or in need of care). (pp. 223-224)

While excusing their lies as being in the immediate best interest of the person lied to, Bok (1978) continues, liars fail to recognize the long-term effects of the lie. One consequence is the liar's own loss of credibility and thus diminished power over others should the lie be discovered. And even an undiscovered lie is stressful for the liar to bear. Additional lies may become necessary, and future temptations to lie are harder to resist.

According to Bok (1978), tolerance of lying also damages the system that allows it. Lies are successful only in an environment where truth is expected, and every lie diminishes the credibility of the truth. Bok notes that many patients have heard stories of deception by health care professionals and have seen deceptions themselves. The result is an expectation that they will be lied to. But all lying is detrimental to health care, where trust is essential.

Bok (1978) is concerned that there is also the risk of exploiting or manipulating the one deceived, especially when the person lied to is in a situation where judgments and actions depend on information from others. Finally, as Zembaty (1981) suggests, a lie robs individuals of their reality and of the opportunity to learn from experience.

Health care professionals have traditionally tolerated lying when they thought the truth would be harmful. The emphasis has been on beneficence and nonmaleficence, not on veracity, as witness the professional codes including the Hippocratic Oath, the World Medical Association Declaration of Geneva, the International Council of Nurses' Code for Nurses, and the 1976 American Nurses' Association Code for Nurses.

Gillon (1985) claims that nurses and physicians often justify lying by saying that in health care the whole and absolute truth is seldom known, making it ridiculous to talk about the truth; or bad news should be withheld to avoid causing additional stress to a severely ill person and thus precipitating death; or patients do not really want to know when their situation is hopeless — they want the truth withheld.

Refuting the first of these reasons for lying, Gillon (1985) argues that the moral question is not whether or not the information is absolutely true, but whether or not the person sharing the information believes it to be true. The second justification may have merit, says Gillon, if the evidence is overwhelming that the news will have harmful effects. The weakness of this argument, however, is that health care providers are not particularly skillful at measuring the benefits and consequences of lying. In addition, Gillon suggests that denial protects people from harmful information that they are unprepared to hear. Bok's (1978) research indicates that the third reason for lying is also faulty. The few studies done have consistently shown that patients want more complete information than nurses and physicians think they do. It may be that health professionals are not always truthful because it is so difficult to share bad news, especially news related to dying. They may also fear the patient's reaction to such information.

Paternalism

Willingness to lie may also be related to the paternalistic attitudes of health care workers toward their patients. According to Zembaty (1981) paternalism is "interference with a person's autonomy justified by reasons referring exclusively to the welfare, good, happiness, needs, interests, or values of the person being constrained." It comes from Fotion's (1979) idea that parents who constrain their children act with the intent of benefiting them. When Mr. Lemay lied to Mrs. Laning, believing it

was in her best interest, he was behaving paternalistically.

Fromer (1981) suggests that hospitalized patients are especially vulnerable to paternalistic behavior from nurses because they have lost much of their autonomy. They must wear hospital gowns; their movements are confined to specific places in the hospital; and they may leave only with permission. Their injury and illness promote dependency and further diminish their autonomy.

Although paternalistic treatment has benevolent motives, Zembaty (1981) warns, it is not always beneficial. Differences in values and inability to judge another's needs may cause paternalistic behavior to fail. Nurses' perception of what is best for a patient is based on their assessment of the situation, but they are also influenced by their role within the system and their attitudes toward sickness and death. The patient's attitudes may differ considerably from those of the nurses. Further, health professionals have insufficient knowledge of patients' psychological makeup to judge their reactions. Bok (1978) adds that health professionals can underestimate patients' abilities to cope with their situation and make judgments based on generalizations that contain a good chance of error. Thus paternalism fails because it is based on false premises and insufficient knowledge.

The paternalistic model of health care is becoming less acceptable to patients as they become more aware of their rights and demand to be actively involved in their treatment with full knowledge of their condition. Moreover, nurses are beginning to support patients' quest for greater autonomy. Recognizing that paternalistic lying interferes with autonomy, Livingston and Williamson (1985) have developed a model for truth telling as a nursing intervention.

The truth-telling model

According to Livingston and Williamson

(1985) nurses have several options including the whole truth, partial truth, silence, lying and decision delay. First, nurses assess whether or not their patients have the age, maturity, and mental competence to make their own decision. If not, the nurses may assume a paternalistic attitude. But if the patients can decide for themselves, the nurses next assess their patients' values regarding health care, their information needs, involvement in decision making and long-term goals.

The nurses then examine their own values, knowledge and interpersonal skills. (They may conclude at this point that it would be best for another person to deliver the information to the patient and will then find someone else to do it.)

Next, the nurses consider the various options for truth telling. The whole truth is given when everyone including patients and family, nurse, physician and institution all value truthfulness; patients have asked specifically to be told the truth; and the risks of knowing the truth are minimal, although the news may be uncomfortable for the patients.

The situation is more difficult should the family and physician wish to protect the patient from bad news, but the nurses believe that the patients want true information and have the right to it. The nurses must then collaborate with the others involved to try to reach a consensus.

A second option is to provide the partial truth, that is, to give only the information requested, without elaborating. Nurses first discover what their patients already know and carefully assess what they want to know. Silence is a third option. There is no intent to deceive, but the nurses delay temporarily giving information.

There are also rare circumstances when lying is necessary to prevent serious risk to the person's health. The final option, decision delay, is used when the nurses have too little

knowledge of their patients' values and prior information or when they believe that their patients are not the appropriate persons to give the information. Nurses promise their patients that they will try to get the information or to find an appropriate person to talk with the patients.

Although Livingston and Williamson describe several options for truth telling, they view anything but the whole truth as only a temporary measure. They also emphasize that all information should be shared using good communication skills, including active listening, empathy and kindness.

These authors also offer suggestions for evaluating the truth-telling intervention. They ask first whether or not the nurse followed personal and professional values. Were ethical principles applied to the decision-making process? Was the client carefully assessed prior to the intervention? Did the nurse collaborate with other primary care givers and the patient's family? Was the intent of the interaction to increase respect and self-determination for the patient, and did the nurse communicate this effectively? Did truth telling enhance the patient's well-being? How do we know? What behavioral and emotional behaviors did the patient demonstrate after the intervention? What self-knowledge has the nurse gained, and how will this affect the practice?

Was the lie justified?

Clearly, Livingston and Williamson (1985) would not have condoned the lie described by Lemay (1985). They emphasized careful assessment of patients' ability to act autonomously, their values regarding health care and their desire for information. The authors encourage nurses who are unfamiliar with their patients to find someone who knows them well enough to communicate the information effectively. In the case described, however, Lemay, the nurse, had never met the dead man's wife and made his decision to lie based on her blindness and his expectation that the lie would contribute to more therapeutic grieving.

Further, Livingston and Williamson consider lying a temporary measure to prevent harm or death. But Lemay never intended to tell Mrs. Laning the truth, although there was no evidence that the truth would have been harmful. Finally, according to Livingston and Williamson, a basic goal of truth telling is to increase the patient's self-determination. But Lemay's intervention decreased Mrs. Laning's autonomy by manipulating the situation and thus her response to it.

Gert and Culver (1979) developed several criteria that can be used to determine whether or not a paternalistic lie is justified.

1. The lie benefits the person lied to; that is, the lie prevents more evil than it causes for that particular individual.

2. It must be possible to describe the greater good that occurs.

3. The individual would have wanted to be lied to: if the evil avoided by the lie were greater than the evil produced by it, the person would be irrational not to want to be lied to.

4. We would always be willing to allow the violation.

These criteria are useful in deciding whether or not Lemay should have lied to Mrs. Laning. The first criterion stipulates that the evil avoided must be greater than the evil produced. In this case Lemay did not consider the possibility that the lie might be harmful. Yet Mrs. Laning's relationship with her husband's family might be damaged if she were ever to discover that they had deceived her. Further, she might never again trust nurses; this trust is especially important when one is hospitalized and dependent on them. Also Lemay told Mrs. Laning that her husband waited for her, implying that he was able to delay his death. If she ever discovered the truth, she might be angry with her husband for not waiting to die. And

even if she never learned of the deception, her fundamental right to experience and control her own life was violated.

The family could also suffer. They participated in the deception for ten long minutes, which must have been distressing. They also must bear the burden of the lie for the rest of Mrs. Laning's life. Lastly, the family members learned that nurses lie, and they would possibly be distrustful if they were ever hospitalized.

Gert and Culver (1979) also stipulate that the benefits of a lie must be describable. Mrs. Laning's statement, "Thank you. I'm so glad George waited for me," suggests that she benefited from the lie. However, knowing that her husband was terminally ill, she may already have realized that she might not be with him when he died. Thus the deception was perhaps unnecessary.

A third criterion is that the individual would have wanted to be lied to. Despite blindness and old age, Mrs. Laning had managed to care for her husband at home and maintain control over her own life. It seems unlikely that she would have wanted someone to take advantage of her blindness and lie to her.

The final criterion is that we would always be willing to allow the violation. The lie was possible only because the woman was blind. If we were willing universally to allow such lies to the blind, their autonomy and ability to cope with their disability would be greatly diminished.

We can only conclude that Lemay should not have deceived the woman. The possible benefits did not outweigh the potential harm, and Mrs. Laning would probably not have approved of the lie. Universal acceptance of this practice could produce abuses, particularly for the elderly and the blind, and further decrease the public's trust of health professionals.

Thus nurses should be committed to telling

the truth and, when faced with situations where they are tempted to lie, should instead seek alternative actions based on honesty. The nurse can share the truth in a caring, supportive way, as suggested by Purtilo and Cassel (1981):

> Underlying the bias towards greater disclosure of information is the conviction that if the health professional, both verbally and through his or her actions, conveys the message that he or she still cares and has the intention and ability to comfort, then it is possible to tell the truth and still maintain the patient's trust and hope. Benevolence is expressed through honesty, rather than played off against it. (pp. 74-75)

REFERENCES

Bok, S. (1978). **Lying: Moral choice in public and private life.** New York: Vintage Books.

Fotion, N. (1979). Paternalism. **Ethics, 89**(2), 191-198.

Frankena, W. (1973). **Ethics.** Englewood Cliffs, NJ: Prentice-Hall, Inc.

Fromer, M.J. (1981). **Ethical issues in health care.** St. Louis: C.V. Mosby.

Gert, B., & Culver, C. (1979). The justification of paternalism. **Ethics, 89**(2), 199-210.

Gillon, R. (1985). Telling the truth and medical ethics. **British Medical Journal, 291,** 1556-1557.

Kant, I. (1981). On a supposed right to lie from altruistic motives. In T. A. Mappes & J. S. Zembaty (Eds), **Biomedical ethics** (pp. 61-64). New York: McGraw-Hill Book Company.

Lemay, C. (1985). No regrets. **Nursing 85, 15**(2), 96.

Livingston, D., & Williamson, C. (1985). In G. Bulechek & M. Aydelotte (Eds.), **Nursing interventions: Treatments for nursing diagnoses** (pp. 365-384). Philadelphia: W.B. Saunders Company.

Purtilo, R., & Cassel, C. (1981). **Ethical dimensions in the health profession.** Philadelphia: W.B. Saunders Company.

Schroeck, R. (1980). A question of honesty in nursing practice. **Journal of Advanced Nursing, 5,** 135-148.

Veatch, R. (1981). Models for ethical medicine in a revolutionary age. In T.A. Mappes & J.S. Zembaty (Eds.), **Biomedical ethics** (pp. 51-55). New York: McGraw-Hill Book Company.

Zembaty, J. (1981). A limited defense of paternalism in medicine. In T.A. Mappes & J.S. Zembaty (Eds.), **Biomedical ethics** (p. 57). New York: McGraw-Hill.

What to do when you suspect incompetence

PAUL L. CERRATO

IN A LAWSUIT-CRAZY WORLD, reporting incompetence can trigger a nasty legal battle with an embittered co-worker. Even without threat of legal action, whistle-blowers may fear being ostracized or may be troubled by the nagging question: What will happen to my colleague's career — or my own — if I speak out?

Given the potentially serious repercussions, how can a nurse fulfill the duty — cited in the profession's code of ethics — to safeguard patients by reporting "incompetent, unethical, or illegal practice by any person"? What criteria distinguish incompetence from a lapse of clinical concentration? Do certain situations justify not reporting a nurse or doctor who's made an error?

Our survey responses and suggestions from our panel may bring our own values into focus, equipping you to handle such questions.

Who's likely to see the shortcomings?

Six nurses in 10 who responded to our survey say they hadn't seen any patients harmed in the past month because of errors or incompetence. This suggests that the majority of nurses and doctors are competent, a notion supported by the general level of care in the U.S. Interestingly enough, though, the tendency to detect incompetence can change radically with a nurse's background.

AD and BSN respondents, for instance, are much more likely than diploma nurses to say they've seen patients harmed in the past month. Is this the result of educational preparation? Perhaps, but bear in mind that diploma nurses as a group have been in practice longest, and the survey respondents with the most experience are also most likely to say they have not seen patients endangered by other caregivers.

If that's the case, are veteran nurses battle-weary, and thus more inclined to ignore what's going on around them because they feel it's futile to try changing the system? Or do their many years of experience bring keener insights into what actually endangers patients — what's worth being concerned about — and what really constitutes incompetence?

What makes the difference?

Members of our panel shed light on the crucial distinction between error and incompetence. Patricia Murphy recalls that "when you're first out of school, you think that everyone is incompetent because they're not perfect. But the longer you're out there on the job, the more you realize the difference between simply making mistakes and real incompetence."

In Phyllis Taylor's experience: "People who are incompetent, physicians and nurses both, are those who repeatedly make the same mistakes. They either have no idea that they are doing something wrong, or they have a rationale that lets them say it's really all right. Those people are very dangerous — and very different from a person who makes a mistake and says 'Oh my God, what have I done? How can I learn from this so I don't do the same thing again?'"

An ICU nurse in a small urban hospital feels the same way. She will report an incident when "the person making the error brushes it off as if it were not a problem at all." Panelist Mila Aroskar adds that if there's an attempt to cover up something that jeopardizes the patient's welfare, you've got a good clue that you are dealing with incompetence and not an isolated mistake.

Many of our survey respondents, too, emphasize that an error is a single event while incompetence is a pattern of events. A nurse from the Great Lakes region puts it this way: "I report any and all acts of incompetence, but I only report the errors that can put patients at risk."

Unfortunately, the law is much less forgiving. Attorney Frank Reardon explains: "What's tough about the law is that it doesn't give you one free bite. You can be the best OB for 50 years, but make one serious mistake, and the law will call it incompetence."

Given that kind of legal system, it's easy to understand why many RNs think twice about reporting their colleagues: Although 91% of survey respondents say they would report an incident that either harms patients or puts them at risk, only half actually reported all the incidents they'd seen. That's a big difference between theory and practice.

Why do nurses keep silent?

Many respondents say the severity of the error is important in deciding whether or not to report a colleague, but an OBG nurse with more than 15 years in practice adds another dimension. Her decision to report errors depends on "the severity of the error and whether or not the person committing it is usually a good provider, or one who acts as though he doesn't care about patients."

Personalities and relationships enter into other nurses' decisions with varying degrees of ethical validity. A nurse who works in a large university hospital on the West Coast considers the impact of an incident report on a colleague's career. On the opposite coast, a med/surg nurse in a suburban community hospital asks the same sort of question: "What will the repercussions be to the persons involved? Will they be suspended, maybe fired?"

An AD graduate at a public hospital admits that she might say nothing about an error that was committed by a close friend of her supervisor. A BSN at a private non-profit hospital factors in the disposition of her supervisor — who, she explains, "can be very moody." An ICU nurse at a university hospital in the Great Lakes region tells us: "I must admit it depends on how much I like the nurse or doctor."

Phyllis Taylor points out that this kind of thinking contradicts a basic tenet of nursing ethics. "My first obligation," she feels, "has to be to the patient; he's most vulnerable; he puts his trust in me. My responsibility to my colleagues comes second."

Fellow panelist Mila Aroskar acknowledges that loyalty can sometimes be a major obstacle to reporting incompetence — particularly in the OR, where team spirit is so strong — and she suggests putting the emphasis back where it belongs: "You're documenting risks to patients, not just labeling someone as incompetent." Taylor adds that the nurse who remains silent may not be doing a colleague any favor: "We have to help people see that it is not being loyal or helpful to the incompetent person to allow that kind of incompetent behavior to continue."

After 11 years in practice, a head nurse at a rural community hospital finds such considerations moot: "I used to encourage the staff to cover themselves with an incident report, but administration is so apathetic that I've given up." This kind of burnout has obviously not hit the nurses at the opposite end of the spectrum: those who report every incident.

Must you tell all?

A number of our survey respondents say they report all errors, regardless of the nature of the mistake, the past performance of the practitioner, or whether a patient suffered any harm. A BSN working at a Southeastern hospital argues persuasively for going strictly by the book:

The incidence of harm to patients

Fortunately, six nurses in 10 report that they'd seen no situations recently where patients were harmed because of the errors or incompetence of doctors or nurses. And the percentages of incidents involving physicians and those involving nurses are virtually identical. Nurses are slightly more likely to report an incident caused by a physician, however, than one that could be laid at a nurse's door. The most notable exceptions: Nurses in hospitals with more than 600 beds are much more likely to say they've seen harm caused by physicians—and much less likely to report harm caused by nurses. Perhaps large hospitals have more residents, who presumably have a lot to learn, and nurses in those hospitals may see little point in getting a nurse in trouble if they see doctors cause more of it.

| | % WHO'VE SEEN INCIDENTS OF HARM TO PATIENTS BECAUSE OF | |
NUMBER OF INCIDENTS	PHYSICIAN ERROR	NURSE ERROR
None	59%	59%
3 or fewer	35	34
4-9	5	6
10 or more	1	1

| | % WHO'VE SEEN NO HARM TO PATIENTS BECAUSE OF | |
NUMBER OF INCIDENTS	PHYSICIAN ERROR	NURSE ERROR
None	22%	17%
Less than half	17	19
More than half	11	15
All	50	49

"An error is an error no matter how minor. It should *always* be reported so that the person responsible can learn from his or her mistake."

An urban diploma nurse is equally adamant: "I've worked 10 years in critical care and have never changed my opinion: *All errors reported.*" Her stance is common among nurses in the ICU or CCU, where relatively small errors of judgment can prove disastrous, but the same kind of adamancy is found on other units as well. A nurse working with geriatric patients in the suburbs speaks from 15 years' experience: "I make no choices. I report all errors."

It's true that hospital policies frequently leave no leeway for choice, but it's also true that professional ethics allow for some selectivity in reporting. In interpreting its own code, the ANA says that a nurse's first move should be to talk directly to the erring caregiver, pointing out the potential danger to patients. "If indicated, the practice should then be reported to the appropriate authority within the institution, agency, or larger system."

When would reporting not be indicated? Survey respondents cite specific instances that, again, reflect the differences between error and incompetence. A med/surg nurse from a suburban hospital, for example, says she might

---

Recognizing error and incompetence

How critical a nurse is of others' performance may depend on the kind of education she's had and the number of years she's been in practice. Diploma nurses are much more likely—and those in practice longest are slightly more likely—to say they haven't seen any harm to patients in the last month because of error or incompetence of doctors or nurses. Whether that's a function of seasoning tempering judgment—diploma nurses tend to have more experience—or differences in course work is hard to say.

| | % WHO'VE SEEN NO HARM TO PATIENTS BECAUSE OF | |
EDUCATIONAL PREPARATION	PHYSICIAN ERROR	NURSE ERROR
Associate degree	55%	52%
Diploma	69	71
BSN	54	56

| | % WHO'VE SEEN NO HARM TO PATIENTS BECAUSE OF | |
YEARS IN PRACTICE	PHYSICIAN ERROR	NURSE ERROR
Less than 2	58%	52%
3-5	54	55
6-10	55	57
11 or more	63	64

---

skip an incident report if "the patient wasn't harmed and the clinician committing the mistake readily admitted to it when approached." An RN at a large proprietary hospital agreed, adding that she wouldn't report someone who was eager to take measures to prevent a recurrence. Others say they might not report a colleague who had been severely overworked when the error was made.

Overall, however, these nurses readily admit that dealing directly with a co-worker is only a first step. A med/surg nurse sums up the situation: "If discussion with the offender doesn't correct the habits that led up to the error, then I'm forced to report the person."

Other RNs counter that not reporting all errors, regardless of how minor they may seem, could set the stage for more serious trouble down the line. Nurses on the next shift, for instance, might not immediately recognize the delayed complications of an error that's left unreported.

That argument is clarified by returning to the idea that reporting is done to protect the patient, not punish the caregiver. In choosing not to report a specific incident, a nurse must have total and well-founded confidence in the clinical judgment that foresees no harmful complications. Without that, there is indeed no ethical choice but to file a report.

What will ease the reporting burden?
The panelists acknowledge that fulfilling the duty to protect patients can cause terrible friction among colleagues. Phyllis Taylor remem-

bers: "That's exactly what happened to me on my very first job. I thought the patients were getting lousy care, and I began to raise questions.

"They said, 'Write it down,' so I did. I lasted seven months as a patient advocate. By the end nobody would eat with me, not one nurse would talk with me, and I finally wound up injuring a patient because nobody would assist me when I asked.

"It was a patient on a Stryker frame who needed to be turned. The other RNs refused to help me — three times — and told me to ask an aide. I finally did, and the patient slipped, lacerating his foot. Their refusal to help came as a direct result of my advocacy for patients. It was just horrendous, and I thought long and hard about leaving nursing."

Instead, though, Taylor left that hospital: "I vowed then that I'd never work again in an institution where the administration wouldn't back me and where I couldn't find allies who'd help and support and care."

Panelist Mila Aroskar believes that kind of support can be provided by incorporating a basic premise of nursing into the system: "We need to create a working environment in which patient welfare is the primary goal — by overpowering the personal agendas and relationships that cause so many repercussions.

That was the idea we tried to get across on the ANA ethics committee. People should not be left out there by themselves. They should feel the freedom — and the obligation as employees — to bring their problems to somebody's attention, and they should expect to have their observations taken seriously. It goes against the grain of nursing to punish people for supporting the patients' welfare and safety."

Taylor agrees but suggests that support should be extended as well to the person who's being reported: "I'll work to make sure that there's a way to help, not just penalize. I'll report caregivers who are drug addicted — whether it is alcohol, or pills, or needles, or whatever — but I also want a program to help the impaired nurses get back on their feet."

Whatever the nature of the support, Taylor emphasizes it cannot be manufactured at a moment's notice: I'd like to see nurses talking *now* about how we can support each other when there are concerns about incompetence — whether it's clinical ignorance, drug addiction, organic brain syndrome, or whatever the issue.

"If we can have structural safeguards in place before we are thrown into a crisis by a colleague's incompetence, none of us will be left out alone and all of us can fulfill our primary responsibility to our patients."

New ANA guidelines on withdrawing or withholding food and fluid from patients

SARA T. FRY, RN, PhD

THE INCREASING USE of life-sustaining technologies in the care of patients has created unprecedented moral and legal questions in health care during the past decade. These questions are central to the reports of legislated public commissions and congressional offices, decision-making guidelines issued by ethics groups, and even the court records of celebrated legal cases. [1-6]

More recently, the question of whether technology-supported nutrition and hydration can be legally and morally withdrawn or withheld from patients has produced professional and public concern. This has been debated by ethicists, lawyers, physicians, and nurses. [7-18]

Of particular concern are the roles of physicians and nurses in decisions to withdraw or withhold food and water from patients. On March 15, 1986, the Council of Ethical and Judicial Affairs of the American Medical Association issued a *Statement on Withholding or Withdrawing Life Prolonging Medical Treatment* declaring that life-prolonging medical treatment and artificially or technologically supplied respiration, including nutrition and hydration, may be withheld from a patient in an irreversible coma even when death is not imminent. [19] In January 1988, the Committee on Ethics of the American Nurses' Association issued its *Guidelines on Withdrawing or Withholding Food and Fluid,* stating, in essence, that there are few instances under which it is morally permissible for nurses to withhold or withdraw food and/or fluid from persons in their care. [20]

These statements/guidelines from both professions will undoubtedly provide direction to physicians and nurses in patient care decisions.

However, neither document is without problems, especially when families are involved in decisions about withdrawing or withholding treatment. This is especially true in decisions involving patients who either did not or cannot make their wishes known. The ANA statement, in particular, may confuse some nurses about their roles in treatment decisions that involve withdrawing or withholding food and fluid from patients *and* the circumstances under which such action might be considered morally permissible.

The purpose of this article is to analyze critically this important document of the ANA Committee on Ethics and to compare its content with the reports and guidelines recently issued by other groups on the subject of terminating life-sustaining technologies, particularly nutrition and hydration, in patient care.

The President's Commission Report, *Deciding To Forego Life-Sustaining Treatment* (1983) focused on the ethical, medical, and legal issues in treatment decisions and made important recommendations for treatment decisions involving vulnerable patient groups such as those who lack decision-making capacity, those with permanent loss of consciousness, seriously ill newborns, and hospitalized patients in need of resuscitation. The report considers life-sustaining treatment broadly and does not discuss nutritional support and hydration separately.

However, the President's Commission report does distinguish between withholding and withdrawing life-sustaining treatment. The term "withholding" refers to not starting treatment, while the term "withdrawing" refers to stopping treatment after it has been started.

While the commission did not make any moral distinction between withdrawing and withholding, it suggested that greater moral justification might be required for withholding treatment because such a decision is made without the knowledge of positive effects from the treatment. In other words, the decision to withhold is always based on surmised effects of the treatment. Withdrawing treatment, on the other hand, is based on actual evidence that a treatment is not helpful to the patient.

This means that stopping a treatment is *not* morally more serious than withholding a treatment and generally has no legal significance in the context of the professional-patient relationship, a common concern of physicians and nurses once treatment has started. As the commission's report points out, "whatever considerations justify not starting should justify stopping as well."[2] Thus, while the terms "withholding" and "withdrawing" have different meanings and there is reason to believe that greater justification ought to be required for withholding than for withdrawing treatment, the report concludes that there is not a morally significant distinction between these types of decision where treatment of patients is concerned.

The commission's reasoning on this point has been cited in several court cases involving treatment decisions since 1983 and has been quite influential on more recent reports on withholding or withdrawing treatments from patients.

Throughout its discussions of decisions on foregoing treatment, the commission's report refers to patients with decision-making capacity and patients who lack decision-making capacity. The terms "capacity" and "incapacity" are viewed as equivalent to the legal terms "competent" and "incompetent." The report recommends that determinations of incapacity be made only when individuals lack the ability to make decisions "that promote their well-being in conformity with their own values and preferences."[1] Such determinations can be made by an informed layperson and should not be viewed as medical categories of decision-making ability. While a legal judgment of "competent" or "incompetent" may be made by a court official, this is comparable to the judgment a layperson might make — it is based on information provided by health personnel or by personal observation of the patient. As a result, the report does not distinguish between "capacity/incapacity" and "competency/incompetency." The equivalent use of these terms was *not* repeated in subsequent reports/studies on decisions on foregoing treatment.

In July 1987, the Office of Technology Assessment (OTA), Congress of the United States, issued an extensive report of its study on the use of life-sustaining technologies with elderly patients.[2] Categorizing its findings as categories of current and future resource use, quality of care, access to care, and decision-making problems and processes, the OTA study specifically notes that "the most controversial life-sustaining technology is nutritional support," and that "the highly emotional reaction to this technology obscures specific clinical, legal, and ethical questions that require resolution."[2]

The OTA study astutely notes that the most troublesome aspect of nutritional support is whether tube and intravenous feeding and hydration are merely "food and water" or a medical treatment. Presumably, if tube and intravenous feeding and hydration are "food and water," they can only be withheld or withdrawn when death of the patient is imminent or it is not medically possible to provide them. If they are "medical treatment," then they can be withdrawn under the same circumstances as other life-sustaining technologies. Indeed, most court cases involving nutritional support and hydration decisions in adult patients have held that tube and intravenous nutrition and hydration are medical treatments that may be "legally withheld or withdrawn from incompetent patients in carefully defined circumstances."[2,5,6] Unfortunately, the OTA report does not discuss or define the "carefully defined circumstances" under which nutrition and hydration might be withheld or withdrawn from elderly patients. It reports on the results of public opinion polls on the subject, the results of the OTA conducted survey on how decisions regarding nutritional support and hydration are made in selected institutions, and reports the decisions of important court cases related to the topic. However, no guidelines for withholding or withdrawing nutritional support and hydration are proposed.

The terms "withholding" and "withdrawing" are defined and the justifications discussed for withholding and withdrawing nutrition and hydration are the same as noted in the 1983 President's Commission report.

However, unlike the President's Commission report, the terms "capacity/incapacity" and "competent/incompetent" are clearly distinguished from one another in discussing patients' decision-making abilities. The terms "competency" and "incompetency" are used only in the legal sense (as determined by court decision) while the terms "capacity" and "incapacity" are used to refer to a patient's mental ability (as determined by any person or group other than a court). The study recognizes that an elderly patient who is not competent might have the capacity to make decisions on foregoing treatment, while those who are presumed competent might not have decision-making capacity.

Two important findings of the OTA study are: in practice, many patients are not involved in decisions about the use of life-sustaining technologies, including nutritional support and hydration; and the assessment of nutritional needs for an elderly patient may be difficult because "nutritional standards for the elderly have not been established."[2] Hence, the effect of deciding to withhold or withdraw nutri-

tional support, when an elderly patient is concerned, is always ambiguous. No one really knows the extent to which withholding or withdrawing nutritional support will, in fact, hasten the patient's demise. More than likely, these findings will compound the ethical and legal confusion concerning the withholding and withdrawing of nutrition and hydration from elderly patients.

The stated purpose of the *Hastings Center's Guidelines on the Termination of Life-Sustaining Treatment* is to provide ethical "guidance on the use of life-sustaining treatments," to "guide moral reflection and judgment" in treatment decisions, and to "provide a framework to structure decision making and to ensure consideration of the relevant facts and values."[3] The *Guidelines* have no legal status but do have normative power in that they clarify what conduct is ethically prohibited, permissible, and/or required.

The *Guidelines* provide clear definitions of key terms and a general guideline to the decision-making process in treatment decisions. Life-sustaining treatment is defined as "any medical intervention, technology, procedure, or medication that is administered to a patient in order to forestall the moment of death, whether or not the treatment is intended to affect the underlying life-threatening disease(s) or biologic processes."[3] Hence, methods of providing nutrition support and hydration to patients are medical interventions that may be foregone in some cases under the same conditions that other life-sustaining medical interventions (ventilators, antibiotics, etc.) may be foregone.

Decision-making capacity is defined as "(a) the ability to comprehend information relevant to the decision; (b) the ability to deliberate about the choices in accordance with personal values and goals; and (c) the ability to communicate (verbally or nonverbally) with caregivers."[3] The *Guidelines* use the terms "capacity" and "incapacity" to refer to the patient's functional ability to make informed health care decisions according to personal values rather than "competence" and "incompetence," which are legal terms applied to patients as a result of a judicial proceeding. Patients may be legally competent but lack decision-making capacity for a particular treatment. Likewise, a patient may be declared legally incompetent but still have decision-making capacity. The same distinctions are used in the OTA study.

The *Guidelines* assert that decision-making capacity is choice-specific (for one treatment choice but not necessarily for another) and is a process standard (patient capacity is assessed during the decision- making process). The use of a process standard of decision-making capacity is clearly one of the best features of the *Guidelines*. It is a standard that respects a patient's self-determination and that recognizes fluctuating levels of patient capacity over time. A patient's decision-making capacity only falls into the incapacity range when caregivers lose certainty about the patient's capacity or when the patient's capacity is clearly inadequate "in light of the gravity of the consequences at stake" for a treatment decision.[3] In terms of the significance of providing nutrition and hydration to patients, the *Guidelines* note that the provision of food and water to individuals has both symbolic and psychological significance and can be the means for a patient to obtain comfort and satisfaction. Yet, the *Guidelines* recognize that such treatment may be foregone while other supportive care measures are provided to keep a patient comfortable and free from pain. Hunger and thirst can be relieved in a patient "without necessarily using medical nutrition and hydration techniques and without necessarily correcting dehydration or malnourishment."[3]

Thus, the *Guidelines* view nutrition and hydration support as medical treatments that must be carefully evaluated on a case-by-case basis in light of each patient's individual values and careful assessment of the benefits and burdens of nutrition and hydration *for that patient.*

To make a careful and thorough assessment of any procedure to administer nutrition and hydration or to forego treatment already started, the *Guidelines* propose "time-limited trials." Presumably, such trials could determine whether a procedure will be effective and what burdens and benefits may result from either starting or stopping treatment. They would be especially helpful under unclear conditions and would enhance decision making in difficult cases where the patient's or the surrogate decision maker's wishes are uncertain.

The *Guidelines* also underscore the value of oral nutrition and hydration whenever the patient is capable of it, even when nutrition and hydration are being received by other means. This means that oral nutrition and hydration may be offered to a patient even when the decision to forego nutritional support and hydration has been made. In other words, the administration of food and water is made in response to patient desire and comfort even when it is known that oral intake will not, in fact, provide adequate nourishment for the patient.

This is a very important point to consider in the debate about treatment decisions that involve foregoing nutritional support and hydration. Many nurses are strongly opposed to such decisions because they view these decisions as prohibiting them from providing sips of water or hand feeding according to the patient's desire and comfort. The *Guidelines* are clear that foregoing treatment does not necessarily involve total abstinence from food and water. Provision of food and water is actually based on the patient's choices and an assessment of their benefits and burdens *to the individual patient.*

As a final point, the *Guidelines* clearly do not consider active euthanasia or assisted suicide under the rubric of "termination of treatment." Even when the motive is compassionate, active euthanasia and assisted suicide are strictly prohibited for the health professional. However, interventions designed to relieve suffering, even though they hasten death, are considered legally and morally permissible "if the intervention proposed serves the patient's needs better than would any alternative, and if the patient or surrogate consents."[3]

Guidelines on Withdrawing or Withholding Food and Fluid, a three-page document issued by the ANA Committee on Ethics earlier this year, focuses on the circumstances under which it is morally permissible for nurses to withhold food and fluid. Pointing out that nurses' professional and moral duties are based on "general moral consensus," the document emphasizes the moral obligation "to provide food and fluid to the needy, sick, and dependent who can be helped by it." Because of this more general moral obligation among members of society, nurses have a specific moral duty to provide food and fluid to patients under their care. As a result, the circumstances under which it is morally permissible for nurses to withhold or withdraw food or fluids from patients are very limited.

The circumstances when these actions are morally permissible are: when patients would clearly be more harmed by receiving than by withholding food and fluid; when competent patients refuse treatment, including food and water, for "good reasons"; when the provision of food and fluid is considered "futile," "severely burdensome" to the patient, sustains life only long enough for the patient to die of other more painful causes, or "inflicts suffering or harm that is not outweighed by an important long-term benefit." In all circumstances, it is expected that nurses will provide nourishment to patients in their care.

The document ends with the injunction that social and economic responsibilities from the nursing profession's position on this matter should be shared by all citizens and not just those patients and their families currently in need of nursing care. It assures the public of nursing's basic obligation to provide food and fluid to those who are most vulnerable in the health care system and the profession's willingness to honor refusals of food and water in some circumstances.

Comparison of terminology

The terms "withholding" and "withdrawing" are never defined in the ANA *Guidelines*. In fact, the withdrawing (or stopping) of nutrition and hydration from patients is discussed only in passing. The *Guidelines'* single comment on withdrawal of nutrition and hydration is that feeding should be discontinued when it is futile or brings about "suffering or harm that is not outweighed by an important long-term benefit."[20] In this comment, "feeding" is seemingly used as equivalent to "food and fluid" and "discontinue feeding" is used as equivalent to "withdrawal of nutrition and hydration."

This loose use of terminology in the *Guidelines* might be confusing to some nurses. First, the decision to withdraw nutritional support and hydration from patients is often more problematic for the nurse than the decision to withhold nutritional support and hydration. As the earlier reports point out, the initiation of a life-sustaining treatment, in general, tends to indicate a promise on the part of the caregiver to continue that treatment and creates expectations, on the part of the patient or his family, that the treatment will be continued. The implied promise and the expectations are derived, in part, from the relationship of loyalty and fidelity that is presumed to exist between the patient and the caregiver. The *Guidelines'* lack of specific discussion on withdrawal of food and fluid from patients might be disappointing to nurses who expect guidance for this often encountered and difficult aspect of care.

Second, the use of the term "feeding" to indicate "food and fluid" is confusing. The provision of fluids to many patients is specifically for purposes of hydration and not "feeding." Does the passing reference to "discontinue feeding" mean that nurses should only discontinue fluids that are, in fact, providing nourishment, or does it extend to measures that are for hydration purposes as well as feeding?

Third, the use of terms "food and fluid" seems to indicate initially that the Committee on Ethics views tube and intravenous feeding and hydration as merely "food and water" rather than medical treatment. Yet the *Guidelines, in toto,* indicate that "food and fluid" can be withdrawn or withheld under the same general circumstances supported by the other reports regarding life-sustaining technologies. This use of terminology is quite opposite the use of terminology in the OTA study, where: "food and water" is used to indicate those measures that can be withheld or withdrawn only when death of the patient is imminent or when it is not medically possible to provide them; and "nutritional support and hydration" is used to indicate medical treatments that can be withheld and withdrawn under the same circumstances as other life-sustaining technologies.

I suspect that the Committee on Ethics meant for the terms "food and fluid" to be interpreted as medical treatment that can be withheld and withdrawn under the same circumstances as other life-sustaining technologies. I also suspect that the use of the term "feeding" in the *Guidelines* really means both nutritional support and hydration rather than nutritional support alone. If this is the case, a more precise use of terms might be warranted in the *Guidelines* to clarify the correct use of the terms for nurses who look to the *Guidelines* for direction.

It would also be helpful if the *Guidelines* used key terms in accordance with their accepted use in the bioethics literature. The ambiguous use of the terms "withdrawing" and

"withholding" is especially confusing because the terms do have different meanings. However, as the earlier reports pointed out, the difference between the two terms does not have moral significance where nutritional support and hydration decisions are concerned. Since the *Guidelines* almost exclusively use the term "withholding" to discuss those circumstances under which it is morally permissible to forego nutrition and hydration, it might be argued that the *Guidelines* are demonstrating the positions of the President's Commission report and the OTA study that whatever considerations justify withholding should also justify withdrawing.

Regardless, it would be helpful for the nurse to know that the terms do have different meanings but that this difference is not morally significant. If the *Guidelines* are indicating that greater justification should be offered by the nurse for withholding treatment than for withdrawing treatment, this indication should be more explicit in the *Guidelines* as well.

The *Guidelines* have also used the legal terms "competent" and "incompetent" to refer to patients' decision-making ability. All of the earlier reports/studies on foregoing life-sustaining treatments have clearly indicated a preference for the more precise terms of "capacity" and "incapacity" in discussing decision- making ability. While the President's Commission report uses them as equivalent terms, all of the previously cited reports and most of the bioethical literature have used the terms "capacity" and "incapacity." I would prefer to see the ANA *Guidelines* use terminology that reflects ethical judgments rather than legal judgments in setting forth what is *morally* permissible for the nurse.

Given the ambiguous use of key terms and the lack of definitions for these terms, the *Guidelines* may raise more questions for the nurse than intended where decisions to forego nutrition and hydration of patients are concerned.

The issue of moral permissibility

According to the ANA *Guidelines*, nurses are expected to provide food and fluid to patients in their care *except* under the following conditions:

1. *When patients would clearly be more harmed by receiving than by withholding food and fluids.*

The concept of harm used in the *Guidelines* is a broad concept that includes not only hurt, pain, and discomfort, but also the loss of valued capacities or pleasures. It is hard to see why this concept of harm was employed in the *Guidelines* for a discussion of the particular circumstances under which food and fluid might be foregone. How would the provision of food and fluid cause the patient to lose valued capacities or pleasures ("harm" him in this sense) and thus warrant a justifiable circumstance for withholding food and fluid (in order to avoid this sense of "harm")? How would the nurse determine that a circumstance indicating harm, in this sense, was occurring? I cannot think of any circumstance in which a patient would be harmed, in this sense, by receiving food and fluid, particularly more than he would be by withholding food and fluid. It is hard to figure out the significance of the broad concept of "harm" employed in the *Guidelines* for this point. It is also the only term and/or concept defined in the *Guidelines*. Why has it been singled out for this significance?

Nevertheless, the narrow concept of harm under which it would be permissible for the nurse to withhold food and fluid from the patient is similar to the concept of harm used in earlier reports and guidelines. As the *Guidelines* note, this type of circumstance is "ethically clearcut and common."

2. *When competent patients refuse treatment, including food and water, for "good reasons."*

The right of the patient with decision-making capacity to refuse life-sustaining treatment, including nutrition and hydration, is upheld in all previous reports and studies on the topic. The ANA *Guidelines* also recognize the right of a competent patient to refuse food and fluid. The difference between the *Guidelines* and previous reports is the *Guidelines'* emphasis on the patient's reasons for refusal of food and fluid. Claiming that it is these reasons that establish the right of refusal, the nurse is obliged to ascertain and weigh the patient's reasons before respecting the patient's choice.

The "good reasons" that might be accepted by the nurse for a competent patient's refusal of food and fluid are: severe physical constraints or intractable pain; way and time to die in the face of an eventually fatal illness; and intent to draw attention to important social causes. The first two reasons are frequently used by patients in their refusals of treatment and are generally respected by caregivers, including physicians and nurses. The third "good reason," however, might be very hard for many nurses to accept and honor. What should nurses consider as an "important social cause"?

Exactly how do "important social causes" provide any patient with a right to refuse food and fluid and an expectation that such a request must be honored by the nurse?

The danger in indicating that "important social causes" constitute "good reasons" for refusal of food and fluid is that nurses might think they are obliged to assist suicide. A footnote in the *Guidelines* on this point claims that suicide attempts do not necessarily entail a refusal of food and water and that suicide intervention by the nurse should include the provision of food and water "until the patient's reasons for the suicide attempt can be ascertained." This footnote, however, does not clear up the ambiguity of whether or not a suicide attempt, in the form of refusal of food and fluid, for an "important social cause" should be honored by the nurse. The *Guidelines* tend to suggest that in the event that a suicidal patient refuses food and water for an important social cause — a "good reason" for refusal — the nurse is obliged to honor the request! I cannot believe that the ANA Committee on Ethics really intends to advocate explicitly that nurses should assist in suicide even though such suicide attempts are for "important social causes."

By leaving the interpretation of what constitutes "important social causes" up to the individual nurse and the individual patient, the ANA Committee on Ethics has seemingly created an opportunity for any patient who is not declared incompetent to expect nurses to honor his refusal of food and fluid if he can convince the nurse that he is doing so for an "important social cause." It is hard to see that refusal of food and water for these reasons can carry the same moral weight as the other cited reasons.

What the Committee on Ethics should have done is make a distinction between termination of treatment, in general, and active euthanasia and assisted suicide. While the line drawn between termination of treatment and active euthanasia and assisted suicide will always be ambiguous, at best, it is important to make the distinction in professional documents. Assisting suicide and active euthanasia are forbidden in our society, even when the motive for such actions is compassionate. The ANA *Code for Nurses* specifically states that the nurse "does not act deliberately to terminate the life of any person."[21] In the *Guidelines*, the distinction should be made clear so that nurses are not confused about the circumstances under which it is morally permissible to participate in treatment decisions involving withholding or withdrawal of food and fluid from patients.

3. *When the provision of food and fluid is considered "futile," "severely burdensome" to the patient, sustains life only long enough for the patient to die of other more painful causes, or inflicts suffering or harm that is not outweighed by an important long-term benefit.*

The President's Commission report argued that life-sustaining treatments are expendable if they are useless or if the burdens of the treatment exceed its benefits.[1] The ANA *Guidelines* seem to use these criteria for circumstances under which it is permissible for the nurse to withhold or withdraw food and fluid.

The circumstances mentioned in the ANA *Guidelines* are similar to the criteria mentioned in the President's Commission report and the circumstances recognized by several court cases for the legal withdrawal or withholding of life-sustaining treatments, including nutrition and hydration.[1,5,6] Yet the *Guidelines* seem to take the position that feeding is almost always more beneficial than burdensome. Emphasizing the general moral obligation of the nurse to provide nurturative actions to patients, the *Guidelines* conclude that the nurse should continue feeding "even when such care is not clearly beneficial so long as it is not harmful." In other words, the nurse should not withdraw nutrition and hydration in circumstances where it is not harmful to the patient even if it is not clearly benefitting him. The consequence of harm (burden), rather than good (benefit), is thus the primary criterion guiding the nurse in decisions to withdraw treatment.

This position in the ANA *Guidelines* certainly goes beyond the criteria noted in the other documents. In fact, The Hastings Center *Guidelines* argue the opposite in claiming "treatments that...simply provide no benefits may justifiably be withheld or withdrawn."[3] The ANA *Guidelines* seem to want the nurse to err on the side of continuing nutrition and hydration even when these measures do not clearly provide benefit to the patient.

Implications
The provision of the *Guidelines* is a significant step for the ANA Committee on Ethics. Treatment decisions involving withholding or with-

drawal of nutrition and hydration from patients have created moral conflict for many practicing nurses and have been some of the most difficult decisions for nurses to make or to participate in. The *Guidelines* will undoubtedly clarify some issues involved in such decisions and offer guidance and comfort to nurses who care for patients without decision-making capacity for whom such decisions will be made.

A significant value in any decision of this type is, of course, the integrity of the health professional. Nurses have a right to remain true to their own conscientious moral and religious beliefs in the face of decisions to forego treatment. Although the *Guidelines* do not mention this fact, it is certainly implied in the *Guidelines* assumption of "the common understanding of nurses' professional and moral duties." Decision making involving the withholding or withdrawal of life-sustaining food and fluid should be flexible enough to accommodate nurses' beliefs without compromising the rights of patients and the standards of care. [3] Thus, although the *Guidelines* do not mention it, nurses should realize that they can withdraw from any patient care situation as a matter of conscience, as long as the care of the patient can be transferred to others in an orderly manner and the nurse does not abandon his or her patient.

Some nurses may not ever want to participate in a decision to withdraw or withhold food and fluid from a patient, as a matter of personal conscience. In these situations, nurses should feel secure in their right to do so as long as the care of the patient is not compromised.

REFERENCES

1. U.S. President's Commission for the Study of Ethical Problems in Medicine and biomedical and Behavioral Research. *Deciding to Forego Life-sustaining Treatment: A Report on the Ethical, Medical, and Legal Issues in Treatment Decisions.* Washington, DC, U.S. Government Printing Office, 1983.

2. U.S. Congress, Office of Technology Assessment. *Life Sustaining Technologies and the Elderly.* Washington, DC, U.S. Government Printing Office, 1987.

3. The Hastings Center. *Guidelines on the Termination of Life Sustaining Treatment and the Care of the Dying.* Bloomington, IN, Indiana University Press, 1987.

4. *In re Quinlan,* 70 N.J. 10, 355 A.2d 647, *cert, denied sub nom., Garger v. New Jersey,* 429 U.S. 9ss (1976).

5. *In re Conroy,* 98 N.J. 321, 486 A.2d 1209 (1985).

6. *Brophy v. New England Sinai Hospital, Inc.,* 398 Mass. 417, 497 N.E. 2d 626 (1986).

7. Callahan, D. On feeding the dying. *Hastings Cent. Rep.* 13:22, Oct. 1983.

8. Brock, D.W. Forgoing life-sustaining food and water: is it killing? In *By No Extraordinary Means: The Choice to Forgo Life-Sustaining Food and Water,* ed. by Joanne Lynne. Bloomington, IN, Indiana University Press, 1986, pp. 118-131.

9. Childress, J.F. When is it morally justifiable to discontinue medical nutrition and hydration? In *By No Extraordinary Means: The Choice to Forgo Life-Sustaining Food and Water,* ed. by Joanne Lynn. Bloomington, IN, Indiana University Press, 1986, pp. 67-83.

10. Meyers, D.W. Legal aspects of withdrawing nourishment from an incurably ill patient. *Arch. Intern. Med.* 145:125-128.

11. Annas, G.J. Fashion and freedom: when artificial feeding should be withdrawn. *Am. J. Public Health* 75:685-688, June 1985.

12. Mishkin, B. Courts entangled in feeding tube controversies. *Nutr. Clin. Pract.* 1:209-215, July-Aug. 1986.

13. Lynn, J., and Childress, J.F. Must patients always be given food and water? *Hastings Cent. Rep.* 13:17-21, Oct. 1983.

14. Micetich, K.S., and others. Are intravenous fluids morally required for a dying patient? *Arch. Intern. Med.* 143:975-978, May 1983.

15. Wanzer, S.H., and others. The physician's responsibility toward hopelessly ill patients. *N. Engl. J. Med.* 310:955-959, Apr. 12, 1984.

16. Zerwekh, J.V. The dehydration question. *Nursing* 13:47-51, Jan. 1983.

17. Fry, S.T. Ethical aspects of decision-making in the feeding of cancer patients. *Semin. Oncol. Nurs.* 2:59-62, Feb. 1986.

18. Mumma, C.M. Withholding nutrition: a nursing perspective. *Nurs. Adm. Q.* 10:31-38, Spring 1986.

19. American Medical Association, Council on Ethical and Judicial Affairs. Opinion. *Withholding or Withdrawing Life Prolonging Treatment.* Mar. 15, 1986.

20. American Nurses' Association, Committee on Ethics. *Guidelines on Withdrawing or Withholding Food and Fluid.* Kansas City, MO, The Association, Jan. 22, 1988. (Photocopied)

21. American Nurses' Association. *Code for Nurses with Interpretive Statements.* (Publ. No. G-56) Kansas City, MO, The Association, 1985.

California Nurses Association position statement on anencephalic infants as organ donors

CNA ETHICS COMMITTEE, 1987-1989

Summary of CNA position

THE CALIFORNIA NURSES Association (CNA) supports efforts to expand the availability of organs for transplantation. However, CNA is opposed to changing California's Determination of Death Act, the Uniform Anatomical Gift Act, or other legislative efforts that would allow the use of live anencephalic infants as organ and tissue donors. It is CNA's position that the possible benefits of allowing the use of these infants as organ donors are far surpassed by the likely negative social, ethical, and professional consequences of such legislative change. The use of live anencephalic infants as donors has legal and ethical implications which have not been addressed sufficiently. CNA supports further study of these issues.

CNA does not oppose the use of anencephalic infants as organ donors when those infants have met the standard criteria for brain death, including "irreversible cessation of all functions of the entire brain, including the brain stem" (President's Commission 1981:73).

CNA opposes on ethical grounds the use of invasive medical procedures, such as ventilatory support, with live anencephalic infants when the sole purpose of the procedure is to benefit the potential organ recipient.

CNA supports further research to document the potential impact of widespread use of anencephalic infants' organs and tissues on (1) society as a whole, (2) the dying process of the anencephalic infant, (3) the pregnant woman who discovers that she is carrying an anencephalic fetus, with particular emphasis on termination of pregnancy decisions and management of labor and delivery, and (4) the impact on the family that chooses to donate and is either successful in that goal or disappointed because the infant's vital organs are unuseable.

If an individual health care institution elects to proceed with the use of anencephalic infants as organ donors while complying with current brain death legislation, CNA recommends that each institution develop a protocol to guide the treatment of these infants which takes into consideration the complex needs of the anencephalic infant, the infant's family, and the hospital staff providing direct care to the donor infant. We also strongly suggest that professional nurses be directly involved in developing the protocol to be used.

Furthermore, we recommend that individual nurses, and other health professionals who disagree on moral grounds with the use of live anencephalic infants as organ donors, be given the option to refuse to participate in the care of the donor infant.

The problem

The shortage of organs available for transplantation is particularly acute in the neonatal and pediatric age range. In order to increase the number of small organs available, the use of anencephalic infants as organ donors has been suggested and attempted in very limited circumstances (Fletcher, Robertson, and Harrison 1986; Holzgreve, et al., 1987; Blakeslee 1987). Because they have a functioning brain stem, anencephalic infants are not dead by current legal standards. If the infants are allowed to die normally, vital organs deteriorate and may become unuseable. Thus in order to harvest organs from anencephalic infants, changes would be required either in current state law, allowing the infants to be declared legally dead by virtue of their anencephaly, or in the clinical management of these infants, such as providing ventilatory support to keep organs from deteriorating.

One legislative remedy under consideration would amend the California Determination of Death Act in order to include a new category, "brain absence," as a legitimate standard for determining that death has occurred. The anencephalic infant would thus be considered legally dead, and organs could be removed. Another possible legislative remedy would be to amend the Uniform Anatomical Gift Act in order to include live anencephalic infants as a new and separate category of organ donor. Others have suggested drastic changes in the clinical management of the anencephalic infant, including treatment with advance life support for a limited time period until true brain death can be ascertained.

The goals of these proposed changes are twofold: first, they would increase the availability of organs for transplantation in newborns and very small infants where these organs are exceedingly scarce, and second, they would allow the parents of an anencephalic infant to donate the child's organs to another infant, ostensibly allowing the parents to find meaning and comfort in the face of personal tragedy. These are highly emotional issues for all concerned. At first glance, the idea of anencephalic infant organ donation seems unproblematic. There is general agreement that the anencephalic infant, if he or she survives to birth, will die within days or weeks. The needs of the potential recipients, such as infants born with hypoplastic left heart syndrome, are great. However, further reflection reveals many potential problems with allowing these infants to be used as organ donors.

Legal issues

Technological interventions may obscure the event of death. As a result, most states have adopted brain death legislation. However, as Alexander Capron (1987) points out, the current determination of death statute was not designed to change societal *definitions* of what death is, rather it was intended to allow for the inclusion of alternate *means* of determining that the same event (i.e. death) has occurred. The current law allows that the complete cessation of all brain functions, including the brain stem, can be used as an alternative means of determining cardio-pulmonary death. This legislation replaces more traditional means of determining that death has occurred — namely when the heart and lungs stop functioning — which had become obsolete because of advances in life-support technology (President's Commission 1981). The anencephalic infant, although lacking higher brain functions, has a functioning brain stem which is capable of sustaining the life of the infant for a period of time. Unlike other organ donors who must be supported by artificial means and then declared "brain dead," the anencephalic infant often breathes on his or her own. Thus functionally this infant does not differ from many other categories of patients in which the suggestion of organ donation would be morally repugnant by current standards, such as patients in a persistent vegetative state state or coma or the severely mentally retarded. Hence CNA believes that amending the Determination of Death Act in this fashion has serious implications, opening the door to abuse and actually changing our legal the door to abuse and actually changing our legal definition of what death is (not simply how death is determined). This magnitude of change in societal definitions of death should not be undertaken lightly and certainly not in connection with the issue of transplantation.

Amending the Uniform Anatomical Gift Act had equally serious consequences. Using living donors who are socially vulnerable and cannot give informed consent would radically change the organ donation process. Such a change could undermine the public trust — that organs will only be removed from the already dead — necessary to maintain an adequate supply or organs. A public policy change of this import should not be undertaken without serious public debate and consideration.

Ethical issues
There are also serious ethical implications of harvesting organs from anencephalic infants. We begin with the assumption that the anencephalic infant is indeed a person, with all the moral rights inherent in personhood. Ethical conflict arises because the desire to "do good" for the potential organ recipient conflict with the desire to respect the personhood of the donor infant. Andrew Jameton summarizes the fundamental ethical principle of respect for persons: "People are not to be treated as tools to achieve one's own or another's benefit" (1984:125). There is a strong tradition in nursing ethics that no person shall ever be used solely as a means to someone else's end, however good that end may be. The *Code for Nurses* states, "Nurses are morally obligated to respect human existence and the individuality of all persons who are the recipients of nursing action" (ANA 1985:2). Attaching a dying anencephalic infant to a ventilator exclusively for the benefit of another child violates that important nursing tradition.

We believe that anencephalic infants, although destined to die, have a right to humane care for the short period of their existence. The *Code for Nurses* dictates a moral obligation to provide care for all patients, including the severely disabled. Treating the anencephalic newborn merely as a potential organ donor

violates the infant's personhood and therefore violates basic nursing ethics.

Potential benefit to the donor infant
Although most commentators on this issue have not considered it, we also believe that it is impossible to consider this problem without "linkage" to the potential recipients of the harvested organs. Many believe that it is an automatic social "good" to make more organs available, especially for infant patients where organs are scarce. As a society we optimistically, albeit unrealistically, assume that all organ recipients will benefit. While this assumption may prove true as experience with pediatric transplants increases, serious concerns arise. First, the number of experimental transplant procedures in newborns and young infants will likely increase rapidly with ready access to harvested anencephalic infant organs. This is a new field with many inherent medical uncertainties. It may actually be preferable for this new field to proceed slowly, in order to allow a careful assessment of the risks and benefits of experimental infant transplant procedures. Secondly, the potential infant recipients of organ transplants are a category of patient that by definition cannot give informed consent to participate in experimental surgical procedures. It is, therefore, especially important to proceed cautiously with this very vulnerable population. Finally, careful evaluation of these procedures is vital because of the high monetary cost of organ transplantation. Serious questions of distributive justice arise when expensive procedures which benefit relatively few individuals are being developed.

Nursing issues
Nursing as a profession is in a unique position to comment on the impact of legislative changes or changes in accepted transplantation practices because of its position at the bedside, caring for the anencephalic infant and family throughout this tragic event. There are special

concerns for the nurses who actually care for these infants, as opposed to physicians and other professionals who may be more remote from the infant. Many nurses have expressed deep concern and have experienced personal conflict about using infants as donors who can breathe on their own. Harvesting the organs requires anesthetizing the infants and then discontinuing ventilatory support. What are the potential negative effects on nurses and other caregivers of being involved in these activities? Further study and consideration are needed.

The moral tradition of nursing, as reflected in the *Code for Nurses,* emphasizes the nurse's role as patient advocate. This advocacy role is of primary importance when considering the needs of vulnerable populations, such as the anencephalic infant.

Impact on the pregnant woman

The widespread use of prenatal screening for neural tube defects, including anencephaly, by measuring the level of alphafeto protein in the pregnant woman's blood, is also relevant to this issue. In the future more and more women carrying anencephalic infants will almost certainly be identified during early pregnancy, rather than at term or late in pregnancy. If these infants are viewed as potential organ donors, the possibility exists that women may be unduly influenced, even coerced, to continue a pregnancy for the sole purpose of donating their infant's organs.

The potential also exists that obstetrical decision-making might be complicated by the desire to maintain organs in a useable condition (Annas 1987). Increased maternal risk (such as the increased morbidity and mortality associated with caesarean delivery) should not be undertaken simply to assure the good condition of the potential donor organs. These issues also require further study. Any protocol governing the use of anencephalic infant's organs must provide adequate safeguards to prevent abuse of the pregnant woman.

The family of the anencephalic infant

Parents facing the personal tragedy of giving birth to an anencephalic infant may feel that this position interferes with their attempts to find meaning in their own infant's death by making organs available for others. This is a compelling concern. However, it is CNA's position that nurses and other health professionals should find other, less potentially negative, means of assisting the grieving family. As nurses we know that tragic events are all too common in health care, particularly in the pediatric and neonatal practice settings. Experience suggests that other means of professional support and concern may also aid the anencephalic infant's family. Finally since many anencephalic infants are stillborn, attempts by families to donate vital organs will often be thwarted (Annas 1987). What impact will this double failure — first failing to produce a normal child and then failing to redeem the tragedy through organ donation — have on families? We do not know if offering the possibility of organ donation might not actually deepen the family's grief.

Recommendations

1) CNA supports existing efforts to increase the availability of donor organs for transplantation. Nursing professional organizations should assist with efforts to increase public awareness of the need for organs.

2) CNA opposes legislation, including changes in the Determination of Death Act, the Uniform Anatomical Gift Act, or any other changes that would allow for the use of live anencephalic infants as organ donors.

3) CNA opposes the use of invasive medical techniques with live anencephalic infants, such as the use of ventilatory support, when the sole aim of treatment is potential benefit to an organ recipient.

4) CNA encourages further study, as well as extensive public debate, of the complex legal and ethical issues surrounding anencephalic infant organ donors. Studies should address the impact of these proposed changes on society as a whole, including the use of health care resources, as well as on the anencephalic infant, the infant's family, and on the health professionals involved.

5) CNA recommends that institutions considering the use of anencephalic infants as organ donors develop rigorous protocols (which incorporate ethical safeguards) to govern the process of organ harvesting and transplantation. Particular consideration should be given to the following issues as protocols are developed: (a) the impact on the dying process of the anencephalic infant, including provisions for routine comfort measures; (b) the impact of organ donation on the pregnant woman; (c) the impact on the family of planned or successful organ donation, and (d) the impact on nurses and other health professionals. And, finally, CNA strongly recommends the involvement of professional nurses in the development of these institutional protocols.

6) Because the use of live anencephalic infants as organ donors represents a significant change in transplantation ethics, some health professionals may object categorically to the practice on moral grounds; others may object in a specific instance, also on moral grounds. CNA recommends that professionals who have serious moral objections to organ harvesting from anencephalic infants, whether categorical or in a specific situation, be excused from the direct care of donor infants without prejudice. Institutional policies should provide a safe mechanism for such refusal.

REFERENCES

American Nurses' Association. (1985). *Code for Nurses*. Kansas City, MO: ANA

Annas, G.J. (1987). From Canada with love: Anencephalic newborns as organ donors? *Hastings Center Report* 17(6):36-38.

Blakeslee, S. (1987). A baby born without her brain is kept alive to donate her heart. *New York Times*, October 19, pp. 1, 10.

Capron, A.M. (1987). Anencephalic donors: Separate the dead from the dying. *Hastings Center Report*, 17(1):5-9.

Fletcher, J.C., Robertson, J.A., & Harrison, M.R. (1986). Primates and anencephalics as sources for pediatric organ transplants. *Fetal Therapy*, 1:150-164.

Holzgreve, W., Beller, F.K., Buchholz, B., et al. (1987). Kidney transplantation from anencephalic infants. *New England Journal of Medicine*, 316:1069-1070.

Jameton, A. (1984). *Nursing practice: The ethical issues*. Englewood Cliffs, NJ: Prentice Hall.

President's Commission for the Study of Ethical Problems in Medicine and Biomedical and Behavioral Research (1981). *Defining Death: Medical, Legal, and Ethical Issues in the Determination of Death*, Washington, DC: U.S. Government Printing Office.

Study questions

Chapter Fifteen

1. What is your opinion about the changes in resource allocations for poor and elderly clients? Do you agree or disagree with Popp's guidelines?

2. How would Fry's recommendations for nursing course content change your preparation for nursing? Do you agree or disagree with her suggestions? Why?

3. What is your response to Oregon's plan for rationing health care to poor clients? How would your nursing practice be affected if such a system were implemented?

4. The rationing of nursing care has an impact on your practice. Explain the ethical and legal problems that will confront nurses where staff and equipment are insufficient.

Chapter Sixteen

Review the legal implications of your practice; then answer the following questions:

5. What are the standards of care for the clients in your clinical practice? How does the nursing staff in your clinical area participate in setting the standards of care?

6. Have you ever been told to follow orders that you felt jeopardized a client's safety? If you have, what have you done to safeguard the client?

7. What would you do if you thought a co-worker was abusing drugs and engaging in unsafe nursing care practices?

8. Do you believe in supporting the efforts to prevent encroachment in your practice, or do you feel that deregulation would allow more individuals to practice nursing?

9. What are your plans for advanced educational preparation? What are your opinions regarding the need for credentialing?

Chapter Seventeen

10. How can nurses be prepared for ethical decision making? What facts are required? What supports are desirable?

11. Based on your review of the nursing research conducted in the area of ethical decision making by nurses, what research do you believe still needs to be done?

12. Does the hospital where you work have an ethics committee? If not, how are ethical decisions made? How are staff supported in making those decisions? If the hospital has an ethics committee, who is on it? Which ethical issues have they confronted?

13. What value does your school of nursing attach to the knowledge and process relevant to ethical decision making? Does it offer a course in ethics? Are students informed about ethical guidelines published by professional nursing organizations? Which prominent ethicists within the nursing profession can you list?

UNIT   FIVE

Additional assignments

1. Review the goals and issues surrounding licensure. Base your review on a historical approach to determine how the current problems developed.

2. Review current legislative activity in the state or territory where you live. Is rationing of health care an issue? How? Will you be active in supporting or defeating such legislation? Prepare a plan of action to implement your position.

3. Review articles in magazines and newspa-

pers relating to the legal and ethical issues involved in rationing health care. Determine the trends and decide how you will be affected. What plan can you initiate to have an impact on the trends?

4. Which ethical issue has troubled you the most in your clinical exposure? What are the issues? How is the hospital to which you are assigned supporting the nursing staff in confronting ethical issues? Is the support adequate? Explain your view.

Acknowledgments

The publisher wishes to acknowledge the following for permission to reprint or excerpt their articles:

UNIT ONE
NURSING AT THE CROSSROADS: LEARNING FROM THE PAST, GROWING TOWARD THE FUTURE
Orlando, Ida J. (1987). Nursing in the 21st century: Alternate paths. *Journal of Advanced Nursing* 12: 405-412.

Schlotfeldt, Rozella M. (1987). Defining nursing: A historic controversy. *Nursing Research* 36(1): 64-67. Copyright 1987, American Journal of Nursing Co. All rights reserved.

Lynaugh, Joan E., and Fagin, Claire M. (1988). Nursing comes of age. *Image: The Journal of Nursing Scholarship* 20(4): 184-190.

Diers, Donna. (1987). To profess—To be a professional. *Journal of Emergency Nursing* 13(1): 4-9, by the C.V. Mosby Co.

Holcomb, Betty. (1988). Nurses fight back. *Ms.* 6: 72-78.

del Bueno, Dorothy. (1988). The promise and the reality of certification. *Image: The Journal of Nursing Scholarship* 20(4): 208-211.

Grimaldi, Carol A. (1987). The nursing scene: A need for specialists. *1988 Health and Medical Annual*. Chicago: World Book, 353-365. Copyright 1988, World Book, Inc.

Peplau, Hildegard. (1987). American Nurses' Association's social policy statement: Part 1. *Archives of Psychiatric Nursing* 1(5): 301-307.

Spitzer, Roxane B., and Davivier, Maryann. (1987). Nursing in the 1990s: Expanding opportunities. *Nursing Administration Quarterly* 11(2): 55-61. Copyright 1987, Aspen Publishers, Inc.

Schlotfeldt, Rozella M. (1987). Resolution of issues: An imperative for creating nursing's future. *Journal of Professional Nursing* 3: 136-142.

Christman, Luther P. (1987). A view to the future. *Nursing Outlook* 35(5): 216-218. Copyright 1987, American Journal of Nursing Co.

Warner, Sandra L., et al. (1988). An analysis of entry into practice arguments. *Image: The Journal of Nursing Scholarship* 20(4): 212-216.

Nurses for the future: The yo-yo ride. (1987). *American Journal of Nursing* 87(12): 1606-1609. Copyright 1987, American Journal of Nursing Co.

Tribulski, Jean A. (1989). How you can use that federal report on nursing. *RN* 2: 61-67. Copyright 1989, Medical Economics Company, Inc.

Ortiz, Marlaine, et al. (1987). Moving to shared governance. *American Journal of Nursing* 87(7): 923-926. Copyright 1987, American Journal of Nursing Co.

Allen, David, et al. (1988). Making shared governance work: A conceptual model. *Journal of Nursing Administration* 18(1): 37-43.

O'Grady, Tim P. (1989). Shared governance: Reality or sham? *American Journal of Nursing* 89(3): 350-351. Copyright 1989, American Journal of Nursing Co.

Miller, Richard. (1988). Staff nurse councils, shared governance, and collective bargaining. Speech given at Wisconsin Nurses Association convention, Green Bay, Wisconsin. October 20, 1988.

McNerney, Walter. (1988). Nursing's vision in a competitive environment. *Nursing Outlook* 36(3), 126-129. Copyright 1988, American Journal of Nursing Co.

Hougaard, Judy. (1988). Clinical ladder program builds self-esteem. *The American Nurse* 20(8): 12.

Hartley, Patricia S., and Cunningham, Diane. (1988). Staff nurses rate clinical ladder program. *The American Nurse* 20(8): 13.

Wintz, Leigh. (1987). Career paths of nurses: When is a nurse no longer a nurse? *Journal of Nursing Administration* 17(4): 33-37.

UNIT TWO
DISCIPLINE ISSUES: NURSING RESEARCH, THEORY, AND PRACTICE
Chinn, Peggy L. (1988). Knowing and doing. *Advances in Nursing Sciences* 10(3): vii-viii. Copyright 1988, Aspen Publishers, Inc.

Curtin, Leah L. (1988). Thought-full nursing practice. *Nursing Management* 19(10): 7-8.

Tanner, Christine A. (1987). Evaluating research for use in practice: Guidelines for the clinician. *Heart & Lung* 16(4): 424-451, by the C.V. Mosby Co.

Lindeman, Carol A. (1988). Research in practice: The role of the staff nurse. *Applied Nursing Research* 1(1): 5-7.

Haller, Karen B., et al. (1979). Developing research-based innovation protocols: Process, criteria, and issues. *Research in Nursing and Health* 2: 45-51. Copyright 1979, John Wiley & Sons, Inc.

Buchda, Vicki. (1987). Loneliness in critically ill adults. *Dimensions of Critical Care Nursing* 6(6): 335-340.

Hathaway, Donna, and Strong, Margaret. (1988). Theory, practice, and research in transplant nursing. *ANNA Journal* 15(1): 9-12.

Goode, Colleen J., et al. (1987). Use of research based knowledge in clinical practice. *Journal of Nursing Administration* 17(12): 11-18.

UNIT THREE
HEALTH CARE DELIVERY ISSUES
Wilson, Thomas A. (1988). Nursing megatrends induced by diagnosis-related groups. *Focus on Critical Care* 15(3): 55-61, by the C.V. Mosby Co.

Joel, Lucille A. (1987). Reshaping nursing practice. *American Journal of Nursing* 87(6): 793-795. Copyright 1987, American Journal of Nursing Co.

Kramer, Marlene, and Schmalenberg, Claudia. (1987). Magnet hospitals talk about the impact of DRGs on nursing care: Part I. *Nursing Management* 18(9): 38-42.

Kramer, Marlene, and Schmalenberg, Claudia. (1987). Magnet hospitals talk about the impact of DRGs on nursing care: Part II. *Nursing Management* 18(10): 33-40.

Final report, volume I, from the Department of Health and Human Services Secretary's Commission on Nursing, December 1988.

Aiken, Linda H., and Mullinix, Connie F. (1987). The nurse shortage: Myth or reality? *New England Journal of Medicine* 317(10): 641-646.

CNA sets forth shortage solutions. (1989). *California Nurse* 85(1): 8-9, by the California Nurses Association.

A look ahead: What the future holds for nursing. (1987). *RN* 50(10): 101-108. Copyright 1987, Medical Economics Company, Inc.

American Medical Association's proposal on introduction of Registered Care Technologists (RCTs). (1988). *Nursing Economics* 6(4): 198-199.

Kassebaum, Donald G. (1989). Coming to terms with the nursing shortage: Asserting the role and initiatives of academic health centers. *Academic Medicine* 64(2): 83.

Pounds, Lois A. (1989). Beyond Florence Nightingale: The general professional education of the nurse. *Academic Medicine* 64(2): 67-69.

Lindeman, Carol A. (1989). Nursing education and practice. *Academic Medicine* 64(2): 70-73.

Parker, Marcie, and Secord, Laura J. (1988). Case managers: Guiding the elderly through the health care maze. *American Journal of Nursing*. 12: 1674-1676. Copyright 1988, American Journal of Nursing Co.

Floyd, Jeanne, and Buckle, June. (1987). Nursing care of the elderly: The DRG influence. *Journal of Gerontological Nursing* 13(2): 20-25.

Sullivan, Toni J., et al. (1987) Nursing 2020: A study of nursing's future. *Nursing Outlook* 35(5): 233-235. Copyright 1987, American Journal of Nursing Co.

Garde, John F. (1988). A case study involving prospective payment legislation, DRGs, and certified registered nurse anesthetists. *Nursing Clinics of North America* 23(3): 521-530.

Schank, Mary J., et al. (1988). The potential of expert systems in nursing. *Journal of Nursing Administration* 18(6): 26-31.

Heaney, Robert P. (1987). Technological imperative and decision support. Proceedings: Inauguration of Dean Sheila A. Ryan, PhD, RN. Rochester, NY: University of Rochester School of Nursing.

UNIT FOUR
THE SOCIOPOLITICAL ENVIRONMENT AND NURSING PRACTICE
Huey, Florence L. (1988). How nurses would change U.S. health care. *American Journal of Nursing* 88(11): 1482-1493. Copyright 1988, American Journal of Nursing Co.

Kovar, Mary G,, and Harris, Tamara. (1988). Who will care for the old? *American Demographics* 10(5): 35-37.

Dimond, Margaret. (1989). Health care and the aging population. *Nursing Outlook* 37(2): 76-77. Copyright 1989, American Journal of Nursing Co.

Lindsey, Ada M. (1989). Health care for the homeless. *Nursing Outlook* 37(2): 78-81. Copyright 1989, American Journal of Nursing Co.

Chow, Marilyn. (1989). Nursing's response to the challenge of AIDS. *Nursing Outlook* 37(2): 82-83. Copyright 1989, American Journal of Nursing Co.

Eck, Sharon A., et al. (1988). Consumerism, nursing, and the reality of the resources. *Nursing Administration Quarterly* 12(3): 1-11. Copyright 1988, Aspen Publishers, Inc.

Aydelotte, Myrtle. (1987). Nursing's preferred future. *Nursing Outlook* 35(3): 114-120. Copyright 1987, American Journal of Nursing Co.

Allen, James P., and Turner, Eugene J. (1988). Where to find the new immigrants. *American Demographics* 10(9): 23-27 + .

Longman, Phillip. (1988). The challenge of an aging society. *The Futurist* 22(5): 33-37.

Rogge, Mary M. (1987). Nursing and politics: A forgotten legacy. *Nursing Research* 36(1): 26-30. Copyright 1987, American Journal of Nursing Co.

Kent, Virginia C., and Canton, Denise S. (1986). Senator Daniel K. Inouye: A champion for nursing in Congress. *Nurse Practitioner* 11(4): 66-78.

White, Diana, and Hamel, Patricia. (1986). National center for Nursing Research: How it came to be. *Nursing Economics* 4(1): 19-22.

Cohen, Wilbur, and Milburn, Lonna. (1988). What every nurse should know about political action. *Nursing and Health Care* 9(6): 295-297, by the National League for Nursing.

White, Suzanne K. (1988). Involvement: Influencing the delivery of health care and the future of critical care nursing. *Focus on Critical Care* 15(4): 59-64, by the C.V. Mosby Co.

UNIT FIVE
LEGAL AND ETHICAL ISSUES
Popp, Sister Rosanne (1988). Health care for the poor: Where has all the money gone? *Journal of Nursing Administration* 18(1): 8-12.

Fry, Sara T. (1987). Rationing health care to the elderly: A challenge to professional ethics. *Nursing Outlook* 35(5): 256. Copyright 1987, American Journal of Nursing Co.

Russell, Sabin. (1988). High cost may lead to rationed medicine. *San Francisco Chronicle*, March 15, 1988. Copyright San Francisco Chronicle.

Collins, Helen L. (1988). When the profit motive threatens patient care. *RN* 10(8): 74-83. CCopyright 1988, Medical Ecnomics Company, Inc.

Encroachment on nursing practice: Position statement. (1988). California Nurses Association.

Northrop, Cynthia E. (1987). Nursing actions in litigation. *Quarterly Review Bulletin* (October): 343-347. Copyright 1989, The Joint Commission on Accreditation of Healthcare Organizations.

Schulmeister, Lisa. (1987). Litigation involving oncology nurses. *Oncology Nursing Forum* 14(2): 25-28.

Yorker, Beatrice C. (1988). Nurses accused of murder. *American Journal of Nursing* 88(10): 1327-1332. Copyright 1988, American Journal of Nursing Co.

Tammelleo, A. David. (February 1988). When nurses must question doctor's orders. *The Regan Report on Nursing Law* 28(9).

Moore, Gary, and Hogan, Richard L. (January/February 1987). Substance abuse and the nurse: A legal and ethical dilemma. *Journal of Professional Nursing*, 5.

Brown, Mary L. (1987). AIDS and ethics: Concerns and considerations. *Oncology Nursing Forum* 14(1): 69-73.

Anderson, David. (October 1988). Death and dying: Ethics at the end of life. *RN*, 42-51. Copyright 1988, Medical Economics Company, Inc.

Schmelzer, Marilee, and Anema, Marion G. (1988). Should nurses ever lie to patients? *Image: Journal of Nursing Scholarship* 20(2): 110-112.

Cerrato, Paul L. (October 1988). What to do when you suspect incompetence. *RN*, 36-41. Copyright 1988, Medical Economics Company, Inc.

Fry, Sara T. (1988). New ANA guidelines on withdrawing or withholding food and fluid from patients. *Nursing Outlook* 36(3): 122-123 +. Copyright 1988, American Journal of Nursing Co.

California Nurses Association position statement on anencephalia infants as organ donors (1988). California Nurses Association.

Index

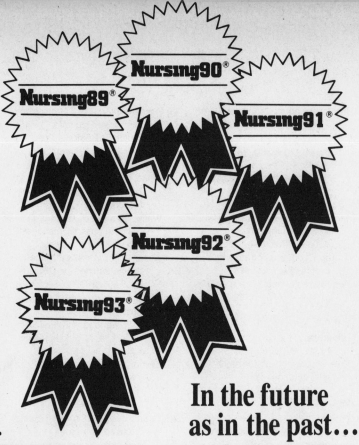

In the future as in the past...

You can rely on *Nursing* magazine to keep your skills sharp and your practice current—with award-winning nursing journalism.

Each monthly issue is packed with expert advice on the legal, ethical, and personal issues in nursing, plus up-to-the-minute...

- Drugs—warnings, new uses, and approvals
- Assessment tips
- Emergency and acute care advice
- New treatments, equipment, and disease findings
- Photostories and other skill sharpeners
- AIDS updates
- Career tracks and trends

Enter your subscription today